S0-ELG-847

RECENT ADVANCES IN CHEMOTHERAPY
Volume II

RECENT ADVANCES
IN
CHEMOTHERAPY

By

G. M. FINDLAY
C.B.E., Sc.D., M.D., F.R.C.P.

Editor, Abstracts of World Medicine and Abstracts of World
Surgery, Gynæcology and Obstetrics, British Medical
Association, London

THIRD EDITION

VOLUME II

THE BLAKISTON COMPANY
Philadelphia
1951

To
M. F.

First Edition 1930
Second ,, . . . 1939
Third Edition in Four Vols.
    Vol. I. 1950
    Vol. II. . . . 1951

ALL RIGHTS RESERVED

*This book may not be reproduced by any
means, in whole or in part, without
the permission of the Publishers.*

*Printed in Great Britain
and published in London by
J. & A. Churchill Ltd.
104 Gloucester Place, W.1.*

615.7
F49r
1950
V. 2

PREFACE TO THE THIRD EDITION

ANCIENT Chinese philosophers believed that the rhythm of the universe and of all things in it was revealed in the principle of Yin and Yang, the alternation of light and darkness, of synthesis and analysis, of growth and rest. The working of this principle can certainly be seen in the history of chemotherapy. For years, by their use of vermifuges and of such drugs as ipecacuanha, cinchona bark, and sulphur, physicians had, without knowing it, been practising chemotherapy. "The cake of custom" was broken by Paul Ehrlich, who first transformed chemotherapy from the Yin to the Yang state. By 1930, when the first edition of this book was published, Ehrlich's original discoveries had, however, ceased to stimulate and there had been a reversion to the Yin condition. Chemotherapy was of interest only to those who dealt with the protozoal diseases of tropical and subtropical countries, and to specialists in venereal diseases. With the discovery of the sulphonamides and of their mode of action, Yin again gave place to Yang and, as a reflection of the more widespread interest thus aroused, the second edition of this work published in 1939 was quickly exhausted. An effort to produce a third edition was abortive as other duties of a more immediate nature intervened, and it was not till 1946 that a serious attempt could be made on the present edition. By then, however, the whole medical world had become interested in Chemotherapy and of the 2,000 reputable medical journals now published only those devoted to the more esoteric forms of psychiatry can be neglected as unlikely to contain papers of chemotherapeutic importance. Despite its ever-growing importance chemotherapy in contradistinction to the older sciences is still largely unprovided with standard text-books which embody general findings and special applications, and up to the present no University in Great Britain has seen fit to provide a chair of chemotherapy although such chairs are urgently needed.

So vast has the scope of chemotherapy now become that to deal at all adequately with recent advances it has become neces-

229426

sary, though with great regret, to divide the present edition into a number of volumes. The first volume thus contains the chemotherapy of scabies and of helminthic and protozoal diseases, with the exception of malaria : the second is devoted wholly to malaria ; the third deals with the chemotherapy of bacterial, rickettsial, and virus infections ; and the fourth contains a survey of sulphonamides and antibiotics, with a discussion of the general principles of chemotherapy. This rearrangement has rendered necessary a complete rewriting of the second edition which must be regarded as now largely of historical interest.

> " Man must pass from old to new
> From vain to real, from mistake to fact,
> From what once seemed good to what now proves the best,
> How could man have progression otherwise ? "

So rapid are the changes that ten years hence it will be surprising if many of the antibiotics now in use are still being employed.

Although the main advance in the past decade has been in the use of antibiotics for the control of bacterial, rickettsial, and some virus infections, very considerable progress, largely stimulated by the War, has also been made in the treatment of helminthic and protozoal diseases. More especially important is the more balanced view now possible of the *rôle* of chemotherapy, in association with other measures, in the control and eradication of malaria and trypanosomiasis in the tropics. The smaller viruses alone resist chemotherapeutic control.

The White Queen was of opinion that " It's a poor sort of memory that only works backwards." It may therefore be hazarded that, if the present rate of advance in chemotherapy continues, within the next hundred years the parasitic infections of man and his domestic animals will have become of little importance and the mortality if not the morbidity which they now cause will have been reduced to almost negligible proportions. Such a change affecting especially the inhabitants of tropical and subtropical countries will have an important bearing on population problems and will intensify the need for an increase in the food supplies available for man. It must, however, be remembered that if Yin can change to Yang the reverse process can also occur and social historians however they may disagree on most points are unanimous that in the past conditions for scientific research have been possible only for very limited periods of time and in particular areas of the civilised world.

Progress may also be hindered by an increasing dominance of drug-fast parasites and the possibilities of mutation among parasites may equal or even defeat the ingenuity of the chemotherapist. Two factors which act as brakes on the progress of chemotherapy may be briefly mentioned. There is at present no wholly satisfactory classification of bacteria : as a result certain bacteria referred to one group by some authorities are placed in another group by others. This obviously leads to considerable confusion when the reactions of bacteria to chemotherapeutic agents are discussed. The second source of confusion is the multiplicity of names given by national pharmacopœial committees and by proprietary firms to one and the same chemical compound. Not only may the same compound have many names, but the same name may be applied to two different chemical compounds. Thus in France nivaquine refers to an antimalarial which is called chloroquine in America, where the name nivaquine is given to another compound. An attempt is at last being made by the World Health Organisation to tackle this very complicated problem.

I owe a deep debt of gratitude to the many friends who have given help and advice and have read the whole or part of this work at various stages of its production. These include Professor G. A. H. Buttle, E. A. Boulter, Mrs. S. Boulter, Dr. L. G. Goodwin, Dr. C. A. Hoare, Miss M. Hollowell, Dr. H. R. Ing, Professor B. G. Maegraith, J. S. Morton, Professor J. M. Watson, and Dr. R. Wien. S. H. Watkins and my elder daughter Anne have given me invaluable assistance in preparing the references and indexes, and my secretary, Miss F. D. I. Rowland, has ably typed the by no means easy manuscript.

Finally, I must again express my thanks to my publishers for their ever-ready help, courtesy, and understanding.

G. M. FINDLAY.

FOREWORD

THIS volume is devoted wholly to the chemotherapy of malaria, a subject which for more than three hundred years has engaged the attention of countless scientists and even now is by no means exhausted. During the Second World War many of the most arduous campaigns were undertaken in highly malarious regions and as a result intensive investigations on the chemotherapy of malaria were carried out throughout the world. These investigations have resulted in important advances in our knowledge of malaria and of malarial chemotherapy. These advances are here described. It is hoped that this survey will be of interest and value to all those working on the malaria problem, whatever their angle of approach.

My thanks are due to the President and Council of the Royal Society of Tropical Medicine and to Colonel H. E. Shortt, F.R.S., for their kindness in permitting the use of the diagram on pages 8 and 9.

G. M. FINDLAY.

CONTENTS

RECENT ADVANCES IN CHEMOTHERAPY

VOLUME II

CHAPTER I

CHEMOTHERAPY AND THE MALARIA PROBLEM

MALARIA is undoubtedly the most prevalent and the most wide-spread of all human diseases, not even excluding gonorrhœa and syphilis. On a conservative estimate there are in the world to-day some 700 million persons infected with malaria and of these at least 100 million are to be found in India. It is believed that between two and three million die directly or indirectly from the disease each year, one million at least of them in India. Since the end of the second world war such factors as the displacement and transfer of populations and the return to Europe of troops from malarious countries have been responsible for spread of the infection and, in some areas, for an increased incidence. In Germany, for instance, of 13,836 cases recorded in the Eastern and Western zones from 1945 to 1947, 3,561 cases were indigenous (Hormann, 1949; Schroeder, 1950). The ill-health which malaria causes, especially in the tropics and sub-tropics, can be compared only with that due to malnutrition, but the extent to which malaria causes miscarriage and a high infant mortality rate probably varies very considerably in different countries : accurate figures are difficult to obtain, but Smith (1943), in Lagos, Nigeria, a hyperendemic area, found that among 500 children dying under one year of age and submitted to autopsy, seventy-two had died from malaria. In Cyprus the virtual eradication of malaria has reduced the infant mortality rate from 185 per 1,000 in 1942 to sixty-seven per 1,000 in 1948 : the malaria incidence was reduced from 18·73 to 0·87 per 1,000 (Shelley, 1950).

The measures taken to overcome the menace of malaria comprise :—

(1) Destruction of the breeding places of anopheline mosquito vectors.

(2) Destruction of larval and adult anopheline mosquitoes.

(3) Drug treatment of persons suffering from malaria and of those exposed to it.

The destruction of anopheline breeding places by drainage and land reclamation is as a rule a costly proceeding which in the tropics, in areas where there is danger of re-entry of mosquitoes from the periphery, necessitates not only a high initial outlay in money and materials but supervision by a trained staff (Gilroy, 1948). In Freetown, Sierra Leone, the eradication of malaria vectors from an area of 35 square miles is said to have cost £150,000 over a period of five years (Walton, 1949). The destruction of anopheline mosquitoes in the larval or adult stages has become easier with the advent of Paris green, D.D.T., and gammexane, but it still requires considerable staff and large supplies of chemicals. In Brazil and in the Nile Valley, where the possibility of reinfection can be guarded against, such measures have met with complete success in eradicating *Anopheles gambiæ*. In islands such as Cyprus, Sardinia, and Mauritius the mosquito population has been reduced to a very low figure, but the problem is more complicated in continental areas, where the introduction of mosquitoes and gametocyte carriers is a constant possibility (Soper and Wilson, 1943 ; Shousha, 1948 ; Lewis, 1949 ; Shelley and Aziz, 1949 ; Aziz, 1948 ; Symes and Hadaway, 1947 ; Giglioli, 1948 ; Soper, 1948). After four years of the most intensive mosquito control in Freetown, Sierra Leone, the parasite rate of school children could not be reduced below 10 per cent., which means that half the child population is still being infected every year (Walton, 1947, 1948, 1949). Residual insecticides are of paramount importance in carrying out these schemes for total eradication. There is, however, growing evidence that insects can become resistant to insecticides. Some races of flies and ticks are now resistant to D.D.T. : certain scale insects and codling moths have become resistant to cyanides. Other insects and birds may be adversely affected by wide use of insecticides. It is therefore possible that in the future it may be necessary to restrict the use of insecticides and to concentrate more on chemotherapeutic methods of control.

The third measure aims at the eradication of malarial infections by the use of drugs having a specific action on malarial plasmodia. During the first quarter of the twentieth century, despite the fact that malaria was known to be transmitted by mosquitoes, the measures which could be taken to control it by chemotherapeutic drugs were inadequate. In the war of 1914–18 whole armies were immobilised in the Balkans because of malaria, while in East Africa, Mesopotamia, and the Jordan Valley the toll of sickness and death was very great. In the war of 1939–45 the malaria rates were at first high in such areas as India, Burma, and West Africa, until synthetic antimalarials were systematically used as suppressives. Even with the increased knowledge available the morbidity from malaria was considerable. In the United States Navy and Army, from 1942 to 1945, there were 575,824 hospital admissions for malaria, with 363 deaths (Coggeshall *et al.*, 1948). In West Africa, from 1940 to 1945, there were among approximately 50,000 Europeans exposed to infection twenty-one deaths from malaria and fifty-nine deaths from blackwater fever. In peace time also malaria may cause sudden devastating outbreaks, as in Ceylon and in Brazil, where the accidental introduction of *Anopheles gambiæ* caused 300,000 cases and 16,000 deaths. In a tropical area where little or no control has been attempted the percentage of the population carrying parasites in the blood is high. Young (1949), in a survey in Liberia in 1948, examined 10,128 persons and found malarial parasites in the blood of 3,104. McLean (1950), in an examination of 200 men, women and children from the vicinity of Lake Victoria, found 184 with parasites in the blood. Although many of these people obviously had some degree of tolerance to malaria they represented a reservior of infection for those who were neither tolerant nor immune.

It may be argued that in the control of endemic malaria greater good will eventually come from engineering schemes and the use of insecticides than from chemotherapeutic control. Nevertheless it would seem that there will for long be a place for chemotherapy in the control of epidemic malaria, and for the present therefore research must be pursued on as broad a front as possible. It is still unfortunately true, as Robert Burton remarked in 1628, that " a common ague sometimes stumbles them all."

The original development of synthetic antimalarials by German workers was primarily the result of the shortage of quinine in the first world war. The first synthetic antimalarial to be produced was pamaquin, formerly known as plasmochin or plasmoquine ; later, mepacrine (atebrin or quinacrine) was synthesised.

Both these compounds have one factor in common with the cinchona alkaloids, they are substitution derivatives of either quinoline or acridine. They may, however, be regarded as alkylamines or, in the case of the natural cinchona alkaloids, as cyclic amines substituted by the quinoline or acridine nucleus. The inclusion of the quinoline or acridine nucleus may be looked on as endowing them with an alkaloidal character, in that they are basic compounds in which at least one nitrogen atom forms part of a cyclic system (Schmidt, 1932).

Despite the advent of mepacrine and pamaquin, very little advance in the chemotherapeutic control of malaria occurred between 1926 and 1940. Mepacrine was considered as valuable in the treatment of malaria but of secondary importance to quinine, whereas pamaquin was thought to have a very limited field of usefulness. It was known, it is true, that pamaquin is gametocytotoxic, that it acts as a true causal prophylactic, and that in combination with quinine it can prevent relapses in vivax malaria : it was considered, however, that the doses required were too large and the toxicity too great for its general use.

When Java, the chief cinchona-growing country, was over-run by the Japanese, the allied nations were faced by the problem of having to maintain armies in highly malarious countries with entirely inadequate supplies of quinine. They were thus forced to reconsider the value of the antimalarial drugs still available, and to find more efficient means of reducing the incidence of malaria. One answer to these problems was the discovery of more effective insecticides, the other was the intensive use of synthetic antimalarials. For the future of malarial chemotherapy it is perhaps fortunate that for long the synthesis of the cinchona alkaloids presented great difficulties to the chemist. Only in 1944 did Woodward and Doering synthesise quinine for the first time, but as at least fifteen different processes are involved, the synthetic production of quinine is not at present a practicable proposition.

The discovery of new synthetic antimalarial drugs depends, as it did in the case of pamaquin and mepacrine, on the experimental evaluation of new compounds in birds and animals infected with various plasmodia and on the clues afforded to the synthetic chemist by the chemical structure of known antimalarial compounds. There are thus two approaches to the production of efficient antimalarials, the chemical and the biological.

References

AZIZ, M., 1948, History of prevention of malaria in Cyprus. *Cyprus med. J.,* 1, No. 3, 21.

BURTON, R., 1628, "The Anatomy of Melancholy," 3rd Edit., Oxford: Henry Cripps.

COGGESHALL, L. T., RICE, F. A., and YOUNT, E. H., Jr., 1948, The cure of recurrent vivax malaria and status of immunity thereafter. *Proc. 4th Int. Congr. trop. Med. and Malar., Wash.,* 1, 749.

GIGLIOLI, G., 1948, "Malaria, filariasis and yellow fever in British Guiana." Georgetown: British Guiana Medical Department.

GILROY, A. B., 1948, "Malaria control by coastal swamp drainage in West Africa." London: Ross Institute of Tropical Medicine.

HORMANN, H., 1949, Malaria in Deutschland 1945 bis 1947. *Z. Tropenmed. Parasit.,* 1, 32.

LEWIS, D. J., 1949, The extermination of *Anopheles gambiæ* in the Wadi Halfa area. *Trans. R. Soc. trop. Med. Hyg.,* 42, 393.

MCLEAN, N., 1950, Malignant tertian malaria. *Brit. Med. J., i,* 189.

SCHMIDT, J., 1932, "A Text-book of Organic Chemistry." London: Gurney and Jackson.

SCHROEDER, W., 1950, Malariaepidemien im östlicher Norddeutschland nach dem zweiten Weltkriege. *Z. Tropenmed. Parasitol.,* 1, 488.

SHELLEY, H. M., 1950, Anopheles eradication in Cyprus. *Med. Offr.,* 83, 27.

SHELLEY, H. M., and AZIZ, M., 1949, Anopheles eradication in Cyprus. *Brit. med. J., i,* 767.

SHOUSHA, A. T., 1948, Species-eradication. The eradication of *Anopheles gambiæ* from Upper Egypt, 1942–45. *Bull. World Hlth. Organ.,* 1, 309.

SMITH, E. C., 1943, Child mortality in Lagos, Nigeria. *Trans. R. Soc. trop. Med. Hyg.,* 36, 287.

SOPER, F. L., 1948, Species sanitation as applied to the eradication of (A) an invading or (B) an indigenous species. *Proc. 4th Int. Congr. trop. Med. and Malar., Wash.,* 1, 850.

SOPER, F. L., and WILSON, D. B., 1943, "*Anopheles gambiæ* in Brazil, 1930–40." New York: Rockefeller Foundation.

SYMES, C. B., and HADAWAY, A. D., 1947, Initial experiments in the use of D.D.T. against mosquitos in British Guiana. *Bull. ento. Res.,* 37, 399.

WALTON, G. A., 1947, On the control of malaria in Freetown, Sierra Leone. I. *Plasmodium falciparum* and *Anopheles gambiæ* in relating to malaria occurring in infants. *Ann. trop. Med. Parasit.,* 41, 380.

WALTON, G. A., 1948, Incidence of malaria in tropical Africa. *Nature, Lond.*, **162**, 114.

WALTON, G. A., 1949, On the control of malaria in Freetown, Sierra Leone. II. Control methods and the effects upon the transmission of *Plasmodium falciparum* resulting from the reduced abundance of *Anopheles gambiæ*. *Ann. trop. Med. Parasit.*, **43**, 117.

WOODWARD, R. B., and DOERING, W. E., 1944, The total synthesis of quinine. *J. Amer. chem. Soc.*, **66**, 849.

YOUNG, M. D., 1949, The incidence of blood parasites in Liberia. *J. Parasit.*, **35** (No. 6, Sect. 2), p. 24.

CHAPTER II

THE BIOLOGY OF MALARIA IN RELATION TO CHEMOTHERAPY

In order to understand the various problems which arise in the chemotherapeutic control of human malaria, as well as the part played by a study of avian malarias in the evaluation of chemotherapeutic remedies, it is necessary briefly to describe what is known of the biology of malaria parasites.

The Life Cycle of Plasmodia

The life cycle of all malaria parasites is closely similar whether they attack man, mammals, birds or saurians. There are two developmental cycles, a sexual cycle which takes place in the mosquito and an asexual cycle which occurs in the vertebrate host. When the mosquito sucks up blood from an infected animal the asexual malaria parasites disintegrate in its stomach, but the male sexual cells, the microgametes, and the female sexual cells, the macrogametes, unite. The fertilised macrogamete then perforates the wall of the mosquito stomach, forming an oöcyst within which sporozoites develop. The ripe oöcyst finally ruptures into the body cavity liberating sporozoites, which migrate to the mosquito's salivary glands. Thence, when the mosquito bites a fresh vertebrate host, sporozoites are injected directly into the blood stream and the asexual cycle begins. After not more than thirty minutes in the peripheral blood stream the sporozoites enter certain liver cells, where they undergo development for from ten to fourteen days, constituting the primary exo-erythrocytic forms of the parasite or cryptozoite of Huff *et al.* (1943) and Huff and Coulston (1944). Huff and Coulston (1946) distinguish between cryptozoites and metacryptozoites. Cryptozoites are the forms resulting from infection of the tissue cells by sporozoites : as they develop they give rise to meta-cryptozoites or metacryptozoic merozoites, which infect the red

LIFE CYCLE OF
Plasmodium cynomolgi.
A type of Mammalian Malaria Parasite.

Explanation of Plate.

1. Sporozoites from salivary glands of mosquito enter liver cells.
2. Liver cell containing early stage of pre-erythrocytic parasite.
3 and 4. Stages in development of the pre-erythrocytic schizont in liver cells.
5. Fully developed pre-erythrocytic schizont rupturing and releasing pre-erythrocytic merozoites.
6. Liver cell containing merozoite of an exo-erythrocytic cycle of schizogony.
7-9. Remaining stages in exo-erythrocytic schizogony ending in second generation of merozoites.
10. Red cell of circulating blood.
11-14. Stages in erythrocytic schizogony in circulating blood.
15. Fully developed erythrocytic schizont rupturing and releasing erythrocytic merozoites and gametocytes.
16-20. Repetition of erythrocytic schizogony.
21 and 22. Development of male gametocyte or microgametocyte in circulating blood.
23 and 24. Development of female gametocyte or macrogametocyte in circulating blood.
25. Wall of stomach of mosquito.
26. Exflagellating microgametocyte producing microgametes in stomach of mosquito.
27. Macrogametocyte extruding polar bodies and so becoming macrogamete.
28. Microgamete free in stomach of mosquito and seeking macrogamete.
29. Zygote, formed by fertilisation of macrogamete by a single microgamete.
30. Oökinete or travelling vermicule formed by elongation of zygote. It is about to penetrate epithelial lining of stomach.
31. Oöcyst, formed by oökinete after penetration of stomach wall of mosquito. It lies under elastic membrane on outer surface of stomach.
32 and 33. Stages in development of oöcyst with production of sporozoites.
34. Rupture of mature oöcyst with dispersion of sporozoites most of which enter salivary glands of mosquito.
35. Salivary gland of mosquito containing mature sporozoites.

(Shortt : *Trans. R. Soc. trop. Med. Hyg.*)

cells. The question of nomenclature is fully discussed by Garnham (1948). At the end of this stage, which is often referred to as the prepatent period, the infected liver cells rupture ; some parasites enter liver cells ; others enter red cells where they develop from small rings, which grow and finally segment into a number of separate merozoites. The red cells then disintegrate and the schizonts are free to infect other red cells. Certain of the asexual parasites, however, develop into gametocytes, male and female, which when taken up by the mosquito during a feed pass into its stomach and there begin once more the sexual cycle.

The presence of exo-erythrocytic, pre-erythrocytic and persisting exo-erythrocytic forms of mammalian malarial parasites within the liver cells has now been conclusively demonstrated in the case of *P. cynomolgi* by Shortt and Garnham (1948a) and Shortt, Garnham and Malamos (1948), and in *P. vivax* by Shortt, Garnham, Covell and Shute (1948). Shortt and his colleagues (1949) have also demonstrated the pre-erythrocytic stages of *P. falciparum* in the liver cells of man. In the majority of species of plasmodia the exo-erythrocytic forms originally produced continue to reproduce themselves as such (Shortt and Garnham, 1948b) : this is certainly true for *P. vivax* and probably for *P. malariæ* in man. In addition, secondary exo-erythrocytic forms or phanerozoites (Huff and Coulston, 1946 ; Huff, 1947) possibly develop from asexual erythrocytic forms. There are thus at least two types of parasite present at any one time, (*a*) exo-erythrocytic forms in fixed tissue cells, and (*b*) erythrocytic forms in the red cells. It is by the exo-erythrocytic forms reinfecting red cells that clinical relapses occur. It is possible, as suggested by Shute (1946), that certain sporozoites, after entering the body, may remain in a resting stage for weeks or months or after going through a portion of their pre-erythrocytic cycle pass into such a resting stage. In the case of *Plasmodium vivax* there is evidence that secondary exo-erythrocytic forms persist for many years in man, in the case of some strains possibly for life. *P. malariæ* may also persist, certainly for eleven years (Boyd, 1947). Secondary exo-erythrocytic forms of *P. falciparum* are almost certainly absent and the primary pre-erythrocytic forms do not persist or else are vulnerable to the commoner antimalarials or to the immune mechanism. An infection due to *P. falciparum* thus burns itself out in from twelve to eighteen months from the date of the original infection. At present no drug is known which destroys sporozoites in the human host, although Clarke and Theiler (1948) have brought forward evidence that a naphthoquinone may destroy the sporozoites of *P. gallinaceum* in fowls with some degree of certainty. This failure to attack sporozoites is probably because they circulate in the blood stream for not more than thirty minutes and in addition, as Davey (1946b) has pointed out, the sporozoite is a resting stage in the life of the parasite : development in the mosquito has been completed and a new phase in the vertebrate host is about to begin. Metabolism is therefore at a low ebb and hence drugs which act by interfering with the metabolism of the parasite have little chance of success.

It is necessary as the result of the knowledge now gained to distinguish the following stages in malaria parasites : sporozoites, pre-erythrocytic forms in the liver, schizonts in the red cells, exo-erythrocytic forms in the liver, gametocytes in the red cells, oöcysts and sporozoites in the mosquito. As Sergent (1949) has put it, the exo-erythrocytic cycle assures the conservation of the plasmodium in the malarial subject in spite of the absence of the malarial vector. The sexual cycle assures the conservation of the plasmodium in the mosquito in the absence of the vertebrate host.

Chemotherapy in Relation to the Life Cycle of Plasmodia

For the experimental investigation of chemotherapeutic drugs, infections can be induced in man or animals by the injection of blood containing a definite number of parasites, by the bites of infected mosquitoes, or by injecting the ground-up salivary glands of infected mosquitoes. By suitable techniques an infecting dose of sporozoites can be standardised so that a definite number of parasites is injected (Porter, 1942 ; Coggeshall *et al.*, 1944). When blood is injected the infection is produced by trophozoites which immediately inaugurate the erythrocytic asexual cycle.

Chemotherapeutic drugs do not as a rule attack all stages of the development cycle with equal intensity. Only a few drugs such as pamaquin, sulphadiazine, metachloride and 2-hydroxy-3-β-decalyl-propyl-1, 4, naphthoquinone, destroy sporozoites, but many are known which attack exo-erythrocytic forms, asexual erythrocytic forms, gametocytes and possibly the developmental forms in the mosquito. A drug which destroys primary exo-erythrocytic forms is a true causal prophylactic ; one which destroys secondary exo-erythrocytic forms is radically curative ; one which attacks asexual forms in the blood is clinically curative or suppressive, although in the case of *P. falciparum*, where secondary exo-erythrocytes do not exist, it may also be radically curative : one which attacks gametocytes is gametocyticidal.

The different reactions shown by the various stages in the life cycle of the parasites to different drugs was first demonstrated by Yorke and Macfie (1924) and Yorke (1925), who showed that quinine was effective when given prior to the injection of blood cells infected with *P. vivax* but ineffective when the infection was induced by sporozoites. Similar results were obtained with pamaquin by Russell (1931a and b) and Russell and Nono (1932) against blood-induced but not against sporozoite-induced infections with *P. cathemerium*, and by Tate and Vincent (1933) working with *P. relictum*. In addition, compounds active against sporozoite-induced malarias are often incapable of sterilising the blood if used against a blood-induced infection (sulphonamides, Coatney and Cooper, 1944 ; Marshall, 1946—metanilamides, Brackett and Waletzky, 1946 ; Hughes and Brackett, 1946—members of the proguanil series, Curd *et al.*, 1945).

The differences exhibited by different stages of a malarial parasite to different drugs are shown in the reaction of *P. gallinaceum*.

To determine whether a plasmodial infection has been entirely eliminated from experimental animals as a result of drug action there must be :—

(1) Failure to observe parasites in repeated blood smears (parasitological relapse).

(2) Failure to observe parasites in the subinoculated animal during a fifteen-day observation period (negative subinoculation).

(3) Ability to produce a normal acute infection in the original

Plasmodium gallinaceum AND CHEMOTHERAPEUTIC DRUGS

Developmental stage.	Drug.	Reference.
Oöcysts Sporozoites	Proguanil, sulphadiazine. 2-Hydroxy-3-β-decalyl-propyl-1, 4-naphthoquinone. Pamaquin, metachloridine, sulphadiazine.	Clarke and Theiler (1948). Terzian *et al.* (1948).
Pre-erythrocytic forms.	Proguanil . . . . Sulphadiazine and more than thirty sulphonamides. Metachloridine and sixteen other metanilamides, aureomycin.	Curd *et al.* (1945). Coatney and Cooper (1944, 1948). Brackett and Waletzky (1946). Coatney *et al.* (1949).
Erythrocytic forms.	Quinine . . . . Mepacrine . . . . Chloroquine 2-Hydroxy-3-β-decalyl-propyl-1, 4-naphthoquinone. Proguanil. Sulphadiazine. Pamaquin . . . . Certuna	Brumpt *et al.* (1937). Brumpt *et al.* (1937). Brumpt *et al.* (1937). Decourt *et al.* (1939).
Secondary exo-erythrocytic forms.	Pamaquin (slight) . . . Sulphadiazine, sulphapyrazine . 2-Hydroxy-3-β-decalyl-propyl-1, 4-naphthoquinone.	Kikuth and Mudrow (1939). Coggeshall *et al.* (1944). Coggeshall *et al.* (1944). Clarke and Theiler (1948).

animal with a second inoculation (in the case of ducks with *P. lophuræ* twenty-three days after the end of therapy). This last is the most reliable proof of cure. Experiments which satisfy these criteria have been carried out by Kelsey *et al.* (1946), Dearborn and Marshall (1946), and Walker *et al.* (1948). These observers agree that pamaquin is able to eradicate *P. lophuræ* from ducks when the infection is blood-induced, doses of 9 mgm. per kgm. of body weight producing a significant number of cures. Pamaquin also eradicates *P. cathemerium* in ducks at the same dose rate. Mepacrine, on the other hand, has no curative action on *P. lophuræ* (Dearborn and Marshall, 1946) but acts on *P. cathemerium* in the duck, though at a dose rate of 9 mgm. per kgm. it cured only 60 per cent. of birds.

In human malarias pamaquin, by destroying pre-erythrocytic forms, is a true causal prophylactic for both *P. vivax* and *P. falciparum*. Since, however, it does not invariably kill off secondary exo-erythrocytes of *P. vivax* it cannot invariably be relied on to produce a radical cure, although when combined with quinine it produces such a result in a high percentage of cases. On the other hand, pamaquin acts on gametocytes, especially those of *P. falciparum*. Quinine, mepacrine, and chloroquine act solely on the asexual erythrocytic forms of *P. vivax* and *P. falciparum*, thus producing a clinical cure and acting as suppressives. Mepacrine and chloroquine, if persisted in, may completely eradicate infections due to *P. falciparum* because they destroy all erythrocytic forms and exo-erythrocytic forms of *P. falciparum* do not persist : these drugs are thus radically curative. Proguanil acts certainly on the majority of strains of *P. falciparum* as a true causal prophylactic, but in established infections it does not invariably destroy all the erythrocytic forms, especially of African strains. Sulphanilamide produces radical cures of *P. knowlesi* infections in rhesus monkeys, as shown by failure of the blood of such cured monkeys to transmit infection to other monkeys and by the possibility of reinfecting monkeys which have been cured by sulphanilamide, once immunity has disappeared. *P. inui* in monkeys is unaffected (Coggeshall, 1940). Proguanil, while it does not kill gametocytes in the blood of the vertebrate host, apparently inhibits the development of the oöcyst in the stomach of the mosquito.

Thus different drugs act on different stages of the developmental cycle of the malarial parasite. In addition the same stages of development of all species of parasite are not equally susceptible to the same drug, and finally there are very considerable differences in the susceptibility to the same drug of different strains of the same species of parasite.

Assessment of Anti-plasmodial Activity

It is obvious that the evaluation of chemotherapeutic remedies for the treatment of human malaria is a matter of very considerable difficulty. The ideal method is of course to test all drugs on healthy human volunteers infected by the bites of mosquitoes with numerous strains of all the species of plasmodia which attack man. The possibility of testing new remedies directly on man became practicable only with the introduction of therapeutic malaria for the cure of syphilis of the central nervous system. Such chemotherapeutic investigations were initiated in Great Britain before the war of 1939–45 by James and his colleagues using patients suffering from tabes or locomotor ataxia. During the war extensive use was made of healthy non-immune human volunteers. However, the supply both of patients with syphilis of the central nervous system and of healthy volunteers is limited ; the experiments can be carried out only in areas where the chances of natural infection with malaria are absolutely excluded and the maintenance of large numbers of human volunteers is expensive and time-consuming, especially when considerable numbers of drugs are to be tested.

Tests of Drugs on Avian Malarias

The use of avian malarial parasites for the study of malarial chemotherapy dates from 1911, when Kopanaris studied the effects of drugs on malaria in canaries. Just after the war of 1914–18 Etienne and Edmond Sergent, with Catanei (1921–25), followed up their original investigations on the plasmodia of birds (Sergent and Sergent, 1907) by investigating the effects of the cinchona alkaloids on *Plasmodium relictum* in canaries. Later, in Germany, bird malaria was used not only to study the action of quinine but of quinine derivatives such as optochin (Morgenroth *et al.*, 1926), and above all of pamaquin, the first synthetic antimalarial, ever to be produced in the laboratory (Röehl, 1926). Antimalarial activity was first determined by lengthening of the incubation or prepatent period : if parasites did not appear in the blood till the tenth day or later it was concluded that the compound was active. Pamaquin was originally selected on the basis of its chemotherapeutic index in producing a clinical cure of *P. relictum* infections in the canary, the chemotherapeutic index being 1 : 32 as compared with 1 : 4 for quinine. The chemotherapeutic index, however as ordinarily determined, is fallacious. A number of investigators (Fourneau *et al.*, 1931, 1933 ; Bovet *et al.*, 1934 ; Albricht and Nieuwenhuyse, 1937) have used *Hæmoproteus orizivoræ* infection in Java sparrows as a means of estimating gametocyticidal action of antimalarial compounds : in addition, Kikuth (1931, 1932, 1935) developed a method by which the schizonticidal action of mepacrine or other compounds could be demonstrated by administering pamaquin as well as the test drug to Java sparrows infected with *H. orizivoræ*. The principle of the method depends on the fact that in *H. orizivoræ* infection only gametocytes appear in the peripheral blood stream, schizogony occurring in the endothelial cells of the inner organs. By giving a gametocyticidal drug such as pamaquin alone the gametocytes disappear from the circulation temporarily, but when mepacrine is given at the same time there is no reappearance of sexual forms in the peripheral blood for a much more prolonged period, if at all, thus indicating that mepacrine has acted on the schizonts. A very considerable number of malarial parasites have now been studied from the point of view of their reaction to chemotherapeutic drugs. The most important are shown in the table.

SPECIES OF PLASMODIA USED IN CHEMOTHERAPEUTIC INVESTIGATIONS

Parasite.	Host.
Plasmodium vivax	Man.
P. malariæ	,,
P. ovale	,,
P. falciparum	,,
P. knowlesi	Rhesus monkey (*Macaca mulatta*).
P. inui	Cercopithecus monkeys.
P. cynomolgi	,, ,,
P. brasilianum	Central American monkeys (*Cebus capucinus ; C. cinus ; Ateles geoffroyi, A. dariensis, Alouata palliata acquatonalis ; A. p. trabéata ; Leontocebus geoffroyi ; Aotus zonalis*).
P. berghei	Mice, Congo tree rat.
P. relictum	Canary.
P. cathemerium	Canary, duck.
P. circumflexum	Canary.
P. gallinaceum	Fowl.
P. lophuræ	Duck, canary, turkey.
P. nucleophilum	Canary.
P. elongatum	,,
P. vaughani	,,
P. hexamerium	,,
P. paddæ	Java sparrow (*Padda orizivora*).
P. floridense	South American lizards (*Sceloporus undulatus ; S. olivaceus ; Anolis carolinensis*).
P. mexicanum	*Crotaphytus c. collaris.*
Hæmoproteus columbæ	Pigeon.
H. orizivoræ	Java sparrow (*Padda orizivora*).

It would obviously be a great advance and would ensure more rapid progress if human malaria parasites could develop in common laboratory animals or if a closely related parasite could be found in one of them. Several species of plasmodium are known to exist in bats (Dionisi, 1899 ; Manwell, 1946 ; McGhee, 1949a), but bats are not suitable laboratory animals. The Congo tree rat *Thamnomys surdaster Surdaster* was found (Vincke and Lips, 1948) to harbour a new species of plasmodium, *P. berghei*, which morphologically bears some resemblance to human plasmodia. This plasmodium is transmitted by *Anopheles dureni* and can be passaged by blood inoculation to mice and tree rats, causing, after intraperitoneal inoculation, parasitæmia in two to three days and death in seven to seventeen days. Schneider *et al.* (1949) have already used this plasmodium in chemotherapeutic studies on the mouse. As it is not yet certain that *P. berghei* belongs to the same genus as the human and simian plasmodia, chemotherapeutic results with this organism must at present be applied with caution to human malaria. McGhee (1949b) has also shown that avian plasmodia, such as *P. lophuræ*, can produce an infection in one-day-old mice. This discovery has not yet been exploited.

In order to overcome the fallacies inherent in the chemotherapeutic index as usually obtained in canaries, Buttle *et al.* (1938) introduced the idea of the quinine index, defined as the ratio of the minimal effective dose of quinine to the minimal effective dose of the drug under test. In addition to the " quinine index " it is sometimes desirable to determine a " pamaquin index," or even a " sulphadiazine index."

The quinine index was very largely employed by American workers in studying during the war years some 14,000 compounds for antimalarial action.

Knoppers and Nieuwenhuyse (1946) have slightly modified the idea of the quinine equivalent and replaced it by what they term " the index of action " of a compound. The dose of the test substance which will produce the same degree of activity as a given dose of quinine in blood-induced malaria in the canary is first determined ; the degree of action of quinine is taken as 1·0. The LD 50 of the compound is then determined, the LD 50 for quinine being taken as 1·0.

$$\text{Index of Action} = \frac{\text{Degree of action of X}}{\text{Degree of toxicity of X}}.$$

By this method, the index of action of quinine being 1·0, the indices of action of the cinchona alkaloids are as follows :—

Alkaloid.	Index of action.
Quinidine	0·6
Cinchonidine	0·3
Cinchonine	0·15
Hydroquinine	0·9
Hydroquinidine	0·55
Hydrocinchonidine . . .	0·16
Hydrocinchonine	0·17
Totaquina Type I . . .	0·44
,, ,, II . . .	0·31

This method of assessing antimalarial activity has not yet been applied to compounds other than the cinchona alkaloids.

The following tests devised by Davey (1946a and b) can be taken as examples of screening tests :—

(1) Tests for drugs used in clinical treatment or clinical suppression. (*a*) Test using *P. gallinaceum* in the chick. Chicks, six days old and weighing 45 to 55 gm., are infected intravenously with approximately 50 million parasitised cells. The inoculum is prepared from the pooled blood of chicks infected four days previously by the intravenous injection of about 100 million parasitised cells. Clotting of the pooled blood is prevented by heparin. A cell count is made and also a stained smear. The pooled blood is diluted with Ringer's solution to give the required 50 million parasitised cells in each 0·2 ml. of inoculum.

Williamson (1948) has prepared a nomogram for obtaining a standard number of infected red cells for intravenous inoculation into six-day-old chicks. Where a = the number of red cells in millions per c.mm. and b = the number of parasitised red cells per 500 red cells in the infected blood from which the dilution is made, the dilution c, required to give a parasitised red cell density of 50×10^6 per 0·2 ml., can be obtained from the relation $ab = 125c$.

Treatment of the chicks with test substances is begun about four hours after they have been infected and is repeated twice daily on each of the following three days. The substances are given orally in solution or suspension through a catheter tube. The strength of the solution is such that a dose for a chick weighing 50 gm. is contained in 1 ml. Six chicks are included for each dose of each drug for the control group. Blood smears from the base of the leg vein are taken on the fifth day about eighteen hours after the last dose. The smears are stained by Giemsa's method. The density of the infection is expressed as the number of parasitised corpuscles in a random sample of 500. The activity of the drug is assessed in the first place by searching for " the critical dose region." The upper limit of this region is approximately the minimum effective dose, the lower limit the lowest dose exerting a measurable effect.

(*b*) Test using *P. lophuræ* in chicks. Chicks are selected as in the test against *P. gallinaceum*. They are inoculated intravenously with 60 to 100 million parasitised red cells. The drug is given as before and is repeated twice daily for four days.

(*c*) Test using *P. lophuræ* in canaries. Nine canaries are each injected intravenously with approximately 40 million parasitised red cells drawn from a chick infected with *P. lophuræ*, 0·2 ml. of fluid being given. Treatment is begun on the ninth day of infection, 0·5 ml. of fluid being given at one feed.

(*d*) Test using *P. cathemerium* in canaries. The canaries should weigh 18 to 22 gm. and three or four are included in each group. Blood drawn from an infected canary is diluted with citrated saline to give eight to twelve parasitised cells in each 0·2 ml. The drug is given orally as before, beginning four hours after inoculation : it is repeated daily on each of the next four days. The peak of the parasitæmia occurs on the fifth to sixth days of the test.

This method has considerable advantages over Röehl's original technique where the parasites are given intramuscularly and the prepatent period often shows considerable variation from bird to bird.

(2) Test for drugs used in causal prophylaxis and radical cure. (*a*) Test using *P. gallinaceum* in chicks. The birds as before are six-day-old chicks weighing 45 to 55 gm. The inoculum of sporo-

zoites is made by grinding up entire mosquitoes with a pestle and mortar with a small amount of heparinised chick blood. This is diluted in Ringer-Locke's solution and lightly centrifuged in a hand centrifuge. The supernatant fluid is diluted to provide one mosquito per 0·2 ml., which is used as the inoculum. The suspension is given intravenously in a dose of 0·2 ml. Treatment is begun about two hours after infection and a second dose is given three to four hours after infection. Doses are then administered twice daily on each of the next five days.

(b) Tests using *P. cathemerium* and *P. relictum* in canaries. The inoculum is prepared as above but only the thoraces of the mosquito *Culex molestus* are ground up and injected intravenously : one half to one infected mosquito is allowed for each canary.

In the majority of screening tests devised in America for assessment of clinical control the drug under investigation was incorporated by weight in the diet and therapy was begun eighteen hours before intravenous inoculation (Wiselogle, 1946). Dietary concentration of drugs which suppresses parasitæmia by 50 per cent. may be used to compare activity (Reilly *et al.*, 1949).

The differences in the response of different species of plasmodium in the same host to the same drug can be explained as due to (1) failure of certain species of plasmodium to absorb the drug : with some compounds this difference can be experimentally determined ; (2) the metabolic reactions with which the drug interferes vary in importance in different species ; (3) some species employ metabolic pathways which are uninfluenced by the particular drug.

As Dearborn and Marshall (1947) point out, pharmacological tests with selected drugs may be of use in differentiating species of avian malaria parasites. Sulphadiazine, for instance, differentiates *P. lophuræ* or *P. circumflexum* from *P. cathemerium* or *P. relictum :* 2, 2', 3, 3'-tetramethyl-1, 1'-diphenyl-[4, 4'-bi-3-pyrazoline]-5, 5'-dione will distinguish *P. cathemerium* or *P. circumflexum* from *P. relictum ;* 3, 7-diacetamido-5-phenyl-phenazinium chloride will differentiate *P. lophuræ* from the other three species ; N'-(5-chloro-2-pyrimidyl) metanilamide will separate *P. cathemerium* from other plasmodia in canaries. Pharmacological tests have not up till now been employed by those interested in the species problem, but they undoubtedly represent a method of species differentiation which requires further study.

In addition to the differences found in the reactions of different parasites to the same drug, there are marked differences between the same parasite's reaction to the suppressive action of the same drug in different hosts. The quinine equivalent of N'-(5-chloro-2-pyrimidyl) metanilamide for suppressing *P. cathemerium* infection in the canary is 30, but in the duck 60 ; similarly, the quinine equivalent of sulphapyrazine in the canary is 0·008, in the duck 3·0 (Wiselogle, 1946). These differences may be due to differences in the metabolism of the same drug by different species of birds. Sulphonamides, for instance, produce higher blood concentrations in ducks than in canaries and are active antimalarials in the duck but not in the canary (Marshall, 1945).

Differences of the same species of plasmodium to the same drug in different hosts may depend not only on differences in the rate of absorption and distribution of the drug, giving different blood concentrations, but on degradation of the drug to an active product in one host and not in another or on degradation of the drug to an inactive compound in one host and not in another (Marshall, 1946). Differences in prophylactic activity of the same drug on different species of parasites in different hosts have been recognised for some time. They have been emphasised especially by Marshall (1946), whose results are shown in the table. In man, the degree of immunity has an important bearing on the suppressive reaction to drugs. In many West Africans with a high degree of acquired immunity to *P. falciparum*, a mild purge and rest in bed alone are enough to bring the temperature down to normal and to cause parasites to disappear from the blood stream. This acquired immunity must be distinguished from natural resistance. The negro both in America and in West Africa has a high degree of natural resistance to *P. vivax* infections.

Tonkin and Hawking (1947) elaborated methods of testing the action of drugs against trophozoite- and sporozoite-induced infections of *P. gallinaceum* in chickens. For trophozoite infections chickens of 60 to 80 gm. body weight are each given an intravenous injection of 10^7 parasitised red cells : the response is read as the percentage of parasitised red cells on the fifth day after

PROPHYLACTIC ACTIVITY IN AVIAN AND HUMAN VIVAX INFECTIONS
(E. K. Marshall, 1946)

Compound.	*P. gallinaceum* in chick.	*P. lophuræ* in turkey.	*P. cathemerium* in canary.	*P. vivax* in man.
Sulphadiazine	+ + +	0	+	0
N¹-(5-Bromo-2-pyrimidyl) sulphanilamide	+ + +	+	+	0
2-Hydroxy-3-(2-methyloctyl)-1, 4-naphthoquinone	+ + +	+	+	0
N¹-(5-Chloro-2-pyrimidyl) metanilamide	+ + +	+ + +	+	0
Pamaquin	0	+	+	+ + +

infection, the fourth day of treatment. Sporozoite infections are induced by the intravenous injection of the supernatant from a suspension of salivary glands equivalent to one infected mosquito per chicken. The minimum effective dose is that which reduces the parasitæmia to less than 2 per cent. on the seventh to ninth day of infection. Since few compounds are completely effective prophylactically, an assessment of value may be made by noting the delay in the appearance of parasites in the peripheral blood stream. The antimalarial activity of a compound, therapeutic or prophylactic, is compared with the maximum tolerated dose in mice, given orally twice daily for four days. For trophozoite-induced infections the maximum effect is obtained when the dose of quinine, mepacrine or pamaquin is concentrated into the first two days of treatment. With sulphadiazine the maximum effect is seen when treatment is spread over four days. Clarke and Theiler (1948) determined the relative efficiency of drugs in malarial infections by taking the ratio of the effective curative dose (ED 50 curative) to the effective suppressive dose (ED 50 suppressive). Thus for instance the curative efficiency of pamaquin against *P. cathemerium* in the duck is 14, of mepacrine 19. For quinine bisulphate the ED 50 (suppressive) against *P. cathemerium* is 75 mgm. per kgm. of body weight daily, but even daily doses of 1,500 mgm. per kgm. are insufficient to produce radical cures. Thus the ratio of ED 50 (curative) to ED 50 (suppressive) is greater than 20 and quinine bisulphate is less efficient than either pamaquin or mepacrine.

Bush (1948) believes that the " 3M " strain of *P. cathemerium*, adapted to the duck, is eminently suitable for routine testing. It is not associated with any virus as is the " 3T " strain used by Wolfson (1943) and it gives a constant parasitæmia peak.

The assessment of the antimalarial activity of drugs by oral administration of the compound in the diet is sometimes complicated by incomplete absorption from the intestine or by varying degrees of destruction of the drug in the alimentary tract : in addition, birds feed only during the hours of light.

Bratton (1945) therefore elaborated a technique by which ducks can be given continuous intravenous injections for three days. The results of single daily intravenous doses of quinine and cinchonine were compared with the results of continuous therapy. The minimum effective dose is taken as that required to reduce parasitæmia in the treated bird to one half that of the control based on third-day blood examinations. By continuous intravenous injection cinchonine was as effective as quinine by a single daily injection, but quinine was about twice as effective on the basis of dosage when given once a day as when given by continuous infusion. Results obtained by continuous intravenous injection of ducks are shown in the table.

ACTIVITY OF ANTIMALARIALS AGAINST *Plasmodium lophuræ* IN THE DUCK WHEN GIVEN IN A CONTINUOUS INTRAVENOUS INFUSION (Bratton, 1945).

Compound.	Minimum effective dose mgm./ kgm. per day.
Quinine hydrochloride dihydrate . .	15
Cinchonine hydrochloride hydrate . .	30
Mepacrine dihydrochloride . . .	6
8-Chloro-5-(2'-diethylaminoethylamino)-2-methoxyacridine dihydrochloride .	18
Pamaquin hydroiodide monohydrate .	0·5
Tartar emetic	16 (toxic)
Sodium antimony thioglycollate . .	16
Oxophenarsine hydrochloride . .	32 (toxic)

In carrying out antimalarial tests with ducks care must be taken to see that intercurrent virus infections are not also transmitted. One such virus infection has been demonstrated by Dearborn (1946).

Assessment of Anti-plasmodial Activity in Tissue Cultures

The possibility that antimalarial action could be studied *in vitro* in tissue cultures of plasmodia was first considered by Ball *et al.* (1945) and Berliner (1946), who used parasitised red cells suspended in Tyrode's solution. The exo-erythrocytic stages of *P. gallinaceum* were grown in tissue culture by Hawking (1945), and this tissue culture technique was adapted by Tonkin (1946) for testing the effect of drugs on this phase of the plasmodium. Ten-day-old chicks are inoculated with sporozoites of *P. gallinaceum* and killed seven to eight days later when heavily infected with tissue forms. The spleen is removed aseptically, minced in Tyrode's solution and set up in Carrel flasks, each of which contains three or four coverslips, arranged on the floor of the flask without touching one another. The fluid phase consists of Tyrode's solution containing 20 per cent. (vol./vol.) chick serum and 3 to 4 per cent. (vol./vol.) chick embryo extract ; 0·05 per cent. phenol red is added to indicate pH changes in the medium and 0·5 units of penicillin per ml. to prevent bacterial growth. Drugs to be tested are dissolved in Ringer's solution, sterilised by boiling, and appropriate concentrations are made by serial dilution ; 2·5 ml. volumes of the fluid phase are then run into the flasks containing the infected spleen explants, followed by 0·5 ml. volumes of the drug solution. Control flasks received 0·5 ml. volumes of sterile Ringer's solution in place of the drug. Flasks are incubated at 37° C. for seven to ten days. Slides are fixed in methyl alcohol, stained with Giemsa, and examined microscopically. Where no parasites can be demonstrated under the microscope the negative result is confirmed by inoculation of the fluid phase into chicks with observation of the presence or absence of subsequent infection.

The concentration of drug necessary to prevent the growth or survival of the exoerythrocytic forms of *P. gallinaceum* is shown in the table.

CONCENTRATIONS OF DRUGS INHIBITING EXO-ERYTHROCYTIC
FORMS OF *P. gallinaceum* IN TISSUE CULTURE (Tonkin, 1946)

Compound.	Concentration.
Sulphathiazole	0·05 mgm./100 ml.
Sulphadiazine	0·2 mgm./100 ml.
2-(*m*-Aminobenzenesulphonamido)-pyrimidine	0·1 mgm./100 ml.
Sontoquin	No activity.
Streptomycin	2·5 mgm./100 ml. (=10 units per ml.).
Streptothricin	250 mgm./100 ml. (=500 units per ml.).
Quinine bisulphate . .	Toxic to macrophages.
Mepacrine hydrochloride .	No activity.
Pamaquin dihydrochloride . .	Toxic to macrophages.
Proguanil acetate (N$_1$-*p*-chlorophenyl-N$_5$-*iso*propyl-biguanidine acetate)	Toxic to macrophages.
M 4430 (N$_1$-*p*-chlorophenyl-N$_5$-methyl*iso*-propylbiguanidine acetate)	No activity.
Stilbamidine	No activity.
p-Anisylguanidine nitrate . .	0·5 mgm./100 ml.

Chemotherapeutic Control of the Sexual Cycle in the Mosquito

A method for examining the effects of antimalarial drugs on the sporogenous cycle of *Plasmodium gallinaceum* in *Aëdes ægypti* has been devised by Terzian (1947). The drugs to be tested are added in various concentrations to a 4 per cent. sugar nutrient solution on which mosquitoes survive for as long as twenty days following an infective meal. The comparative effect of various drugs is shown in the table on p. 26.

With concentrations of sulphadiazine of 0·1 per cent. level, oöcysts are formed in large numbers but rarely grow beyond the medial point of development. With concentrations of 0·3 per cent. there is more complete inhibition of oöcyst development. If sulphadiazine is delayed until sporozoites have developed it has little or no action in preventing infection of chicks. Pamaquin, on the other hand, has a direct action on sporozoites (Terzian *et al.*, 1948). Similar studies have been made with *P. falciparum* (Terzian and Weathersby, 1949).

Dietary factors may influence the development of sporozoites,

COMPARISON OF THE EFFECTS OF VARIOUS DRUGS ON THE
SPOROGENOUS CYCLE OF *P. gallinaceum* IN *A. ægypti* AS
DETERMINED BY SUBSEQUENT INOCULATION INTO CHICKS
(Terzian *et al.*, 1948)

Drug.	Sporozoite density in mosquitoes.	Drug concentration, gm. per 100 ml.	Average per cent. red cells parasitised. (Days after inoculation.)					Number of survivors (out of six).
			8	10	12	14	16	
Quinine . . .	4 +	0·05	+	20·2	28·0	2·0		1/6
Mepacrine . .	4 +	0·02	+	36·5	46·1			0/6
Sontoquin (nivaquine)	4 +	0·05	1·6	33·4	28·0			1/5
Chloroquine . .	4 +	0·03	3·2	11·8	23·0			0/6
1-(7'-Chloro-4'-quino-lyl)-3-diethylamino-2-propanol . .	4 +	0·1	2·7	26·8	32·0	12·0		1/6
7-Chloro-4(3'-diethyl-aminopropylamino) quinoline . .	4 +	0·05	+	15·9	26·2			0/6
4-(7'-Chloro-4'-quino-lylamino)-α-diethyl-amino-o-cresol .	4 +	0·05	3·0	22·1	48·0			0/6
Pamaquin . .	2 +	0·03	0	+	9·3	18·6	13·1	2/6
Metachloridine . .	0	0·01	0	0	0	0		6/6
Proguanil . .	0	0·01	0	0	0	0		6/6
Sulphadiazine . .	0	0·1	0	0	0	0		6/6
Controls . . .	4 +		+	35·8	24·0			2/6

for their numbers are steadily depleted when the mosquitoes are
given only carbohydrate food (Mackerras and Ercole, 1948).

Proguanil, although it has no direct action on gametocytes of
P. vivax or on their fertilisation processes, appears to inhibit the
development of the oöcyst in the stomach wall of the mosquito.
There is also evidence that sulphamezathine stimulates the
formation of gametocytes of *P. falciparum*. Such gametocytes,
however, are unable to give rise to sporozoites in *Anopheles
gambiæ* (Findlay *et al.*, 1946).

The Response of Different Avian Plasmodia to Drugs

Even before 1939 it was realised that there were quantitative
differences in susceptibility to drugs of various avian malarias.
Manwell (1930a, b, 1932, 1934) studied five species, *P. relictum*,

P. cathemerium, P. circumflexum, P. elongatum and *P. rouxi*, and found that they varied in their responses to quinine and pamaquin. Kikuth (1931), using the same two drugs, observed differences in the first four species, and Manwell (1933) found that mepacrine radically cured *P. rouxi* infections in the canary but did not prevent or radically cure infections with *P. cathemerium* or *P. circumflexum*. Manwell *et al.* (1941) observed that sulphapyridine was without effect on *P. relictum* or *P. nucleophilum* infection but was active against *P. circumflexum* in the canary. Many of the earlier investigations were qualitative rather than quantitative in nature and it is therefore difficult to arrive at any valid conclusion as to the susceptibility of avian plasmodia to the suppressive activity of drugs (Curd, 1943). Later observations have been

SUSCEPTIBILITY OF AVIAN MALARIAS TO DRUGS (QUININE EQUIVALENTS REFERRED TO LOPHURÆ MALARIA IN DUCKS) (Dearborn and Marshall, 1947)

Compound.	Species of Plasmodium.			
	Lophuræ.	*Cathemerium.*	*Relictum.*	*Circumflexum.*
Quinine (base)	1	1/2	1/4	1/2
Sulphadiazine	3	1/64	1/128	1
Pamaquin (base)	64	64	64	32
Mepacrine hydrochloride . . .	4	6	3	2
8-(3'-Aminopropylamino)-6-methoxyquinoline dihydrochloride	2	4	4	4
2, 2', 3, 3'-Tetramethyl-1, 1'-diphenyl-[4, 4'-bi-3-pyrazoline]-5, 5'-dione . .	1/2	1/32	2	< 1/32
Dimethyldithiocarbamic acid methylene diester	1	1/2	1	1/2
3, 7-Diacetamido-5-phenylphenazinium chloride	1/8	2	2	4
4-tert-Butyl-α-diethylamino-6-phenyl-*o*-cresol hydrochloride . . .	2	2	1	1
Chloroquine diphosphate . . .	8	16	4	8
1-(7'-Chloro-4'-quinolylamino)-3-diethylamino-2-propanol diphosphate . .	2	3	2	2
7-Chloro-2-phenyl-α-2-piperidyl-4-quinolyl-2'-piperidyl methanol dihydrochloride .	8	8	4	4
N¹-(5-Chloro-2-pyrimidyl) metanilamide .	32	32	8	< 1/32
7-Chloro-2-(*p*-chlorophenyl)-4-quinolyl-dibutylaminomethyl methanol monohydrochloride	16	8	8	8

on a quantitative basis. Thus, for instance, the minimal effective dose of quinine base capable of suppressing lophuræ malaria in the duck averages about 26 mgm. per kgm. per day, according to Dearborn and Marshall (1947). The quinine equivalents relative to lophuræ malaria of a number of other compounds on avian malarias show considerable variation; the results are shown in the table on p. 27.

Although much has been learnt from a study of malarial parasites in animals it must be confessed that the results of " screening" compounds in avian malaria have been difficult to apply directly to man since there is no direct correlation between the effects of drugs on avian and human malarias. No one species of avian parasite and no one avian host is satisfactory for the assessment of chemical compounds of possible value in human malarias. Even between *P. knowlesi* in rhesus monkeys and human malarial parasites there are wide differences in the reaction to chemotherapeutic compounds, although, broadly speaking, it may be said that any compound which is active against *P. knowlesi* will show some activity against human parasites. It is, however, impracticable to use large numbers of rhesus monkeys for the preliminary examination of possible antimalarial drugs. The true evaluation of drugs for the treatment of human malarias can be made only in man and in such an evaluation strains of parasites of varying geographical provenance must be employed unless highly fallacious results are to be obtained.

References

ALBRICHT, I. C., and NIEUWENHUYSE, C., 1937, De werkzaam-heid van methyleenblauw op vogelmalaria. *Ned. Tijdschr. Geneesk.*, 81, 483.

BALL, E. G., ANFINSEN, C. B., GEIMAN, Q. M., McKEE, R. W., and ORMSBEE, R. A., 1945, *In vitro* growth and multiplication of the malaria parasite *Plasmodium knowlesi*. *Science*, 101, 542.

BERLINER, R. W., 1946, The *in vitro* assay of suppressive antimalarial activity : *P. falciparum. Fed. Proc.*, 5, 164.

BOVET, D., BENOIT, G., and ALTMAN, R., 1934, Action thérapeutique de quinoléines à poids moléculaire élevé, homologues de la plasmoquine, sur les hématozoaires des calfats et des serins. *Bull. Soc. Path. exot.*, 27, 236.

BOYD, M. F., 1947, A note on the chronicity of a quartan malaria infection. In, Societé belge de Médecine tropicale, "Liber jubilaris J. Rodhain," p. 99. Bruxelles. A. Goemaere.

BRACKETT, S., and WALETZKY, E., 1946, Antimalarial activity of meta-chloridine (2-*meta*-nilamido-5-chloropyrimidine) and other metanilamide derivatives in test infections with *Plasmodium gallinaceum*. *J. Parasit.*, 32, 325.

BRATTON, A. C., Jr., 1945, Continuous intravenous chemotherapy of *Plasmodium lophuræ* infection in ducks. *J. Pharmacol.*, **85**, 103.

BRUMPT, E., BOVET, D., and BRUMPT, L., 1937, Action des médicaments antipaludiques sur l'infection de la poule par le *Plasmodium gallinaceum*. In, " Festschrift Bernhard Nocht zum 80 Geburtstag," p. 61. Hamburg. Augustin.

BUSH, D. L., 1948, Experimental transmission of the " 3M " strain of *Plasmodium cathemerium* to the duck and its chemotherapeutic suitability for routine antimalarial screening. *J. Parasit.*, **34**, 321.

BUTTLE, G. A. H., HENRY, T. A., SOLOMON, W., TREVAN, J. W., and GIBBS, E. M., 1938, The action of the cinchona and certain other alkaloids in bird malaria. *Biochem. J.*, **32**, 47.

CLARKE, D. H., and THEILER, M., 1948, Studies on parasite-host-interplay between *Plasmodium gallinaceum* and the chicken as influenced by hydroxynaphthoquinone. *J. infect. Dis.*, **82**, 138.

COATNEY, G. R., and COOPER, W. C., 1944, Prophylactic effect of sulfadiazine and sulfaguanidine against mosquito-borne *Plasmodium gallinaceum* infection in domestic fowl (preliminary report). *Publ. Hlth. Rep., Wash.*, **59**, 1455.

COATNEY, G. R., GREENBERG, J. G., COOPER, W. C., TREMBLEY, H. L., 1949, Antimalarial activity of aureomycin against *Plasmodium gallinaceum* in the chick. *Proc. Soc. exper. Biol., N.Y.*, **72**, 586.

COGGESHALL, L. T., 1940, The selective action of sulfanilamide on the parasites of experimental malaria in monkeys *in vivo* and *in vitro*. *J. exp. Med.*, **71**, 13.

COGGESHALL, L. T., PORTER, R. J., and LAIRD, R. L., 1944, Prophylactic and curative effects of certain sulfonamide compounds on exoerythrocytic stages in *Plasmodium gallinaceum* malaria. *Proc. Soc. exp. Biol., N.Y.*, **57**, 286.

CURD, F. H. S., 1943, The activity of drugs in the malaria of man, monkeys and birds. *Ann. trop. Med. Parasit.*, **37**, 115.

CURD, F. H. S., DAVEY, D. G., and ROSE, F. L., 1945, Studies on synthetic antimalarial drugs. Some biguanide derivatives as new types of antimalarial substances with both therapeutic and causal prophylactic activity. *Ann. trop. Med. Parasit.*, **39**, 208.

DAVEY, D. G., 1946a, The use of avian malaria for the discovery of drugs effective in the treatment and prevention of human malaria. I. Drugs for clinical treatment and clinical prophylaxis. *Ann. trop. Med. Parasit.*, **40**, 52.

DAVEY, D. G., 1946b, The use of avian malaria for the discovery of drugs effective in the treatment and prevention of human malaria. II. Drugs for causal prophylaxis and radical cure or the chemotherapy of exoerythrocytic forms. *Ann. trop. Med. Parasit.*, **40**, 453.

DEARBORN, E. H., 1946, Filtrable agents lethal for ducks. *Proc. Soc. exp. Biol., N.Y.*, **63**, 48.

DEARBORN, E. H., and MARSHALL, E. K., Jr., 1946, Curative action of drugs in lophuræ malaria of the duck. *Proc. Soc. exp. Biol., N.Y.*, **63**, 46.

DEARBORN, E. H., and MARSHALL, E. K., Jr., 1947, The susceptibility of different species of avian malarial parasites to drugs. *Amer. J. Hyg.*, **45**, 25.

DECOURT, P., BELFORT, J., and SCHNEIDER, J., 1939, Etude de l'action de l'oxy(diméthylaminobutyl-amino) quinoléine sur *Plasmodium gallinaceum* et *Plasmodium falciparum*. *Bull. Soc. Path. exot.*, **32**, 419.

DIONISI, A., 1899, Un parasite du globule rouge dans une espèce de chauvesouris (*Miniopterus Schreibersii Kuhl*). *Arch. ital. Biol.*, **31**, 151.

FINDLAY, G. M., MAEGRAITH, B. G., MARKSON, J. L., and HOLDEN, J. R., 1946, Investigations in the chemotherapy of malaria in West Africa. V. Sulphonamide compounds. *Ann. trop. Med. Parasit.*, **40**, 358.

FOURNEAU, E., TRÉFOUEL, J., TRÉFOUEL, Mme., BOVET, D., and BENOIT, G., 1931, Contribution à la chimiothérapie du paludisme : essais sur les calfats. *Ann. Inst. Pasteur*, **46**, 514.

FOURNEAU, E., TRÉFOUEL, J., TRÉFOUEL, Mme., BOVET, D., and BENOIT, G., 1933, Contribution à la chimiothérapie du paludisme : essais sur les calfats (Deuxième mémoire). *Ann. Inst. Pasteur.*, **50**, 731.

GARNHAM, P. C. C., 1948, Exo-erythrocytic schizogony in Malaria. *Trop. Dis. Bull.*, **45**, 831.

HAWKING, F., 1945, Growth of protozoa in tissue culture. I. *Plasmodium gallinaceum* exoerythrocytic forms. *Trans. R. Soc. trop. Med. Hyg.*, **39**, 245.

HUFF, C. G., 1947, Life cycle of malarial parasites. *Ann. Rev. Microbiol.*, **1**, 43.

HUFF, C. G., and COULSTON, F., 1944, The development of *Plasmodium gallinaceum* from sporozoite to erythrocytic trophozoite. *J. infect. Dis.*, **75**, 231.

HUFF, C. G., and COULSTON, F., 1946, Relation of natural and acquired immunity of various avian hosts to cryptozoites and metacryptozoites of *Plasmodium gallinaceum* and *Plasmodium relictum*. *J. infect. Dis.*, **78**, 99.

HUFF, C. G., COULSTON, F., and CANTRELL, W., 1943, Malarial cryptozoites. *Science*, **97**, 286.

HUGHES, C. O., and BRACKETT, S., 1946, Prevention of sporozoite-induced infections of *Plasmodium cathemerium* in canary by metachloridine. *J. Parasit.*, **32**, 340.

KELSEY, F. E., OLDHAM, F. K., and GITTELSON, A. L., 1946, Curative effect of plasmoquin in *Plasmodium lophuræ* infections. *Fed. Proc.*, **5**, 185.

KIKUTH, W., 1931, Immunobiologische und chemotherapeutische Studien an verschiedenen Stämmen von Vogelmalaria. *Zbl. Bakt. Abt. 1. Orig.*, **121**, 401.

KIKUTH, W., 1932, Atebrin ein neuss synthetisches malariaheitmittel. *Riv. Malariol.*, **11**, 157.

KIKUTH, W., 1935, Die experimentelle chemotherapie der Malaria. *Dtsch. med. Wschr.*, **61**, 573.

KIKUTH, W., and MUDROW, L., 1939, Chemotherapeutische Untersuchungen an den endothelialen Formen (E-Stadien) des *Plasmodium cathemerium*. *Z. ImmunForsch.*, **95**, 285.

KNOPPERS, A. T., and NIEUWENHUYSE, C. T., 1946, The combinations of cinchona alkaloids and bird malaria. Summation or synergism ? (in connection with the cinchona problem). *Arch. int. Pharmacodyn.*, **73**, 260.

KOPANARIS, P., 1911, Die Wirkung von Chinin, Salvarsan und Atoxyl auf die *Proteosoma* (*Plasmodium præcox*). Infektion des Kanarienvogels. *Arch. Schiffs.-u. TropenHyg.*, **15**, 586.

MACKERRAS, M. J., and ERCOLE, Q. N., 1948, Observations on the development of human malarial parasites in the mosquito. *Aust. J. exp. Biol. med. Sci.*, **26**, 439.

McGHEE, R. B., 1949a, The occurrence of bat malaria in the New Hebrides and Philippine Islands. *J. Parasit.*, **35**, 545.

McGHEE, R. B., 1949b, Infection of the immature white mouse with the avian malaria parasite. *J. Parasit.*, **35**, 123.

MANWELL, R. D., 1930a, Further studies on the effect of quinine and plasmochin on the avian malarias. *Amer. J. trop. Med.*, **10**, 379.

MANWELL, R. D., 1930b, The varying effects of quinine and plasmochin therapy on the different avian malarias. *J. Parasit.*, **17**, 110.

MANWELL, R. D., 1932, Quinine and plasmochin therapy in *Plasmodium rouxi* infections, with further notes on the effects of these drugs on the other avian malarias. *Amer. J. trop. Med.*, **12**, 123.

MANWELL, R. D., 1933, Effect of atebrin on avian malarias. *Proc. Soc. exp. Biol.*, *N.Y.*, **31**, 198.

MANWELL, R. D., 1934, Quinine and plasmochin therapy in infections with *Plasmodium circumflexum*. *Amer. J. trop. Med.*, **14**, 45.

MANWELL, R. D., 1946, Bat malaria. *Amer. J. Hyg.*, **43**, 1.

MANWELL, R. D., COUNTS, E., and COULSTON, F., 1941, Effect of sulfanilamide and sulfapyridine on the avian malarias. *Proc. Soc. exp. Biol.*, *N.Y.*, **46**, 523.

MARSHALL, E. K., Jr., 1946, Symposium on advances in pharmacology resulting from war research ; chemotherapy of malaria, 1941–45. *Fed. Proc.*, **5**, 298.

MARSHALL, P. B., 1945, The absorption of sulphonamides in the chick and the canary and its relationship to antimalarial activity. *J. Pharmacol.*, **84**, 1.

MORGENROTH, J., ABRAHAM, L., and SCHNITZER, R., 1926, Experimentelle Studien zur Malariabehandlung. Die Wirkung des Hydrochinins und Optochins auf die Vegelmalaria. *Dtsch. med. Wschr.*, **52**, 1455.

PORTER, R. J., 1942, The tissue distribution of exoerythrocytic schizonts in sporozoite-induced infections with *Plasmodium cathemerium*. *J. infect. Dis.*, **71**, 1.

REILLY, J., CHEN, G., and GEILING, E. M. K., 1949, An evaluation of antimalarials with *Plasmodium lophuræ* in the chick. *J. infect. Dis.*, **85**, 205.

RÖEHL, W., 1926, Die Wirkung des Plasmochins auf die Vogelmalaria. *Arch. Schiffs-u. TropenHyg.*, **30**, Beiheft., 311.

RUSSELL, P. F., 1931a, Avian malaria studies : prophylactic plasmochin in inoculated avian malaria. *Philipp. J. Sci.*, **46**, 305.

RUSSELL, P. F., 1931b, Avian malaria studies ; prophylactic plasmochin *versus* prophylactic quinine in inoculated avian malaria. *Philipp. J. Sci.*, **46**, 347.

RUSSELL, P. F., and NONO, A. M., 1932, Avian malaria studies : plasmochin as prophylactic drug in sporozoite infections of avian malaria. *Philipp. J. Sci.*, **49**, 595.

SCHNEIDER, J., DECOURT, P., and MONTÉZIN, G., 1949, Sur l'utilisation d'un nouveau plasmodium (*Pl. berghei*) pour l'étude et la recherche de medicaments antipaludiques. *Bull. Soc. Path. exot.*, **42**, 449.

SERGENT, ED., 1949, Contribution à l'étude du second cycle evolutif insexue des Plasmodium chez les paludeens. *Arch. Inst. Pasteur Algér.*, **27**, 211.

SERGENT, EDM., and SERGENT, ET., 1907, Etudes sur les hématozoaires d'oiseaux. *Plasmodium relictum, Leucytozoon ziemanni et Hæmoproteus noctuæ, Hæmoproteus columbæ*, trypanosome de l'hirondelle. *Ann. Inst. Pasteur*, **21**, 251.

SERGENT, ET. and SERGENT, EDM., 1921a, Avantages de la quininisation préventive démonstrés et précisés experimentalement (paludisme des oiseaux). *Ann. Inst. Pasteur*, **35**, 125.

SERGENT, ET., and SERGENT, EDM., 1921b, Etude expérimentale du paludisme ; paludisme des oiseaux (*Plasmodium relictum*). *Bull. Soc. Path. exot.*, **14**, 72.

SERGENT, ET., and SERGENT, EDM., 1921c, Etude expérimentale du paludisme (paludisme des oiseaux à *Plasmodium relictum*, transmis par *Culex pipiens*). *Arch. Inst. Pasteur Afr. N.*, **1**, 1.

SERGENT, ET., and SERGENT, EDM., 1922, Etude expérimentale du paludisme des oiseaux (*Plasmodium relictum*). *Arch. Inst. Pasteur Afr. N.*, **2**, 320.

SERGENT, ET., SERGENT, EDM., and CATANEI, A., 1923, Etude expérimentale de paludisme des oiseaux (*Plasmodium relictum*) : cinchonidine. *Arch. Inst. Pasteur Algér.*, **1**, 270.

SERGENT, ET., SERGENT, EDM., and CATANEI, A., 1924a, Etude expérimentale du paludisme des oiseaux (*Plasmodium relictum*) : cinchonine. *Arch. Inst. Pasteur Algér.*, **2**, 443.

SERGENT, ET., SERGENT, EDM., and CATANEI, A., 1924b, Etude expérimentale du paludisme des oiseaux (*Plasmodium relictum*). Résumé des essais de traitement préventif ou curatif par les alcaloides du quinquina. *Arch. Inst. Pasteur Algér.*, **2**, 455.

SERGENT, ET., SERGENT, EDM., and CATANEI, A., 1925a, Etude expérimentale du paludisme des oiseaux (*Plasmodium relictum*) : action de la cinchonine sur le Plasmodium pendant la période aiguë. *Arch. Inst. Pasteur Algér.*, **3**, 122.

SERGENT, ET., SERGENT, EDM., and CATANEI, A., 1925b, Etude expérimentale du paludisme des oiseaux (*Plasmodium relictum*): le stovarsol. *Arch. Inst. Pasteur Algér.*, **2**, 124.

SHORTT, H. E., 1948, The life cycle of *Plasmodium cynomolgi* in its insect and mammalian hosts. *Trans. R. Soc. trop. Med. Hyg.*, **42**, 227.

SHORTT, H. E., FAIRLEY, N. H., COVELL, G., SHUTE, P. G., and GARNHAM, P. C. C., 1949, The pre-erythrocytic stage of *Plasmodium falciparum* : a preliminary note. *Brit. med. J.*, ii, 1006.

SHORTT, H. E., and GARNHAM, P. C. C., 1948a, Pre-erythroytic stage in mammalian malaria parasites. *Nature, Lond.*, **161**, 126.

SHORTT, H. E., and GARNHAM, P. C. C., 1948b, Demonstration of a persisting exo-erythrocytic stage in *Plasmodium cynomolgi* and its bearing on the production of relapses. *Brit. med. J.*, i, 1225.

SHORTT, H. E., GARNHAM, P. C. C., COVELL, G., and SHUTE, P. G., 1948. The pre-erythrocytic stage of human malaria *Plasmodium vivax*. *Brit. med. J.*, i, 547.

SHORTT, H. E., GARNHAM, P. C. C., and MALAMOS, B., 1948, The pre-erythrocytic stage of mammalian malaria. *Brit. med. J.*, i, 192.

SHUTE, P. G., 1946, Latency and long-term relapses in benign tertian malaria. *Trans. R. Soc. trop. Med. Hyg.*, **40**, 189.

TATE, P., and VINCENT, M., 1933 Susceptibility of autogenous and anautogenous races of *Culex pipiens* to infection with avian plasmodium (*Plasmodium relictum*). *Parasitology*, **25**, 96.

TERZIAN, L. A., 1947, A method for screening antimalarial compounds in the mosquito host. *Science*, **106**, 449.

TERZIAN, L. A., STAHLER, N., and WEATHERSBY, A. B., 1948, The action of antimalarial drugs in mosquitoes infected with *Plasmodium gallinaceum*. *J. infect. Dis.*, **84**, 47.

TERZIAN, L. A., and WEATHERSBY, A. B., 1949, Action of antimalarial drugs in mosquitoes infected with *Plasmodium falciparum*. *Amer. J. trop Med.*, **29**, 19.

TONKIN, I. M., 1946, The testing of drugs against exoerythrocytic forms of *P. gallinaceum* in tissue culture. *Brit. J. Pharmacol.*, 1, 163.

TONKIN, I. M., and HAWKING, F., 1947, The technique of testing chemotherapeutic action on *Plasmodium gallinaceum*. *Brit. J. Pharmacol.*, 2, 221.

VINCKE, I. H., and LIPS, M., 1948, Un nouveau plasmodium d'un rongeur sauvage du Congo, *Plasmodium berghei* n. sp. *Ann. Soc. belge Méd. trop.*, **28**, 97.

WALKER, H. A., STAUBER, L. A., and RICHARDSON, A. P., 1948, Curative action of pamaquine naphthoate, quinacrine hydrochloride and quinine bisulphate in *Plasmodium cathemerium* infections of the duck. *J. infect. Dis.*, **82**, 187.

WILLIAMSON, J., 1948, A nomogram for the preparation of standard inocula in the Davey chick test for antimalarial activity. *Ann. trop. Med. Parasit.*, **42**, 238.

WISELOGLE, F. Y., edited by, 1946, " A survey of antimalarial drugs, 1941–45." 2 vols. Ann Arbor, Michigan. J. W. Edwards.

WOLFSON, F., 1943, Further studies of the " 3T " strain of *Plamodium cathemerium* in white Pekin ducks. *Amer. J. Hyg.*, **37**, 325.

YORKE, W., 1925, Further observations on malaria made during treatment of general paralysis. *Trans. R. Soc. trop. Med. Hyg.*, **19**, 108.

YORKE, W., and MACFIE, J. W. S., 1924, Observations on malaria made during treatment of general paralysis. *Trans. R. Soc. trop. Med. Hyg.*, **18**, 13.

CHAPTER III

THE CHEMICAL APPROACH TO ANTIMALARIAL COMPOUNDS (I)

I. The Cinchona Alkaloids and their Modifications

ANY consideration of the chemical structure of synthetic anti-malarials must inevitably go back to the structure of the cinchona alkaloids.

The following general formula is now assigned to this group of alkaloids (Rabe, 1909 ; Rabe, Huntenburg, Schultze, and Volger, 1931) :—

Quinoline Group.   Secondary Alcohol Group.   Quinuclidine Group.

QUININE ALKALOIDS GENERAL FORMULA (I)

In quinine and quinidine $R = OCH_3$. $R' = CH : CH_2$.
In cinchonine and cinchonidine $R = H$. $R' = CH : CH_2$.
In cupreine $R = OH$. $R' = CH : CH_2$.
In the hydro bases R' becomes $CH_2 . CH_3$.
In the alkylcupreines R becomes OAlk (homologues of quinine).
In the alkylhydrocupreines and alkylhydrocupreidines R becomes OAlk and R' becomes $CH_2 . CH_3$ (homologues of dihydroquinine and dihydroquinidine).

The four chief crystallisable alkaloids derived from cinchona bark are, as is well known, quinine, quinidine, cinchonine and cinchonidine, but over twenty other alkaloids have been isolated from various species of cinchona and cuprea. The majority of these alkaloids, the non-crystallisable and amorphous alkaloids, are sometimes described collectively as quinoidine : strictly speaking, however, quinoidine is the pitch-like residue left after the removal of the commercially valuable alkaloids from the total alkaloids of cinchona bark. The four alkaloids, quinine, quinidine, cinchonine and cinchonidine, form two pairs of iso-merides of which each member of the first pair differs from each member of the second by the residue of a methoxy group. In addition, the members of each pair yield for the most part products furnished by the two pairs from parallel series differing constantly by the residue of a methoxy group. From the general formula it will be noted that it includes four centres of asymmetry, numbered 3, 4, 8 and 9. The differences between the members of each pair of isomerides are due to differences in configuration at certain of these centres and from a considerable body of evidence (Lapp, 1935 ; Henry *et al.*, 1937 ; Solomon, 1938), the direction of rotation at each of these centres for each of the principal cinchona alkaloids is now known and is shown in the following table (Solomon, 1938) :—

STEREOCHEMICAL PICTURE OF THE CINCHONA ALKALOIDS

Compound.		Relative configurations at C atoms.			
		3	4	8	9
Cinchonine . .	⎫ dextro-				
Dihydrocinchonine .	⎬ rotatory	+	−	+	+
Quinidine . .	⎬ series				
Dihydroquinidine .	⎭				
Cinchonidine . .	⎫ lævo-				
Dihydrocinchonidine	⎬ rotatory	+	−	−	−
Quinine . . .	⎬ series.				
Dihydroquinine	⎭				

The first successful synthesis of quinine was carried out by Woodward and Doering (1944).

Modification of the Cinchona Alkaloids

Modification of the cinchona alkaloids gives rise to a number of compounds of therapeutic interest, for with hydrogenation of the vinyl group and replacement of the methoxy group of quinine and quinidine by higher alkyloxy groups the following compounds are produced. When the alkyloxy group is

—OCH₃	there is formed Methylhydrocupreine.

—OCH$_3$ there is formed Methylhydrocupreine.
—OC$_2$H$_5$,, ,, ,,   Ethylhydrocupreine (Optochin).
—OCH(CH$_3$)$_2$,, ,, ,,   *iso*Propylhydrocupreine.
—OCH$_2$. CH(CH$_3$)$_2$,, ,, ,,   *iso*Butylhydrocupreine.
—OCH$_2$. CH$_2$. CH(CH$_3$)$_2$,, ,, ,,   *iso*Amylhydrocupreine (Eukupin).
—O . (CH$_2$)$_5$. CH(CH$_3$)$_2$,, ,, ,,   *iso*Octylhydrocupreine (Vuzin).

Optochin has a curative action in pneumococcal infections in mice and was one of the first compounds to destroy bacteria *in vivo* ; vuzin is toxic *in vitro* to *Corynebacterium diphtheriæ* whereas eukupin and vuzin possess local anæsthetic properties.

A red azo dye, 6'-methoxyquinoline-8'-azodihydrocupreine, was prepared by Giemsa and Oesterlin (1933). In human malaria it was found by Green (1934) to act like quinine on the parasites of malignant tertian and quartan malaria but to be inferior in vivax infections. According to Missiroli and Mosna (1934), however, it is free from toxic effects and does not produce deafness or buzzing in the ears.

Considerable attention has been paid to modifications of the cinchona alkaloids with a view to obtaining more active compounds. Some of the changes undergone by quinine are as yet but little understood. Solutions of quinine, for instance, are known to decrease in antimalarial activity when exposed to ultra-violet light. The amount of decomposition varies with the *p*H of the solution and with the concentration of the alkaloidal salt (Kyker *et al.*, 1946), but the chemical changes produced by ultra-violet light are still unknown. Kyker *et al.* (1947) believe that one of the active antimalarial substances resulting from exposure to ultra-violet light cannot be quinine, Roskin and Romanowa (1929) having originally demonstrated that the irradiation of solutions of quinine by ultra-violet light decreased the antimalarial action. Incidentally, Delperdange (1948) has reported a new crystalline form of quinine hydrochloride which is less sensitive to light than the fine needles of the basic hydrochloride : the newly described form resembles sugar candy and may be a mixture of isomers.

The effects of hydrogenation on antimalarial activity were studied by Buttle, Henry, and Trevan (1934), using *Plasmodium relictum* infections in canaries. If the antimalarial activity of quinine were taken as 1, the quinine activities or the therapeutic efficiency of the four main cinchona alkaloids and their dihydrogen derivatives were :—

Quinine	1
Dihydroquinine	1–2
Quinidine	less than 0·5
Dihydroquinidine	0·5–1
Cinchonine	less than 0·2
Dihydrocinchonine	,, ,, 0·2
Cinchonidine	0·5
Dihydrocinchonidine . . .	less than 0·2

The antimalarial activity of modified cinchona alkaloids has also been investigated. Quinine chloride is lacking in activity (Giemsa *et al.*, 1926), a result confirmed by Buttle *et al.* (1934), and Cohen and King (1938), who found that other cinchona alkaloidal chlorides and the corresponding hydro compounds also are inactive. Antimalarial activity thus disappears in these alkaloids when the —CHOH group is replaced by —CHCl. A similar loss of activity (Giemsa and Oesterlin, 1933) is associated with replacement by —CH₂ (desoxyquinine, desoxydihydrocinchonine, desoxydihydrocinchonidine, desoxycinchonine, desoxycinchonidine); —CH— (hydroquinine and cinchine); —CO— (quininone); CH . OAc— (acetyldihydroquinine).

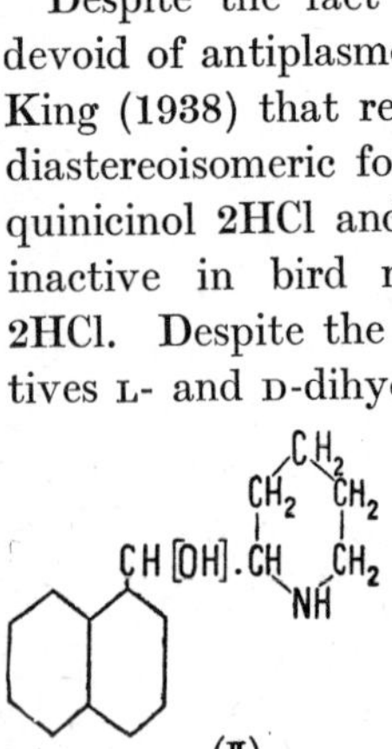

Despite the fact that quinicine, an isomeride of quinine, is devoid of antiplasmodial action, it seemed possible to Ainley and King (1938) that reduction to the carbinol which occurs in two diastereoisomeric forms might restore activity. Both L-dihydroquinicinol 2HCl and D-dihydroquinicinol 2HCl, however, proved inactive in bird malaria as did α-N-methyldihydroquinicinol 2HCl. Despite the close resemblance of the γ-piperidine derivatives L- and D-dihydroquinicinols to dihydroquinine this did not confer antimalarial activity on them : when, however, the piperidine ring was attached at its α-position through the carbinol group to the methoxyquinoline nucleus as in (II ; R = OMe), two diastereoisomerides were obtained both of which showed antiplasmodial activity. The toxicity of this group of substances was comparable with that of the cinchona alkaloids and not with substances of the type of pamaquin, which are much more toxic.

As these bases, however, were difficult of access and modification by conversion into the tertiary bases led to loss of activity it seemed desirable to prepare a more accessible series of simple carbinolamines (III) in which the strongly basic nitrogen centre is still separated from the quinoline nucleus by two carbon atoms as in quinine or hydroquinine.

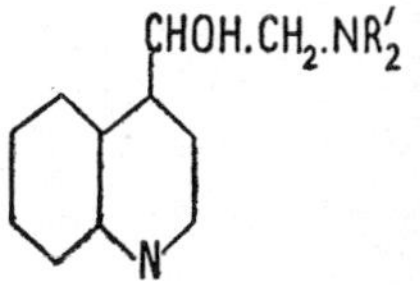

Compounds of type (III) may be looked upon as derived from quinine or more correctly dihydroquinine by fission of the quinuclidine portion of the molecule.

Although Schönhöfer (1938) had reported that such bases prepared by Kaufmann's method were inactive in bird malaria, King and Work (1940) found that certain carbinolamines were active against *P. relictum* when $R' = C_4H_9$, C_5H_{11} or C_6H_{13}. While no naphthyl, methoxynaphthyl or quinolyl derivative had any noticeable activity, in the methoxyquinolyl series there was a zone of activity, the three bases dibutyl-, diamyl- and dihexyl-aminomethyl-6-methoxy-4-quinolyl-carbinols all being active whereas the higher and lower homologues were inactive. The dibutyl compound, it may be noted, differs in its molecular structure from dihydroquinine only by having four extra hydrogen atoms. The results when some of these compounds were given prophylactically against *P. relictum* to canaries were as follows, the first dose being given four hours after injection of parasites :—

Compound.	Dose.	Day of appearance of parasites in peripheral blood.
Untreated controls	—	5
Quinine	6 × 2·5 *	12–14
Dibutylaminomethyl-6-methoxy-4-quinolyl-carbinol	6 × 2·5	9
Diamylaminomethyl-6-methoxy-4-quinolyl-carbinol	6 × 10	10–11
Dihexylaminomethyl-6-methoxy-4-quinolyl-carbinol	6 × 10	13

* Dose in mgm. given daily per 20 gm. body weight.

These results proved that compounds of this type possess weak antiplasmodial properties and, as had previously been suggested by Magidson and Rubtsov (1937), that activity is not completely dependent on the nature of the quinuclidine half of compounds related to the cinchona alkaloids.

Following on the work of Ainley and King (1938) and King and Work (1940), a number of quinoline methanols were prepared in America and tested for suppressive and prophylactic activity in man (Wiselogle, 1946 ; Lutz *et al.*, 1946 ; Brown *et al.*, 1946 ; Koepfli, 1946 ; Rapport *et al.*, 1946 ; Buchman *et al.*, 1946). The most important of the compounds are :—

No.	Compound.	Suppressive activity *P. vivax* (blood induced) (McCoy). Quinine equivalent.
SN 2157	6-Methoxy-4-quinolyl-2^1-piperidyl-carbinol . .	0·2
SN 2549	4-Quinolyl-2^1-piperidyl-carbinol	0·3
SN 8538	2-Phenyl-4-quinolyl-2^1-piperidyl-carbinol . .	1·0
SN 9849	6-Methoxy-2-phenyl-4-quinolyl-2^1-piperidyl-carbinol	1·0
SN 10275	6 : 8-Dichloro-2-phenyl-4-quinolyl-2^1-piperidyl-carbinol.	3·0
SN 10525	6-Methoxy-2-phenyl-4-quinolyl-dibutylaminomethyl-carbinol.	0·2
SN 10527	6-Methoxy-2-phenyl-4-quinolyl-dioctylaminomethyl-carbinol.	0·3
SN 11441	7-Chloro-2-phenyl-4-quinolyl-dihexylaminomethyl-carbinol.	0·3

All these compounds showed activity against blood-induced *P. vivax* infection. In both types derived from 4-quinoline methanol the incorporation of other substituents into the aromatic nucleus increased activity in bird malaria. Thus against *P. lophuræ* in ducks, or *P. cathemerium*, SN 10,275 is twenty to eighty times as active as quinine (Marshall, 1946). SN 2,157 and SN 2,549 were also tested against blood-induced infections due to *P. falciparum* (McLendon strain). None of the compounds tested in bird malaria had prophylactic activity. Some of the compounds were poorly absorbed when given by mouth and SN 8,538 and SN 10,275 were toxic. In doses of 1 gm. of the salt per day SN 10,275 was found by Pullman *et al.* (1948) to produce symptoms associated with photosensitivity, varying from a slight tingling of the skin of the face to severe burning accompanied by erythema : in one individual desquamation of the skin over the nose was seen, and another had mild labial œdema. These symptoms appeared only after exposure to sunlight for periods of at least fifteen minutes. The sensitivity to sunlight persisted for from one half to ten months after ceasing to take the drug. Two subjects manifested increased sensitivity to light mechanical trauma, such as rubbing or shaving, and a third noted smarting and burning of the eyes after exposure to sunlight. Mild gastro-intestinal symptoms, cramps, nausea, and diarrhœa occasionally developed. In view of these symptoms it is satisfactory to know that SN 10,275 does not possess any marked activity in controlling acute attacks, for relapses of vivax malaria occurred when the plasma concentrations fell to 59 and 80 μgm. per litre ; neither does SN 10,275 have any action on sporozoites.

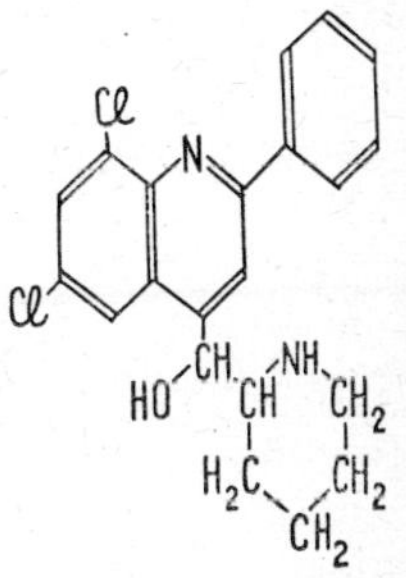

isoAlloxazines

In view of the possibility that the antiplasmodial action of quinine and mepacrine might be due to an antagonism between the drug and the riboflavin-containing enzyme systems almost certainly present in malarial parasites (Madinaveitia, 1944, 1946), attempts were made by King and Acheson (1946) to build isoalloxazines of the type of (I) but with basic side-chains in place of the ribityl group.

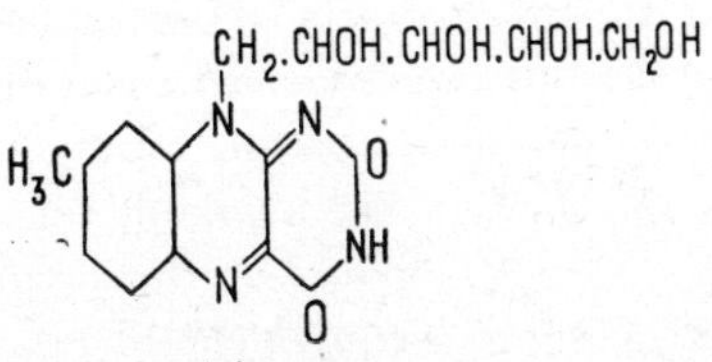

(I)

Some antimalarial activity was found.

As a continuation of the work suggesting that quinine inactivated riboflavin-containing enzymes in the malarial parasite,

King and Wright (1948) prepared a series of bases of the type (II) containing a 6 : 7-dimethyl quinoline nucleus with methyl groups structurally spaced as in riboflavin. The antiplasmodial properties of these compounds were compared with those of corresponding bases without the methyl groups but with the 6-methoxy group.

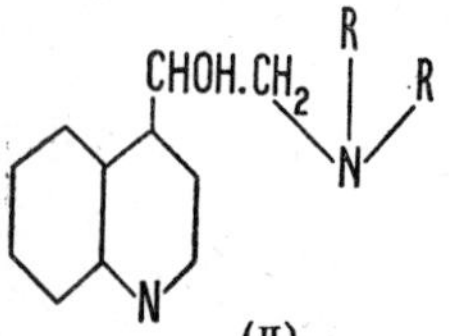

(II)

The starting material was 3 : 4-xylidine. The results are shown in the table on the opposite page.

No piperidinomethyl or morpholinomethyl derivative in either series was active. The dibutylaminomethyl, diamylaminomethyl and dihexylaminomethyl derivatives H, I, and J in the 2-phenyl-quinoline series were, however, active, having chemotherapeutic indices of 1 : 4, 1 : 8 and 1 : 4 respectively. In the series without the 2-phenyl groups the dibutylaminomethyl derivative C showed no activity, whereas the diamylaminomethyl and dihexylamino-methyl derivatives D and E showed activity.

A comparison of these active bases with their 6-methoxy-quinolyl analogues is of interest. King and Work (1940) had shown that dibutylaminomethyl, diamylaminomethyl and dihexylaminomethyl-6-methoxy-4-quinolylcarbinols were all active against *P. relictum* in canaries, but, apart from the inactivity of dibutylaminomethyl-6 : 7-dimethyl-4-quinolylcarbinol C and the slight activity of the dibutylaminomethyl-6-methoxy-4-quinolylcarbinol there is nothing to choose between the activities of the two series of bases.

The replacement therefore of the 6-methoxy group by two methyl groups in the 6 : 7-positions, corresponding to those in riboflavin, does not lead to any enhanced chemotherapeutic action. The three 6-methoxyquinolyl bases in the 2-phenyl series, corresponding to H, I, and J, were not available for comparison on *P. relictum* in canaries. On *P. lophuræ* in ducks and *P. gallinaceum* in chicks they had a quinine equivalent about unity (Wiselogle, 1946).

The *iso*alloxazine nucleus has been substituted by Neeman (1946) for the acridine nucleus of mepacrine by condensation of N-(*w*-diethylaminoalkyl)phenylenediamines with alloxan.

ANTIMALARIAL ACTION OF CARBINOLAMINES
AGAINST *P. relictum* IN CANARIES

(King and Wright, 1948)

Compound.	Number of days × dose in mgm. per 20 gm. body weight.	Day of appearance of parasitæmia.	Maximum tolerated dose: Chemotherapeutic Index.
A. Piperidinomethyl-6 : 7-dimethyl-4-quinolylcarbinol.	6 × 5	5	M.T.D.
	6 × 5	5	
	5 × (2 × 5) + 5	7	
B. Morpholinomethyl-6 : 7-dimethyl-4-quinolylcarbinol.	6 × 2·5	5	M.T.D.
	6 × 2·5	7	
	5 × (2 × 2·5) + 2·5	7	
C. Dibutylaminomethyl-6 : 7-dimethyl-4-quinolylcarbinol.	6 × 1·25	7	M.T.D.
	6 × 1·25	7	
D. Diamylaminomethyl-6 : 7-dimethyl-4-quinolylcarbinol.	6 × 2·5	12	M.T.D.
	6 × 2·5	5	
E. Dihexylaminomethyl-6 : 7-dimethyl-4-quinolylcarbinol.	4 × 10 + 2 × 5	14	M.T.D.
	2 × 10 + 4 × 5	9	
	1 × 10 + 3 (2 × 10) + (2 × 5)	16	
F. Piperidinomethyl-2-phenyl-6 : 7-dimethyl-4-quinolylcarbinol.	6 × 1·25	7	M.T.D.
	6 × 1·25	8	
G. Morpholinomethyl-2-phenyl-6 : 7-dimethyl-4-quinolylcarbinol.	6 × 2·5	7	M.T.D.
	6 × 2·5	7	
H. Dibutylaminomethyl-2-phenyl-6 : 7-dimethyl-4-quinolylcarbinol.	6 × 10	sterile	M.T.D.
	6 × 10	19	
	6 × 5	30	
	6 × 5	sterile	
	6 × 2·5	30	
	6 × 2·5	21	
	6 × 1·25	9	
	6 × 1·25	7	C.I.—1:4
I. Diamylaminomethyl-2-phenyl-6 : 7-dimethyl-4-quinolylcarbinol.	6 × 10	sterile	M.T.D.
	6 × 10	,,	
	6 × 5	,,	
	6 × 5	,,	
	6 × 2·5	16	
	6 × 2·5	12	
	6 × 1·25	9	
	6 × 1·25	14	C.I.=1·8
J. Dihexylaminomethyl-2-phenyl-6 : 7-dimethyl-4-quinolylcarbinol.	6 × 10	sterile	M.T.D.
	6 × 10	,,	
	6 × 5	23	
	6 × 5	23	
	6 × 2·5	16	
	6 × 1·5	30	
	6 × 1·25	10	
	6 × 1·25	9	C.I.=1·4
Control birds		5 to 7	

Haworth and Robinson (1948) showed that 2-6-dichloro-3-β-diethylaminoethylaminoquinoxaline was possessed of considerable antimalarial activity. Crowther *et al.* (1949) found that increasing the complexity of the side-chain has a dystherapeutic effect and the same is true if the 2-chlorine atom is removed and replaced by other groups such as hydroxyl, ethoxyl or thiol. In the simple 2-chloro-3-dialkylaminoalkylaminoquinoxalines replacement of the chlorine atom by a methyl group has a similar effect in reducing activity against *P. gallinaceum.* The effect of variation in the substituents in 2-chloro-3-β-diethylaminoethylaminoquinoxaline showed that no variant was as good as the original 6-chloro-compound. The most active derivative was 2 : 6-dichloro-3-β-diethylaminoethylamino-6 (or 7) methoxyquinoxaline (Curd, Davey and Stacey, 1949).

Substituted Methanols

That the quinoline nucleus is not essential for antimalarial activity is once again demonstrated by the fact that the introduction of a dialkylaminomethylene group into the α position of substituted methanols produces substances with antimalarial activity (May and Mosettig, 1946). Thus α-diamylaminomethyl-1, 2, 3, 4-tetrahydro-phenanthrene-9-methanol (SN 1,796), and α-dinonylaminomethyl-1, 2, 3, 4-tetrahydro-phenanthrene-9-methanol (SN 5,241) have about one-quarter the efficiency of quinine against *P. gallinaceum :* in many respects they equal quinine against blood-induced vivax infections, but unfortunately they both produce toxic reactions (Wiselogle, 1946). Chemical methods for the preparation of quinoline methanols have been recorded by Campbell and Kerwin (1946) and Campbell *et al.* (1946a, b, c).

Some significance had been attached by Fourneau *et al.* (1933) to the facts that substances showing antimalarial activity, cinchona alkaloids, pamaquin, mepacrine, and numerous allied bases, all have molecular weights between 300 and 400, and that structural specificity is not great provided that the molecular weight is above a certain limiting value. Work (1940) therefore produced a wide variety of carbinolamines and polyamines without a quinoline nucleus. None of these compounds showed any activity against *P. relictum* in canaries. These observations thus bring out the true *rôle* of the quinoline nucleus for antimalarial activity in the cinchona alkaloids and related synthetic anti-malarials. Fulton (1940) claimed that such a simple base as 1-diethylamino-4-aminopentane was active, a finding which would run contrary to this conclusion. Work (1940), however, was unable to confirm his results. As King and Work (1940) had examined quinoline derivatives bearing carbinolamine side-chains, Mathieson and Newberry (1949) similarly studied a series of mono- and di-substituted phenylcarbinolamines : none had any significant action on *P. gallinaceum* in chicks.

The activity of *epi*-C^9-bases was first investigated by Dirscherl and Thron (1935), who found a loss of activity. Epimerisation at C^9 (*cf.* Formula IV) was shown by Buttle *et al.* (1938) to reduce the activity of quinine from 1 to 0·1 in *epi*-C^9-quinine and that of quinidine from 0·5 to 0·1 in *epi*-C^9-quinidine ; whilst dihydro-quinine has a quinine ratio of 1·35, *epi*-C^3-dihydroquinine has the same activity as quinine.

Alkylquitenines

The antimalarial activities of the alkylquitenines were investi-gated by Goodson, Henry, and Macfie (1930). On oxidation of quinine the inactive acid quitenine is formed. Activity is restored to quitenine and the other analogous carboxylic acids derived from quinidine, cinchonidine, and cinchonine by esterification. As the molecular weight of the alcohol used for esterification increases, so does the antimalarial activity, the maximum being reached at butyl- or amylquitenine, after which there is a fall.

Cohen and King (1938) showed that methylquitenine dihydro-chloride was slightly active, thus confirming the results obtained by Goodson, Henry, and Macfie (1930) ; methylcinchotenine and methylcinchotenidine dihydrochloride were inactive therapeuti-cally, as were quitenamide and quitenmethylamide, 2-methyl-4-(β-pyridino) quinoline 2HCl, and 2-styryl-4-β-pyridino-quinoline 2HCl.

Since the alkylquitenines are easily hydrolysed, Buttle *et al.* (1938) prepared a series of *apo*quinine and *apo*quinidine ethers.

These complex compounds have been investigated chemically by Henry and Solomon (1934) and Henry *et al.* (1935 and 1937).

When a series of ethers of the phenolic base *apo*quinine (Formula V, R = H) and of its reduction product dihydrocupreine (Formula VII, R = H) were tested therapeutically in canaries it was found that if each series is divided into members containing odd and even numbers of carbon atoms there is, with some anomalies, a definite tendency in the four series so produced for the quinine ratio to rise to a maximum and then to fall as the series is ascended :—

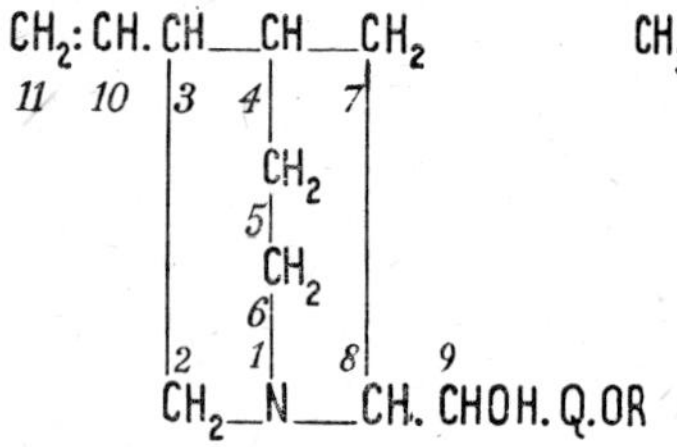

CH_2:CH.CH——CH——CH_2
11 10 |3 4| 7|
            CH_2
          5|
            CH_2
          6|
|2 1| 8| 9
CH_2——N——CH.CHOH.Q.OR

(Formula iv)

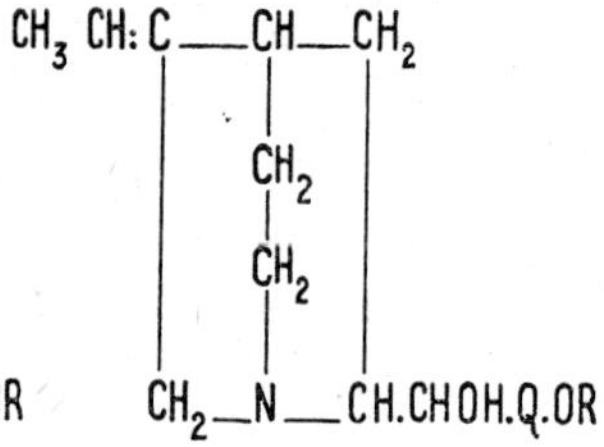

CH_3 CH:C ——CH——CH_2
| |
           CH_2
           |
           CH_2
| |
CH_2——N——CH.CHOH.Q.OR

(Formula v)

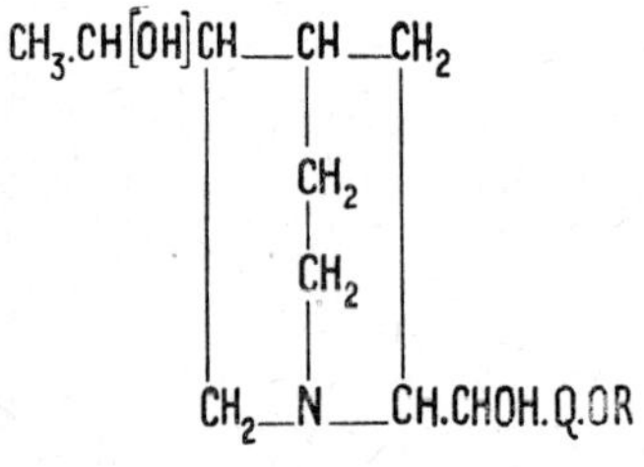

CH_3.CH[OH]CH——CH——CH_2
| |
           CH_2
           |
           CH_2
| |
CH_2——N——CH.CHOH.Q.OR

(Formula vi)

CH_3 CH_2.CH——CH——CH_2
| |
           CH_2
           |
           CH_2
| |
CH_2——N——CH.CHOH.Q.OR

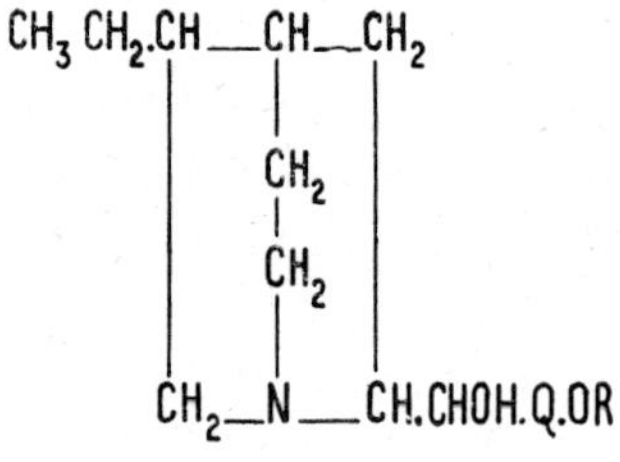

(Formula vii)

Q=Quinolyl residue

R=Alkyl group or hydrogen

A similar curious alternation in the parasiticidal activity of members of a homologous series was first noted by Magidson and Strukow (1933a and b), Magidson *et al.* (1935), in testing the anti-malarial activity in infected siskins of a series of 6-methoxy-quinolines substituted in position 8 (Formula IV) by the chain —NH—$[CH_2]_n$—NEt_2—, the chemotherapeutic indices (i) for different values of n being :—

n	2	3	4	5	6	7	8	9	10	11
i	—	26	—	25	—	34	—	40	—	5
i	6	—	11	—	13	—	—	—	—	—

This alternation was confirmed by Bovet *et al* (1934), who tested the same series of compounds on the Java sparrow, *Padda oryzivora*. It was also observed that as the series was ascended the drugs acquired schizontocidal action in addition to their original gametocyticidal character.

Alternation, however, is not always observed in such tests with homologous series, for Magidson and Strukow (1933b) found that when the chain in position 8 was kept constant at —NH—$[CH_2]NEt_2$ and the group in 6 varied from HO— to $C_5H_{11}O$—, there was a continuous but irregular fall in the chemo-therapeutic index from 1 : 13 to 0. Similarly, Magidson and Grigorowsky (1936) showed that in a short series of substituted acridines with methoxy at position 7, chlorine at position 3, and at position 5 the chain —NH—$[CH_2]_n$NEt where $n = 2$ to 6, the chemotherapeutic index began at 1 : 8, rose to 1 : 20 at $n = 4$ and fell to 1 : 6 and 1 : 5 at $n = 5$ and 6 respectively.

These observations show that changes in action *in vivo* of a homologous series of parasiticidal drugs cannot yet be satis-factorily correlated with chemical structure, solubility or other known physical factors. Possibly it is a combination of factors which leads to alternation in the effect of length of chain on activity.

A study of antimalarial activity in a short series of dihydro-cupreidine ethers (Formula VII : R = Alkyl) by Buttle *et al.* (1938) shows that in the dextrorotatory series a rise in activity against *P. relictum* occurs as the side-chain is increased in length with a maximum at the ethyl compound. In the case of the hydroxy-

ANTIMALARIAL ACTIVITY IN HOMOLOGOUS SERIES OF *apo*QUININE AND DIHYDROCUPREINE ETHERS
(Buttle *et al.*, 1938)

Quinine ratio.		apoQuinine ethers.	Name of ether.	Dihydrocupreine ethers.	Quinine ratio.	
Even.	Odd.				Odd.	Even.
0·69	—	$C_{20}H_{24}O_2N_2$	Methyl	$C_{20}H_{26}O_2N_2$	—	1·35
—	1·18	$C_{21}H_{26}O_2N_2$	Ethyl	$C_{21}H_{28}O_2N_2$	1·05	—
1·23	—	$C_{22}H_{28}O_2N_2$	n-Propyl	$C_{22}H_{30}O_2N_2$	—	1·49
—	1·10	$C_{23}H_{30}O_2N_2$	n-Butyl	$C_{23}H_{32}O_2N_2$	1·87	—
1·47	—	$C_{24}H_{32}O_2N_2$	n-Amyl	$C_{24}H_{34}O_2N_2$	—	1·33
—	1·72	$C_{25}H_{34}O_2N_2$	n-Hexyl	$C_{25}H_{36}O_2N_2$	1·50	—
1·21	—	$C_{26}H_{36}O_2N_2$	n-Heptyl	$C_{26}H_{38}O_2N_2$	—	1·70
—	1·6	$C_{27}H_{38}O_2N_2$	n-Octyl	$C_{27}H_{40}O_2N_2$	1·43	—
0·98	—	$C_{28}H_{40}O_2N_2$	n-Nonyl	$C_{28}H_{42}O_2N_2$	—	1·12
—	1·18	$C_{29}H_{42}O_2N_2$	n-Decyl	$C_{29}H_{44}O_2N_2$	1·6	—
0·75	—	$C_{30}H_{44}O_2N_2$	n-Undecyl	$C_{30}H_{46}O_2N_2$	—	1·25
—	0·58	$C_{35}H_{54}O_2N_2$	Cetyl	—	—	—

-*apo*-bases (Formula VI : R = H or Me), antimalarial activity is reduced since the presence of a phenolic hydroxyl group in the quinoline nucleus and an additional hydroxyl group attached to carbon atom 10 combine to reduce the basic character which seems to be essential for antimalarial activity. Studies of hydroxyethyl*apo*cupreine in avian malarias by Hegner *et al.* (1941a and b) show that it destroys the asexual forms of *P. lophuræ* in ducks and *P. cathemerium* in canaries.

In general it may be said that no obvious relationship can be traced between optical activity and antimalarial action in the cinchona alkaloids, for while the L-bases, quinine and cinchonidine, are more active than the D-bases, quinidine and cinchonine (Buttle *et al.*, 1934), *apo*quinidine methyl ether (+ 334·2°) is more active than either of its L-isomerides α- or β-*iso*quinine. The conversion of the phenolic L-bases, *apo*quinine and *isoapo*quinine, into their methyl ethers, β- and α-*iso*quinines, results in a reduction of antimalarial action ; the converse is the case when the D-phenolic base, *apo*quinidine, is methylated.

(II) Pamaquin and other 8-Aminoquinolines

During the 1914–18 war the shortage of quinine led to experiments in Germany the object of which was to obtain some new

synthetic drug which could be used in place of the naturally occur-
ing cinchona alkaloids. Apart from the cinchona alkaloids and
arsenicals, the only compound then known to be active in malaria
was methylene blue, the value of which had been demonstrated
in 1891 by Guttman and Ehrlich.

Methylene blue (I)   (II)

By changing the alkyl groups attached to the extra-nuclear
nitrogen atoms it was found that the antimalarial activity varied.
By introducing a basic dialkylamino group into the side-chain as
in (II) antimalarial activity was much increased (Schulemann,
1932).

Having discovered that the attachment of a basic side-chain
to the thiazine nucleus of methylene blue led to an enhancement
of antimalarial activity, the effect of attaching the same and
similar groupings to other heterocyclic nuclei was investigated.

After a wide variety of these had been tested, eventually
pamaquin (plasmoquin, plasmochin, beprochin, præquine,
quipenyl) was discovered by Schulemann *et al.* (1932).

The constitution of pamaquin was stated by Hörlein (1926) to
be 6-methoxy-8-diethylamino-*iso*pentylaminoquinoline, or as it
may also be described, 8-(4'-di-
ethylamino-1'-methylbutylamino)-6-
methoxy quinoline. It is conven-
tionally manufactured by condensation of 6-methoxy-8-aminoquinoline
with 1-diethylamino-4-bromopentane
(Schulemann *et al.*, 1930).

Pamaquin (III)

Although derived originally from methylene blue, the constitu-
tional formula of pamaquin has analogies with that of quinine.
By means of a new analytical technique which involves the use of
counter-current extractions (Craig, 1944 ; Craig *et al.*, 1945) it has

been possible to show that commercial samples of pamaquin are contaminated with an isomeric entity due to an unexpected rearrangement of the side-chain of the compound in the course of synthesis. The main contaminant, present to the extent of 12 to 30 per cent., has been termed *iso*plasmochin, 6-methoxy-8-(3'-diethylamino-1'-ethylpropylamino)-quinoline : the melting-point is 130°–139° C. Pure pamaquin was first prepared by Elderfield *et al.* (1946), but according to Schmidt (1947) the toxicity and antimalarial action of pure pamaquin does not differ significantly from that of the ordinary commercial product.

Homologues of Pamaquin

The discovery of pamaquin, the characteristic feature of which is a dialkylaminoalkylamino side-chain, $HN(CH_2)_n . NRR'$, naturally stimulated interest in the side-chains which could be attached to a methoxyquinoline nucleus.

Barber and Wragg (1946b) prepared an isethionate of tetrahydropamaquin. This compound was two and a half times as active as pamaquin against schizonts of *P. gallinaceum* in chicks and as active as pamaquin against the schizonts of *P. lophuræ* in ducks. When given to hens in the highest tolerated doses it prolonged the incubation period of sporozoite-induced *P. gallinaceum*. The LD 50 for 200-gm. rats was 30 mgm. per day, given for four weeks : the corresponding LD 50 for pamaquin was 7·5 mgm.

Thirteen synthetic quinoline derivatives were synthesised by Barger and Robinson (1929) and were subsequently tested by Tate and Vincent (1933) for their action in curing bird malaria. The chemotherapeutic indices of two, 8-γ-aminopropylamino-6-ethoxyquinoline (R 25) and the corresponding methoxy-quinoline (R 36), were 1 : 16, as compared with 1 : 30 for pamaquin. R 36 was first prepared by Baldwin (1929).

R 36 is probably also the active constituent of phthalobis-[γ-(6-methoxy-8-quinolylamino)propyl]-amide since the hydrochloride of this base is hydrolysed in aqueous solution and probably also in the body to 8-γ-aminopropylamino-6-methoxyquinoline (R 36). 8-γ-Phthalimidopropylamino-6-methoxyquinoline, which is not similarly hydrolysed, is completely inactive (Gray and Hill,

1949). The action of these compounds closely resembled that of pamaquin while 8-γ-aminopropylamino-6-*n*-butoxyquinoline had a sterilising action on *P. relictum* equal to, if not greater than, that of pamaquin, although its chemotherapeutic action was only 1 : 8. Those compounds in this series which have been tested clinically have, however, been found to be inactive in infections due to *P. falciparum* and in addition they are very liable to cause methæmalbumin formation.

Of the other homologues of pamaquin that have been tested clinically the majority are 6-methoxyquinolines with a dialkylamino-alkylamino side-chain in position 8, and, as pointed out by Henry and Gray (1935), it is the length and nature of this side-chain which is the principal source of variation. Of forty-eight compounds of this character prepared by Fourneau *et al.* (1931, 1933), no less than thirty-eight possessed some curative action in bird malaria. The majority, however, were unstable and soon became toxic. The compounds listed in the table were found to have low toxicity combined with a considerable degree of curative action.

Compound.	Name of Drug.	Character of side-chain.
6-methoxy-8-diethylamino-*iso*-pentylaminoquinoline .	Pamaquin	$NH . CH(CH_3) . CH_2CH_2CH_2 . N(C_2H_5)_2$
6-methoxy-8-dimethylamino-*n*-propylaminoquinoline .	Fourneau 574	$NH . CH_2 . CH_2 . CH_2 . N(CH_3)_2$
6-methoxy-8-diethylaminoamyl-aminoquinoline . . .	Fourneau 664	$NH . CH_2 . C(CH_3)_2 . CH_2 . N(C_2H_5)_2$
6-methoxy-8-diethylamino-*n*-propylaminoquinoline . .	Fourneau 710 (Rhodoquine)*	$NH . CH_2 . CH_2 . N(C_2H_5)_2$
8-diethylamino-*n*-propylamino-quinoline	Fourneau 728	$NH . CH_2 . CH_2CH_2 . N(C_2H_5)_2$
6-methoxy-8-diethylamino-*n*-amylaminoquinoline . .	Fourneau 735	$NH . CH_2CH_2CH_2CH_2 . CH_2 . N(C_2H_5)_2$
8-diethylamino-undecylamino-6-methoxyquinoline . .	Fourneau 852	$NH . (CH_2)_{11}N(C_2H_5)_2$

According to Fourneau and his colleagues, these compounds are less toxic than pamaquin for laboratory animals, and in Java sparrows infected with *Hæmoproteus paddæ* they have chemotherapeutic indices superior to that of pamaquin (C.I. = 1 : 40) ; rhodoquine (No. 710) has a chemotherapeutic index of 1 : 100, No. 735, 1 : 150 ; No. 664, 1 : 40. As a result of these observations it was believed that the methoxy group in position 6 in the quino-

[* The term " rhodoquine " was originally applied to all the oxyquinolines prepared by Fourneau and his colleagues ; it is now restricted to 710.]

line nucleus is not essential for antimalarial action, while the substitution of —OCH_3— for OC_2H_5— appears always to exert an unfavourable action, as does the group —C . CH_2—O—R placed in the diamino chain. In at least one compound replacement of dimethylamino by diethylamine reduced toxicity ten times.

Fourneau 574 was found to be less toxic in man than rhodoquine, which tends to produce vertigo : it is also very stable in a tropical climate. Massias (1933), who treated forty-three patients with this drug combined with 1 gm. of " quiniostovarsol " (quinine and acetarsol), found that only two patients showed toxic symptoms and vomited. When given without quinine, however, early relapses occurred both in benign and malignant tertian infections (Massias, 1934a and b).

Fourneau 664 was tested in vivax infections by Monier (1931), who found that daily doses of 0·1 gm. were toxic and doses of 0·04 gm. insufficient to remove parasites from the blood. Doses of 0·06 to 0·08 gm. daily injected intramuscularly as a 1 per cent. solution gave good immediate results and all parasites were removed from the peripheral blood stream by total doses of 0·3 gm. Relapses were prevented by the administration of 0·5 gm. The therapeutic activities of rhodoquine (Fourneau 710) are discussed on p. 336. The Russian product, plasmocide, is described as being chemically identical with rhodoquine. Fourneau 852 is said to be much less toxic for man than pamaquin, whereas it is claimed that it acts as powerfully as mepacrine on the asexual stages of *P. relictum* in canaries and of *Hæmoproteus paddæ* in Java sparrows. In the treatment of human malarial infections Fourneau 852 has been combined with sodium acetarsol. This compound, termed rhodoquine V (Fourneau 915), was found by Sergent and Vogt (1933) to cause complete disappearance of asexual forms from the peripheral blood within five days when given in a daily dose of 0·6 gm. ; relapses, however, were not infrequent, while occasionally vomiting occurred. With daily doses of 0·9 gm. severe toxic symptoms were seen.

The action of a series of homologues of pamaquin with unbranched chains, where $n = 2$ to 11, was studied by Bovet, Benoit and Altman (1934). *Hæmoproteus* infections in the Java sparrow and *P. relictum* in canaries were employed. For *Hæmoproteus* infections the graph obtained by plotting minimal effective doses of the various compounds against values of n is roughly parabolic with summits at $n = 3$ and $n = 5$: it may be taken as a measure of activity against the sexual forms of the parasites, when, however, the action of the same set of compounds is tested on avian malaria in canaries the anti-plasmodial activities for the higher values of n are almost as great as for the lower values of n in the Java sparrow. Thus when $n = 11$ the chemotherapeutic index is 1 : 100 for the canary and 1 : 3 for the Java sparrow : it is assumed that the higher activity in the canary must be due to action on both the sexual and asexual forms of the parasites. If this assumption be correct any increase in molecular complexity as in the replacement of quinoline by acridine or by lengthening the side-chain in pamaquin must cause a change from activity against sexual to activity against asexual forms. There is thus no theoretical reason why, by synthesis, compounds should not be prepared with high activity against both sexual and asexual forms of malaria parasites.

Further modifications of the pamaquin molecule were examined in Germany prior to 1939 : of these Certuna or Cilional (IV), which differs from pamaquin in having a 6-hydroxy instead of a 6-methoxy group and one less methyl group in the side-chain, was believed by Kikuth (1938) to have a more powerful gametocyti-cidal action than pamaquin.

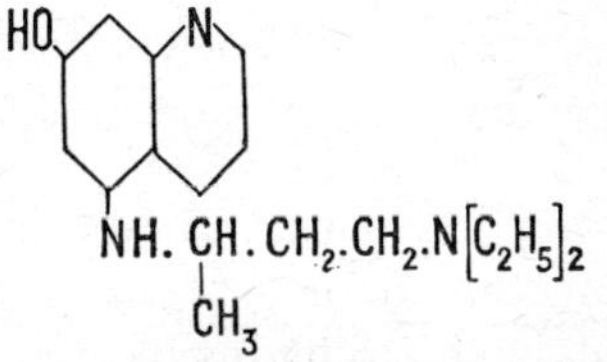

Certuna (IV)

It has no action on relapsing vivax malaria (Mühlens, 1938 ; Sioli, 1938) but was used to some extent by the Italians during the war of 1939–45, mixed with mepacrine. Field (1939) and Decourt *et al.* (1939) found that in doses of 0·03 gm. daily for five days, or even 0·06 gm. daily for ten days, it had no action on the asexual forms of *P. vivax* or *P. falciparum*. Sexual forms of *P. falciparum*, however, are rapidly destroyed. Chopra *et al.* (1938) obtained similar results in India.

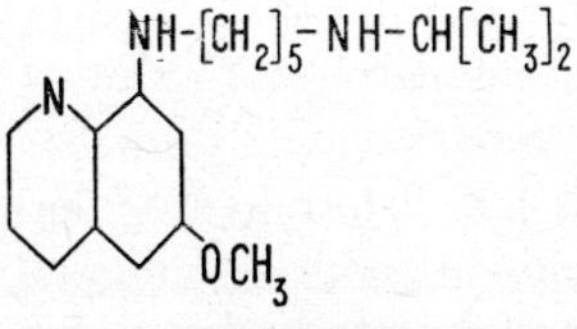

Pentaquine

Many other 8-aminoquinoline derivatives were investigated

during the war in America. Of those of which descriptions are given by Wiselogle (1946) the most interesting is pentaquine (SN 13,276), 6-methoxy-8-(5'-*iso*propylaminoamylamino)quinoline. It is prepared by condensation of 6-methoxy-8-aminoquinoline with 5-*iso*propylaminoamylchloride (Drake *et al.*, 1946a and b), and is now used as the diphosphate, the salt containing 75·5 per cent. of the base. It crystallises in the form of yellow needles, melts at 180°–190° C., is moderately soluble in water and slightly soluble in alcohol. Assays by the Craig countercurrent method show that less than 5 per cent. of impurities is present. *iso*-Pentaquine (SN 13,274) is 8-(4'-*iso*propylamino-1'-methylbutyl-amino)-6-methoxyquinoline : it is usually employed as the oxalate which contains 74 to 79 per cent. of the base. The cost of manufacture is, however, so great that *iso*pentaquine is not at present available except for experimental purposes.

The synthesis of a number of 8-(5'-alkylamino-1'-methylpentyl-amino)-derivatives of quinoline is described by Elderfield *et al.* (1947).

The compound known during the war as R 63 (Robinson and Tomlinson, 1934 ; Crum and Robinson, 1943 ; Glen and Robinson, 1943 ; and Quin and Robinson, 1943) has been shown by Mosher (1946) and Barber and Wragg (1946a) to be a mixture containing a high proportion of 8-γ-aminopropylamino-6-methoxyquinoline dihydrochloride (R 36). The antimalarial activity of R 63 can be accounted for on the basis of the 8-γ-aminopropylamino-6-methoxy-quinoline dihydrochloride which it contains (Barber and Wragg, 1947). According to Coatney and Cooper (1948), 8-(5'-*iso*propyl-amylamino)-6-methoxylepidine has some action as a casual prophylactic in avian malarias.

Antimalarial action is still retained if the quinoline nucleus of either pamaquin or pentaquine is reduced with the formation of 8-(δ-diethylamino-α-methylbutylamino)-6-methoxy-1 : 2 : 3 : 4-tetrahydroquinoline), termed tetrahydropamaquin ; 8-(ω-*iso*-propylaminoamylamino)-6-methoxy-1 : 2 : 3 : 4-tetrahydroquino-line, termed tetrahydropentaquin ; 8-γ-aminopropylamino-6-methoxy-1 : 2 : 3 : 4-tetrahydroquinoline, the tetrahydro-deriva-tive of R 36, 8-γ-aminopropylamino-6-methoxyquinoline hydro-chloride.

The action of these compounds against trophozoite-induced avian infections has been studied by Gray and Hill (1949).

Compound.	Antimalarial activity against P. gallinaceum. P. relictum.		Toxicity for mice. LD 50 mgm./kgm.
	Minimum effective dose (as base).		
Tetrahydropamaquin hydrochloride	2·0	2·5	90
,, naphthoate .	2·5	2·5	200
Pamaquin hydrochloride . .	0·5	0·5	16
,, naphthoate . . .	0·625	0·5	50
Tetrahydropentaquin diphosphate .	0·5	4·0	300
Pentaquin monophosphate . .	0·25	0·5	150
8-γ-Aminopropylamino-6-methoxy-1 : 2 : 3 : 4-tetrahydroquinoline hydrochloride	0·5	4·0	200
8-γ-Aminopropylamino-6-methoxy-quinoline hydrochloride . .	0·25	2·0	200

The reduction products were all less active than the parent compounds, but in the case of tetrahydropamaquin and tetrahydropentaquin the toxicity was reduced. Tetrahydropamaquin isethionate has the same activity as pamaquin against *P. falciparum* gametocytes but little or no activity against the trophozoites of *P. vivax*. In man also it is less toxic than pamaquin. Tetrahydropamaquin naphthoate was tested clinically in North Africa and was well tolerated, but its gametocyticidal activity is less than that of pamaquin.

Primaquine is the name assigned by the Council on Pharmacy and Chemistry of the American Medical Association (1949) to 8-(4'-amino-1'-methylbutylamino)-6-methoxyquinoline. Its action appears to be similar to that of pentaquine, but whether it possesses any advantage over pentaquine or *iso*pentaquine is still uncertain.

(III) Mepacrine

Following the production of pamaquin, further work, using the principle of attachment of a basic alkyl group to a heterocyclic nucleus, led, in 1932, to the compound first termed erion, and later plasmoquine E, atebrin, atabrine, methoquine, crinodora, palusan (Italian), arichin, haffkinine, acriquine (Indian), and finally mepacrine or quinacrine (Mauss and Mietszch, 1933; Mietszch and Mauss, 1934). Comparatively little was known about the potentialities of this compound before 1939, but during the Second World War it received intensive study. According to Mauss and Mietszch (1933) mepacrine is 2-chloro-5-diethylamino-*iso*pentylamino-7-methoxy-acridine dihydrochloride. It thus contains the same side-chain as pamaquin with the 6-methoxy-quinoline nucleus of the latter replaced by a 2-chloro-7-methoxy acridine nucleus.

In the Union of the Soviet Republics the name arichin 8 (acriquine) has been given to a closely allied compound which, according to Rubinstein (1936), is 2-chloro-7-methoxyl-5-diethyl-aminobutylaminoacridine. Exposure to ultra-violet light is said to be essential for the formation of this compound.

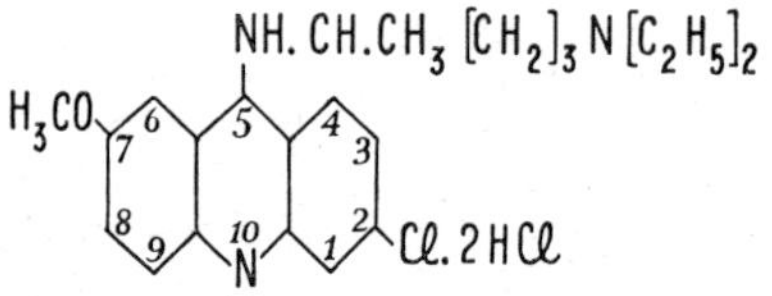

Mepacrine (I) 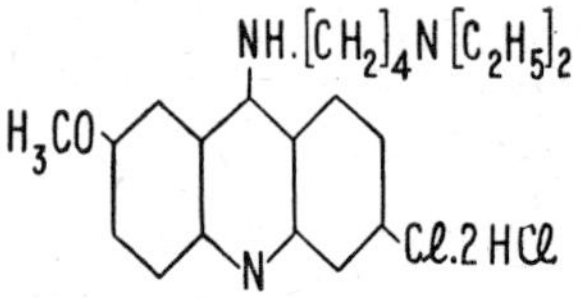   Acriquine (II)

Several other acridine derivatives have been prepared but have either not been tested at all in man or the testing has been inadequate (Mauss, 1942).

In compounds of the mepacrine type the important substituents for antimalarial activity appear to be halogen, alkyl, alkoxyl, and alkylthio, while the work of Kritschewski *et al.* (1934), Magidson and Grigorowsky (1936) and Magidson and Trawin (1936) has added nitro and cyano groups.

Schönhöfer (1942) had suggested that the antimalarial activity of mepacrine was connected with the capacity of the molecule to exhibit a form of tautomerism involving the lability of a hydrogen atom which can assume two alternative positions in the molecule.

The effects of simplification of the mepacrine molecule were further studied by Work (1946a and b), it having already been recognised from the work of Schönhöfer (1942) that compounds of types (III) and (IV), where R = dialkylaminoalkyl, possess antimalarial activity, which, as in mepacrine, may be associated with the possession of a tautomeric system. For the further

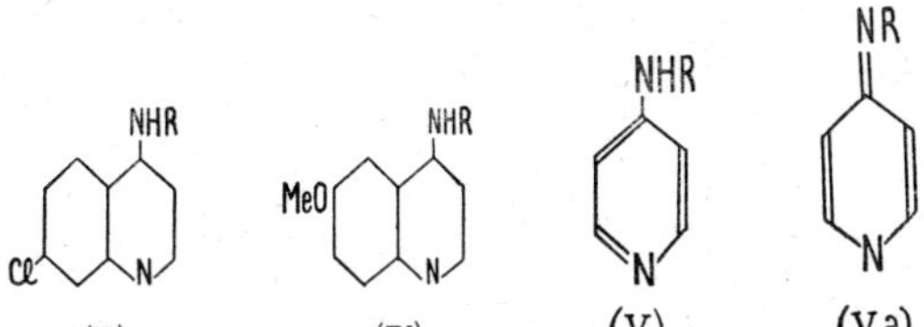

(III)   (IV)   (V)   (Va)

simplification of types (III) and (IV) retention of a similar tautomeric system seemed desirable as (V) or (Va).

Unfortunately such compounds were without antimalarial activity, as were compounds such as N′-*p*-chlorophenyl-N-β-diethylaminoethyl-*p*-methoxybenzamidine.

Of the four possible isomers of mepacrine which have the methoxy group in position 7 of the acridine nucleus and the chlorine atom in the opposite, nitrogen-free ring, there have been prepared, in addition to mepacrine, the related 3-chloro-isomer (Feldman and Kopeliowitsch, 1935), and 7-methoxy-4, chloro 5-[(4-diethylamino-2-amyl)-amino]-acridine (Grigorovskii and Terent'eva, 1947 ; Dauben, 1948), and 2-methoxy-5, 9-[(4′-diethylamino*iso*amyl)-amino]-acridine (Dauben, 1948). The only experiments on antimalarial activity have so far been carried out with the 4-chloro-isomer : in 50 mgm. amounts per day per 65 gm. of body weight chickens infected with *P. gallinaceum* showed a prolongation of the incubation period. Mepacrine, in similar experiments, was effective in doses of 8 mgm.

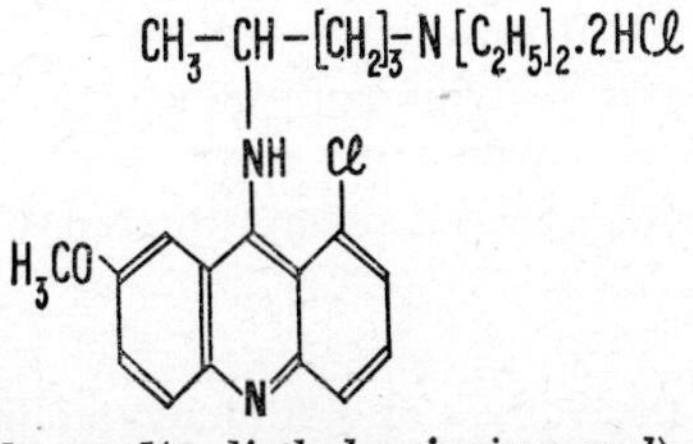

7-Methoxy-4-chloro-5-[(4-diethylaminoisoamyl)-amino]-acridine.

Gilman and Benkeser (1947) have developed a series of 7-chloroquinolines patterned as " open models " for mepacrine.

One of these has a methoxyphenyl group in place of the fused methoxybenzol group in mepacrine.

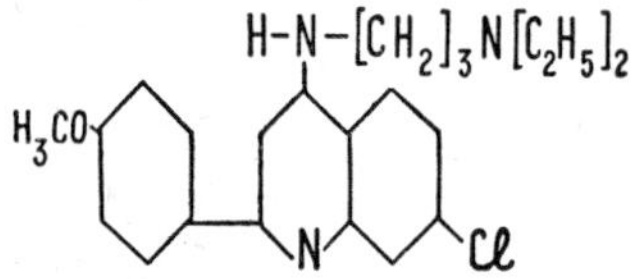

A homologue is obtained by opening the opposite benzene ring. Gilman and Spatz (1944) similarly reported antimalarial activity in certain 4-dialkylaminoalkylamino-2-arylquinolines which they considered to be " open chain models " of mepacrine. They can as well be regarded as modified 4-dialkylaminoalkylamino-quinolines.

Mepacrine Analogues

Humphlett *et al.* (1948) prepared a number of ketones from γ-diethylaminobutyronitrile and aromatic Grignard reagents and converted them into the corresponding oximes, these in their turn being reduced to the corresponding diamines. The quinine equivalents of these mepacrine analogues are shown in the table.

Mepacrine Analogues.

Aryl-$CH(NH_2)CH_2CH_2CH_2NEt_2$.					Quinine equivalent.
α-Naphthyl	.	.	.	.	0·16
p-Chlorophenyl	.	.	.	.	0·16
p-Fluorophenyl	.	.	.	.	1·2
m-Trifluoromethylphenyl	.	.	.	1·2
α-Thienyl	.	.	.	.	0·16

All these compounds, it may be noted, showed a slight *in vitro* action against an avirulent human strain of tubercle bacilli, the minimum active dosage being 0·2 mgm. per 10 ml. of culture. The compound in which aryl is phenyl showed a minimum active dose of 1 mgm.

(IV) Derivatives of 4-Aminoquinoline

The fact that antimalarial activity is present when a dialkyl-aminoalkylamino side-chain is attached to position 4 of the quinoline nucleus and that this activity is enhanced by the introduction of appropriate substituents into positions 6 or 7 of the quinoline nucleus was exploited by Andersag *et al.* (1939 and 1941) and by Russian workers (Magidson and Rubtsov, 1937). Some derivatives of this class were shown by Galperin (1940) and Schönhöfer (1942) to be active in bird malaria, though, unlike isomeric derivatives of 8-aminoquinoline, they have no action on gametocytes (Galperin, 1940). Like the derivatives of amino-acridine, only the asexual stages of malarial parasites are attacked, and exo-erythrocytic forms are unaffected. This is not surprising for, as Blanchard (1947) has emphasised, acridine is 2, 3-benzo-quinoline and position 5 of the acridine nucleus is strictly comparable to position 4 of the quinoline nucleus.

Work continued for some years in Germany on these derivatives and its direction was to some extent ascertainable from a study of the relevant patent literature (D.R.P. 683692, Nov. 13, 1939). In addition to the methods previously studied, another device was largely used, namely the breaking down of the mepacrine molecule into its constituent parts with a view to throwing further light on the relations between chemical structure and antimalarial activity. In this way compounds of types I and II, which repre-

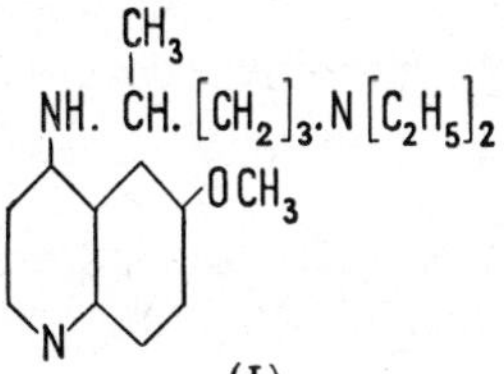

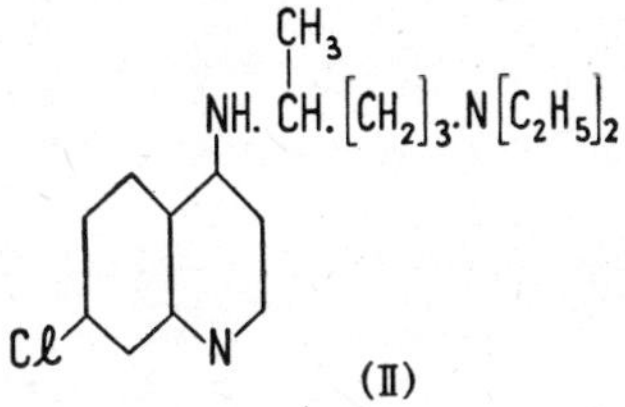

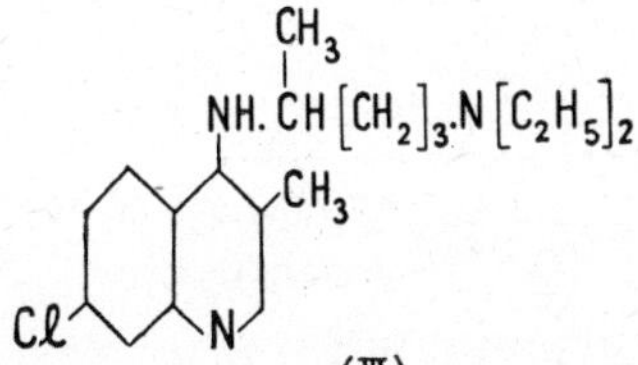

sent portions of the mepacrine molecule, were produced (Andersag *et al.*, 1939 and 1941). 7-Chloro-4-(4′-diethylamino-1′-methyl-butylamino)-3-methylquinoline (III), later known as sontoquine (sontochin, santoquine, nivaquine), was given limited clinical trials in Germany and in North Africa, where some of it was captured by the Americans (Kikuth, 1945). The antimalarial activity of sontoquine (termed in America nivaquine) is practically the same both quantitatively and qualitatively as that of mepacrine except that sontoquine does not stain the tissues. It is, however, not easy to produce in large amounts. On the other hand, the hydrochloride is more soluble than mepacrine and the toxicity is less. Sontoquine has been employed by Decourt and

Choroquine

Schneider (1947). The usual dose is 0·3 gm. daily, but 1 gm. can be given without causing gastric symptoms.

Stimulated by the possession of sontoquine, a great many other 4-aminoquinoline derivatives were synthesised and studied in America (Wiselogle, 1946 ; Steck et al., 1948). The majority of the 4-aminoquinolines prepared by Steck et al. (1948) carry an hydroxyl group in the basic side-chain. The only one with antimalarial activity is 7-chloro-4-(4′-diethylamino-1′-methylbutylamino)-6-methoxyquinoline and this compound is too toxic for general use. Chloroquine, 7-chloro-4-(4′-diethylamino-1′-methylbutylamino)-3-methylquinoline (resochin, aralen, SN 7,618), which differs from sontoquine only by the absence of a methyl group, proved the most effective in experimental animals. It was easier to synthesise than sontoquine and improvements have since been introduced into its synthesis (Riegel et al., 1946, Surrey and Hammer, 1946 ; Drake et al., 1946a and b), and also into the synthesis of 4, 7-dichloroquinoline, an important intermediate product in its preparation (Price and Roberts, 1946).

Gilman and Spatz (1944) and Gilman et al. (1946) found that 2-(3′-chlorophenyl)-4-[(α-methyl-δ-diethylaminobutyl)-amino]-6-methoxyquinoline which has a chlorophenyl group in place of the fused chlorobenzene group in mepacrine retains antimalarial action. The methoxy group in mepacrine is partially replaceable by a methyl group (Magidson and Grigorowsky, 1936) and in some open models the methyl group has been substituted for the methoxy group. One of these compounds, 2-(3′-chlorophenyl)-4-[α-methyl-δ-diethylaminobutylamino]-6-methylquinoline was shown by Gilman *et al.* (1946a, b), to be active in avian malaria but the two isomers, 2-(4'-chlorophenyl)-4-[(α-methyl-δ-diethylamino-butyl)-amino]-6-methylquinoline and 2-(4'-chlorophenyl)-4-[(α-methyl-δ-diethylaminobutyl)-amino]-7-methylquinoline, were both inactive.

The antimalarial activity of a number of sontoquine derivatives was studied by Gray and Hill (1949). The chemical relationship of these compounds, their antimalarial activity against tropho-zoite-induced infections of *P. gallinaceum*, and their toxicity for mice is shown in the table in association with the generic formula.

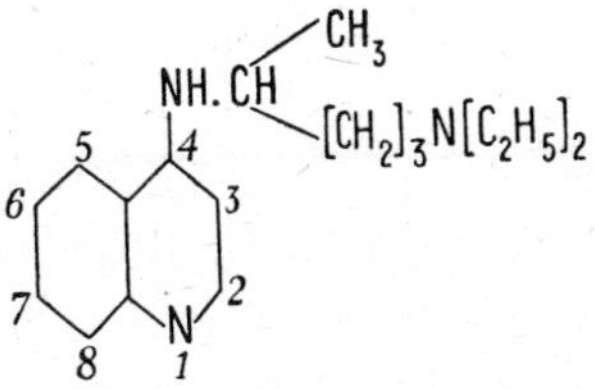

Compound.	Substitution in quinoline nucleus.					Activity against *P. gallinaceum.* MED. in mgm./kgm.	Toxicity for mice. LD 50 mgm./kgm.
	3	5	6	7	8		
Chloroquine . .	—	—	—	Cl	—	1·0	250
Sontoquine . . .	CH_3	—	—	Cl	—	5·0	450
Nivaquine, Compound I	CH_3	—	—	—	—	10·0	500
,, II	CH_3	—	Cl	—	—	20·0	400
,, III	CH_3	Cl	—	—	—	50·0	800
,, IV	CH_3	—	—	—	Cl	200·0	800
,, V	CH_3	—	—	Cl	CH_3	Inactive	600

All doses are in terms of the hydrochloride.

Compound I was prepared by Andersag *et al.* (1941), compounds II and IV were prepared by Steck *et al.* (1946a, b), and III and V by Gray and Hill (1949). Position 7 in the quinoline nucleus, as in chloroquine, is the optimum one for the chlorine atom, while the presence of a methyl group in position 3 (sontoquine) reduces activity, and a second methyl group in position 8 results in complete inactivity.

Another quinoline derivative tested clinically in man is 7-chloro-4-(3'-diethylaminomethyl-4'-hydroxyanilino)-quinoline dihydrate dihydrochloride.

This compound, which has been used under the name Cam Aqi, or camoquin (Halawani *et al.*, 1947), is a yellow crystalline powder and very soluble in water, since 1 gm. dissolves in 5 ml. of water at 25° C. It causes little or no staining of the skin, and is said to

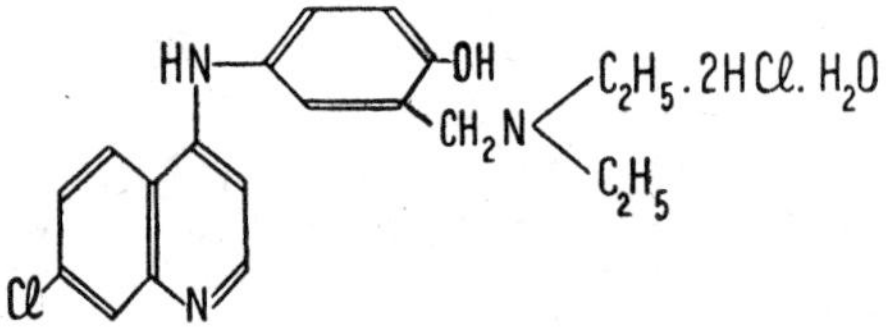

Camoquin

be readily absorbed from the gastro-intestinal tract. It was first synthesised by Burckhalter *et al.* (1946). Curiously enough, *o*-methyl camoquin, synthesised by Burckhalter *et al.* (1943), where the OH of camoquine is replaced by OCH₃, has the same quinine equivalent, 25. Burckhalter (1949) suggests that in the chick the *o*-methyl derivative is demethylated. Demethylation of mepacrine has been observed to occur in man (Hammick and Firth, 1944 ; Hammick and Mason, 1945).

Funke *et al.* (1946) studied the effects of condensing 6-methoxy-8-aminoquinoline with the halogen derivative prepared from an aliphatic-aromatic amino alcohol to give compounds of the type

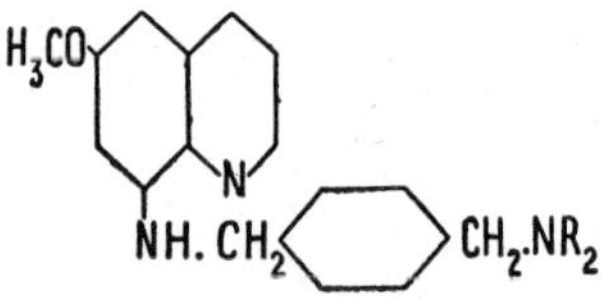

They thus obtained 4′-diethylaminomethyl-8-benzylamino-6-methoxyquinoline (2236 F), in which the side-chain is of a novel type. The corresponding primary amine and the next higher homologue were also prepared, as well as the *ortho-* and *meta-*isomers, besides compounds with two substituent methyl groups in the aromatic ring. In the acridine series two analogous derivatives were prepared. The results are shown in the table : 2236 F was the most satisfactory against *P. relictum* in the canary, and would seem worthy of clinical tests in man.

Activity of Quinoline and Acridine Derivatives against
Plasmodium relictum

(Funke *et al.*, 1946)

Compound.	Chemotherapeutic index.
4'-diethylaminomethyl-8-benzylamino-6-methoxyquinoline (2236 F) . . .	1 : 50
3'-diethylaminomethyl-8-benzylamino-6-methoxyquinoline (3128 F) . . .	1 : 50
2'-diethylaminomethyl-8-benzylamino-6-methoxyquinoline (2389 F) . . .	Inactive
4'-aminomethyl-8-benzylamino-6-methoxyquinoline (2409 F) . . .	1 : 10
4'-dimethylaminomethyl-8-benzylamino-6-methoxyquinoline (2244 F) . . .	1 : 20
4'-diethylaminomethyl-8-phenylethyl-6-methoxyquinoline (2349 F) . . .	1 : 20
4'-diethylaminomethyl-3'-4'-dimethyl-8-benzylamino-6-methoxyquinoline .	1 : 40
4'-diethylaminomethyl-9-benzylamino-2-methoxy-6-chloroacridine . . .	1 : 4
5-diethylaminomethyl-9-phenylethylamino-2-methoxy-6-chloroacridine . . .	Inactive

Steck *et al.* (1948) prepared certain 4-aminoquinolines with an hydroxyl group in the side-chain : the only compound showing antimalarial activity was 7-chloro-4-(4'-diethylamino-1'-methyl-butylamino)-6-methylquinoline : it was, however, extremely toxic and therefore could not be used.

The chemistry of the 4-hydroxyquinolines has been fully reviewed by Reitsema (1948).

Methods of determining the purity of aminoquinolines used as antimalarials have been worked out by Goetz-Luthy (1949), employing the technique of fusion analysis, in association with the polarising microscope.

(V) Acridone Derivatives

Under certain conditions mepacrine can be cleaved into an aliphatic diamine and an acridone which can be represented as the desmotropic 5-hydroxyacridine.

Kikuth and Mudrow-Reichenow (1947) tested the effects on malaria in the canary of compounds having the general formula.

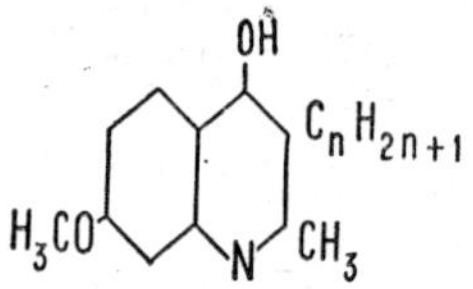

Canaries were infected both by intramuscular injection and by mosquito bites. The results are shown in the table.

Aliphatic chain.	Number of carbon atoms.	Chemotherapeutic index.	
		Blood infection.	Mosquito infection prophylaxis.
$(CH_2)_2$—CH_3 . .	3	1 : 8	1 : 1
$(CH_2)_3$—CH_3 . .	4	1 : 16	1 : 2 ?
$(CH_2)_4$—CH_3 . .	5	1 : 30	1 : 4 ?
$(CH_2)_5$—CH_3 . .	6	1 : 120	1 : 4
$(CH_2)_6$—CH_3 (endochin)	7	1 : 120	1 : 16
$(CH_2)_7$—CH_3 . .	8	1 : 30	1 : 2
$(CH_2)_9$—CH_3 . .	10	1 : 2	0
$(CH_2)_{11}$—CH_3 . .	12	1 : 2	0

The best of these compounds is the white water-insoluble powder 7 - methoxy - 4 - hydroxy - 3 - *n* - heptyl - 2 - methylquinoline named endochin, which appears to be a true causal prophylactic against *P. relictum*, where its chemotherapeutic index is 1 : 120. Six daily doses of 0·3 mgm. per 20 gm. of body weight were sufficient.

The compound is soluble in a mixture of diglycol monomethylether and water and can be mixed with oil or gum arabic. With oral doses of 0·05 to 0·2 gm. per kgm. cats and rabbits show no toxic symptoms, but 0·1 to 0·5 gm. per kgm. causes no symptoms in rats. A single dose of 2 gm. per kgm.

Endochin

kills instantly, and with 1 gm. per kgm. a proportion of animals die after some days without characteristic symptoms.

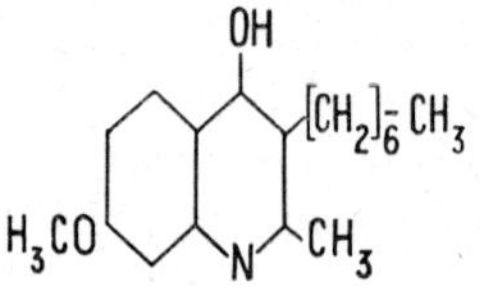

In clinical trials on induced malaria in man this compound has not been of value.

The first of these compounds to be produced was 3-allyl-4-hydroxy-2-methylquinoline and, according to Salzer *et al.* (1948), more than one hundred closely related compounds were studied, using the Roehl test, between 1939 and 1942. The relationship between chemical constitution and therapeutic activity may be briefly summarised as follows. A 7-MeO substituent greatly increases activity but other substituents at C-7 or MeO at other positions on the benzene ring decrease activity and may lead to completely inactive compounds. Activity is lowered in the 7-EtO compound and has disappeared in the BuO and $C_6H_{13}O$ compounds ; on the other hand, the 7-MeS compound is again active. Changing the 4-HO group, except replacement by MeS, caused complete loss of activity : both etherification and introduction of basic or acid groups, such as COOH, SO_3H or halogens, gave inactive compounds. The chemotherapeutic indices of the 4-HS compounds were in general lower than those of the corresponding 4-HO compounds. Variation of the 3-substituent also caused changes in activity. The 3-Me and 3-Et compounds were inactive but activity increased from the propyl to the heptyl derivative and then from the octyl to the dodecyl derivative became poorer. Unsaturated are as effective as saturated alkyl groups, but branching decreases and usually destroys the activity. The aliphatic chain can, however, be interrupted by an O or S atom without decreasing activity. Thus a butoxyethyl or an ethoxybutyl compound is as active as a hexyl compound, but the chemotherapeutic index is less because of the greater toxicity. Attempts to impart water solubility by introducing COOH into a 3-alkyl substituent caused complete inactivation : the esters and hydrazides of such COOH compounds are almost inactive.

Stephen *et al.* (1945, 1947) investigated the action against *P. gallinaceum* infections in chickens of a number of closely related tetrahydroacridones (I ; $n = 2$) ; hydroxydihydro-β-quinindenes (I ; $n = 1$) and 4-hydroxyquinolines. Prophylactic action has been found in certain compounds, conforming to type (II), R′ and R″ being saturated hydrocarbon residues.

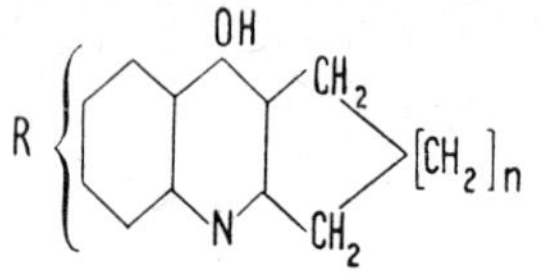

(I) 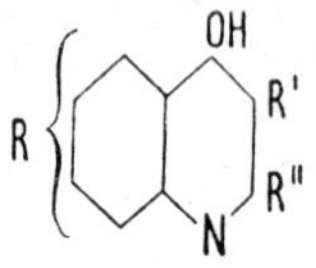   (II)

7-Methoxyacridone is inactive, but its $1 : 2 : 3 : 4$-tetrahydro derivative has considerable action. 3-Methoxy-6, 7, 8, 9-tetrahydro-5(10)-acridone is twice as active as endochin or sulphadiazine in the prophylaxis of *P. gallinaceum* infection in the chicken.

ACRIDONE DERIVATIVES HAVING ACTION ON EXO-ERYTHROCYTIC FORMS OF *P. gallinaceum* (Coatney and Cooper, 1948)

Chemical name.	Empirical formula.	Other designations.
3-Heptyl-7-methoxy-2-methyl-4-quinolinol	$C_{18}H_{25}NO_2$	Endochin
3-Methoxy-6, 7, 8, 9-tetrahydro-5(10)-acridone	$C_{14}H_{15}NO_2$	
2-Methoxy-7-methyl-6, 7, 8, 9-tetrahydro-5(10)-acridone . .	$C_{15}H_{18}NO_2$	
7-Ethyl-2-methoxy-6, 7, 8, 9-tetrahydro-5(10)-acridone . .	$C_{16}H_{19}NO_2$	
2-Methoxy-9-methyl-6, 7, 8, 9-tetrahydro-5(10)-acridone . .	$C_{15}H_{17}NO_2$	

Certain other acridone derivatives have been found by Coatney and Cooper (1948) to have some action on the exo-erythrocytic forms of *P. gallinaceum*.

(VI) Pyridoacridines and Benzacridines

Derivatives of $1 : 2 : 2' : 3'$-pyridoacridine were prepared by Dobson and Kermack (1946), who found that $3 : 4 : 2' : 3'$-pyridoacridine, carrying in position 5 of the acridine nucleus a basic side-chain of the type present in mepacrine, was active against *P. gallinaceum* in chicks. Certain derivatives of $3 : 4 : 2' : 3'$-pyridoacridine carrying a basic side-chain in the 5 position such as

8-chloro-5-(γ-diethylaminopropylamino)-3 : 4 : 2′ : 3′-pyridoacridine were highly active : the presence of a chlorine atom in the 8 position enhanced activity : the corresponding 1 : 2 : 2′ : 3′-pyridoacridine was inactive. The results suggested that the additional pyridine ring has considerable effect on antimalarial activity. Bachman and Picha (1946) prepared certain benzacridine bases which, however, were not possessed of antimalarial action. Hutchison and Kermack (1947), and Dobson, Hutchison and Kermack (1948) synthesised further benzacridines : 8-chloro-5-(γ-diethylaminopropylamino)-1 : 2-benzacridine was without action in a dose of 160 mgm. per kgm. of body weight but 8-chloro-5-(δ-diethylamino-α-methylbutylamino)-3 : 4-benzacridine was active in a dose of 120 mgm. per kgm. This suggests that the position in which the extra ring is fused is of greater importance than the actual nature of the ring, whether pyridine or benzene. Further information on the relation between chemical structure and chemotherapeutic activity was obtained by testing certain derivatives of 1 : 2 : 3′ : 2′-pyridoacridine and 3 : 4 : 3′ : 2′-pyridoacridine. The most active base was that derived from 3 : 4 : 2′ : 3′-pyridoacridine : the analogous 3 : 4-benzacridine was also active but the base derived from 3 : 4 : 3′ : 2′-pyridoacridine was doubtfully active. Benzacridine and pyridoacridine compounds in which the extra ring is fused in the 1 : 2 position of the acridine nucleus are devoid of activity. The failure of the 3 : 4 : 3′ : 2′-pyridoacridine base shows that the geometrical form of the heterocyclic nucleus, though important, is only one factor of several which determines chemotherapeutic action.

Various derivatives of *m*- and *p*-phenanthrolines with basic side-chains of the type present in mepacrine have been synthesised while Halcrow and Kermack (1946) have described a method of preparing *o*-phenanthroline derivatives. Further derivatives of *p*-phenanthroline with appropriate amines have been prepared by Douglas *et al.* (1947). The antimalarial activities of these various compounds have not been studied.

p-Phenanthroline derivatives with a basic group in the 4 position have no antimalarial action, but Douglas and Kermack (1949) found that 4-(4′-diethylamino-1′-methylbutylamino)- and 9-chloro-4-(3′-diethylaminopropylamino)-*p*-phenanthroline both have some suppressive action in doses of 10 mgm. per 20 gm. of body weight. Whereas the *p*-phenanthroline derivative with the *iso*amyl side-chain was active against the blood forms of *P. gallinaceum* in chicks, 4-(3'-diethylaminopropylamino)-*p*-phenanthroline was quite inactive against *P. relictum* in canaries.

(VII) α-Aminocresols and *ortho*-cresols

Many derivatives of α-amino-*o*-cresol were prepared by Burckhalter *et al.* (1946) by means of the Mannich reaction, the condensation of phenols with formaldehyde and dialkylamines. Some of these compounds have an action in avian malaria : thus 6, 6'-dialkyl-α, α'-bis-dimethylamino-4, 4'-bi-*o*-cresol (SN 8,316) and α, α'-bis-diethylamino-5, 5'-bi-*o*-cresol (SN 10,271) have a quinine equivalent of 4. The closely allied 4-(6-chloro-2-methoxy-9-acridylamino)-α-diethylamino-*o*-cresol (SN 8,617) has against *P. gallinaceum* in the chick a quinine equivalent of 3, against *P. lophuræ* in the duck of 4, and against *P. cathemerium* in the canary of 2. It is also active against blood-induced falciparum and vivax infections in man, having a quinine equivalent of 2. It has, however, no curative action in a daily dose of 0·36 gm. combined with 30 mgm. of pamaquin (Wiselogle, 1946).

Among compounds described by Wiselogle (1946) was 6, 6'-diallyl-α, α'-bis(diethylamino)-4, 4'-bi-*o*-cresol (SN 6,771).

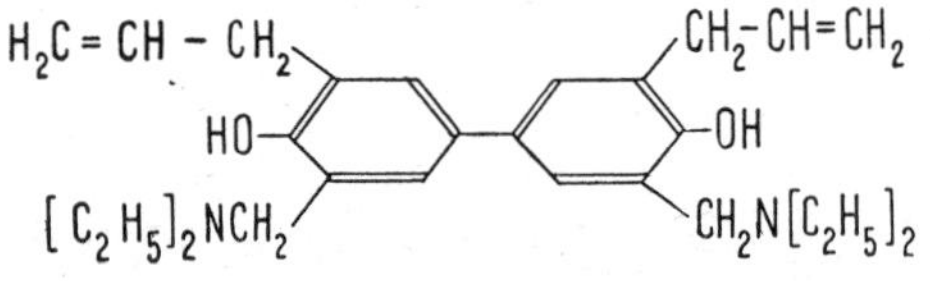

SN 6771

Studies by Butter, summarised by Wiselogle (1946), showed that the drug had a quinine equivalent of less than 0·2, on the basis of total oral dosage against the erythrocytic forms of the McCoy strain of *P. vivax*. Partial or complete suppression of parasites was found to be associated with plasma concentrations of 1·2 to 5·6 mgm. per litre maintained for four days. These results have been confirmed by Cooper *et al.* (1949), using the St. Elizabeth strain of *P. vivax*. Late attacks, beginning more than six months after exposure, were brought to an end by doses of 2 gm. of SN 6,771 per day (0·5 gm. every six hours) for six days. Although parasitæmia and fever were terminated the action was by no means rapid. In nineteen attacks from two to ten days (mean 5·3 days) were required for blood smears to become negative, whereas as many as five days (mean 2·4 days) were required for patients to become and remain afebrile. Relapses followed all the eight primary late attacks in from ten to sixteen days (average 13·3 days) after cessation of therapy. Relapses likewise occurred after four of seven second late attacks in from eighteen to twenty-nine days after stopping therapy.

The suppressive action of SN 6,771 was also tested against the St. Elizabeth strain of *P. vivax*. Five volunteers were given 3 gm. per day (1·5 gm. every twelve hours) for four days before, on the day of biting and for six days after exposure to the bites of ten *Anopheles quadrimaculatus* mosquitoes. Malaria occurred in two of the volunteers sixteen days after exposure, two others showed low-grade parasitæmia (days sixteen and nineteen, and days eighteen and nineteen), but did not have typical primary attacks till 282 and 291 days after the day of bites ; the remaining volunteer did not have any manifestations of malaria till 285 days following exposure. When administration was continued for twenty days after exposure in a dose of 0·75 gm. twice daily, as well as for four days before and on the day of infection, the five subjects had their primary attacks delayed until 258 to 304 days (8·5 to ten months) after infection.

There is thus no evidence of suppressive action on the part of SN 6,771. Toxic reactions were very slight. One patient given therapeutic courses had nausea, and among those given the compound as a suppressive, six out of ten persons had nausea, in one instance accompanied by diarrhœa.

(VIII) Cinnoline Derivatives

While much attention has been directed to the discovery of antimalarials derived from either quinoline or acridine, comparatively little attention has been directed to the effectiveness of other structural types, though such attention has resulted in the discovery of proguanil.

Quinazoline compounds such as the 4-basic alkylaminoquinazo-lines (formula I; $R = NO_2$ or Cl) prepared by Magidson and Golovchinskaya (1938) were devoid of activity. Activity however was found by Schönhöfer (1942) in certain 6-substituted 4-basic

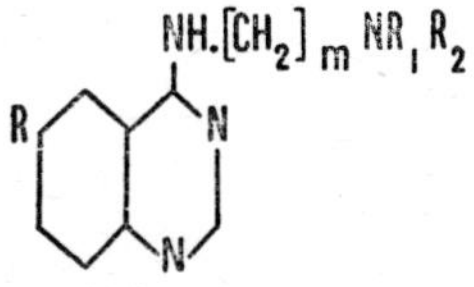

(I) 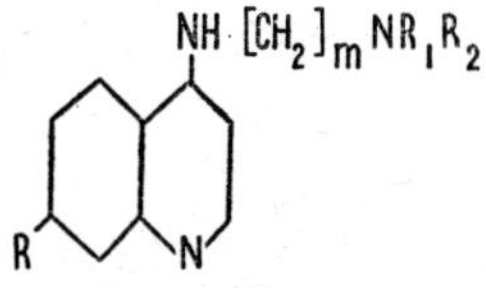   (II)

alkylaminoquinolines, and the closely analogous 7-substituted derivatives (Type II) are, according to the Patent Literature (1938), active. In view of these considerations, Simpson and Schofield (1946) investigated the cinnoline-ring system for antimalarial activity.

Compounds of Type III were tested for activity against *P. gallinaceum* in chicks. Results are shown in the table.

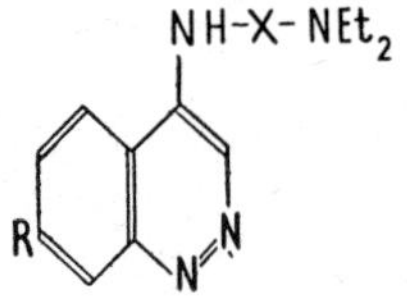

(III)

Compound.	Dose (mgm./kgm.).	Activity.
(1) $R = H$; $X = CH(Me)(CH_2)_3$ . .	250	+ + +
	120	+
(2) $R = OMe$; $X = CH(Me)(CH_2)_3$.	80	—
(3) $R = H$; $X = (CH_2)_3$ . . .	200	±
	120	—

These results lend support to the hypothesis of Schönhöfer (1942) that antimalarial activity is related to the formal possibility of prototropy between the "normal" molecule (amino-aromatic) and the imino-quinonoid form.

CINNOLINE COMPOUNDS (Keneford and Simpson, 1947)

Compounds of type

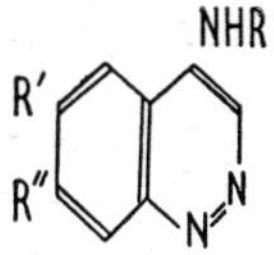

R	R′	R″	Dose (mgm./kgm.).	Activity.
CHMe . [CH$_2$]$_3$NEt$_2$	H	H	250	+ +
			120	+
	H	Cl	80	+ +
			40	+ +
	Cl	H	160	+ to + +
			80	−
	Br	H	160	+ to + +
			80	−
	OMe	H	80	−
	Cl	Cl	160	+ +
			80	+ to + +
			40	−
	Cl	Me	160	+ to + +
			80	+
[CH$_2$]$_2$. NEt$_2$	H	H	200	±
			120	−
	H	Cl	80	+
	Cl	Cl	80	−
[CH$_2$]$_3$. NEt$_2$	H	Cl	80	+ +
			40	+
	Cl	Cl	80	+
[CH$_2$]$_3$. NMe$_2$	H	Cl	80	+ to + +
			40	+
	Cl	Cl	160	+ to + +
			80	±
	Cl	Me	160	+ to + +
			80	+
[CH$_2$]$_3$. NBu$_2$^{a}	H	Cl	80	+
	Cl	Cl	80	−
[CH$_2$]$_3$. N . C$_5$N$_{10}$.	H	Cl	80	+
	Cl	Cl	80	−

Keneford and Simpson (1947) subsequently prepared a series of derivatives of type (IV) substituted at C_6 and C_7. The results are shown in the table on p. 69. The following conclusions can be drawn:

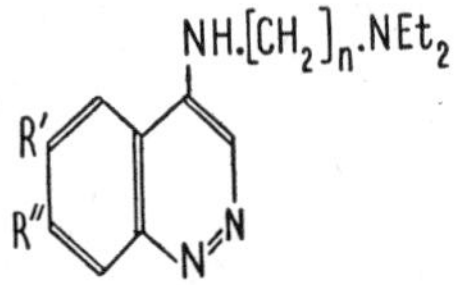

(IV)

(1) combination of the side-chain characteristic of mepacrine and pamaquin with a suitably substituted nucleus results in greater activity than does the combination of other side-chains with the same nuclei : (2) substitution at C_7, *ceteris paribus*, increases antimalarial activity ; (3) substitution at C_6 exerts a dystherapeutic effect. Chapman, Gibson and Mann (1947) investigated six series of 4-dialkylamino-alkylaminoquinazolines having 6-chloro-, 7-chloro-, 7-nitro, 6-methoxy-, and 7-methoxy- substituents. The highest activity was found in the compound containing the α-diethylamino-α-methylbutylamino side-chain : in addition substitution by a chlorine atom in the 7 position led to the highest activity.

The antimalarial activity of a number of quinoxaline derivatives has been studied by Haworth and Robinson (1948) : the most active compound was 2 : 6-dichloro-3-β-diethylaminoethyl-aminoquinoxaline which had a considerable action against *P. gallinaceum* in chicks in a dose of 20 mgm. per kgm. of body weight.

(IX) Carbamates

Certain carbamates show antimalarial action against *P. lophuræ* in ducks : *p*-carbobutoxyphenyl carbanilate (SN 1,285) appears to have an activity about one-tenth that of quinine. Leffler and Matson (1948) varied the substituents on the carbamate moiety as follows :—

$$R - N - C - OR''$$

R and R' are hydrogen, alkyl, aryl or heterocyclic groups, whereas R'' is usually a substituted aryl group.

It was found that the introduction of carbobutoxy or sulphamyl groups on the phenyl in R″, and the *p*-methoxy substitution in the phenyl R′ when R was hydrogen increased the activity against *P. lophuræ*. Other groups were less effective. However, highly active compounds were not found in this series. A quinine equivalent of 0·6 was reached with *p*-carbobutoxyphenyl *p′*-methoxy-carbanilate (SN 1,048) ; *p*-sulphamylphenyl *p′*-methoxy-carbanilate (SN 4,178) had a quinine equivalent of 0·33. In both instances this activity fell to less than 0·1 when tests were carried out in monkeys against *P. knowlesi*.

(X) Thio and Dithio Compounds

In 1945 Christian and Jenkins synthesised 5, 5′-diacetamido-8, 8′-diquinolyl disulphide. This compound (SN 9,583) was found to have a quinine equivalent against *P. lophuræ* in ducks of four. Since then a number of thio and dithio compounds have been synthesised by Christian *et al.* (1946), Wetzel *et al.* (1946), and Cheng *et al.* (1946). Only a small number have been tested for antimalarial activity and of these the only one active against *P. lophuræ* in ducks is 5, 5′-diamino-8, 8′-diquinolyl disulphide (SN 8,167) with a quinine equivalent of 1·07.

(XI) Guanidines

The action of a number of guanidines on *P. gallinaceum* was studied by King and Tonkin (1946) : *p*-tolylguanidine nitrate was found to have a slight retarding action on a sporozoite-induced infection in chicks. The most active compound was *p*-anisyl guanidine nitrate, which is active also against the exo-erythrocytic forms in tissue culture : *p*-tolylguanidine nitrate, N-*p*-tolyl-N-methylguanidine nitrate, *o*-xylyldiguanidine nitrate, *p*-phenethylguanidine nitrate and N-*p*-anisyl-N′-ethylguanidine hydrochloride were also slightly active. These compounds, because of their low molecular weight, have considerable penetrating power. Gupta and Guha (1948) have prepared a number of aromatic and aliphatic substituted guanidines which require biological study. Basu *et al.* (1950) find that N^1 (6-methoxy-8-aminoquinolyl)-N^5-*p*-methoxyphenyl biguanide has a gametocyticidal action on *Hæmoproteus columbæ*.

References

AINLEY, A. D., and KING, H., 1938, Antiplasmodial action and chemical constitution. Part II. Some simple synthetic analogues of quinine and cinchonine. *Proc. roy. Soc. B*, **125**, 60.

AMERICAN MEDICAL ASSOCIATION, 1949, Report of Council on Pharmacy and Chemistry. Primaquine, generic designation for the drug SN 13,272 (8-[4-amino-1-methylbutylamino]-6-methoxyquinioline. *J. Amer. med. Ass.*, **141**, 26.

ANDERSAG, H., BREITNER, S., and JUNG, H., 1939, German Patent 683,692 (October 26th, 1939).

ANDERSAG, H., BREITNER, S., and JUNG, H., 1941, U.S. Patent 2,233,970 (March 4th, 1941).

BACHMAN, G. B., and PICHA, G. M., 1946, Synthesis of substituted aminobenzacridines. *J. Amer. chem. Soc.*, **68**, 1599.

BALDWIN, A. W., 1929, Attempts to find new antimalarials. Part III. Some substituted aminoalkylamino quinolines. *J. chem. Soc.*, 2959.

BARBER, H. J., and WRAGG, W. R., 1946a, Composition of the antimalarial drug R.63 and the Ing and Manske hydrazine hydrolysis of N-substituted phthalimides. *Nature, Lond.*, **158**, 514.

BARBER, H. J., and WRAGG, W. R., 1946b, Contributions to the chemistry of synthetic antimalarials. Part II. Tetrahydropamaquin. *J. chem. Soc.*, 610.

BARBER, H. J., and WRAGG, W. R., 1947, Contributions to the chemistry of synthetic antimalarials. Part IV. Hydrazine hydrolysis and radical exchange reactions of N-substituted phthalimides in relation to the constitution of the antimalarial R.63. *J. chem. Soc.*, 1331.

BARGER, G., and ROBINSON, R., 1929, Attempts to find new antimalarials. *J. chem. Soc.*, 2947.

BASU, U. P., SEN GUPTA, A. R., and BOSE, A. N., 1950, Synthesis of 8-aminoquinolines. Part I. 8-Biguanide derivatives. *J. Sci. ind. Res.*, **9**, 57.

BLANCHARD, K. C., 1947, Antimalarial drugs. *Ann. Rev. Biochem.*, **16**, 587.

BOVET, D., BENOIT, G., and ALTMAN, R., 1934, Action thérapeutique de quinoleines à poids moléculaire élevé, homologues de la plasmoquine, sur les hématozoaires des calfats et des serins. *Bull. Soc. Path. exot.*, **27**, 236.

BROWN, R. F., JACOBS, T. L., WINSTEIN, S., KLOETZEL, M. C., SPAETH, E. C., FLORSHEIM, W. H., ROBSON, J. H., LEVY, E. F., BRYAN, G. M., MAGNUSSON, A. B., MILLER, S. J., OTT, M. L., and TEREX, J. A., 1946, α-(2-Piperidyl)-2-aryl-4-quinolinemethanols. *J. Amer. chem. Soc.*, **68**, 2705.

BUCHMAN, E. R., SARGENT, H., MYERS, T. C., and HOWTON, D. R., 1946, Potential antimalarials (chloro-2-phenylquinolyl-4)-α-piperidylcarbinols. *J. Amer. chem. Soc.*, **68**, 2710.

BURCKHALTER, J. H., 1949, The anomalous antimalarial activity of o-methyl camoquin. *J. Amer. pharm. Ass.*, **38**, 658.

BURCKHALTER, J. H., TENDICK, F. H., JONES, E. M., HOLCOMB, W. F., and RAWLINS, A., L , 1946, Aminoalkylphenols as antimalarials. I. Simply substituted α-aminocresols. *J. Amer. chem. Soc.*, **68**, 1894.

BURCKHALTER, J. H., TENDICK, F. H., JONES, E. M., JONES, P. A., HOLCOMB, W. F., and RAWLINS, A. L., 1948, Aminoalkyphenols as antimalarials. II. (Heterocyclic-amino)-α-amino-o-cresols. The synthesis of camoquin. *J. Amer. chem. Soc.*, **70**, 1363.

BUTTLE, G. A. H., HENRY, T. A., SOLOMON, W., TREVAN, J. W., and GIBBS, E. M., 1938, The action of the cinchona and certain other alkaloids in bird malaria. III. *Biochem. J.*, **32**, 47.

BUTTLE, G. A. H., HENRY, T. A., and TREVAN, J. W., 1934, The action of the cinchona and certain other alkaloids in bird malaria. II. *Biochem. J.*, **28**, 426.

CAMPBELL, K. N., HELBING, C. H., and KERWIN, J. F., 1946a, Studies in the quinoline series. V. The preparation of some α-dialkylaminomethyl-2-quinoline methanols. *J. Amer. chem. Soc.*, **68**, 1840.

CAMPBELL, K. N., and KERWIN, J. F., 1946, Studies in the quinoline series. II. The preparation of some dialkylamino-methyl-4-quinoline methanols. *J. Amer. chem. Soc.*, **68**, 1837.

CAMPBELL, K. N., KERWIN, J. F., LAFORGE, R. A., and CAMPBELL, B. K., 1946b, Studies in the quinoline series. VII. The preparation of some α-dialkylaminomethyl-8-quinoline methanols. *J. Amer. chem. Soc.*, **68**, 1844.

CAMPBELL, K. N., SOMMERS, A. H., KERWIN, J. F., and CAMPBELL, B. K., 1946c, Studies in the quinoline series. VI. The preparation of some α-dialkylaminomethyl-8-quinoline methanols. *J. Amer. chem. Soc.*, **68**, 1851.

CHAPMAN, N. B., GIBSON, G. B., and MANN, F. G., 1947, Synthetic antimalarials. Part XVI. 4-Dialkylaminoalkylamino quinolines. Variations of substituents in the 6- and 7- positions. *J. chem. Soc.*, 890.

CHENG, YUEN-FU, CHRISTIAN, J. E., and JENKINS, G. L., 1946, The synthesis of chemotherapeutic agents. III. The synthesis of certain thio compounds. *J. Amer. pharm. Ass.*, **35**, 334.

CHOPRA, R. N., DAS GUPTA, B. M., and SEN, B., 1938, Studies on the action of synthetic antimalarial drugs on Indian strains of malaria : cilional in the treatment of " crescent carriers." *Indian med. Gaz.*, **73**, 667.

CHRISTIAN, J. E., and JENKINS, G. L., 1945, The synthesis of derivatives of 5-aminoquinoline. *J. Amer. pharm. Ass.*, **34**, 147.

CHRISTIAN, J. E., JENKINS, G. L., KEAGLE, L. C., and CRUM, J. A., 1946, The synthesis of chemotherapeutic agents. I. The synthesis of certain thio and dithio compounds. *J. Amer. pharm. Ass.*, **35**, 328.

COATNEY, G. R., and COOPER, W. C., 1948, Symposium on exoerythrocytic forms of malarial parasites. III. The chemotherapy of malaria in relation to our knowledge of exoerythrocytic forms. *J. Parasit.*, **34**, 275.

COHEN, A., and KING, H., 1938, Antiplasmodial action and chemical constitution. Part I. Cinchona alkaloidal derivatives and allied substances. *Proc. roy. Soc. B.*, **125**, 49.

COOPER, W. C., RUHE, D. S., COATNEY, G. R., JOSEPHSON, E. S., YOUNG, M. D., and BURGESS, R. W., 1949, Studies in human malaria. XI. The protective and therapeutic action of SN. 6771 against St. Elizabeth strain vivax malaria. *Amer. J. Hyg.*, **49**, 60.

CRAIG, L. C., 1944, Identification of small amounts of organic compounds by distribution studies. II. Separation by counter-current distribution. *J. biol. Chem.*, **155**, 519.

CRAIG, L. C., GOLUMBIC, C., MIGHTON, H., and TITUS, E., 1945, Identification of small amounts of organic compounds by distribution studies. *J. biol. Chem.*, **161**, 321.

CROWTHER, A. F., CURD, F. H. S., DAVEY, D. G., and STACEY, G. J., 1949, Synthetic antimalarials. Part XXXIX. Dialkylaminoalkylamino-quinoxalines. *J. chem. Soc.*, 1260.

CRUM, J., and ROBINSON, R., 1943, Attempts to find new antimalarials. Part XX. *J. chem. Soc.*, 561.

CURD, F. H. S., DAVEY, D. G., and STACEY, G. J., 1949, Synthetic antimalarials. Part XL. The effect of variation of substituents in 2-chloro-3-β-diethylamino-ethylaminoquinoxaline. *J. chem. Soc.*, 1271.

DAUBEN, W. G., 1948, The synthesis of nuclear isomers of quinacrine. *J. Amer. chem. Soc.*, **70**, 2420.

74 CHEMICAL APPROACHES

DECOURT, P., BELFORT, J., and SCHNEIDER, J., 1939, Etude de l'action de l'oxy (diméthylaminobutyl amino) quinoléine sur *Plasmodium gallinaceum* et *Plasmodium falciparum*. *Bull. Soc. Path. exot.*, **32**, 419.

DECOURT, P., and SCHNEIDER, J., 1947, Traitement curatif du paludisme par divers sels du 3-méthyl-4-(diethylaminopentyl)-amino-7-chloroquinoleine (nivaquine). *Bull. Soc. Path. exot.*, **40**, 14.

DELEPERDANGE, G. R., 1948, Forme crystalline non décrite du chlorhydrate basique de quinine. (Note préliminaire.) *Rev. Palud.*, **6**, 103.

DIRSCHERL, W., and THRON, H., 1935, Das Vorkommen von Epi-chinin und Epichinidin in der Chinarinde. Ein Beitrag zur Chemie des Chinoidins. *Liebigs Ann.*, **521**, 48.

DOBSON, J., HUTCHISON, W. C., and KERMACK, W. O., 1948, Attempts to find new antimalarials. XXVII. Derivatives of various benzacridines and pyridoacridines. *J. chem. Soc.*, 123.

DOBSON, J., and KERMACK, W. O., 1946, Attempts to find new antimalarials. Part XXIII. Derivatives of 3 : 4 : 2′ : 3′-pyridoacridine and 1 : 2 : 2′ : 3′-pyridoacridine. *J. chem. Soc.*, 150.

DOUGLAS, B., JACOMB, R. G., and KERMACK, W. O., 1947, Attempts to find new antimalarials. Part XXVI. Further derivatives of *p*-phenanthroline. *J. chem. Soc.*, 1659.

DOUGLAS, B., and KERMACK, W. O., 1949, Attempts to find new antimalarials. XXVIII. *p*-Phenanthroline derivatives substituted in the 4-position. *J. chem. Soc.*, 1017.

DRAKE, N. L., CREECH, H. J., DRAPER, D., GARMAN, J. A., HAYWOOD, S., PECK, R. M., WALTON, E., and VAN HOOK, J. O., 1946a, Synthetic antimalarials. The preparation and properties of 7-chloro-4-(4′-diethylamino-1′ methylbutylamino)-quinidine (SN. 7,618). *J. Amer. chem. Soc.*, **68**, 1214.

DRAKE, N. L., VAN HOOK, J., GARMAN, J. A., HAYES, R., JOHNSON, R., KELLEY, G. W., MELAMED, S., and PECK, R. M., 1946b, Synthetic antimalarials. 8 - (5 - *iso*propylaminoamylamino) - 6 - methoxyquinoline (SN. 13,276) and some related compounds. *J. Amer. chem. Soc.*, **68**, 1529.

ELDERFIELD, R. C., CRAIG, L. C., LAUER, W. M., ARNOLD, R. T., GENSLER, W. J., HEAD, J. D., BEMBRY, T. H., MIGHTON, H. R., TINKER, J., GALBREATH, J., HOLLEY, A. D., GOLDMAN, L., MAYNARD, J. T., and PICUS, N., 1946, A study of plasmochin and the occurrence of rearrangements in the preparation of certain plasmochin analogs. *J. Amer. chem. Soc.*, **68**, 1576.

ELDERFIELD, R. C., KREMER, C. B., KUPCHAN, S. M., BIRSTEIN, O., and CORTES, G., 1947, Synthesis of certain 8-(5-alkylamino-1-methylpentylamino)-derivatives of quinoline. *J. Amer. chem. Soc.*, **69**, 1258.

FELDMAN, J. C., and KOPELIOWITSCH, E. L., 1935, Synthesen in der Acridinreihe. (Die Erforschung von Malariaheilmitteln.) *Arch. Pharm. Berl.*, **273**, 488.

FIELD, J. W., 1939, " Malaria " in *Rept. Inst. med. Res. F.M.S.* for the year 1938, p. 97.

FOURNEAU, E., TRÉFOUEL, J., TRÉFOUEL, Madame, BOVET, D., BENOIT, G., 1933, Contribution à la chimiothérapie du paludisme. Essais sur les calfats (deuxième mémoire). *Ann. Inst. Pasteur*, **50**, 731.

FOURNEAU, E., TRÉFOUEL, J., TRÉFOUEL, Madame, BOVET, D., and BENOIT, G., 1931, Contribution à la chimiothérapie du paludisme. Essais sur les calfats. *Ann. Inst. Pasteur*, **46**, 514.

FULTON, J. D., 1940, The course of *Plasmodium relictum* infection in canaries and the treatment of bird and monkey malaria with synthetic bases, *Ann. trop. Med. Parasit.*, **34**, 53,

FUNKE, A., BOVET, D., and MONTÉZIN, G., 1946, Quinoléines à chaine latérale arylalophatique douées de propriétés antimalariques. *Ann. Inst. Pasteur*, **72**, 264.

GALPERIN, E. P., 1940, Quinoline compounds with sidechain in position 4, *Amer. Rev. Soviet Med.*, 1944, **1**, 220.

GIEMSA, G., and OESTERLIN, M., 1933, Chemotherapeutische Studien auf dem Gebiete der Chinaalkaloide. *Arch. Schiffs-u. Tropenhyg.*, **37**, *Beiheft* 4, 217.

GIEMSA, G., WEISE, W., and TROPP, C., 1926, Chemotherapeutische Studien mit Vogelmalaria (*Plasmodium præcox*). *Arch. Schiffs-u. Tropenhyg.*, **30**, 334.

GILMAN, H., and BENKESER, R. A., 1947, Some 7-chloro-quinolines patterned as " open models " for atebrin. *J. Amer. chem. Soc.*, **69**, 123.

GILMAN, H., CHRISTIAN, R. V., and SPATZ, S. M., 1946a, Some quinolines patterned as " open models " of a modified atebrin. *J. Amer. chem. Soc.*, **68**, 979.

GILMAN, H., and SPATZ, S. M., 1944, Some quinolines patterned as " open models " of atebrine. *J. Amer. chem. Soc.*, **66**, 621.

GILMAN, H., TOWLE, J. L., and SPATZ, S. M., 1946b, Some methylquinolines patterned as " open models " of atebrin. *J. Amer. chem. Soc.*, **68**, 2017.

GLEN, W. L., and ROBINSON, R., 1943, Attempts to find new antimalarials. Part XIX. *J. chem. Soc.*, 557.

GOETZ-LUTHY, N., 1949, Fusion analysis, a rapid method for identification of organic compounds. *J. chem. Educ.*, **26**, 159.

GOODSON, J. A., HENRY, T. A., and MACFIE, J. W. S., 1930, The action of the cinchona and certain other alkaloids in bird malaria. *Biochem. J.*, **24**, 874.

GRAY, A., and HILL, J., 1949, Antimalarial studies in the quinoline series. *Ann. trop. Med. Parasit.*, **43**, 32.

GREEN, R., 1934, Lectures on the development and use of the synthetic antimalarial drugs. *Bull. Inst. med. Res. F.M.S.*, No. 2.

GRIGOROVSKII, A. M., and TERENT'EVA, E. M., 1947 [Syntheses in the acridine series. Study of acridine compounds as a source of antimalarials]. *J. gen. Chem., Moscow*, **17**, 517.

GUPTA, P. R., and GUHA, P. C., 1948, Studies in antimalarials. Some R- and R'-disubstituted guanidines. *Curr. Sci.*, **17**, 238.

GUTTMAN, P., and EHRLICH, P., 1891, Über die Wirkung des Methylenblau bei Malaria. *Berl. klin. Wschr.*, **28**, 953.

HALAWANI, A., BAZ, II., and MORKOS, F., 1947, A preliminary report on the antimalarial CAM-AQI. *J.R. Egypt. med. Ass.*, **30**, 99.

HALCROW, B. E., and KERMACK, W. O., 1946, Attempts to find new anti-malarials. Part XXIV. Derivatives of *o*-phenanthroline (7 : 8 : 3' : 2'-pyridoquinoline). *J. chem. Soc.*, 155.

HAMMICK, D. L., and FIRTH, D., 1944, Mepacrine derivatives in urine. *Nature, Lond.*, **154**, 461.

HAMMICK, D. L., and MASON, S. F., 1945, Primary degradation products of mepacrine in human urines. *Nature, Lond.*, **156**, 718.

HAWORTH, R. D., and ROBINSON, S., 1948, Synthetic antimalarials. Part XXVII. Some derivatives of phthalazine, quinoxaline and *iso*-quinoline. *J. chem. Soc.*, 777.

HEGNER, R., WEST, E., and DOBLER, M., 1941a, Further studies of hydroxy-ethylapocupreine against bird malaria. *Amer. J. Hyg.*, **34C**, 132.

HEGNER, R., WEST, E., RAY, M., and DOBLER, M., 1941b, A new drug effective against bird malaria. *Amer. J. Hyg.*, **33C**, 101.

HENRY, T. A., and GRAY, W. H., 1935, Trypanocidal and antimalarial drugs. *Trop. Dis. Bull.*, **32**, 385.

HENRY, T. A., and SOLOMON, W., 1934, Modified cinchona alkaloids. Part I. Apoquinine and apoquinidine. *J. chem. Soc.*, 1923.

HENRY, T. A., SOLOMON, W., and GIBBS, E. M., 1935, Modified cinchona alkaloids. Part II. The action of sulphuric acid on quinine and quinidine. *J. chem. Soc.*, 966.

HENRY, T. A., SOLOMON, W., and GIBBS, E. M., 1937, Modified cinchona alkaloids. Part IV. Constitution. *J. chem. Soc.*, 592.

HÖRLEIN, H., 1926, Über die chemischen Grundlagen und die Entwicklungsgeschichte des Plasmochins. *Arch. Schiffs-u. Tropenhyg.*, **30**, *Beiheft No. 3, 5.*

HUMPHLETT, W. J., WEISS, M. J., and HAUSER, C. R., 1948, Preparation of ketones from γ-diethylaminobutyronitrile and aromatic Grignard reagents and their conversion to diamines. Synthesis of quinacrine analogs. *J. Amer. chem. Soc.*, **70**, 4020.

HUTCHISON, W. C., and KERMACK, W. O., 1947, Attempts to find new antimalarials. XXV. Some derivatives of 3 : 4 : 2′ : 3′-pyridoacridine substituted in the 2-position. *J. chem. Soc.*, 678.

KENEFORD, J. R., and SIMPSON, J. C. E., 1947, Synthetic antimalarials. Part XX. Cinnolines. Part XIII. Synthesis and antimalarial action of 4-aminoalkylamino-cinnolines. *J. chem. Soc.*, 917.

KIKUTH, W., 1938, Zur Weiter Entwicklung der Chemotherapie der Malaria : " Certuna "—ein neues Gametenmittel. *Klin. Wschr.*, **17i**, 524.

KIKUTH, W., 1945, Zur Weiter Entwicklung der Malariatherapie, Sontochin ein neues synthetisches Malariaheitmittel. Appendix 4. Pharmaceuticals : Research and Manufacture at I. G. Farbenindustrie. Final Report No. 116. British Intelligence Objectives Sub-Committee. London : H.M. Stationery Office.

KIKUTH, W., and MUDROW-REICHENOW, L., 1947, Über kausalprophylaktisch bei Vogelmalaria wirksame Substanzen. *Z. Hyg. Infektkr.*, **127**, 151.

KING, H., and ACHESON, R. M., 1946, New potential chemotherapeutic agents. Part V. Basically substituted *iso*alloxazines. *J. chem. Soc.*, 681.

KING, H., and TONKIN, I. M., 1946, Antiplasmodial action and chemical constitution. Part VIII. Guanidines and diguanidines. *J. chem. Soc.*, 1063.

KING, H., and WORK, T. S., 1940, Antiplasmodial action and chemical constitution. Part III. Carbinolamines derived from naphthaleine and quinoline. *J. chem. Soc.*, 1307.

KING, H., and WRIGHT, J., 1948, Antiplasmodial action and chemical constitution. IX. Carbinolamines derived from 6 : 7-dimethyl-quinoline. *Proc. roy. Soc. B.*, **135**, 271.

KOEPFLI, J. B., 1946, The synthesis of potential antimalarials 2-phenyl-α-(2-piperidyl)-4-quinolinemethanols. *J. Amer. chem. Soc.*, **68**, 2697.

KRITSCHEWSKI, I. L., MAGIDSON, O. Y., HALPERIN, E. P., and GRIGOROWSKI, A. M., 1934, Die Synthese chemotherapeutischer Verbindung. Akridin-derivate gegen Malaria. *G. Batt. Immun.*, **13**, 685.

KYKER, G. C., CORNATZER, W. E., and McEWEN, M. M., 1946, The ultra-violet irradiation of quinine. *J. biol. Chem.*, **162**, 353.

KYKER, G. C., McEWEN, M. M., and CORNATZER, W. E., 1947, The formation of antimalarial agents by ultraviolet decomposition of quinine. *Arch. Biochem.*, 12, 191.

LAPP, C., 1935, Le pouvoir rotatoire spécifique des sels de quinine, quinidine, cinchonine et cinchonidine. *C.R. Acad. Sci., Paris*, **201**, 80.

LEFFLER, M. T., and MATSON, E. J., 1948, Carbamate antimalarials. *J. Amer. chem. Soc.*, **70**, 3439.

LUTZ, R. E., BAILEY, P. S., CLARK, M. T., CODINGTON, J. F., DEINET, A. J., FREEK, J. A., HARNEST, G. H., LEAKE, N. H., MARTIN, T. A., ROWLETT, R. J. Jr., SALSBURY, J. M., SHEARER, N.H. Jr., SMITH, J. D., and WILSON, J. W. 3rd, 1946, Antimalarials. α-Alkyl and dialkylamino-methyl-2-phenyl-4-quinoline-methanols. *J. Amer. chem. Soc.*, **68**, 183.

CHEMICAL APPROACHES 77

MADINAVEITIA, J., 1944, The antagonism of some antimalarial drugs by
riboflavine. *Biochem. J.*, **38**, Proc. xxvii.
MADINAVEITIA, J., 1946, The antagonism of some antimalarial drugs by
riboflavin. *Biochem. J.*, **40**, 373.
MAGIDSON, O. Y., and GOLOVCHINSKAYA, E. S., 1938 [Quinazoline compounds
as a source of medicinal products. I. Alkylamino derivatives of 6-nitro-
and 6-chloro-quinazoline]. *J. gen. Chem., Moscow*, **8**, 1797.
MAGIDSON, O. Y., and GRIGOROWSKY, A. M., 1936, Acridin-Verbindungen
und ihre Antimalaria-Wirkung (I. Mitteil). *Ber. dtsch. chem. Ges.*, **69**,
396.
MAGIDSON, O. Y., MADAJEWA, O. S., and RUBZOW, M. W., 1935, Die Derivate
des 8-Aminocholins als Antimalariapräparate. Mitt. IV. Verbindungen-
mit langen Ketten in 8-Stellung. *Arch. Pharm., Berl.*, **273**, 320.
MAGIDSON, O. Y., and RUBTSOV, M. V., 1937 [Quinoline compounds as sources
of medicinal products. VI. Antimalarial compounds with the side-chain
in the four-position]. *J. gen. Chem., Moscow*, **7**, 1896.
MAGIDSON, O. Y., and STRUKOW, I. T., 1933a, Die Derivate des 8-Amino
chinolins als Antimalariapräparate. Mitt. I. Die Wirkung von Alkyl
in Stellung 6 auf chemotherapeutische Eigenschaften. *Arch. Pharm.,
Berl.*, **271**, 359.
MAGIDSON, O. Y., and STRUKOW, I. T., 1933b, Die Derivate des 8-Amino-
chinolins als Antimalariapräparate. Mitt. II. Der Einfluss der Länge
der Kette in Stellung 8. *Arch. Pharm., Berl.*, **271**, 569.
MAGIDSON, O. Y., and TRAWIN, A. L., 1936, Über Acridin Verbingungen und
ihre Antimalaria-Wirkung. II. Mitteil. Verbindungen mit Cyanund
Methylmercapto-Gruppen. *Ber. dtsch. chem. Ges.*, **69**, 537.
MARSHALL, E. K., Jr., 1946, Chemotherapy of malaria, 1941–45. *Fed. Proc.*,
5, 298.
MASSIAS, C., 1933, Le " 574 " associé au quiniostovarsol dans le traitement
du paludisme à *Plasmodium vivax* et à *Plasmodium præcox*. *Bull. Soc.
Path. exot.*, **26**, 590.
MASSIAS, C., 1934a, Nouvelles observations de 48 paludéens traités par un
dérivé quinoléique associé au quiniostovarsol. *Bull. Soc. Path. exot.*,
27, 641.
MASSIAS, C., 1934b, Dérivé quinoléinique employé seul contre le paludisme à
P. vivax et à *P. præcox*. *Bull. Soc. Path. exot.*, **27**, 644.
MATHIESON, D. W., and NEWBERRY, G., 1949, Contributions to the chemistry
of synthetic antimalarials. VIII. Aromatic carbinolamines. *J. chem.
Soc.*, 1133.
MAUSS, H., 1942, Acridinverbindungen als Malariamittel. *Medizin und
Chemie*, **4**, 60. Berlin, Verlag Chemie G.M.B.H.
MAUSS, H., and MIETSZCH, F., 1933, Atebrin, ein neues Heilmittel gegen
Malaria. *Klin. Wschr.*, **12**, 1276.
MAY, E. L., and MOSETTIG, E., 1946, Attempts to find new antimalarials.
I. Amino alcohols derived from 1, 2, 3, 4-tetrahydrophenanthrene.
J. Org. Chem., **11**, 1.
MIETSZCH, F., and MAUSS, H., 1934, Gegen Malaria Wirksame Acridinver-
bindungen. *Z. Angew. Chem.*, **47**, 633.
MISSIROLI, A., and MOSNA, E., 1934, Sulle proprietà terapeutiche di un
prodotto derivato della chinina : C. 77-Giema. *Riv. Malariol.*, **13**, 148.
MONIER, H. M., 1931, Essai d'un dérivé de la quinoléine (664 Fourneau) dans
la malarie expérimentale. *Bull. Soc. Path. exot.*, **24**, 93.
MOSHER, H. S., 1946, Heterocyclic basic compounds. VIII. 8-[3-(3′-amino-
propylamino)-propylamino]-6-methoxyquinoline. *J. Amer. chem. Soc.*,
68, 1565.
MÜHLENS, P., 1938, " Certuna " ein neues Tropikagametenmittel. *Dtsch.
med. Wschr.*, **64**, 295.

NEEMAN, M. E., 1946, Syntheses of 9-substituted flavins as antimalarials. *J. chem. Soc.*, 811.

PRICE, C. C., and ROBERTS, R. M., 1946, The synthesis of 4-hydroxy-quinolines. I. Through ethoxymethylenemalonic ester. *J. Amer. chem. Soc.*, **68**, 1204.

PULLMAN, T. N., EICHELBERGER, L., ALVING, A. S., JONES, R. Jr., CRAIGE, B. Jr., and WHORTON, C. M., 1948. The use of SN.10,275 in the prophylaxis and treatment of sporozoite-induced vivax malaria (Chesson strain). *J. clin. Invest.*, **27**, Suppl. p. 12.

QUIN, D. C., and ROBINSON, R., 1943, Attempts to find new antimalarials. Pt. XVIII. *J. chem. Soc.*, 555.

RABE, P., 1909, Zur Kenntriss der Chinaalkaloide. X. *Liebigs Ann.*, **365**, 353.

RABE, P., HUNTENBURG, W., SCHULTZE, A., and VOLGER, G., 1931, Die Totalsynthese der China-Alkaloide, Hydrochinin und Hydrochinidin. *Ber. dtsch. chem. Ges.*, **64**, 2487.

RAPPORT, M. M., SENEAR, A. E., MEAD, J. F., and KOEPFLI, J. B., 1946, The synthesis of potential antimalarials. 2-Phenyl-α-(2-piperidyl)-4-quinolinemethanols. *J. Amer. chem. Soc.*, **68**, 2697.

REITSEMA, R. H., 1948, The chemistry of 4-hydroxy-quinolines. *Chem. Rev.*, **43**, 43.

RIEGEL, B., LAPPIN, G. R., ALBISETTI, C. J., ADELMAN, B. H., DODSON, R. M., GINGER, L. G., and BAKER, R. H., 1946, The preparation of some 4-aminoquinolines. *J. Amer. chem. Soc.*, **68**, 1229.

ROBINSON, R., and TOMLINSON, M. L., 1934, Attempts to find new antimalarials. XII. *J. chem. Soc.*, 1524.

ROSKIN, G., and ROMANOWA, K., 1929, Arzneimittel und ultraviolette Strahlen. I. Mitt. Die Chininwirkung auf die Zelle bei gleichzeitiger Bestrahlung derselben mit ultravioletten Strahlen. *Z. ImmunForsch.* **62**, 147.

RUBINSTEIN, B. N., 1936, Die Behandlung der Impfmalaria bei Paralytikern mit dem neuen synthetischen Präparet Acrichin. *Arch. Schiffs.-u. Tropenhyg.*, **40**, 167.

SALZER, W., TIMMLER, H., and ANDERSAG, H., 1948, Ueber einen neuen, gegen Vogelmalaria wirksamen Verbindungtypus. *Chem. Berichte*, **81**, 12.

SCHMIDT, L. H., 1947, quoted by Blanchard, K. C., Antimalarial drugs. *Ann. Rev. Biochem.*, **16**, 587.

SCHÖNHÖFER, F., 1938, Studies in the series of the aliphatic-basic substitution compounds of quinoline. In : *Medicine in its Chemical Aspects*, **3**, 62, Leverkusen, "Bayer."

SCHÖNHÖFER, F., 1942, Ueber die Bedeutung der chinoiden Bindung in Chinolinverbindungen für die Malaria-wirkung. *Hoppe-Seyl. Z.*, **274**, 1.

SCHULEMANN, W., 1932, Synthetic antimalarial preparations. *Proc. R. Soc. Med.*, **25**, 897.

SCHULEMANN, W., SCHÖNHÖFER, F., and WINGLER, A., 1930, U.S.A. Patent 1,747,531 (February 18th).

SCHULEMANN, W., SCHÖNHÖFER, F., and WINGLER, A., 1932, Synthese des Plasmochin. *Klin. Wschr.*, 11i, 381.

SERGENT, A., and VOGT, P., 1933, Essais de traitement de la tierce maligne par le " 915 Fourneau " ou rhodoquine. *Bull. Soc. Path. exot.*, **26**, 1255.

SIMPSON, J. C. E., and SCHOFIELD, K., 1946, Antimalarial action of cinnoline derivatives. *Nature, Lond.*, **157**, 439.

SIOLI, F., 1938, Prüfung des neuen Malariamittels " Certuna " bei der Impfmalaria der Paralytiker. *Klin. Wschr.*, 17i, 527.

SOLOMON, W., 1938, Modified cinchona alkaloids. Part V. β-*iso*Quinotoxin and the stereochemistry of the parent bases. *J. chem. Soc.*, 6.

STECK, E. A., HALLOCK, L. L., and HOLLAND, A. J., 1946a, Quinolines. I. The synthesis of 3-methyl-4-(1′-methyl-4′-diethylaminobutyl amino)-quinoline and some 6-substituted derivatives. *J. Amer. chem. Soc.*, **68**, 129.

STECK, E. A., HALLOCK, L. L., and HOLLAND, A. J., 1946b, Quinolines. II. The synthesis of 8-substituted 3-methyl-4-(1′-methyl-4′-diethyl-amino-butylamino)-quinolines. *J. Amer. chem. Soc.*, **68**, 132.

STECK, E. A., HALLOCK, L. L., and SUTER, C. M., 1948, Quinolines. VI. Some 4-aminoquinoline derivatives. *J. Amer. chem. Soc.*, **70**, 4063.

STEPHEN, J. M. L., TONKIN, I. M., and WALKER, J., 1945, Antimalarial activity in tetrahydroacridones and related substances. *Nature, Lond.*, **156**, 629.

STEPHEN, J. M. L., TONKIN, I. M., and WALKER, J., 1947, Tetrahydroacri-dones and related compounds as antimalarials. *J. chem. Soc.*, 1034.

SURREY, A. R., and HAMMER, H. F., 1946, Some 7-substituted 4-amino-quinoline derivatives. *J. Amer. chem. Soc.*, **68**, 113.

TATE, P., and VINCENT, M., 1933, The action of synthetic quinoline compounds on avian malaria. *Parasitology*, **25**, 411.

WETZEL, J. W., WELDTON, D. E., CHRISTIAN, J. E., JENKINS, G. L., and BACHMAN, G. B., 1946, The synthesis of chemotherapeutic agents. II. The synthesis of certain thio and dithio compounds. *J. Amer. pharm. Ass.*, **35**, 331.

WISELOGLE, F. Y., edited by, 1946, "A survey of antimalarial drugs, 1941 1945." 2 vols. Ann Arbor, Michigan. J. W. Edwards.

WOODWARD, R. B., and DOERING, W. E., 1944, The total synthesis of quinine. *J. Amer. chem. Soc.*, **66**, 849.

WORK, T. S., 1940, Antiplasmodial action and chemical constitution. Part IV. The synthesis of some complex carbinolamines and polyamines. *J. chem. Soc.*, 1315.

WORK, T. S., 1946a, The synthesis of antimalarial compounds related to niquidine. Part I. Model experiments on the synthesis of quinolyl carbinols. *J. chem. Soc.*, 194.

WORK, T. S., 1946b, The synthesis of antimalarial compounds related to niquidine. Part II. Synthesis of a dihydro-x-niquidine. *J. chem. Soc.*, 197.

CHAPTER IV

THE CHEMICAL APPROACH TO ANTIMALARIAL COMPOUNDS (II)

(XII) Proguanil (Paludrine)

SEVERAL reasons prompted Curd and Rose (1946a) to begin an investigation of pyrimidine derivatives for antimalarial action, the first being a consideration of the antimalarial activity of the sulphonamides, an activity originally discovered by Díaz de León (1937). As the sulphonamides do not conform to the general chemical structure characteristic of the older antimalarial drugs it was concluded that either their activity must be completely unrelated to that of the other antimalarials or that some other relationship must be sought. Before the demonstration by Marshall et al. (1942) that the antimalarial activity of sulphonamides is similar to their antibacterial action in that it is inhibited by p-aminobenzoic acid, it was thought that the sulphonamides must be regarded as aniline derivatives in which the sulphonamide or substituted sulphonamide group performs the same pharmacological function as Magidson et al. (1934), and Magidson and Grigorowsky (1936) had suggested for the basic side-chain in the older type of antimalarial. Since the attainment of very high blood levels is characteristic of the sulphonamide derivatives of 2-aminopyrimidine and 2-amino : 4 : 6-dimethyl-pyrimidine, it was considered that the introduction of these residues into other structures might confer similar properties on them.

The second reason for studying the pyrimidines was the similarity between the formulæ of mepacrine and riboflavin : the activity of mepacrine might be due to a competition for certain enzyme systems in the malarial parasite.

The third reason was the characteristic of resonance possessed by the pyrimidines, mepacrine also having a resonance system.

Compounds of type (I) and (II) were first prepared : they can be regarded as pyrimidine derivatives of aniline.

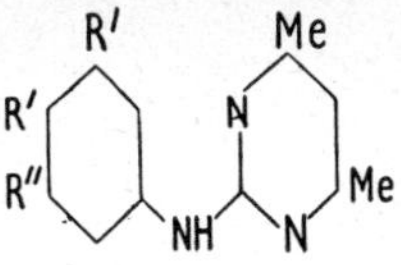

(I) 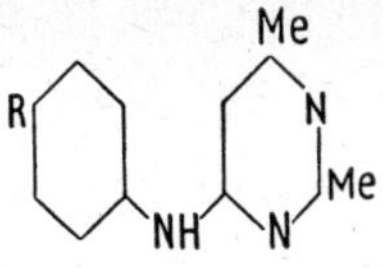   (II)

Pyrimidine derivatives carrying dialkylaminoalkylamino groups which are characteristic of mepacrine and pamaquin were then studied. The 4-dialkylaminoalkylamino derivatives were of particular interest since one tautomeric possibility in this type of compound (III ⇌ IV) is exactly analogous to that which can occur in mepacrine to which Schönhöfer (1942) has attributed the antimalarial activity of mepacrine (V ⇌ VI).

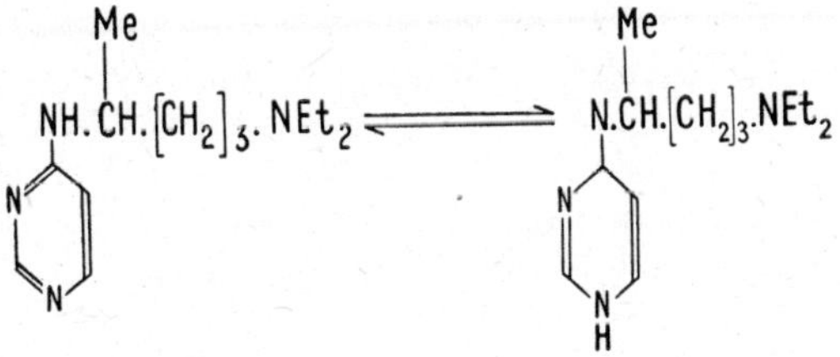

(III)   (IV)

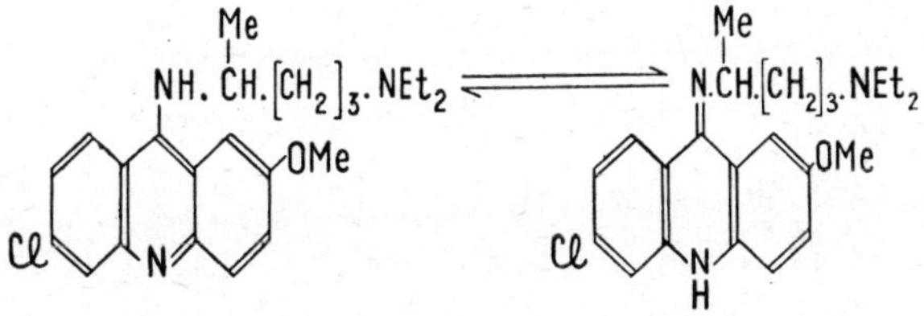

(V)   (VI)

Compounds of the general formula VII (R' = dialkylamino-alkyl) were also prepared because they combine in a different manner two of the structural features of mepacrine : a basic alkylamino heterocyclic system and a chlorine—or methoxyl-substituted anilino residue which can be identified as fused components of the mepacrine molecule in one of its tautomeric forms (VI). Furthermore Schönhöfer (1942) has suggested that the antimalarial activity of pamaquin may be due to the possibility, which exists in a molecule of this orientation, that in the body compounds of quinonoid character may be formed. The same possibility existed in 2-p-anisidino-4-β-diethylaminoethyl-amino-6-methylpyrimidine (VII ; R = OMe, R′ = $CH_2CH_2NEt_2$). This compound 2665 was in fact active against *P. gallinaceum* in a dose of 200 mgm./kgm.

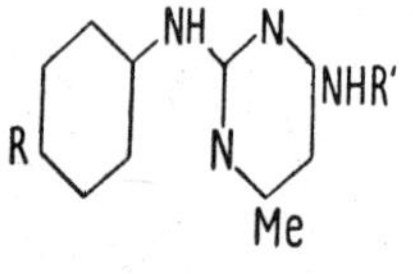

(VII) 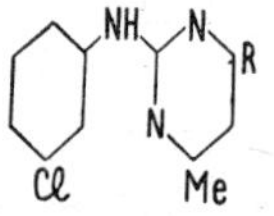   (VIII) 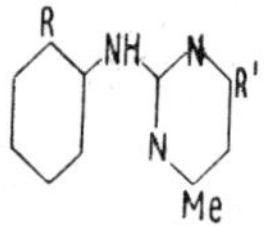   (IX)

Another compound, 2-p-chloroanilino-4-β-diethylaminoethyl-amino-6-methylpyrimide (VII ; R = Cl, R′ = $CH_2CH_2NEt_2$) (2666) was also found to be active in a dose of 100 mgm./kgm. These were antimalarial compounds of an entirely new type.

ANTIMALARIAL ACTIVITY OF 2-ARYLAMINO-4-DIALKYL-AMINO-ALKYLAMINO-6-METHYLPYRIMIDINE DIHYDROCHLORIDES
(Curd, Davis, Owen, Rose and Tuey, 1946a)

No.	Formula of base.	Dose mgm./kgm.	Activity.
2665	VII ; R = OMe, R′ = $[CH_2]_2 . NEt_2$	200	+ +
2666	VII ; R = Cl, R′ = $[CH_2]_2 . NEt_2$	100	+ +
		80	+ +
		40	+
3299	VII ; R = Cl, R′ = $[CH_2]_3 . NEt_2$	80	+ +
		40	+
3711	VII ; R = Cl, R′ = $[CH_2]_3 . NMe_2$	40	+ +
		20	+
3338	VII ; R = Cl, R′ = $[CH_2]_4 . NEt_2$	200	+ +
		80	+
3300	VII ; R = Cl, R′ = CHMe . $[CH_2]_3 . NEt_2$	200	+ +
		100	—
3381	IX ; R = Cl, R′ = NH . $[CH_2]_2 . NEt_2$	200	±
		150	—
3466	IX ; R = Cl, R′ = NH . $[CH_2]_3 . NEt_2$	200	—
3554	VIII ; R = NH . $[CH_2]_3 . NEt_2$	200	+
		150	±
		80	—
3382	IX ; R = OMe, R′ = NH . $[CH_2]_2 . NEt_2$	200	—
		100	—
2725	VII ; R = H, R′ = $[CH_2]_2 . NEt_2$	80	—

+ + = Active. + = Slightly active. ± = very slightly active. — = inactive.

The effect of varying the 4-dialkylaminoalkylamino group was also investigated in view of the finding by Fourneau *et al.* (1933) and Magidson and Grigorowsky (1936) that in other series of anti-malarial drugs significant variations in activity occur with variation of the basic alkyl side-chain.

The antimalarial activity of these compounds, as tested against *P. gallinaceum* by the method of Curd, Davis, Owen, Rose and Tuey (1946a), is shown in the table on the opposite page, based on Formulæ VII, VIII and IX.

Series of 2-anilino-4 : 6-dimethylpyrimidines, 4-anilino-2 : 6-dimethylpyrimidines, and 4-β-diethylamino-2-aryl-6-methyl-pyrimidines were all inactive.

Highest activity against *P. gallinaceum* was in fact shown by those compounds in which the substituent occupied the *para*-position of the anilino residue (X ; R = Cl or OMe, R' = dialkylaminoalkyl) ; transference to the *meta*- or *ortho*-positions gave compounds with only a trace of activity. Variation of the dialkylaminoalkyl-amino group and replacement of the original chlorine and methoxyl substituents in the anilino residue by other groupings did not entirely abolish antimalarial activity as seen in the table on pages 84 and 85, (Curd, Davis and Rose, 1946).

Hull *et al.* (1946) prepared pyrimidine derivatives bearing no aryl or arylamino substituents. Derivatives of 2- and 6-methyl-pyrimidine containing basic groups were inactive as antimalarials. Similar lack of antimalarial activity was encountered in a series of derivatives of 2 : 6-dimethylpyrimidine bearing a basic substituent in position 4. Only one derivative of 4 : 6-dimethyl-pyrimidine, 2-(δ-diethylamino-α-methylbutylamino)-4 : 6-dimethyl pyrimidine was examined but it too was inactive. Antimalarial activity was first encountered when basic side-chains were introduced at position 4 in 2-amino-5 : 6-dimethylpyrimidine. Thus 2 - amino - 4 - (δ - diethylamino - α - methyl - butylamino) - 5 : 6-dimethylpyrimidine (XI ; R = CHMe . [CH$_2$]$_3$. NEt$_2$) and 2-amino - 4 - γ - diethylaminopropylamino - 5 : 6 - dimethylpyrimidine (XI ; R = [CH$_2$]$_3$. NEt$_2$) were active against *P. gallinaceum* at a dose of 4 mgm. per 50 gm. but were toxic to the host (maximum

ANTIMALARIAL ACTIVITIES (Curd, Davis and Rose, 1946)

No.	Nature of R.	Dose mgm./kgm.	Activity.

(a) 2 - Arylamino - 4 - β - diethylaminoethylamino - 6 - methyl - pyrimidine dihydrochloride.

General formula :

3383	4'-Phenetidino-	200	+ +
3527	4'-Methylthioanilino- . . .	80	+ to + +
		60	+ to + +
3464	4'-Toluidino	100	+ +
		80	+ +
3375	3'-Toluidino	160	—
3528	2'-Toluidino	120	+
		80	±

(b) 2 - Arylamino - 4 - γ - diethylaminopropylamino - 6 - methylpyrimidine dihydrochloride.

General formula :

3748	4'-Butylanilino	80	±
3643	4'-Bromoanilino-	100	+ +
		80	+ +
		40	+
3830	4'-Nitroanilino	80	+ +
		40	+
3905	4'-Cyanoanilino	80	+ +
		40	+
3507	4'-Phenetidino	200	+
		80	—
3693	4'-Dimethylaminoanilino(trihydrobromide)	80	+
3782	4'-Carbomethoxyanilino-	160	+ to + +
		80	+
3840	4'-Phenylanilino-	200	+ to + +
		80	+
3564	3' : 4'-Dichloroanilino- . . .	200	+ to + +
		150	+ to + +
		120	+ to + +
		80	±
3668	3'-Chloro-4'-methylanilino- . . .	200	+ +
		120	+
		80	+
3694	3' : 4'-Dimethylanilino- . . .	120	+
3621	2' : 4'-Dichloroanilino- . . .	120	+ to + +
		80	+ to + +
		40	±

PROGUANIL PRECURSORS

No.	Nature of R.	Dose mgm./kgm.	Activity.
3598	4′-Chloro-2′-methylanilino- . . .	80	+ +
		40	+ to + +
3685	2′ : 5′-Dichloroanilino-	200	—
		120	—
3620	4′-Chloro-2′-methyanilino-γ-dibutylamino-	200	+ +
	propylamino-derivative . . .	120	+
		80	—
		40	—

(c) 2-p-Chloroanilino-4-alkylamino-6-methylpyrimidine dihydrochlorides.

General formula :

3906	NH . [CH₂]₂ . NMe₂	40	+
		20	±
4413	NH . [CH₂]₂ . N <[CH₂]₃> CH₂ . .	160	+ +
		80	+
		40	—
4412	NH . [CH₂]₂ . N <[CH₂]₄> CH₂. . .	240	+ +
		160	+ +
		80	—
		40	—
3557	NH . [CH₂]₃ . N <[CH₂]₄> CH₂ . .	80	+ to + +
		60	+
4438	NH . CHMe . CH₂ . N <[CH₂]₄> CH₂. .	160	+
		80	—
3578	NH . [CH₂]₃ . Buα₂-(γ-dibutylaminopropyl-	200	+ +
	amino-derivative)	80	—
		40	—
3671	NH . [CH₂]₃ . NHBu-(γ-butylaminopropyl-	80	+ to + +
	amino-derivative)	40	+
4439	NH[CH₂]₃ . O . [CH₂]₂ . NEt₂ . . .	120	+
		40	—
4440	NH . [CH₂]₃ . NMe[CH₂]₃ . NEt₂ trihydro-	160	+ to + +
	chloride	80	+
4414	NMe . [CH₂]₂ . NEt₂	160	+ +
		80	—
4499	N([CH₂]₂ . NEt₂)₂ trihydrobromide .	160	±
4498	NH . CH(CH₂ . NEt₂)₂ trihydrobromide .	240	—
		120	—
4667	NH . [CH₂]₃ . NMePrβ	80	+ to + +
		40	+ to + +
		20	—
3542	p-NH . C₆H₄ . O . [CH₂]₂ . NEt₂ . .	80	+ to + +
3654	p-NH . C₆H₄ . NMe₂ . . .	320	±
		120	—
4874	NH . [CH₂]₂ . NH₂	40	+ +
		20	+

tolerated dose of XI (R = $[CH_2]_3 . NEt_2$) was 4 mgm./50 gm. : MLD for mice per os 250 to 500 mgm./kgm.).

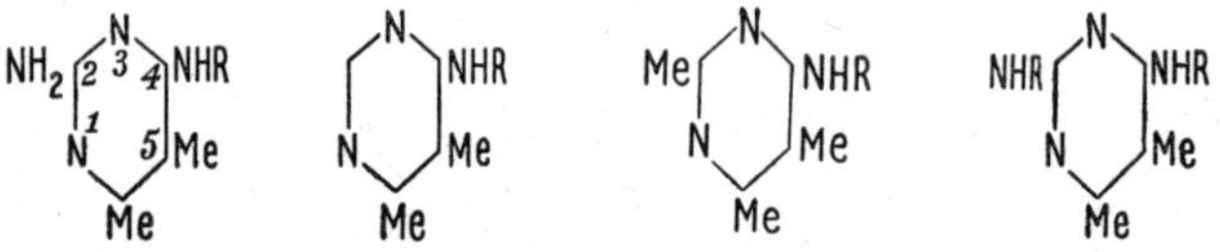

(XI) (XII) (XIII) (XIV)

Omission of the 2-amino-group, giving compounds of type XII or its replacement by methyl (type XIII), reduced the activity very markedly without greatly affecting toxicity : replacement of the 2-amino-group by a second dialkylaminoalkyl group (type XIV) destroyed antimalarial activity. These findings led to a study of the effect of varying the nature of the basic side-chain and the alkyl groups at C_5 and C_6. No compounds showed higher antimalarial activity than the two compounds of type XI, while many showed increased toxicity.

Antimalarial activity is thus present in comparatively simple pyrimidine derivatives.

A series of 2-phenylguanidino-4-amino-alkylamino-6-methylpyrimidines was prepared by Curd and Rose (1946b). It was thought that a diguanidine such as (XV) might give rise to compounds of type (XVI) having similar tautomeric potentialities

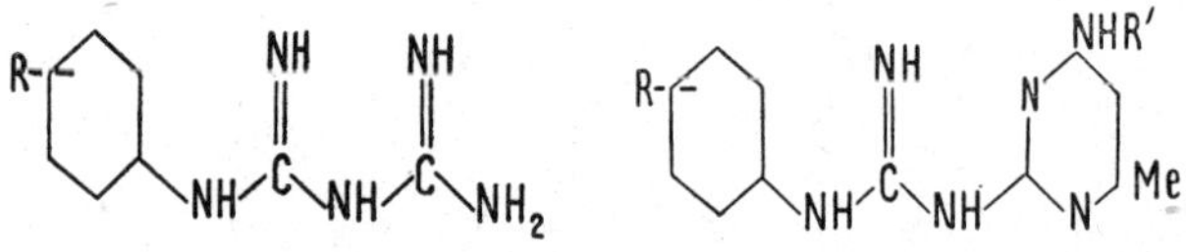

(XV) (XVI)

to type (XVII), and when formulated as a planar figure having some slight structural resemblance to riboflavin.

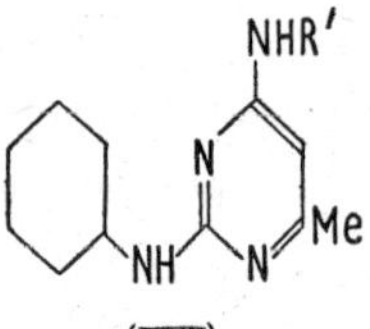

(XVII)

The first preparation in this series was 2-p-chlorophenyl-guanidine-4-β-diethylaminoethylamino-6-methylpyrimidine (XVI; R = p-Cl, R' = $CH_2 . CH_2 . NEt_2$) (3349).

ANTIMALARIAL ACTIVITY OF 2-PHENYLGUANIDINO-4-AMINOALKYL-AMINO-6-METHYLPYRIMIDINES AGAINST *P. gallinaceum*
(Curd and Rose, 1946b)

Formula of Base XVI.

No.	R	R'	Dose mgm./kgm.	Activity
3688	p-Cl	$CH_2 . CH_2 . CH_2 . NEt_2$	300	+
3349	p-Cl	$CH_2 . CH_2 . NEt_2$	40	+ +
			20	+
3916	p-Cl	$CH_2 . CH_2 . CH_2 . NC_5H_{10}$	160	+
3907	p-Cl	$CH_2 . CH_2 . CH_2 . CH_2 . NEt_2$	200	+
3833	m-Cl	$CH_2 . CH_2 . NEt_2$	80	+
3836	o-Cl	$CH_2 . CH_2 . NEt_2$	160	+
4510	p-F	$CH_2 . CH_2 . NEt_2$	40	+ +
			20	+
3779	p-Br	$CH_2 . CH_2 . NEt_2$	50	+
3831	p-I	$CH_2 . CH_2 . NEt_2$	40	+
			40	+ +
3822	p-CN	$CH_2 . CH_2 . NEt_2$	20	+
3747	p-NO_2	$CH_2 . CH_2 . NEt_2$	40	+ +
			20	+
3742	p-MeO	$CH_2 . CH_2 . NEt_2$	200	—

The formal planar similarity of mepacrine and of 2-p-chloro-anilino-4-β-diethylaminoethylamino-6-methylpyrimidine (XVII, R' = $[CH_2]_2 . NEt_2$, R = Cl) to riboflavin and the inhibition of the antibacterial activity of the first two compounds for *Lactobacillus casei* by the vitamin (Madinaveitia, 1946) led to the belief that there might be some connection between mepacrine and the pyrimidine antimalarials of type (XVII), the activity of both types of compound possibly due to an interference with the functioning of a riboflavin-containing enzyme system in the malaria parasite. Modifications in the mepacrine molecule investigated by other workers, excluding simple changes in substituents, were taken by

Curd, Raison and Rose (1946) as a guide for further variations in the 2-substituted anilino-4-dialkylaminoalkylamino-6-methylpyrimidine structure (XVIII).

Magidson and Rubtsov (1937) and Schönhöfer (1942) found that 4-dialkylaminoalkylamino derivatives of 6-methoxyquinoline (XIX) have antimalarial activity. The 7-halogen-substituted-4-

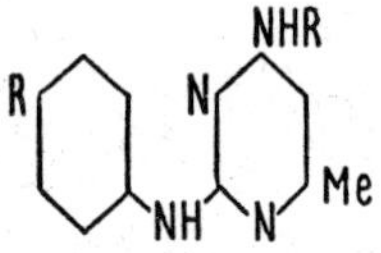

(XVIII) 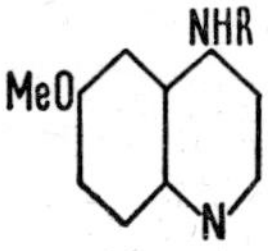   (XIX) 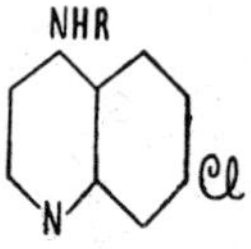   (XX)

dialkyl-aminoalkylaminoquinolines (XX) of D.R.P. 683,692 are also known to be active. These compounds represent portions of the mepacrine molecule, as can be seen from the appended formulæ: they may thus owe their activity to this relationship and act in a similar manner to mepacrine. According to E. P. 481,874, benzoquinoline derivatives, carrying an aminoalkylamino group in the 4 position, also have antimalarial activity. The permissible variations include not only derivatives of 5 : 6-benzoquinoline (XXI) but also of 7 : 8-benzoquinoline (XXII).

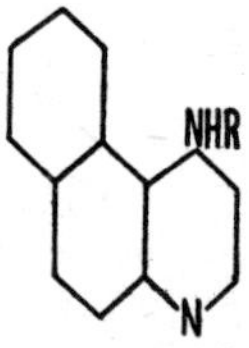

(XXI) 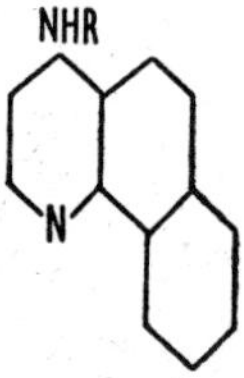   (XXII)

The former compound may be regarded as derived from those of type (XIX), the third ring of mepacrine being attached to the benzene nucleus instead of the pyridine nucleus so that the 6-methoxy group of (XIX) is replaced by a fused benzene nucleus in the 5 : 6 position. The latter are similarly related to type (XX), the 7-chlorino atom being replaced by a benzene ring fused in the 7 : 8 position. A corresponding variation of the 2-*p*-substituted-anilino-4-aminoalkylamino-6-methylpyrimidines (XVIII) was

therefore indicated, and a series of 2-β-naphthylamino-4-amino-
alkylamino-6-methylpyrimidines (XXIII ; R = H, R′ = alkylene. N(alkyl)$_2$) were therefore prepared by Curd, Raison and
Rose (1946).

All compounds of type (XXIII) showed antimalarial activity
when tested against *P. gallinaceum* in chicks, although none was
outstandingly active.

For comparison with compounds of type (XXIII), 2-α-naphthyl-
amino - 4 - β - diethylaminoethylamino - 6 - methyl - pyrimidine
(XXIV ; R = H) was prepared but was without demonstrable
activity. In (XXIV ; R = H) neither of the points of attachment
of the second benzene nucleus in the naphthylamino residue corresponds to the *para* position of the anilino residue in the prototype

(XXIII)   (XXIV)

(XVIII). To explore this relationship further, the synthesis of the
corresponding 4-chloro-α-naphthylamino compound (XXIV ;
R = Cl) was undertaken; antimalarial activity had been largely
restored.

These results were taken to support the belief that the mode of
action of the 2-β-naphthylamino compounds of type (XXIII) was
not fundamentally different from that of the simple anilino
derivatives of type (XVIII), probably involving a riboflavin
antagonism.

Curd, Richardson and Rose (1946) then continued their studies
of 2-arylamino-4-aminoalkylamino-6-methylpyrimidines by preparing compounds having (1) no substituent in the 6 position,
(2) a 6-phenyl group, and (3) various substituents in the 5 position,
with and without a 6-methyl group.

According to Krichevskiï *et al.* (1935) and Magidson and Rubtsov
(1937), the introduction of a methyl group into the 2 position of
compounds of type (XIX) appears to have a dystherapeutic

ANTIMALARIAL ACTIVITY OF 2-NAPHTHYLAMINO-4-AMINOALKYL-
AMINO-6-METHYLPYRIMIDINES AGAINST *P. gallinaceum*
(Curd, Raison and Rose, 1946)

No.	Formula of base.	Dose mgm./ kgm.	Activity.
3301	XXIII ; R = H, R′ = [CH₂]₂ . NEt₂	200 80 40	$+ +$ $+$ to $+ +$ $\pm$
3581	XXIII ; R = H, R′ = [CH₂]₃ . NEt₂	80 40	$+$ $+$
3582	XXIII ; R = H, R′ = [CH₂]₄ . NEt₂	160 80	$+$ $-$
3583	XXIII ; R = H, R′ = CHMe . [CH₂]₃ . NEt₂	120 80	$+$ $-$
3584	XXIII ; R = H, R′ = p-C₆H₄O . [CH₂]₂ . NEt₂	160 80	$+$ $-$
3501	XXIII ; R = OCH₃, R′ = [CH₂]₂ . NEt₂	80 40 20	$+ +$ $+ +$ $+$
3502	XXIII ; R = Br, R′ = [CH₂]₂ . NEt₂	80 40 20	$+ +$ $+ +$ $+$
4009	XXIII ; R = Br, R′ = [CH₂]₂ . NMe₂	40 20	$+ +$ $\pm$
4008	XXIII ; R = Br, R′ = [CH₂]₃ . NMe₂	40 20	$+ +$ $+$
4007	XXIII ; R = Br, R′ = [CH₂]₃ . NEt₂	80 40	$+ +$ $+$
4466	XXIII ; R = Br, R′ = [CH₂]₃ . NBuᵃ₂	160 40	$+$ $-$
4605	XXIII ; R = Br, R′ = [CH₂]₃ . NMePrᵝ .	80 40	$+ +$ $+$
4977	XXIII ; R = Br, R′ = CHMe[CH₂]₃ . NEt₂	40 80	$\pm$ $-$
3585	XXIV ; R = H	80	$-$
3764	XXIV ; R = Cl	80 40	$+$ $+$

effect, while according to D.R.P. 683,692 the same is true of compounds of type (XX). By analogy it seemed possible that removal of the 6-methyl group in type (XVIII) might lead to increased activity. 2-*p*-Chloroanilino-4-β-diethylaminoethylamino-pyrimidine (XXV ; R = Cl, R′ = H, R″ = [CH₂]₂. NEt₂) and the corresponding diethylaminopropylamino derivative (XXV ; R = Cl, R′ = H, R″ = [CH₂]₃ . NEt₂) were also found to be

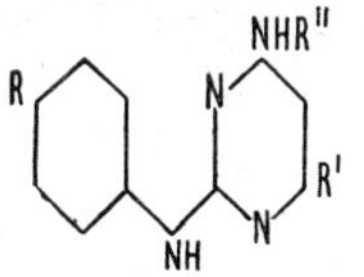

NHR"

R ... N ... R'

NH ... N

(XXV)

possessed of a much smaller degree of antimalarial activity than the corresponding 6-methyl derivatives.

Similar low antimalarial activity was found with 2-p-toluidino-4-p-diethylaminoethylaminopyrimidine.

The importance of the 6-methyl group in (XVIII; R = Cl, R' = dialkylaminoalkyl) led to examination of the effect of replacing the 6-methyl group by a variety of other groups: 2-p-chloro-anilino-4-β-diethylaminoethylamino-6-phenylpyrimidine was devoid of antimalarial activity.

The formal resemblance of compounds of type (XVII) to riboflavin (XXVI) was a guiding thread in these investigations, it being supposed that the pyrimidine ring of (XVII) corresponds to the same ring of the vitamin.

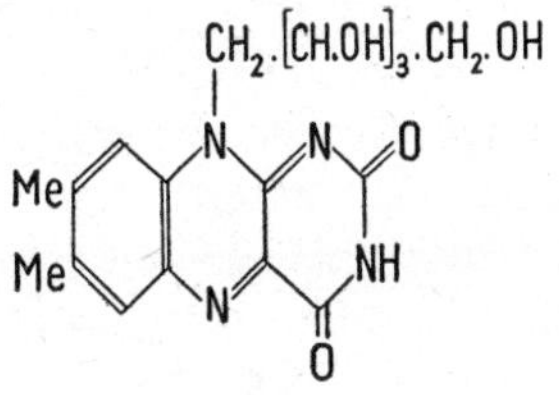

$CH_2.[CH.OH]_3.CH_2.OH$

Me ... N ... N ... O

Me ... N ... NH ... O

(XXVI)

NHR'

Me ... N ... R

N ... NH

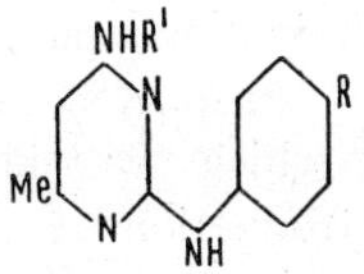

(XVIIa)

It was also possible that the observed antagonism between (XVII; R = Cl, R' = $[CH_2]_2$. NEt_2) and riboflavin (Madinaveitia, 1946) might be accounted for by a correspondence of the pyrimidine ring of the former with the benzene ring of riboflavin, thus correlating the 6-methyl group of (XVII) with the 6-methyl group of the vitamin. This is illustrated in (XVIIa).

The introduction of an additional methyl group into the 5 position of the pyrimidine ring of (XVII) to correspond to the 7-methyl group of riboflavin appeared to be of interest, while an additional reason was provided by the investigations of Hull *et al.* (1946), who found that while 2 - amino - 4 - amino-alkylamino-6-methylpyrimidines of type XXVII, corresponding to the anilino derivatives of type XVII, were without antimalarial activity at tolerated doses, the introduction of alkyl substituents into the 5 position of the pyrimidine ring to give (XXVIII; R = dialkylaminoalkyl, R′ = alkyl) restored activity.

This dissimilarity between compounds of type (XXVII) and type (XVII), and the fact that no antagonism could be demonstrated between riboflavin and (XXVIII; R = CHMe[CH₂]₃ . NEt₂, R′ = Me), using *Lactobacillus casei* as a test organism, suggested a mode of action for compounds of type (XXVIII) different from that responsible for the activity of compounds of type (XVII). The hypothesis was then advanced that compounds of type

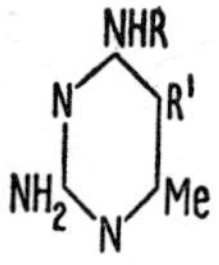

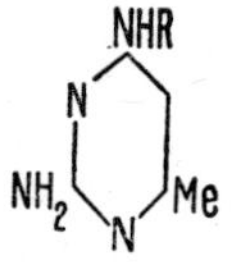

(XXVIII) might be capable of interference with either the synthesis or function of purine nucleotides, particularly those such as adenosine, which are widely distributed coenzyme constituents. By the introduction of a substituent into the 5 position of the pyrimidine ring of compounds of type (XVII) potentiation of activity might occur since such compounds should theoretically act as riboflavin antagonists and also purine nucleoside antagonists. Thus an enzyme system of which riboflavin-adenosine dinucleotide is a constituent should readily be actively attacked. Compounds of type (XXIX) might also be capable of interference, not only with riboflavin-containing enzymes but also with other enzyme systems having a purine nucleoside as a coenzyme constituent. A series of compounds of types (XXIX) and also (XXX), however, all showed a low-grade antimalarial activity. The activity of these compounds is shown in the table (Curd, Richardson and Rose, 1946).

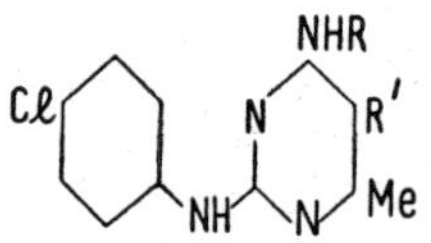

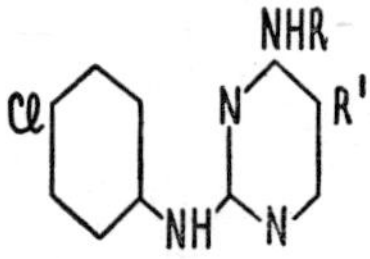

ANTIMALARIAL ACTIVITIES OF PYRIMIDINE DERIVATIVES AGAINST
P. gallinaceum IN CHICKENS (Curd, Richardson and Rose, 1946)

No.	Compound.	Dose mgm./ kgm.	Activity.
3780	2-*p*-Chloroanilino-4-γ-diethylaminopropylamino-pyrimidine.	160 80	+ −
3839	2-*p*-Chloroanilino-4-β-diethylaminoethylamino-pyrimidine.	160 80	+ to + + −
3834	2-*p*-Toluidino-4-β-diethylaminoethylamino-pyrimidine.	120 80	± ±
4145	2-*p*-Chloroanilino-4-β-diethylaminoethylamino-6-phenylpyrimidine.	160 80	± −
3687	2-*p*-Chloroanilino-4-γ-diethylaminopropylamino-5 : 6-dimethylpyrimidine.	160 80 40	+ + + + + to + +
3903	2-*p*-Chloroanilino-4-β-diethylaminoethylamino-5 : 6-dimethylpyrimidine.	40 20	+ ±
4410	2-*p*-Chloroanilino-4-γ-dimethylaminopropyl-amino-5 : 6-dimethylpyrimidine.	40 20	+ + +
4065	2-*p*-Chloroanilino-4-β-diethylaminoethylamino-6-methyl-5-ethylpyrimidine.	120 80 40	+ to + + + ±
4119	2-*p*-Chloroanilino-4-β-dimethylaminoethylamino-6-methyl-5-ethylpyrimidine.	80 40	+ −
4120	2-*p*-Chloroanilino-4-γ-diethylaminopropylamino-6-methyl-5-ethylpyrimidine.	80 40	+ −
4146	2-*p*-Chloroanilino-4-β-diethylaminoethylamino-5-phenylpyrimidine.	160 80	± −
4208	2-*p*-Chloroanilino-4-γ-diethylaminopropylamino-5-phenylpyrimidine.	80 40	− −
4064	2-*p*-Anisidino-4-β-diethylaminoethylamino-5-phenylpyrimidine.	160 80	− −
4260	2-*p*-Chloroanilino-4-β-diethylaminoethylamino-5-phenoxypyrimidine.	160 80 40	− − −
2666	2-*p*-Chloroanilino-4-β-diethylaminoethylamino-6-methylpyrimidine.	80 40	+ + +
3711	2-*p*-Chloroanilino-4-γ-dimethylaminopropylamino-6-methylpyrimidine.	40 20	+ + +
3884	NH . [CH₂]₂ . NEt₂ . .	80 40	− −
4787	NH . [CH₂]₃ . NEt₂	80 40	± −
4788	NH . [CH₂]₃ . NBu₂ᵃ	80 60 40	+ to + + − −
5063	NH . CHMe . [CH₂]₃NEt₂ . . .	80 40	− −
5041	NH . [CH₂]₃ . N<[CH₂]₄>CH₂ . .	80 40	+ −
5152	NH . [CH₂]₃ . NHBuᵃ	80	−

Following the discovery of antimalarial activity in compounds of the type (XVIII; $R = Cl$, OMe, $R' = [CH_2]_2 . N(dialkyl)_2$) by Curd and Rose (1946a), compounds of the two possible isomeric structures were studied (XXXI and XXXII).

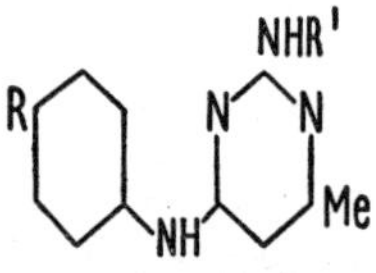

$$\text{NHR'} \qquad\qquad \text{NHR'}$$

(XXXI) 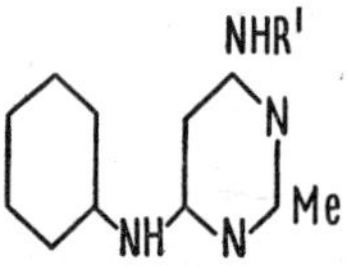　　　　　　　(XXXII)

In compounds of type (XXXI) the positions of the substituted anilino and aminoalkylamino residues in (XVIII) are interchanged.

If in compounds of type (XVIII) antimalarial activity is dependent on riboflavin antagonism, it seemed possible that compounds of type (XXXI) might also display antimalarial properties. The hypothesis of Schönhöfer (1942) that antimalarial activity was related to the possibility of the formation of a p-quinonoid structure in the molecule was confined to quinoline and acridine derivatives, but on the basis of work on compounds of type (XVIII) it was thought that it might also be applicable to pyrimidine derivatives provided other structural requirements were satisfied.

The activity of 2-aminoalkylamino-6-methoxyquinolines (Magidson and Rubtsov, 1937 ; Schönhöfer, 1942) would seem to exclude *o*-quininoid tautomerism from any significance for antimalarial activity. Curd, Raison and Rose (1946), however, suggested that the activity of the 4-dialkylaminoalkylamino-6-methoxyquinolines is due to their structural relationship to mepacrine. On structural grounds it is difficult to see how the isomeric 2-dialkylaminoalkylamino compounds can act in this way ; it is therefore conceivable that their inactivity may be due to inability to function as riboflavin antagonists rather than to the fact that tautomerism to give a p-quinonoid structure is not possible. Compounds of type (XXXI) are likewise incapable of exhibiting the p-quinonoid type of tautomerism, the aminoalkylamino group not being in the *para* position to either of the heterocyclic nitrogen atoms.

In addition an investigation of compounds of type (XXXI)

involved varying the aminoalkylamino side-chain in position 2 while having a *p*-chloroanilino group in position 4, the *p*-chloroanilino group being selected because previous work on compounds of type (XVIII) had shown that the highest antimalarial activity was obtained with the chlorine substituent (Curd and Rose, 1946a ; Curd, Davis and Rose, 1946).

The results of antimalarial tests, shown in the table on p. 96, indicate that the effect of variation of the basic side-chain was different from that which had been obtained in the isomeric series (XVIII).

In view of the high activity exhibited by 2-(6'-bromo-β-naphthylamino)4-β-diethylamino-ethylamino-6-methylpyrimidine (Curd, Raison and Rose, 1946) in the initial study of compounds of type (XXXI), a number of substances of the general formula (XXXIII) were included.

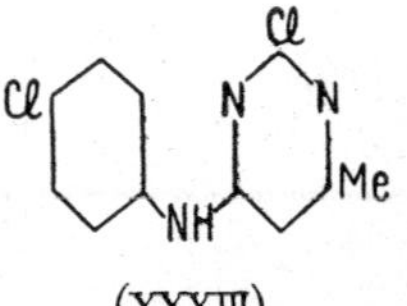

(XXXIII)

Further investigations on 4-arylamino-2-aminoalkylamino-6-methylpyrimidines by Curd, Davis, Owen, Rose and Tuey (1946b) involved variation in the dialkylamino group : 4-*p*-nitroanilino-2-aminoalkylamino- and 4-*p*-cyanoanilino-2-aminoalkylamino-6-methylpyrimidines of the type (XXXI ; R = NO_2 or CN) with a variety of different aminoalkylamino groups in the 2 position : variations of the substituents in the anilino residue and variations of the substituents in the 5 and 6 positions. The antimalarial activity of these compounds is considerably less, as shown in the table, than that of the corresponding compounds carrying a methyl group in the 6 position. A possible explanation which is applicable not only to compounds of type **XXXI** but to type **XXXIV** and is reconcilable with any theory relating to the antimalarial activity of both types of tautomeric changes is that the 6-methyl group merely functions as a blocking group. Kelsey *et al.* (1944) have shown that quinine is enzymatically altered by the *in vitro* action of rabbit liver to give a degradation product which from the work of Mead and Koepfli (1944) seems to be obtained by the introduction of a hydroxyl group into the α position of the quinoline nucleus. Thus in compounds of types (**XXXI**)

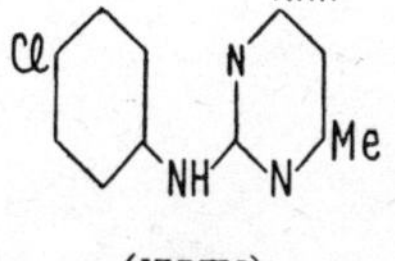

(XXXIV)

Antimalarial Activity of Pyrimidine Derivatives against
P. gallinaceum in Chicks.

(Curd, Davis, Owen, Rose and Tuey, 1946a)

No.	Nature of R.	Dose mgm./kgm.	Activity.

(a) Compounds of the type $Et_2N.[CH_2]_2-NH-$

No.	Nature of R.	Dose mgm./kgm.	Activity.
3883	4'-Chloroanilino	120	+
		80	+
		40	—
3885	4'-Toluidino	160	—
		40	—
3886	4'-Anisidino	160	—
		40	—
3887	3':4'-Dichloroanilino	200	—
		40	—
3888	Anilino	160	—
		80	—
4317	4'-Nitroanilino	120	+ +
		80	+
		40	—
4346	4'-Cyanoanilino	160	+ +
		80	+ to + +
		40	+

(b) Compounds of the type

No.	Nature of R.	Dose mgm./kgm.	Activity.
3743	NH.[CH₂]₃.NEt₂	120	+ +
		80	+ +
		80	+
4561	NH.[CH₂]₄.NEt₂	240	+ +
		120	+ to + +
		80	+ to + +
		40	—
5052	NH.CHMe.[CH₂]₃.NEt₂ dihydrobromide	80	—
		40	—
4345	NH.[CH₂]₃.NMe₂	160	+ +
		80	+ +
		40	+
		20	—
4508	NH.[CH₂]₃.NHBuα	40	+ to + +
		20	—
4190	NH.[CH₂]₃.N <[CH₂]₄>CH₂ . .	80	+ +
		40	+
4316	NH.[CH₂]₃.NBuα [base] . .	80	+ +
		40	+ +
		20	+
4786	NH.[CH₂]₃.NMePrβ . .	40	+
4668	NH.[CH₂]₄.NMe₂ (base) . .	40	—
4669	NH.[CH₂]₄.NBuα₂ (base) . .	80	+ +
		40	±
5149	NH.[CH₂]₃.N(C₅H₁₁α) base . .	80	+ +
		20	±

No.	Nature of R.	Dose mgm./kgm.	Activity.

(c) Compounds of the type

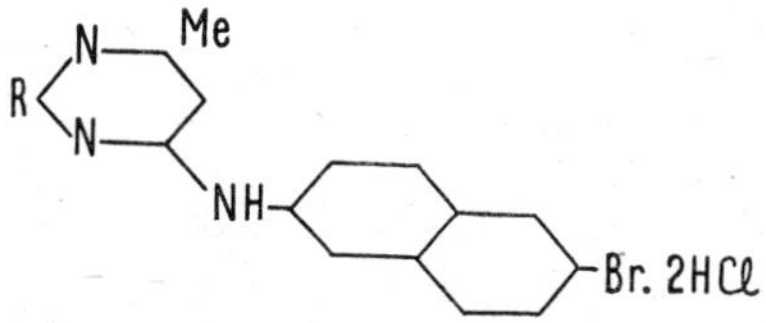

No.	Nature of R.	Dose mgm./kgm.	Activity.
4118	2-p-Chloroanilino-4-γ-dimethylaminopropyl-amino-6-methyl-5-ethylpyrimidino.	80 40	+ + +
4396	2-p-Chloroanilino-4-δ-diethylamino-α-methylbutylamino-6-methyl-5-ethyl-pyrimidine.	160 120 80	+ — —
4209	2-p-Chloroanilino-4-β-diethylamino-5-benzyl-6-methylpyrimidine.	160 40	+ to + + +
4231	2-p-Chloroanilino-4-γ-diethylaminopropyl-amino-5-benzyl-6-methylpyrimidine.	160 80	+ to + + —
4288	2-p-Chloroanilino-4-γ-dimethylamino-propylamino-5-benzyl-6-methylpyrimidine.	160 80	+ ±
4253	2-p-Chloroanilino-4-δ-diethylamino-α-methylbutylamino-5-benzyl-6-methyl-pyrimidine.	160 80	— —
3563	5-Bromo-2-p-chloroanilino-4-γ-diethyl-aminopropylamino-6-methyl-pyrimidine.	400 80	+ —
4343	2-p-Chloroanilino-4-β-diethylaminoethyl-amino-5 : 6-cyclohexenopyrimidine.	200 120 80 40	+ + + + —
4356	2-p-Chloroanilino-4-γ-diethylaminopropyl-amino-5 : 6-cyclohexenopyrimidine.	80 40	+ to + + +
4355	2-p-Chloroanilino-4-γ-dimethylaminopropyl-amino-5 : 6-cyclohexenopyrimidine.	80 40 20 10	+ + + + + to + + +
4557	2-p-Chloroanilino-4-γ-dimethylaminopropyl-amino-5 : 6-cyclopentenopyrimidine.	80 40	+ to + + —
3815	2-p-Chloroanilino-4-β-diethylaminoethyl-amino-5-methylpyrimidine.	80 40	— —

ANTIMALARIAL ACTIVITIES AGAINST *P. gallinaceum* IN CHICKS.
(Curd, Davis, Owen, Rose and Tuey, 1946b)

No.	R	Dose mgm./kgm.	Activity
	(a) Compounds of the type 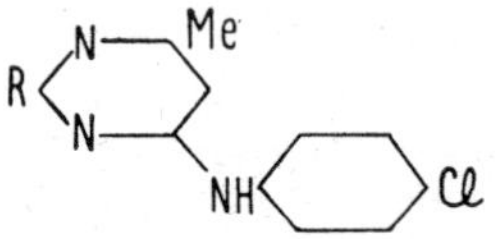		
5153	NH . [CH$_2$]$_3$. NMe . [CH$_2$]$_2$. NEt$_2$ (trihydrochloride).	240 / 120	— / —
5132	NH . [CH$_2$]$_3$. O . [CH$_2$]$_2$. NEt$_2$.	160 / 80	— / —
5096	NMe . [CH$_2$]$_2$. NEt$_2$	160 / 80	— / —
5154	NH . [CH$_2$]$_2$. NH$_2$.	120 / 80 / 40	+ + / — / +
	(b) Compounds of the type 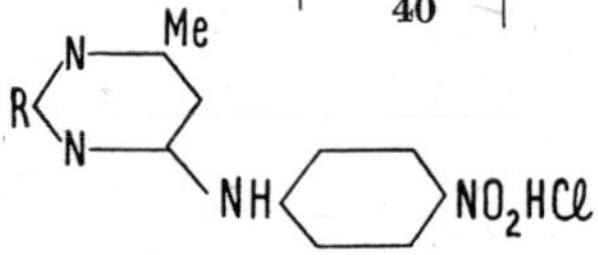		
4950	NH . [CH$_2$]$_3$. NEt$_2$	80 / 40 / 20	+ + / + to + + / ±
4631	NH . [CH$_2$]$_3$. N<[CH$_2$]$_4$>CH$_2$	40 / 20	+ + / + to + +
4630	NH . [CH$_2$]$_3$. NBu$_2$^{a}	40 / 20	+ to + + / +
5094	NH . [CH$_2$]$_3$. NMe$_2$ (base)	80 / 40	+ + / +
5054	NH . CHMe . [CH$_2$]$_3$. NEt$_2$	80 / 40	+ to + + / +
5189	NH . [CH$_2$]$_3$. NHBu^a (base)	40 / 20	+ to + + / +
5133	NH . [CH$_2$]$_3$. O . [CH$_2$]$_2$. NEt$_2$ (base)	120 / 80	+ + / +
	(c) Compounds of the type		
5001	NH . [CH$_2$]$_3$. NEt$_2$	40 / 20	+ / —
4971	NH . [CH$_2$]$_3$. N<[CH$_2$]$_4$>CH$_2$.	80 / 40	+ + / +
5043	NH . [CH$_2$]$_3$. NBu$_2$^{a}	20	+ +
5053	NH . CHMe . [CH$_2$]$_3$. NEt$_2$ (dihydrobromide).	160 / 120 / 80	+ + / + + / ±

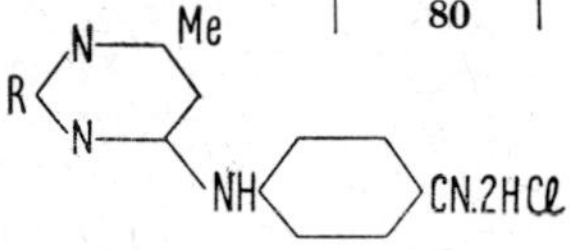

No.	R	Dose mgm./ kgm.	Activity.

(d) 4-Arylamino-2-aminoalkylamino-6-methylpyrimidines.
Variation of substituents in the anilino residue.

No.	R	Dose mgm./kgm.	Activity.
4951	4-*m*-Chloroanilino-2-γ-di-*n*-butyl-amino-6-methylpyrimidine dihydrochloride.	120	+
5042	4-*m*-Nitroanilino-2-γ-piperidinopropylamino-6-methylpyrimidine dihydrochloride.	160	±
		80	—
5002	4-(3′ : 4′-Dichloroanilino)-2-γ-di-*n*-butyl-amino-propylamino-6-methylpyrimidine dihydrochloride.	40	±
		20	—
5000	4-(2′ : 4′-Dichloroanilino)-2-γ-di-*n*-butyl-aminopropylamino-6-methylpyrimidine dihydrochloride.	80	+
		40	±
4929	4-*p*-Hydroxyanilino-2-γ-diethylamino-propylamino-6-methylpyrimide dihydrochloride.	160	±
		80	—
4930	4-*p*-Hydroxyanilino-2-γ-di-*n*-butylamino-propylamino-6-methylpyrimidine dihydrochloride.	160	—
		80	—

(e) 4-Arylamino-2-aminoalkylaminopyrimidines.
Variation of the substituents in the 5 and 6 positions.

No.	R	Dose mgm./kgm.	Activity.
4811	4-*p*-Chloroanilino-2-γ-di-*n*-butylamino-propylaminopyrimidine dihydrochloride.	80	Toxic
		40	—
5049	4-*p*-Nitroanilino-2-γ-di-*n*-butyl-amino-pyrimidine.	80	+ +
		40	±
5004	4-*p*-Chloroanilino-2-γ-di-*n*-butylamino-5 : 6-dimethylpyrimidine dihydrochloride.	80	+
		40	±
4230	4-*p*-Chloroanilino-2-γ-diethylaminopropyl-amino-6-methyl-5-ethylpyrimidine dihydrochloride.	40	+
		20	—
5050	4-*p*-Nitroanilino-2-γ-diethylaminopropyl-amino-6-methylpyrimidine dihydrochloride.	80	+ to + +
		40	+
		20	—
5057	4-*p*-Cyanoanilino-2-γ-diethylaminopropyl-amino-6-methyl-5-ethylpyrimidine.	80	+ to + +
		40	+ to + +
		20	±
5100	4-*p*-Chloroanilino-2-γ-di-*n*-butylamino-propylamino-6-methyl-5-ethylpyrimidine dihydrochloride.	80	+ +
		40	—
		20	—

and (**XXXIV**) the presence of a methyl group in the 6 position merely renders the substances of greater stability *in vivo* than the corresponding unmethylated compounds.

While the hypothesis that the pyrimidine compounds acted against malarial plasmodia because they interfered like mepacrine with the metabolism of riboflavin cannot be entirely rejected,

4—2

there were difficulties in its acceptance. Curd and Rose (1946c), therefore modified the Schönhöfer theory, which seeks to relate antimalarial activity in the mepacrine molecule to the possible formation of a *p*-quinonoid tautomer involving the ring nitrogen atom and the 5-alkyl-amino group in the manner shown in (XXXIV). Reference to types (X) and (XXXV) shows that a similar *p*-quinonoid structure is possible only in the former yet both provide active antimalarial substances.

The Schönhöfer hypothesis was therefore modified to embrace tautomerism leading to an *o*-quinonoid structure, it being concluded that antimalarial activity might be expected when both arylamino and alkylamino substituents were present each of which permitted the formulation of either *o*- or *p*-quinonoid-like tautomers. The inactivity of the isomeric type (XXXII) as shown by Basford *et al.* (1946, 1947) necessitated some modification of this generalisation : in addition, it was further postulated that the tautomeric systems associated with the substituent arylamino and alkylamino groups should be capable of independent function. In (XXXII) the tautomeric systems are interdependent in that positioning of the bonds in the RNH—C=N— system in the manner formulated prevents tautomerism elsewhere in the molecule. This point can be further illustrated by referring to tautomer (XXXVI), which has no equivalent among the variants of (XXXII) except the unlikely (XXXIX).

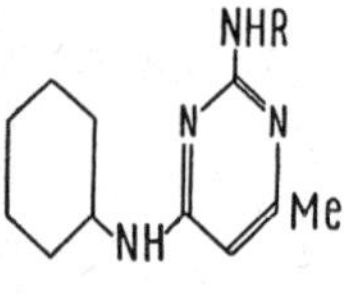

(XXXV) 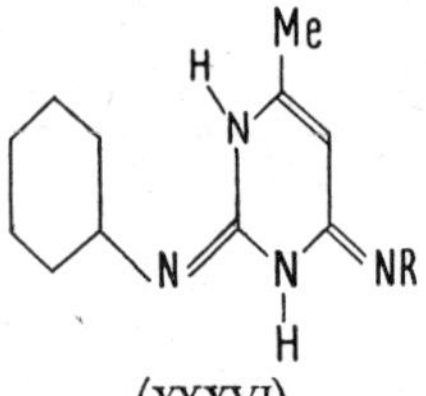   (XXXVI) 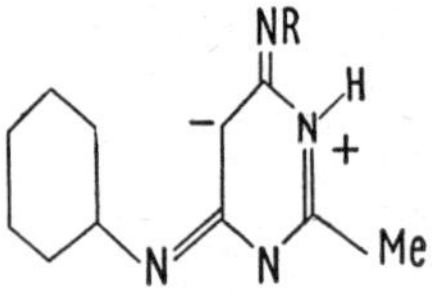   (XXXIX)

The guanidine (XVI) is similar to (X) and provides still another system, that of the guanidine linkage, capable of tautomeric modification.

In addition to the prototropic changes inherent in the molecules now being considered, a like number of resonance possibilities are conceivable. The pyrimidine moiety of (X) may be a hybrid between the several zwitterion forms (Xa) to (Xe) and the Kékulé forms.

(xa)   (xb)   (xc)   (xd)   (xe)

Protrotropy or resonance, or both, may be associated with anti-malarial activity.

Further consideration suggested that while a pyrimidine ring provided a convenient means for testing out these possible relationships between structure and antimalarial action, a ring system *per se* need not be essential and any heteroenoid system of the type might be expected to function in the same manner.

The diguanide ("biguanide") molecule provided the necessary structural features around which active drugs might be prepared. Initially drugs of type (XL) were prepared in which R = [CH$_2$]$_2$NEt$_2$, [CH$_2$]$_3$NEt$_2$, and CHMe[CH$_2$]$_3$NEt$_2$, The first of these compounds proved quite inactive, possibly due to

(XL)   (XLI)

the highly basic character of the molecule and the possible influence on tautomerism and resonance of the ionic charges which it would carry under physiological conditions. To minimise any such effect one of the basic groups was left out and simpler molecules typified by (XLI) were synthesised.

Variations in the aryl substituents and in the terminal alkyl groups were then introduced. Compounds 4430 and 4888, the latter now known as proguanil or paludrine, were the most active compounds.

Proguanil is N_1-*p*-chlorophenyl-N_5-*iso*propyl biguanide.

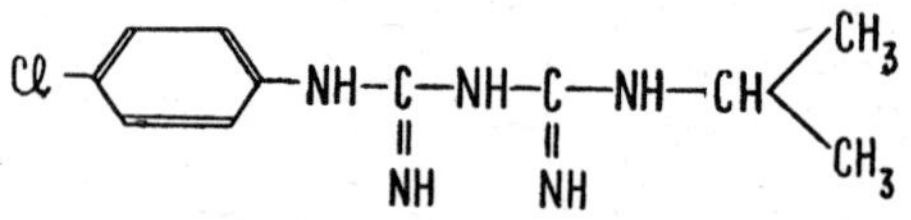

While a wide range of mono- and di-alkyl derivatives corresponding to (XL) and (XLI) were active, highest activity thus occurred with a total of 3 or 4 carbon atoms in the alkyl groups with a maximum at mono-*iso*propyl (XL; $R = Pr^\beta$). The parent *p*-chlorophenylguanide and its monomethyl derivative were ineffective. Replacement of the alkyl group by a further aryl residue to give, for instance, (XLII), greatly reduces antimalarial action as does the introduction of a methyl group as in (XLIII).

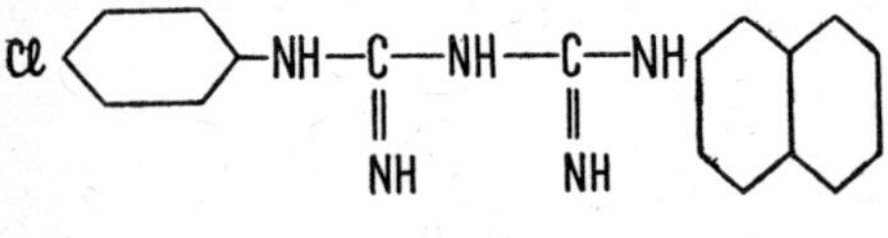

(XLII)

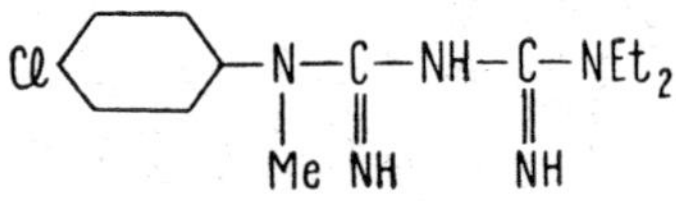

(XLIII)

The influence of the substituent in the benzene ring appears to be similar to that in the earlier pyrimidine drugs, chlorine in the *para* position being the most effective of the few variants examined. Some differentiation of the effects of resonance and tautomerism becomes possible in the light of these findings. Structure (XL) can be formulated in seven " zwitterion " modifications, of which (XLa), (XLb) and (XLc) are examples, and the same number of

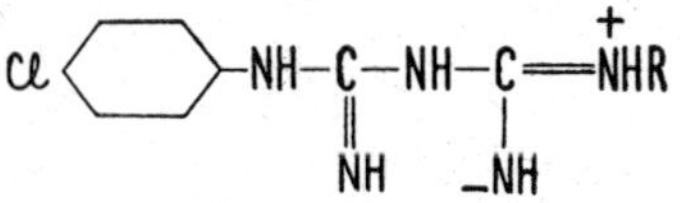

(XLa)

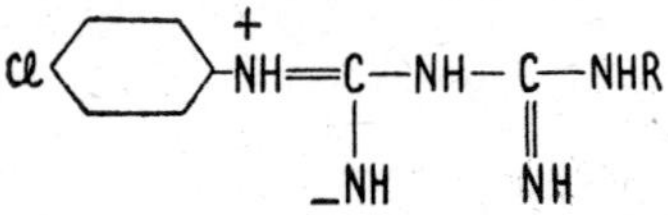

(XLb)

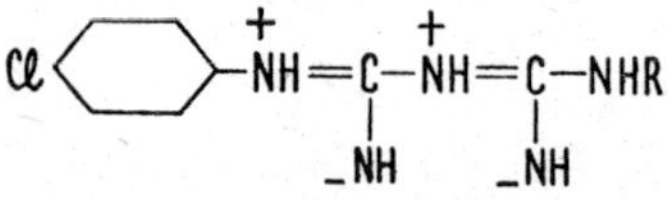

(XLc)

possibilities exists for the dialkyl and trialkyl derivatives (XLI) and (XLIII), active and almost inactive respectively.

It may therefore be significant that in the feebly active (XLIII) the positioning of the alkyl groups does not permit of the existence in the molecule of the two independent tautomeric systems originally postulated as essential for antimalarial activity. Similar limitations apply to the simple guanidine (XLIV), which is inactive.

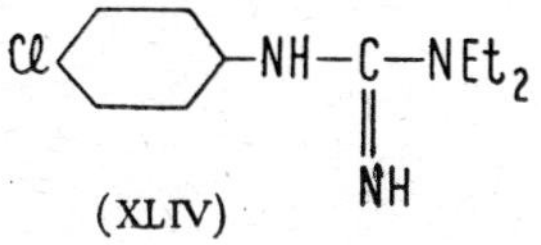

$$\text{Cl} \langle \bigcirc \rangle - \text{NH} - \underset{\underset{\text{NH}}{\|}}{\text{C}} - \text{NEt}_2$$

(XLIV)

An additional feature of the diguanide structure which requires consideration is the possibility that the molecule may be modified by hydrogen bonding leading to cyclic structures such as (XLV), the existence of which may influence biological properties.

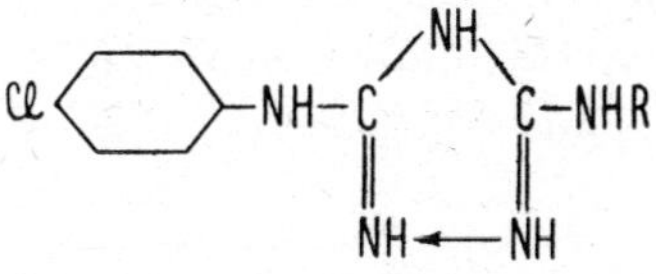

$$\text{Cl} \langle \bigcirc \rangle - \text{NH} - \underset{\underset{\text{NH} \leftarrow}{\|}}{\text{C}} \overset{\diagup \text{NH} \diagdown}{\underset{\text{NH}}{\|}} \underset{\underset{\text{NH}}{\|}}{\text{C}} - \text{NHR}$$

(XLV)

To summarise very briefly, therefore, it may be said that the molecule of proguanil reveals a benzene ring linked to an *iso*-propylamino group $\left(-\text{NH} - \text{CH} \diagup_{\diagdown \text{CH}_3}^{\text{CH}_3} \right)$ through two amidine groups joined " in series."

A characteristic of the amidine group is its capacity to be involved in resonance, that is for electrons to move from one nitrogen atom to the other and back again, with a consequent displacement of electrical charge and the appropriate shift of the double bond, thus :—

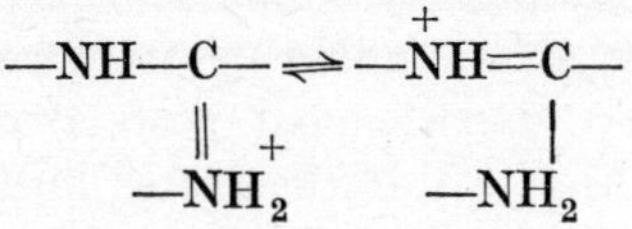

$$-\text{NH}-\text{C}- \rightleftharpoons -\overset{+}{\text{N}}\text{H}=\text{C}- $$
$$\underset{-\text{NH}_2}{\overset{\|\,+}{}} \qquad \underset{-\text{NH}_2}{|}$$

Proguanil has certain chemical features in common with mepacrine. Both are strong bases and form stable salts with acids; both contain a chlorine-substituted benzene ring and both carry alkyl groups attached to nitrogen, that in mepacrine being the more complex. Mepacrine also has a resonance system across the middle of the molecule; not the simple amidine group that appears twice in proguanil, but an extended amidine system with an unsaturated carbon chain ($-C'=C'-$) interposed which nevertheless permits the drift of electrons from one nitrogen atom to the other, thus :—

$$-NH-C'=C'-C- \rightleftharpoons -\overset{+}{N}H=C'-C'=C-$$

$$\underset{-NH}{\overset{\parallel}{}}{}^{+} \qquad\qquad \underset{-NH}{\overset{|}{}}$$

The evolution of proguanil was not, however, directly from mepacrine. The first compound really active in bird malaria was 2666 (XLVI). This contained the substituted benzene ring and the alkyl group attached to a nitrogen atom and close inspection shows both extended and true amidine systems.

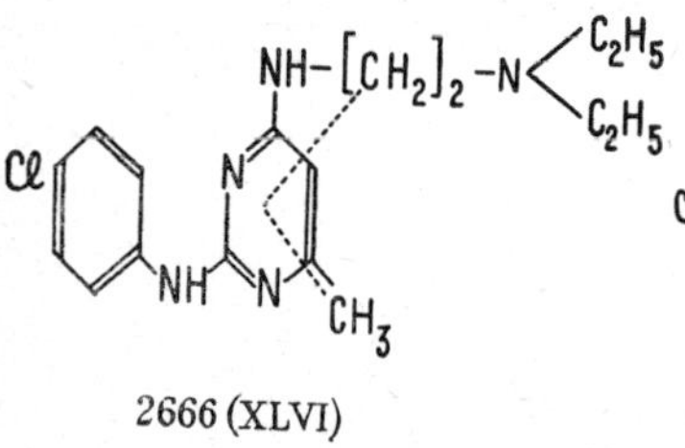

2666 (XLVI) 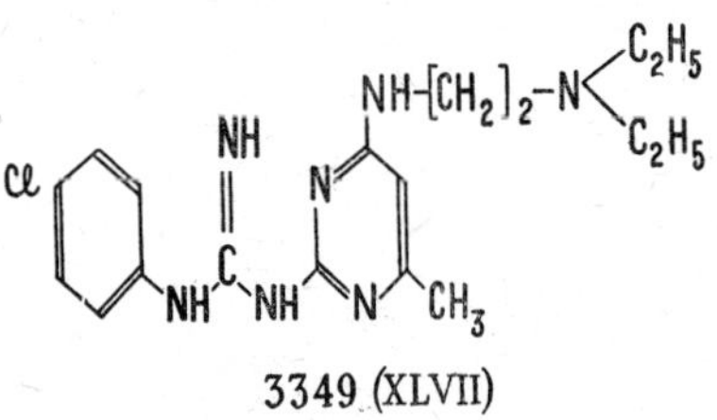   3349 (XLVII)

The compound 3349 is a guanidine derivative of 2666 and is even richer in amidine groups; it was more active in experimental malaria and was the first of the new type to show activity in human malaria.

Eventually, in attempting to simplify the 2666 molecule, it was assumed that there was a minimal structural requirement for antimalarial activity, the fragment postulated as inessential in 2666 (XLVI) being that within the dotted line. The residue was then seen to resemble the arrangement of the atoms found in the biguanide molecule (NH_2—C—NH—C—NH_2)

$$NH_2-\underset{\underset{NH}{\|}}{C}-NH-\underset{\underset{NH}{\|}}{C}-NH_2$$

Eventually the highest antimalarial activity was found in proguanil, where the terminal alkyl group is simple *iso*propyl, in place of the more complex diethylaminoethyl group in the 2666 molecule.

ANTIMALARIAL ACTIVITY OF DIGUANIDINES AGAINST *Plasmodium gallinaceum* IN CHICKENS

(1) 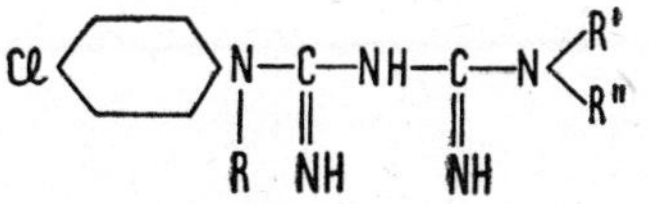
$$Cl\text{—}C_6H_4\text{—}\underset{\underset{R}{|}}{N}\text{—}\underset{\underset{NH}{\|}}{C}\text{—}NH\text{—}\underset{\underset{NH}{\|}}{C}\text{—}N\Big<\!\!\begin{array}{l}R'\\R''\end{array}$$

No.	R	R'	R''	Dose mgm./kgm.	Activity.
3374	H	$[CH_2]_2 . NEt_2$	H	250	—
	H	$[CH_2]_3 . NEt_2$	H	—	—
5114	H	$CHMe[CH_2]_3 . NEt_2$	H	—	—
4172	H	$[CH_2]_2 . NEt_2$	Et	200	—
3327	H	H		125	—
5093	H	Me		80	—
4134	H	Me		80	—
4967	H	Et		20	+ +
3926	H	Et		80	+ +
4094	Me	Et		160	+
4887	H	Prα		20	+ + +
4888	H	Prβ		10	+ + +
4329	H	Prα		40	+ +
4430	H	Prβ		16	+ + +
5393	Me	Prβ			
4968	H	$CH_2CH : CH_2$		20	+ +
4565	H	Buα		80	+ +
4567	H	Buβ		320	+
4568	H	Buγ		40	+ +
4095	H	Buα	Buα	200	—
				400	+
4635	H	$C_5H_{11}\alpha$	H	80	+ +
5596	H	$CH<[CH_2]_4>CH_2$	H	—	
4204	H	$[CH_2]_4 = R'R''$		80	+
3926	H	$[CH_2]_5 = R'R''$		80	—
5157	H	$[CH_2]_2 . O . [CH_2]_2 = R'R''$		40	—
5234	H	OMe	H	80	—
4171	H	Me	$[CH_2]_2$ Me	60	—

(2) Aryl—NH—C—NH—C—NH—N$\begin{smallmatrix}\diagup R' \\ \diagdown R''\end{smallmatrix}$
$\qquad\qquad\ \ \|\qquad\ \ \|$
$\qquad\qquad NH\qquad NH$

No.	Formula of Diguanidine			Dose mgm./ kgm.	Activity.
	Aryl	R'	R''		
4461	Ph	Me	Prβ	—	
4210	Ph	Et	Et	160	—
4492	Ph	Buα	Buα	160	—
4175	p-C$_6$H$_4$Me	Me	Me	200	—
4969	3 : 4-C$_6$H$_3$Me$_2$	Et	Et	200	+
				80	ǀ
4174	p-C$_6$H$_4$. OMe	Me	Me	200	—
4125	p-C$_6$H$_4$. OMe	Et	Et	120	—
3781	p-C$_6$H$_4$. OMe	[CH$_2$]$_5$ = R'R''		200	+
—	p-C$_6$H$_4$. NO$_2$	Me	Me	—	
4376	p-C$_6$H$_4$. NO$_2$	Et	Et	80	+
4566	p-C$_6$H$_4$. NHAc	Me	Prβ	80	—

(3) Aryl'—NH—C—NH—C—Aryl''
$\qquad\qquad\quad\ \|\qquad\ \ \|$
$\qquad\qquad\ NH\qquad NH$

No.	Aryl'	Aryl''	Dose	Activity
4202	Ph	Ph	80	—
—	p-C$_6$H$_4$Cl	Ph	—	—
4123	p-C$_6$H$_4$Cl	p-C$_6$H$_4$. OMe	120	—
4970	p-C$_6$H$_4$Cl	C$_{10}$H$_7\beta$	80	+
4124	p-C$_6$H$_4$. OMe	p-C$_6$H$_4$. OMe	200	—
—	p-C$_6$H$_4$Me	p-C$_6$H$_4$Me	—	

Some further investigations have been made on the antimalarial activity of the pyrimidines.

The relationship between the structure of certain other homologues of proguanil and their activities against blood forms of *P. gallinaceum* in the chick is discussed by Spinks (1948). Substances as closely related as 5093 and 4134 are completely inactive even in high doses.

Guanylureas and biurets corresponding to proguanil and related diguanides were prepared by Curd, Davey, and Richardson (1949) and dithiobiurets and 1 : 2 : 4-triazoles by Curd, Davey, Richardson and Ashworth (1949). None of these compounds had any prophylactic action against sporozoite-induced infections of *P. gallinaceum* and 1-*p*-chlorophenyl-5-*iso*propyldithiobiuret and a number of related compounds had no suppressive action.

ACTIVITY OF HOMOLOGUES OF PROGUANIL AGAINST BLOOD FORMS
OF *P. gallinaceum* (Spinks, 1948)

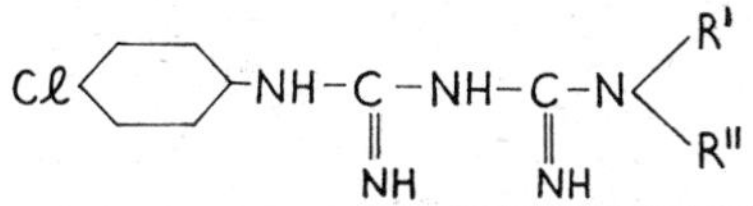

Compound.	R'.	R''.	Dose (mgm./kgm.)	Activity.
5093 . .	H	CH_3	80	—
4134 . .	CH_3	CH_3	80	—
4967 . .	H	C_2H_5	20	+ +
4430 . .	CH_3	iso-C_3H_7	16	+ + +
3963 . .	C_2H_5	C_2H_5	80	+ +
4565 . .	H	n-C_4H_9	80	+ +
Proguanil . .	H	iso-C_3H_7	10	+ + +

However, some guanylureas showed suppressive activity in doses of 40 to 160 mgm. per kgm. of body weight.

Having found that certain 2-amino-4-dialkylaminoalkylamino-5 : 6-dialkyl-pyrimidines of type (XLVIII) possess antimalarial activity (Hull *et al.*, 1946), it was suggested that interference with an adenosine-containing enzyme system was responsible for the biological activity of this group of substances.

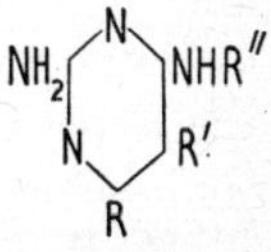

(XLVIII)

Hull *et al.* (1947) proceeded to prepare further modifications of this type structure as well as other pyrimidine derivatives, having different orientations of amino-, alkyl, and dialkylaminoalkylamino substituents. The results are shown in the table on p. 110.

While a 5-alkyl group is necessary to promote activity in compounds of type (XLVIII), the presence of a 6-substituent in (XLVIII) is not essential, for 2-amino-4-β-diethylaminoethyl-amino-5-methylpyrimidine (XLVIII ; R = H, R' = Me, R'' = [CH_2]_2 . NEt_2) and 2 - amino - 4 - γ - diethylaminopropylamino - 5-methylpyrimidine (XLVIII ; R=H, R'=Me, R''=[CH_2]_3 . NEt_2) are both highly active against *P. gallinaceum*. Substitution of a phenoxy-group for the methyl group in these compounds reduced but did not entirely destroy the activity.

Of the six possible isomerides (XLIX to LIV) of the type structure (XLVIII) representatives of five (XLIX to LIII) were

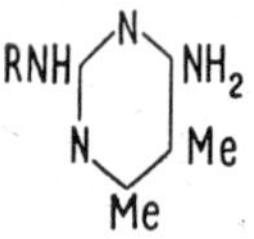

described by Hull *et al.* (1947), and in addition some monomethyl pyrimidines (types LV and LVI) allied to (XLIX) and (L). The results of tests for antimalarial activity are shown in the table on p. 111.

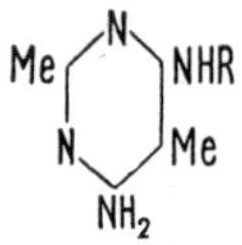

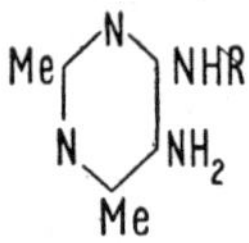

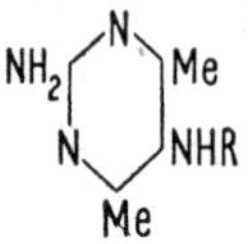

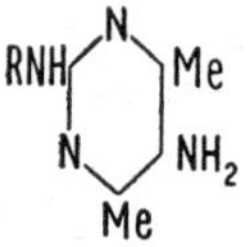

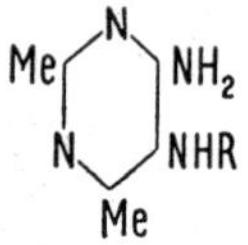

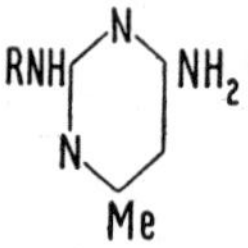

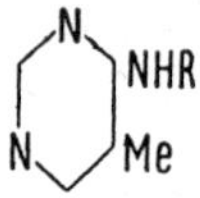

Only among compounds of type (L) is marked activity present, 4 - amino - 6 - γ - diethylaminopropylamino - 2 : 5 - dimethylpyrimidine (L ; R = $[CH_2]_3 . NEt_2$) being highly active. The most active compounds thus have structures which are compatible with the hypothesis that they act by interference with an adenosine-containing enzyme system. The weak activity shown by (LII ; R = $[CH_2]_2 . NEt_2$) is of interest in view of the theories on the relation of chemical structure to antimalarial activity put forward by Schönhöfer (1942) and modified by Curd and Rose (1946c).

Curd, Landquist and Rose (1947) extended their investigation to corresponding and related 1 : 3 : 5 1-triazine derivatives prepared either by acylation and ring-closure of N^1-aryl-N^5-alkyl diguanidines, otherwise by stepwise reaction of cyanuric chloride with aryl- and alkyl-amines. All compounds in the series were without activity. In addition, Curd and Raison (1947) found that if the heterocyclic structure of mepacrine were dispensed with as in a series of N-β-diethylamino-ethylarylamidines and N-β-diethylaminoethyl-N^1-arylamidines, antimalarial activity was again lost.

Kalthod and Linnell (1947 and 1948) have prepared derivatives of 4-aminopyridine with the general formula

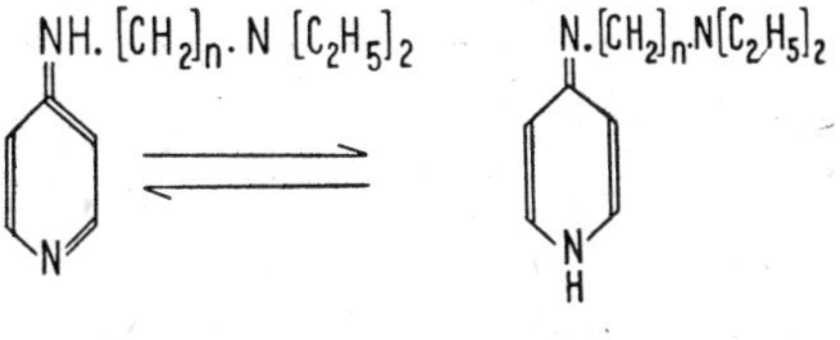

where the alkylene bridge possesses an unbranched structure : these compounds are capable of exhibiting tautomerism similar to that encountered in mepacrine. Compounds in which the substituent aminoalkyl groups possess branched structure have also been prepared, the terminal group being represented by the piperidino radical.

A number of sulphanilamidopyridines, as well as derivatives of 2, 6-diaminopyridine have been synthesised by Bernstein *et al.* (1947a, b, c). Sulphanilamidopyridines were inactive against *P. lophuræ* in ducks, but some derivatives showed slight activity against *P. cathemerium* in ducks : 2, 6-diaminopyridine was active, but of a number of acylated, alkylated, ring-substituted, and fused-ring derivatives only 2-amino-6-acetylamidopyridine ; 2, 6-diacetylamidopyridine ; and 2, 5-diaminopyrido-[2, 3-D]-thiazole exhibited an activity about one-third that of quinine. 2-Amino-5-iodopyridine showed slight activity against *P. lophuræ* in ducks, but derivatives of this compound were inactive.

The chain of investigations which had thus led to the discovery of two biguanidine derivatives with high prophylactic activity in man began with the study of the mepacrine molecule and proceeded by logical deductions from the results of causal prophylactic experiments on birds (Curd, Davey and Rose, 1945). At first proguanil was considered to be a true causal prophylactic not only against *P. gallinaceum* in the hen but also against *P. cathemerium* and *P. relictum* in the canary, and possibly against *P. lophuræ* in the chick. Davey (1946) later modified the previous report, describing complete prophylaxis against *P. gallinaceum* and *P. lophuræ* in the chick but only low-grade activity against *P. cathemerium* and *P. relictum* in the canary. Hawking (1947) confirmed the results

ANTIMALARIAL ACTIVITY OF DERIVATIVES OF 2-AMINOPYRIMIDINE (TYPE XLVIII) (Hull *et al.*, 1947) AGAINST *P. gallinaceum* IN CHICKS

\t\t\tSubstituents at positions.			Dose mgm./ kgm.	Activity.
4	5	6		
$NH.[CH_2]_2.NEt_2$ Me	H	. . .	160	+ +
			80	+ +
			40	—
$NH.[CH_2]_3.NEt_2$ Me	H	. . .	160	Toxic
			80	+ +
			40	+
$NH.[CH_2]_2.NEt_2$ OPh	H	. . .	120	+
			60	±
$NH.[CH_2]_3.NEt_2$ OPh	H	. . .	240	Toxic
			120	±
			40	—
$NH.[CH_2]_2.NEt_2$ Br	Me	. . .	120	—
			80	—
$NH.[CH_2]_3.NEt_2$ Br	Me	. . .	120	—
			80	—
$NH.[CH_2]_2.NEt_2$ H	NH_2	. . .	240	—
$NH.[CH_2]_3.NEt_2$ H	NH_2	. . .	240	Toxic
			120	—
$NH.[CH_2]_2.NEt_2$ H	$NH.[CH_2]_2.NEt_2$		160	±
			40	—
$NH.[CH_2]_2.NEt_2$ Me	NH_2	. . .	80	Toxic
			40	—
$NH.[CH_2]_3.NEt_2$ Me	NH_2	. . .	80	Toxic
			40	—
$NH.[CH_2]_2.NEt_2$ Me	Cl	. . .	160	Toxic
			80	—
$NH.[CH_2]_3.NEt_2$ Me	Cl	. . .	160	Toxic
			40	Toxic
			20	—

against *P. gallinaceum* in tissue cultures : though proguanil itself did not exhibit this activity the blood of a fowl given proguanil was active, suggesting that the action against exo-erythrocytic forms is the result of a metabolic product of proguanil formed by

Antimalarial Activity of Derivatives of 2-Aminopyrimidine (Types XLIX and LIII) and Monomethyl Pyrimidines (Types LV and LVI) against *P. gallinaceum* in Chickens.
(Hull *et al.*, 1947)

Type.	R	Dose mgm./kgm.	Activity.
L	$[CH_2]_2 . NEt_2$	80	+ +
		40	+ +
L	$[CH_2]_3 . NEt_2$	80	+ +
		40	+ +
		20	+
L	$[CH_2]_3 . NMe_2$	160	+ +
		80	+
XLIX	$[CH_2]_2 . NEt_2$	160	−
XLIX	$[CH_2]_3 . NEt_2$	80	±
		40	−
XLIX	$[CH_2]_3 . NBu_2{}^a$	80	Toxic
		40	−
LV	$[CH_2]_2 . NEt_2$	160	Toxic
		80	−
LV	$[CH_2]_3 . NEt_2$	160	Toxic
		80	−
LV	$[CH_2]_3 . NBu_2{}^a$	80	Toxic
		40	+
		20	−
LV	$[CH_2]_3 . NMe_2$	160	±
		80	−
LI	$[CH_2]_3 . NEt_2$	160	−
LI	$[CH_2]_3 . NEt_2$	160	−
LI	$[CH_2]_3 . NBu_2{}^a$	80	Toxic
LII	$[CH_2]_2 . NEt_2$	160	+
		80	−
LVI	$[CH_2]_3 . NEt_2$	120	−
LVI	$[CH_2]_2 . NEt_2$	160	Toxic
		80	−

the animal host. Gingrich (1946) found no activity against the exo-erythrocytic forms of *P. cathemerium* in the canary, and Coatney and Cooper (1948) found that though proguanil was a true causal prophylactic against *P. gallinaceum* the drug had to be administered at toxic levels.

Attempts to cure established infections of the avian malarias with proguanil have been universally unsuccessful.

Proguanil does not act as a causal prophylactic in infections in monkeys due to *P. knowlesi* or *P. cynomolgi*, nor does it eradicate these infections once they are established.

(XIII) Other Pyrimidine Derivatives

A very large number of other pyrimidine derivatives have been synthesised and tested for antimalarial action against *P. gallinaceum*.

No compound of high activity has been found, but considerable light has been thrown on the relation between chemical constitution and antimalarial activity. Cliffe *et al.* (1948) attempted to study the effects on 2-arylguanido-4-aminoalkylaminopyrimidines of changing the nature and position of the substituent in the aryl group, and of variations in the complexity of the basic side-chain, as well as of the introduction of substituents into position 5 of the pyrimidine ring and of different groups in position 6. No notable increase in therapeutic activity occurred, the most active compounds being as follows :—

Compound.	Dose mgm. per kgm.	Activity.
2-*p*-Chlorophenylguanidino-4-γ-diethylaminopropylamino-5 : 6-dimethylpyrimidine.	120 40	+ + +
2-*p*-Methylthiophenylguanidino-4-β-diethylaminoethylamino-6-methyl pyrimidine.	200 120	+ + +
2-(3′ : 5′-Dichlorophenyl)guanidino-4-β-diethylaminoethyl-amino-6-methylpyrimidine.	160 80	+ + + +
2-*p*-Chlorophenylguanidino-4-β-piperidino-α-methylethyl-amino-6-methylpyrimidine.	80 40	+ + +
2-*p*-Chlorophenylguanidino-4 : 6-dimethylpyrimidine.	160	+ +

2-Arylureido- and 2-arylthioureido-pyrimidines with dialkyl-amino-groups in the 4-positions were without significant activity against *P. gallinaceum* in chicks, a rather curious finding in view of the activity of the corresponding 2-arylguanidino-4-dialkyl-amino-alkylamino-6-methylpyrimidines (Ashworth *et al.*, 1948).

Crowther *et al.* (1948) found, on the other hand, that activity against *P. gallinaceum* was shown by the isomeric 4-arylguanidino-2-dialkylamino-alkylamino-6-methyl- and 4-arylguanidino-6-dialkylamino-alkylamino-2-methylpyrimidines : activity was also present in 2-arylguanidino-4-dialkylamino-alkylamino-6-methyl-pyrimidines in which the guanidino-linkage carries an additional alkyl group. The most active compounds were :—

Compound.	Dose mgm. per kgm.	Activity.
4-*p*-Chlorophenylguanidino-2-β-diethylaminoethylamino-6-methylpyrimidine.	40	+ to + +
4-*p*-Chlorophenylguanidino-2-γ-di-*n*-butylaminopropyl-amino-6-methylpyrimidine.	80 40 20	+ to + + + ±
4-*p*-Chlorophenylguanidino-6--diethylaminopropyl-amino-2-methylpyrimidine.	120 40 20	+ + + + +
2-N^1-*p*-Chlorophenyl-N^2-methylguanidino-N^3-4-β-diethylaminoethylamino-6-methylpyrimidine.	40 20	+ + +
2-N^1-*p*-Chlorophenyl-N^2-ethylguanidino-N^3-4-β-diethyl-aminoethylamino-6-methylpyrimidine.	40 20 10	+ + + + —

Several pyrimidylamino- and pyridylamino-pyrimidines, analogous to the anilinopyrimidines, were inert when tested against *P. gallinaceum* in chicks (Curd, Graham and Rose, 1948).

Curd, Graham, Richardson, and Rose (1947) examined series of 2-quinolylamino-4-dialkylaminoalkylamino and 4-quinolylamino-2-dialkylaminoalkylamino-6-methylpyrimidines. The former series showed some activity in chickens infected with *P. gallinaceum* and the latter none. This finding was particularly surprising in the case of 2-(8′-methoxy-6′-quinolyamino)-4-β-diethylaminoethyl-amino-6-methylpyrimidine, since this was derived from an active compound. However, it may also be regarded as a 3′ : 4′-5′-trisubstituted anilinopyrimidine and the introduction of one additional substituent into a *m*-position of the active 2-*p*-substi-tuted anilino-4-dialkylaminoalkylamino-6-methylpyrimidines of type (I) has a dystherapeutic effect (Curd, Davis and Rose, 1946).

To determine whether the activity of 2-anilino-4-dialkylamino-alkylaminopyridines of type **II** was determined by their general

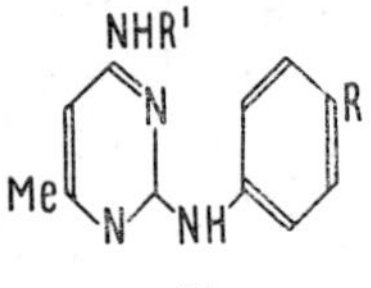

(I) 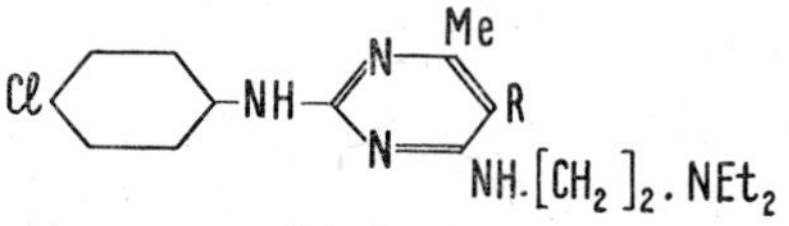   (II)

structure, Mann and Porter (1947) examined the corresponding compounds in which the pyrimidine ring is replaced by a benzene ring (diphenylamines of type **III**). The similar benzene analogues of the active 2-amino-4-dialkylaminoalkylaminopyrimidine of type **IV** were also synthesised. All these compounds containing the benzene ring were quite inactive. The activity of the pyrimidines must, it would seem, be associated with the pyrimidine ring itself or with the tautomerism which this ring allows.

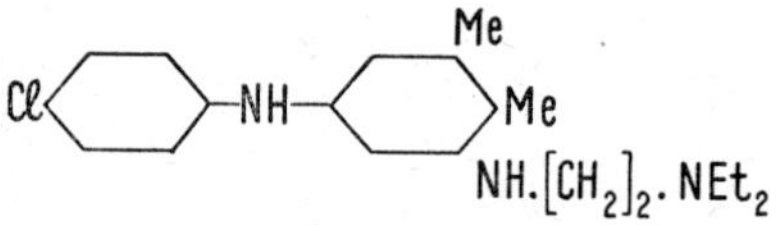

(III) 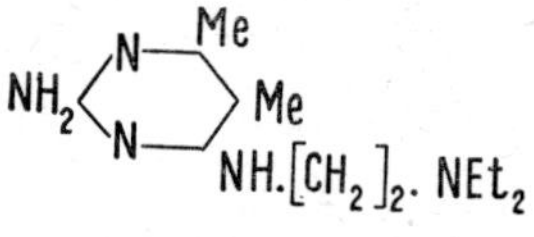   (IV)

To investigate the relationship between antimalarial action and chemical constitution still further, Mann *et al.* (1947) prepared compounds in which the pyrimidine ring of the 2-*p*-chloro-anilino-4-dialkylaminoalkylamino-6-methylpyrimidines was replaced by a benzene ring. Compounds so prepared, of the general type 4'-chloro - 3 - dialkylaminoalkylamino - 4 : 5 - dimethyl - diphenyl-amine were without antimalarial action.

Much of the investigation into pyrimidines had been guided by the idea that such compounds might act by interfering with riboflavin. Curd, Raison and Rose (1947), for instance, studied the

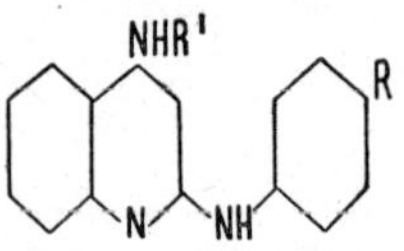

(V) 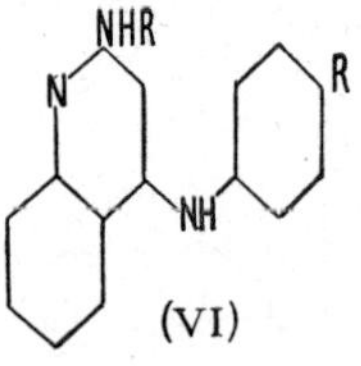   (VI)

differential reactivities of the substituent groups in 2 : 4-dihydroxy and 2 : 4-dichloroquinoline by preparing a series of 2-arylamino-4-aminoalkylaminoquinolines of type (V) and their isomers (VI).

Compounds of type (V) show on the whole a higher degree of antimalarial activity than those of type (VI) and the former also show a greater resemblance to the riboflavin molecule. Other investigations, however, have failed to substantiate the view that pyrimidines and mepacrine acted by interfering with the utilisation of riboflavin by the malaria parasites (*cf.* p. 524). Hull, Lovell, Openshaw, Payman and Todd (1946) suggested that 5-methylpyrimidines might block purine synthesis because of the 5-substituent. King and King (1947) therefore carried out experiments on the synthesis of 8-aminopurines : 6-chloro-8-methylthio-2-methylpurine hydrochloride and the corresponding guanidine were completely lacking in antimalarial activity.

(XIV) Quinazolines

Curd, Landquist and Rose (1948), in continuing their work on 2-arylamino-4-aminoalkylaminoquinazolines prepared a series of 2-p-chloroanilino-4-β-diethylaminoethylaminoquinazolines carry-

ANTIMALARIAL ACTIVITY OF 2-p-CHLOROANILINO-4-β-
DIETHYLAMINOETHYLAMINOQUINAZOLINES

Substituent.	Dose mgm./ kgm.	Activity.	Substituent.	Dose mgm./ kgm.	Activity.
3756	40	+ to + +	7-Methyl	160	+ to + +
	20	−		80	+
6-Chloro-	80	+ +		40	−
	40	+	5-Methoxy-	80	±
7-Chloro-	200	+ to + +	6-Methoxy-	80	+ to + +
	40	−		40	+
6-Nitro-	80	+ +		20	−
	40	+ to + +	7-Methoxy-	120	+ to + +
7-Nitro-	120	+ +		80	±
	80	±	8-Methoxy	160	+
	40	−		80	−
6-Amino-	160	+ to + +	6 : 7-Dimethoxy	80	+ to + +
	80	+		40	±
7-Amino-	160	+ to + +	6 : 7-Benzo	400	+ +
	80	+		200	+ to + +
				120	+

ing various substituents in one or more positions of the quinazoline nucleus. The activity of the parent substance 2-*p*-chloroanilino-4-β-diethylaminoethylaminoquinazoline (3756) and the effect of the various substituents is shown in the table on page 115.

It will be seen that none of the substituted compounds prepared was more active than the parent substance and most were less. The fact that the introduction of substituents into the benzene-ring of the quinazoline nucleus is without effect is of interest in view of the disclosure (B.P. Appln. 27673/38) of the influence of analogous substitution such as the substitution of halogen in the 7-position of the 4-dialkylaminoalkylaminoquinolines.

Hall and Turner (1945a and b) prepared a number of basic derivatives of various heterocyclic systems as possible antimalarials.

In addition Hall and Turner (1948) synthesised benziminazoles such as 5 (or 6)-chloro-2-diethylamino (or piperidino) methylbenziminazoles and 5 (or 6)-chloro-2-diethylamino-methylbenziminazoles.

Curd, Hoggarth, Landquist and Rose (1948) prepared some 4-arylamino-2-aminoalkylaminoquinazolines and some related derivatives carrying arylthio- and dialkylaminoalkylamino-groups in either the 2 : 4- or the 4 : 2-positions (type II). None of these types exhibited any activity against *P. gallinaceum*.

These results would seem to indicate a different mode of action for the quinazolines of type (I) as compared with the pyrimidines of type (III) (X = NH) despite the obvious structural resemblance

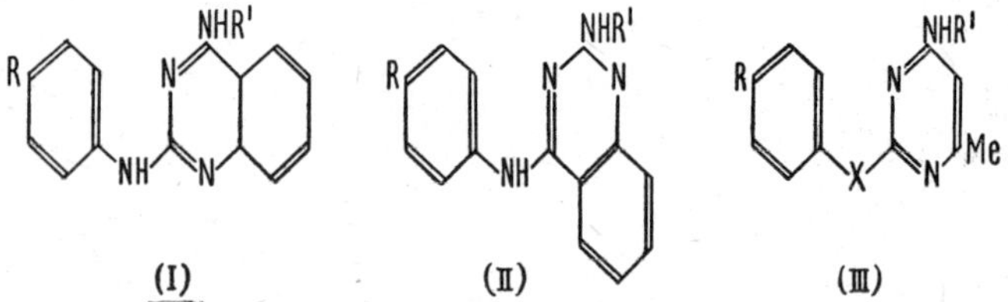

(I)   (II)   (III)

of the two types. It was suggested by Curd, Landquist and Rose (1947) that in certain antimalarial compounds positive activity was associated with the possibility of conjugation of a terminal alkylamino- or aminoalkylamino- group and an anilino-residue through a system made up of alternate carbon and nitrogen atoms.

Such an arrangement would be provided in the case of the quinazolines by the polarised forms (or the tautomers corresponding
thereto) represented by (Ia) and (IIa).   If   the   conjugation

hypothesis were applicable in the present instances then in type (I)
the form (Ia) provides a major contribution to a resonance hybrid
whereas (IIa) is insignificant with respect to type (II).

Alternatively, the biological results with type (II) may be
compared with those yielded by the isosteric 4-arylamino-2-
aminoalkylaminoquinolines (Curd, Raison and Rose, 1947) which
exhibit only feeble activity.   In this respect then the quinazoline
system may be regarded from the biological standpoint as a
quinoline derivative, and further evidence in support of this view
is provided by the considerable antimalarial activities found in
the 4-dialkylaminoalkylaminoquinazolines and the corresponding
substituted quinolines, activities which are enhanced in both
instances by the introduction of chlorine into the 7-position.

It may be noted that 2-(6'-quinolylguanidino-4-β-diethylamino-
ethylamino-, and 4-(6'-quinolylguanidino)-2-β-diethylaminoethyl-
amino-6-methylpyrimidines are quite devoid of antimalarial action
(Gulland and Macey, 1949).

A series of 2 : 4-diaminopyrimidines was synthesised by Falco
et al. (1949).   Of these compounds the most active is 2 : 4-diamino-
5-*p*-chloro-phenoxy-6-methyl pyrimidine.   When tested in chicks
against blood-induced infections due to *P. gallinaceum* it had a
quinine equivalent of 4·3 and against blood-induced infections due to
P. berghei in the mouse a quinine equivalent of 4·7 (Goodwin, 1949).

The extensive investigations on pyrimidines as antimalarials
have undoubtedly thrown much light on the relationship between
chemotherapeutic action and chemical structure.   They have not,
so far, given rise to the synthesis of any compound with a
striking action in human malaria.   When, however, the pyrimidine

nucleus was discarded for a biguanidine structure, far more active compounds were obtained. Nevertheless there is still uncertainty as to the mode of action of these compounds since all the evidence points to the fact that proguanil is not in itself active but is changed in the body into some highly active product. How far this active substance owes its potency to interference with an essential metabolite of the malarial parasites and what the essential metabolite is is still uncertain though there are a number of suggestions for further investigation.

References

ASHWORTH, R. DE B., CROWTHER, A. F., CURD, F. H. S., and ROSE, F. L., 1948, Synthetic antimalarials. Part XXIV. Some 2-phenylureido- and 2-phenylthioureido-4-dialkylaminoalkylamino-6-methylpyrimidines. *J. chem. Soc.*, 581.

BASFORD, F. R., CURD, F. H. S., HOGGARTH, E., and ROSE, F. L., 1947, Synthetic antimalarials. Part XXI. 4-Aryl-amino-6-aminoalkylamino-pyrimidines. Further variations. *J. chem. Soc.*, 1354.

BASFORD, F. R., CURD, F. H. S., and ROSE, F. L., 1946, Synthetic antimalarials. Part VIII. Some 4-arylamino-6-aminoalkylamino-2-methyl-pyrimidines. *J. chem. Soc.*, 713.

BERNSTEIN, J., PRIBYL, E. J., LOSEE, K., and LOTT, W. A., 1947a, III. Some substituted sulfanilamidopyridines. *J. Amer. chem. Soc.*, **69**, 1158.

BERNSTEIN, J., STEARNS, B., DEXTER, M., and LOTT, W. A., 1947b, I. Derivatives of aminopyridines. *J. Amer. chem. Soc.*, **69**, 1147.

BERNSTEIN, J., STEARNS, B., SHAW, E., and LOTT, W. A., 1947c, II. Derivatives of 2, 6-diaminopyridine. *J. Amer. chem. Soc.*, **69**, 1151.

CLIFFE, W. H., CURD, F. H. S., ROSE, F. L., and SCOTT, M., 1948, Synthetic antimalarials. Part XXIII. 2-Arylguanidino-4-aminoalkylaminopyrimidines. Further variations. *J. chem. Soc.*, 574.

COATNEY, G. R., and COOPER, W. C., 1948, The chemotherapy of malaria in relation to our knowledge of exoerythrocytic forms. *J. Parasit.*, **34**, 275.

CROWTHER, A. F., CURD, F. H. S., and ROSE, F. L., 1948, Synthetic antimalarials. Part XXV. Some 4-arylguanidino-2- and -6-dialkylamino-alkylaminopyridines. *J. chem. Soc.*, 586.

CURD, F. H. S., DAVEY, D. G., and RICHARDSON, D. N., 1949, Synthetic antimalarials. Part XLII. The preparation of guanylureas and biurets corresponding to paludrine and related diguanidines. *J. chem. Soc.*, 1732.

CURD, F. H. S., DAVEY, D. G., RICHARDSON, D. N., and ASHWORTH, R. DE B., 1949, Synthetic antimalarials. Part XLIII. Some dithiobiurets and 1 : 2 : 4-triazoles related to proguanil. *J. chem. Soc.*, 1739.

CURD, F. H. S., DAVEY, D. G., and ROSE, F. L., 1945, Studies on synthetic antimalarial drugs. X. Some biguanide derivatives as new types of antimalarial substances with both therapeutic and causal prophylactic activity. *Ann. trop. Med. Parasit.*, **39**, 208.

CURD, F. H. S., DAVIS, M. I., OWEN, E. C., ROSE, F. L., and TUEY, G. A. P., 1946a, Synthetic antimalarials. Part VI. Some 4-Arylamino-2-amino-alkylamino-6-methyl-pyrimidines. *J. chem. Soc.*, 370.

CURD, F. H. S., DAVIS, M. I., OWEN, E. C., ROSE, F. L., and TUEY, G. A. P., 1946b, Synthetic antimalarials. Part IX. 4-Arylamino-2-aminoalkyl-amino-6-methyl-pyrimidines. Further variations. *J. chem. Soc.*, 720.

CURD, F. H. S., DAVIS, M. I., and ROSE, F. L., 1946, Synthetic antimalarials. Part II. 2-Substituted-anilino-4-amino-alkylamino-6-methylpyrimidines. *J. chem. Soc.*, 351.

CURD, F. H. S., GRAHAM, W., RICHARDSON, D. N., and ROSE, F. L., 1947, Synthetic antimalarials. Part XXII. Some quinolylamino-substituted pyrimidine derivatives. *J. chem. Soc.*, 1613.

CURD, F. H. S., GRAHAM, W., and ROSE, F. L., 1948, Synthetic antimalarials. Part XXVI. Pyridyl- and pyrimidylaminopyridines. *J. chem. Soc.*, 594.

CURD, F. H. S., HOGGARTH, E., LANDQUIST, J. K., and ROSE, F. L., 1948, Synthetic antimalarials. Part XXXII. Some 4-arylamino and 4-arylthio-2-aminoalkylaminoquinazolines and 2-arylthio-4-aminoalkylamino-quinazolines. *J. chem. Soc.*, 1766.

CURD, F. H. S., LANDQUIST, J. K., and ROSE, F. L., 1947, Synthetic anti-malarials. Part XII. Some 1 : 3 : 5-triazine derivatives. *J. chem. Soc.*, 154.

CURD, F. H. S., LANDQUIST, J. K., and ROSE, F. L., 1948, Synthetic anti-malarials. Part XXXI. 2-*p*-Chloroanilino-4-*β*-diethylaminoethylamino-quinazolines containing various substituents in the quinazoline nucleus. *J. chem. Soc.*, 1759.

CURD, F. H. S., and RAISON, C. G., 1947, Synthetic antimalarials. Part XIII. Some *N*-dialkylaminoalkyl-amidines. *J. chem. Soc.*, 160.

CURD, F. H. S., RAISON, C. G., and ROSE, F. L., 1946, Synthetic antimalarials. Part V. 2-Naphthylamino-4-aminoalkylamino-6-methylpyrimidines. *J. chem. Soc.*, 366.

CURD, F. H. S., RAISON, C. G., and ROSE, F. L., 1947, Synthetic antimalarials. Part XVII. Some arylamino-aminoalkylaminoquinoline derivatives. *J. chem. Soc.*, 899.

CURD, F. H. S., RICHARDSON, D. N., and ROSE, F. L., 1946, Synthetic anti-malarials. Part VII. 2-Arylamino-4-dialkylaminoalkylaminopyrimidines. Variation of substituents in the 5- and the 6-position. *J. chem. Soc.*, 378.

CURD, F. H. S., and ROSE, F. L., 1946a, Synthetic antimalarials. Part I. Some derivatives of arylamino and aryl substituted pyrimidines. *J. chem. Soc.*, 343.

CURD, F. H. S., and ROSE, F. L., 1946b, Synthetic antimalarials. Part IV. 2-Phenylguanidino-4-aminoalkyl-amino-6-methylpyrimidines. *J. chem. Soc.*, 362.

CURD, F. H. S., and ROSE, F. L., 1946c, Synthetic antimalarials. Part X. Some aryl-diguanidine (-biguanidine) derivatives. *J. chem. Soc.*, 729.

DAVEY, D. G., 1946, The use of avian malaria for the discovery of drugs effective in the treatment and prevention of human malaria. II. Drugs for causal prophylaxis and radical cure or the chemotherapy of exoery-throcytic forms. *Ann. trop. Med. Parasit.*, 40, 453.

DÍAZ DE LEÓN, A., 1937, Primeros casos de paludismo tratados pur un derivado de la sulfanilamida. *Bol. Ofic. sanit. pan-amer.*, 16, 1039.

FALCO, E. A., HITCHINGS, G. H., RUSSELL, P. B., and VAN DER WERFF, H., 1949, Antimalarials as antagonists of purines and pteroylglutamic acid. *Nature, Lond.*, 164, 107.

FOURNEAU, E., TRÉFOUEL, J., TRÉFOUEL, Madame, BOVET, D., and BENOIT, G., 1933, Contribution à la chimiotherapie due paludisme : essais sur les calfats. Deuxième Memoire. *Ann. Inst. Pasteur*, 50, 731.

GINGRICH, W., 1946, in " A survey of antimalarial drugs, 1941–1945," edited by F. Y. WISELOGLE, Vol. I, p. 503. Ann Arbor, Michigan, J. W. Edwards.

GOODWIN, L. G., 1949, Response of *Plasmodium berghei* to antimalarial drugs. *Nature, Lond.*, 164, 1133.

GULLAND, J. M., and MACEY, P. E., 1949, Synthetic antimalarials. Part XXXVIII. 2-(6'-Quinolylguanidino)-4-*β*-diethylaminoethylamino, and 4-(6'-quinolylguanidino)-2-*β*-diethylaminoethylamino-6-methylpyri-midines. *J. chem. Soc.*, 1257.

120 *CHEMICAL APPROACHES*

HALL, D. M., and TURNER, E. E., 1945a, Structure and antimalarial activity. Part I. Some acridine derivatives. *J. chem. Soc.*, 694.
HALL, D. M., and TURNER, E. E., 1945b, Structure and antimalarial activity. Part II. *iso*Alloxazines, quinoxalines, and quinoxalo*cyclo*pentadienes. *J. chem. Soc.*, 699.
HALL, D. M., and TURNER, E. E., 1948, Structure and antimalarial activity. Part III. Some benziminazoles. *J. chem. Soc.*, 1909.
HAWKING, F., 1947, Activation of paludrine *in vitro*. *Nature, Lond.*, 159, 409.
HULL, R., LOVELL, B. J., OPENSHAW, H. J., PAYMAN, L. C., and TODD, A. R., 1946, Synthetic antimalarials. Part III. Some derivatives of mono- and di-alkylpyrimidines. *J. chem. Soc.*, 357.
HULL, R., LOVELL, B. J., OPENSHAW, H. J., and TODD, A. R., 1947, Synthetic antimalarials. Part XI. The effect of variation of substituents in derivatives of mono- and di-alkylpyrimidines. *J. chem. Soc.*, 41.
KALTHOD, G. G., and LINNELL, W. H., 1947, Chemotherapeutic exploration of the pyridine nucleus : substituted amines. Part I. *Quart. J. Pharm.*, 20, 546.
KALTHOD, G. G., and LINNELL, W. H., 1948, Chemotherapeutic exploration of the pyridine nucleus : substituted amines. Part II. *Quart. J. Pharm.*, 21, 63.
KELSEY, F. E., GEILING, E. M. K., OLDHAM, F. K., and DEARBORN, E. H., 1944, Studies on antimalarial drugs. The preparation and properties of a metabolic derivative of quinine. *J. Pharmacol.*, 80, 391.
KING, F. E., and KING, T. J., 1947, New potential chemotherapeutic agents. Part VII. Experiments on the synthesis of 8-aminopurines. *J. chem. Soc.*, 943.
KRICHEVSKÍI, I. L., SHTERNBERG, E. Y., and HAL'PERIN, E. P., 1935, [Synthetic chemotherapeutic compounds. IV. Quinoline and acridine antimalarials]. *J. Microbiol. Moscow*, 14, 642.
MADINAVEITIA, J., 1946, The antagonism of some antimalarial drugs by riboflavin. *Biochem. J.*, 40, 373.
MAGIDSON, O. Y., DELEKTORSKAYA, N. M., and LIPOWITSCH, I. M., 1934, Die Derivative des 8-Aminochinolins als Antimalariapräparate. Mitt. III. Der Einfluss der Verzweigung der Kette in Stellung 8. *Arch. Pharm. Berl.*, 272, 74.
MAGIDSON, O. Y., and GRIGOROWSKY, A. M., 1936, Acridin-Verbindungen und ihre Antimalaria-Wirkung. (I Mitt). *Ber. dtsch. chem. Ges.*, 69, 396.
MAGIDSON, O. Y., and RUBTSOV, M. V., 1937, [Quinoline compounds as sources of medicinal products. VI. Antimalarial compounds with the side-chain in the four-position]. *J. gen. Chem. Moscow*, 7, 1896.
MANN, F. G., NAYLOR, F. T., and PORTER, J. W. G., 1947, Synthetic antimalarials. Part XIX. Dialkylaminoalkylaminodiphenylguanidines. *J. chem. Soc.*, 914.
MANN, F. G., and PORTER, J. W. G., 1947, Synthetic antimalarials. Part XVIII 3-Dialkylaminoalkylaminodiphenylamines. *J. chem. Soc.*, 910.
MARSHALL, E. K., Jr., LITCHFIELD, J. T., Jr., and WHITE, H. J., 1942, Sulfonamide therapy of malaria in ducks. *J. Pharmacol.*, 75, 89.
MEAD, J., and KOEPFLI, J. B., 1944, The structure of a new metabolic derivative of quinine. *J. biol. Chem.*, 154, 507.
SCHÖNHÖFER, F., 1942, Über die Bedentung der chinoiden Bindung in Chinolinverbindungen für der Malarialwirkung. *Hoppe-Seyl. Z.*, 274.
SPINKS, A., 1948, Studies on synthetic antimalarial drugs. XX. The blood concentrations and physiological distribution of some homologues of paludrine in relation to their antimalarial activities. *Ann. trop. Med. Parasit.*, 42, 190.

CHAPTER V

THE PHARMACOLOGY OF ANTIMALARIAL DRUGS

The Pharmacology of Cinchona Alkaloids

DURING the years of the Second World War much fresh light was thrown on the pharmacology of quinine and of the other cinchona alkaloids.

When taken by mouth, the cinchona alkaloids are rapidly and almost completely absorbed from the intestinal tract. When, for instance, 2 or 3 gm. of cinchonine or of the 2-hydroxy derivative is given in serial doses daily by mouth only 2 to 3 per cent. can be recovered from the stools. The presence in the intestine of sodium chloride in concentrations up to 4 per cent. does not affect the rate of absorption of quinine sulphate ; the amount of quinine salt absorbed does not bear a linear relationship to time, since the rate of absorption decreases after the first thirty minutes. Fæces do not destroy the cinchona alkaloids, for cinchonine, for instance, can be incubated with fæces at 37° C. for some hours and recovered quantitatively. Basu *et al.* (1947) believe that bile salts play an important part in facilitating the absorption of quinine from the intestine. Four hours after an oral dose the concentrations of quinine or cinchonine in the plasma are approximately the same as four hours after intravenous injection. Peak plasma concentrations after oral doses of all the four alkaloids are obtained in from one to four hours. Hiatt (1944) came to the conclusion that cinchonine base was absorbed less readily than the other cinchona alkaloids given by mouth as bases. Cornatzer and Andrews (1944), on the other hand, using isolated intestinal loops in dogs, believed that cinchonine as the dihydrochloride was absorbed more rapidly than the dihydrochlorides of the other alkaloids. Single oral doses of the alkaloids as bases frequently yield plasma drug concentrations considerably lower than those obtained with soluble salts. On maintenance regimens, however, the equilibrium plasma concentration is the same with either alkaloidal base or salt.

In the plasma it is probable that the alkaloids are bound to non-diffusible elements, presumably in the albumin fraction. This certainly holds good for cinchonine and 2-hydroxycinchonine (Earle *et al.*, 1948). The red cell concentration of quinine is greater than that in the plasma, but both red cell and plasma concentrations, after rising to a peak usually one hour after dosing, rapidly fall (Marshall, 1945b). Taggart *et al.* (1948), however, found that both for quinine and cinchonine the concentration in the cellular elements in the blood is 20 per cent. less than in plasma. It is possible that the cellular permeability of the red cells is altered during the malarial process. Overman (1948), for instance, has shown that malaria causes a fall in the red cell content of potassium ions but a rise in sodium and chlorine ions. In monkeys infected with *P. knowlesi* there is a high degree of correlation between the severity of the parasitæmia and the extent of the ionic shift. The abnormalities in cellular permeability are corrected by destruction of the malaria parasites by chemotherapeutic drugs.

Hiatt (1944), in comparing the plasma concentrations of the four cinchona alkaloids given by mouth to man as free bases, found that low concentrations of cinchonine were present in the plasma as compared with the other cinchona alkaloids. This difference is not due to differences in the rate of absorption, and, as Hiatt and Quinn (1945) have emphasised, distribution of all four alkaloids in the body after intravenous injection is very similar.

The effect of different dose-schedules on the resulting plasma concentrations of the four cinchona alkaloids has been further studied in detail by Taggart *et al.* (1948). Therapy consisted of an initial priming dose, usually one half the total daily dose, followed by small maintenance doses at four to eight hourly intervals. Mean plasma drug concentrations were the averages of individual daily mean concentrations. The results are shown in the table on the opposite page.

With corresponding oral doses cinchonine, quinidine, and cinchonidine give plasma concentrations approximately 5, 25, and 40 per cent. of the corresponding quinine levels. Considerably higher plasma levels are achieved by 2-hydroxy cinchonine than by equal doses of cinchonine (Earle *et al.*, 1948). The very low plasma levels with cinchonine given by mouth would appear to

DOSAGE SCHEDULES OF CINCHONA ALKALOIDS AND RESULTANT
PLASMA DRUG CONCENTRATIONS (Taggart *et al.*, 1948)

Drug.	Total daily dose (gm. base).	Number of subjects.	Mean plasma drug concentration.	
			Range, mgm./litre.	Average, mgm./litre.
Quinine .	0·20	20	1·9– 5·1	3·3
	0·50	6	2·9– 6·5	4·9
	0·75	9	5·5– 9·5	6·3
	1·50	44	7·0–12·9	9·6
Cinchonine .	0·50	6	<0·05	<0·05
	1·00	13	0·1– 0·5	0·2
	2·00	16	0·3– 2·7	1·0
Quinidine .	0·1	10	0·2– 1·3	0·7
	0·6	4	1·4– 3·3	2·0
	1·5	3	2·6– 5·0	3·5
Cinchonidine	0·3	6	0·8– 3·2	1·7
	1·0	13	1·2– 3·8	2·2
	2·0	6	2·3– 9·2	5·5

be due to a higher rate of metabolic breakdown for cinchonine
than for the other cinchona alkaloids (Taggart *et al.* 1946;
Andrews and Cornatzer, 1947), at any rate in man, for in the dog
cinchonine is broken down far more slowly. In metabolic experiments with cinchonine it must be remembered that almost all
specimens of " pure " cinchonine contain some quinine and
dihydrocinchonine. A second important difference between
cinchonine and the other cinchona alkaloids is that with increasing
doses of cinchonine the resultant plasma concentrations are
increased out of all proportion to the increments of dosage. With
the other alkaloids the increases are disproportionately small in
relation to the dose.

The plasma concentrations of all four cinchona alkaloids fall
rapidly in man after cessation of administration. In animals,
the rate of disappearance of quinine from the plasma is also very
rapid. In the dog, rabbit, and hen, according to Chen and Geiling
(1944), 95 per cent. has disappeared from the circulation in three
minutes. The rate of disappearance is not affected by blockade of

the reticulo-endothelial system. Few direct observations have been made in man on the extent to which the cinchona alkaloids are localised in tissues. In animals, quinine is selectively concentrated by several organs in the body. After oral or intravenous administration the drug is found in considerable amounts in pancreas, liver, spleen, lung, and kidney. Blood, muscle, connective and nervous tissues contain relatively little (Kelsey *et al.* 1943 ; Burton and Kelsey, 1943 ; Kelsey *et al.*, 1945 ; Hiatt and Quinn, 1945). Neither the cellular components involved nor the mechanism of the concentration is fully understood. Several explanations have been suggested, including specific adsorption by the cells of the blood capillaries, by cell membranes or by cytoplasmic or nuclear colloids (Chen and Geiling, 1944 ; Hiatt and Quinn, 1945). The process of selective absorption of quinine by normal tissues is not unlike that found to occur with certain dyes in and around tumours : in fact Kelsey and Brunschwig (1947) have reported that quinine is selectively concentrated by human neoplastic tissues. Possibly quinine is adsorbed by the nondialysable constituents of the cell. Burton and Kelsey (1943) find that when quinine is injected intravenously into pregnant rabbits the amount fixed in the maternal liver increases as term approaches.

Concentrations of quinine in cerebrospinal fluid are less than in plasma, the ratio being 1 : 20 to 1 : 50. The concentration of quinine in cerebrospinal fluid varied from 19 to 260 μgm. when the plasma concentrations ranged from 1,290 to 6,820 μgm. per litre (Lippincott *et al.*, 1946).

Fresh light on the metabolism of the cinchona alkaloids was thrown by the discovery of Kelsey and Oldham (1943) that animal tissues contain an enzyme capable of catalysing the oxidation of quinine. The oxidation of the other cinchona alkaloids, of quinoline and some of its derivatives, and of N-methylnicotinamide is also affected (Brodie *et al.*, 1946 ; Knox, 1946). The rate of destruction of quinine may be rapid, for Chen and Geiling (1944) found that 70 per cent. of quinine was destroyed in five minutes by a heart-lung preparation. The most important decomposition product formed from quinine is, according to Mead and Koepfli (1944), lævorotatory 2'-hydroxy-6'-methoxy-3-vinylruban-9-ol, or quinine with a hydroxyl group substituted in position 2 of the quinoline ring. The LD 50 of the degradation product, quinine carbostyril, given intravenously to chicks is 100 to 120 mgm. per kgm., that of quinine being 30 to 40 mgm. per kgm. (Kelsey *et al.*, 1946). The quinine degradation product (QDP) is unextractable with sodium hydroxide but can be extracted from ammoniacal solution (Kelsey *et al.*, 1944). Marshall and Rogers (1948) have described a method for its estimation in the presence of quinine. In man the 6'-desmethoxy analogue of 1, 2'-hydroxy, 6'-methoxy-3-vinylruban-9-ol, as well as a more highly oxidised derivative, has been obtained from human urine by Brodie and Udenfriend (1945) after the ingestion of cinchonine, and somewhat similar products have been isolated after the ingestion of quinidine and cinchonidine, although their exact structure is still uncertain. Marshall (1945a) believed that the degradation product of quinine lacked anti-plasmodial action, but Kelsey *et al.* (1946) have denied this.

The distribution of the enzyme responsible for destroying the cinchona alkaloids varies somewhat in different animals : it is present in the liver of the rabbit but absent or at any rate undemonstrable in the liver of the hen (Kelsey and Oldham, 1943). Nevertheless quinine is destroyed by the fowl liver, the rate of destruction being more rapid in young than in old birds. The activity of the rabbit liver is decreased during the later stages of pregnancy, probably because of the reduction in enzyme rather than because of the presence of an inhibitory substance (Oldham and Kelsey, 1943). Knox (1946) has found that the oxidase from rabbit liver contains 0·6 gm. of riboflavin per unit of activity : it is associated with flavoprotein liver aldehyde oxidase and appears to be a duo-functioning flavoprotein analogous to xanthine oxidase. Under anaerobic conditions the oxidase is reduced by cinchonine, but under aerobic conditions hydrogen peroxide is formed as the oxidation of the substrate proceeds. A study of the point of attack of the oxidase on cinchona alkaloids suggested to Mead *et al.* (1946) that a compound such as 2'-phenyldihydro-cinchonine would be impervious to the attack of the enzyme and thus able to exert a more prolonged antimalarial action. Although 2'-phenyldihydrocinchonine is more active than cinchonine in avian malaria, there are technical difficulties in producing this compound on a large scale.

The enzymatic degradation of quinine is inhibited by mepacrine and pamaquin, the inhibitory action being on the enzyme rather than on the substrate (Chen, 1947).

It seems probable that the cinchona alkaloids may be metabolised differently in hens and ducks (Kelsey *et al.*, 1943 ; Waletsky and Brown, 1943). Ducks undoubtedly metabolise both quinine and quinidine more slowly than do hens : in the latter the drug concentration is higher in the plasma than in the red cells up to four hours after administration, whereas in the duck the concentration in the red cells is higher than in the plasma (Kelsey *et al.*, 1945).

The metabolism of cinchonine has received considerable attention. After an oral dose of cinchonine less than 0·5 per cent. of the original alkaloid appears as such in the urine, but 2′-hydroxycinchonine and a more highly oxygenated derivative, probably 2′, 6′-dihydroxycinchonine, are present to the extent of 55 and 25 per cent. of the original alkaloid administered. The renal clearance of 2′-hydroxycinchonine is higher than that of cinchonine itself and very close to that of the renal plasma flow, but despite this rapid excretion, some at least of this substance undergoes further oxidation (Earle, 1946 ; Earle *et al.*, 1948). After oral or intravenous administration of 2′-hydroxycinchonine it disappears rapidly from the blood and only negligible concentrations are found in the plasma twelve hours after the last dose. Quinidine is metabolised in a similar manner, and Brodie *et al.* (1946) have found two compounds in urine, one of which is 2′-hydroxyquinidine while the other differs from quinidine in the possession of an additional oxygen atom in the quinuclidine portion of the molecule. Quinine and cinchonidine also give rise to 2′-hydroxy derivatives. The relationship of antimalarial activity to the rate of absorption of cinchona alkaloids has been studied by Marshall (1945b).

Quinine in the normal animal decreases the motility of the intestine to a slight degree, but in the rat suffering from the syndrome due to vitamin B-complex deficiency it increases the motility considerably (Kyker *et al.*, 1946). The antipyretic action of quinine is of course due to its effect on the central temperature-regulating mechanism, resulting in peripheral vasodilation. Intraperitoneal injection of 10 to 15 mgm. per kgm. of body weight of quinine chloride reduced the electrical activity of the cerebral cortical cells of rats (Ten Cate and Boeles, 1948). Quinine, like mepacrine and proguanil, diminishes the inhibitory action of the vagus on the heart (Babkin and Ritchie, 1945 ; Gertler and Karp, 1947). According to Burn and Dutta (1948), quinine and also quinidine antagonise the action of acetylcholine on heart, gut, and skeletal muscle. The effect of quinine on the isolated frog heart increases with alkalinisation in the pH range 6·5 to 8·0. This is ascribed by Goljachowski (1934) to the formation of the undissociated free base which is bound by the heart tissue. Adenosine triphosphate in man, cat, and guinea-pig slows the sinus rhythm. This effect is decreased by quinine and quinidine (Wayne *et al.*, 1949). Babkin and Karp (1947) and Karp (1948) have found that quinine bisulphate in doses of 10 to 30 mgm. per kgm. of body weight does not effect the response of the gastric secretion to histamine but does reduce the volume of gastric secretion as well as the output of pepsin produced by vagal stimulation. In 1945 Driesbach and Hanzlik found that epinephrine counteracted the depressor effects of intravenously injected quinine. Hiatt (1949) reported that cinchona alkaloids are capable of antagonising the pressor effects and changes in cardiac rhythm caused by injections of adrenaline. Cinchona alkaloids cause renal vasodilatation and decrease of the blood pressure in dogs with experimental neurogenic hypertension, possibly due to an inhibitory effect on the adrenergic sympathetic endings. Since Hiatt *et al.* (1945) proved that these alkaloids can inhibit certain parasympathetic nerve endings as well as the motor fibres to skeletal muscles it is possible that these have an inhibitory action on all motor nerve endings. When quinine is given intravenously the toxic dose is much lower if there is hæmorrhage, shock, asphyxia or hyperthermia. In the normal rabbit the median fatal dose given intravenously is 208 mgm. per kgm., but after hæmorrhage it is only 146 mgm. per kgm. Adrenaline antagonises the effects of shock, hæmorrhage, and hyperthermia in the rabbit and hyperthermia and hæmorrhage in the cat ; when rabbits or cats are asphyxiated adrenaline does not reduce quinine toxicity. Calcium chloride is less effective (Dreisbach, 1949).

Although the greater part of the cinchona alkaloids are destroyed in the body and the end-products appear in the urine, a small amount of quinine may be found in the bile (Bernardbeig and Caujolle, 1935). The various metabolic products recoverable from the urine account for 65 per cent. of the total oral dose in the case of cinchonine, 20 per cent. in the case of quinine, and less than 5 per cent. in the case of quinidine and cinchonidine (Craig, 1944 ; Brodie *et al.*, 1946). The renal clearance of cinchonine may be depressed by the concomitant administration of large doses of sodium bicarbonate although the clearance of 2-hydroxycinchonine is not significantly altered. Haag *et al.* (1943) showed that quinine is excreted more rapidly in acid than in alkaline urine. Acton and Chopra (1925) believed that alkalies given with quinine increased the rate of absorption of the alkaloid by the intestinal mucosa, diffusion being increased by an excess of OH ions on the cell membranes and decreased by an excess of H ions. This claim has not been confirmed. Hookworm damage to the intestine does not influence the plasma concentration or the rate of urinary excretion following a single dose of quinine sulphate (Andrews and Webb, 1942).

In the treatment of malaria in man cinchona alkaloids may be given by mouth, intravenously, intramuscularly or per rectum. The last route, which was popular when only cinchona bark was available, is now rarely, if ever, used. In cases of acute cerebral malaria intravenous injections of quinine bihydrochloride are of value, and provided the injections are given very slowly there is little risk of collapse. There still exists a widespread belief, more especially in Africa, that the intramuscular route possesses some esoteric advantage over every other route of administration. The evidence for any such advantage is not apparent. If an immediate effect is desired this is obtained without delay by intravenous injection : if a prolonged effect is desired this can be readily obtained by repeated oral administration. Mariani (1903) showed that after intramuscular injection 60 per cent. of quinine hydrochloride was still present in rabbit muscle seventeen hours after injection. Intramuscular injection does not delay excretion for, as Clark (1937) has pointed out, the amount of quinine excreted and the rate of excretion are about the same whether the drug is given orally, intravenously or intramuscularly. McLay (1922) in fact showed, and his results have not been contradicted, that parasites disappeared more rapidly from the blood stream after oral administration than after the intramuscular injection of the same amount of alkaloid. On the other hand, all observers are agreed that even when diluted 1 in 150 quinine salts cause considerable necrosis if injected into the muscle. This necrosis may also involve nerve or artery while paralysis and even tetanus may follow. Dutch workers claim that the hydrochloride of quinine causes less necrosis than the bihydrochloride when injected intramuscularly because of its less acid reaction ; its pH is about 6·0 as compared with pH 3·0. Urethane is often injected intramuscularly with the quinine bihydrochloride. Quinine carbonate is poorly absorbed from the gut but the ethyl carbonate is quickly absorbed (Winckel *et al.*, 1950).

Attempts to delay the excretion of quinine are claimed by Quevauviller (1946) following the injection of subtosan, a 20 per cent. aqueous solution of polyvinyl-pyrrolidine. When injected intravenously in rabbits together with quinine it is said not only to slow the rate of excretion in the urine but to decrease the amount excreted. Rogers (1918) and Silvestri (1923) claim that after intramuscular injection of cinchonine dihydrochloride in rabbits the alkaloid enters the circulation more rapidly than in the case of quinine. Muscle necrosis is said to be less with cinchonine than with quinine, although Acton and Chopra (1924) were unable to confirm this finding. Nevertheless, the amount of cinchonidine and cinchonine base precipitated at the site of an intramuscular injection is less than with quinine and quinidine.

Pirk and Engelberg (1945) and Wahi (1947) have shown that doses of 0·3 gm. daily cause a significant rise in the prothrombin time : this rise is inhibited by the administration of vitamin K. Quinine and mepacrine increase reticulocyte counts in malarial and non-malarial subjects (Dähne, 1943). The pharmacology of quinidine is discussed by Ployé (1950).

Estimation of Cinchona Alkaloids

In following the metabolism of the cinchona alkaloids, methods of estimating the drug are obviously of considerable importance. Older methods, such as those described by Ramsden *et al.* (1918), have for the most part been discarded and more accurate methods are now available (Prudhomme, 1940 ; Kelsey and Geiling, 1942 ; Chen and Geiling, 1944 ; Brodie and Udenfriend, 1943a, 1945 ; Marshall and Rogers, 1945). The method devised by Brodie and Udenfriend (1943a) is of advantage as it allows for the determination of other organic bases and by combination with an extraction procedure permits the estimation of the cinchona alkaloids and their metabolic degradation products in the same specimen.

For those who do not possess an instrument such as the Coleman electronic fluorimeter, Spinks and Tottey (1946a) have devised a method of estimating quinine in plasma which is four to five times more active than that devised by Chen and Geiling (1944), though it has the disadvantage that it cannot be applied to whole blood.

Plasma (1 ml.) is treated with N/1 sodium hydroxide (1 ml.) and warmed at 55° C. for twenty minutes. After cooling, benzene (10 ml.) containing 2 per cent. of ethanol is added and the mixture is shaken vigorously for five minutes and centrifuged for fifteen minutes at 4,000 revolutions per minute. An aliquot of the solvent, 8–9 ml., is withdrawn and shaken with N/12 sulphuric acid (12 ml. for three minutes). After centrifuging for five minutes at 2,000 revolutions per minute the lower layer is removed and read in a modified spekker fluorimeter, using a blue filter, against a series of standards containing 0, 0·2, 0·5, 1·0, 2·0, 3·0 and 5·0 μgm. of quinine base in 12 ml. of N/12 sulphuric acid. Normal plasma gives no fluorescence. The mean recovery after adding different amounts of quinine to plasma was 102 per cent. $\pm$ 3·7 (p$=$0·05).

The Pharmacology of Mepacrine

With the failure of the quinine supplies during the war of 1939–45 the Allies were forced to study intensively the anti-malarial compounds which remained. Of these compounds mepacrine appeared the most important. Much work had already been carried out before the war, especially in Germany, on the pharmacology of mepacrine, and later observations have served to confirm these earlier findings, extending them, however, in certain directions. Mepacrine is a yellow powder with a somewhat bitter taste, soluble in water to the extent of 2 or 3 per cent. at room temperature, or 7 per cent. in water at 40° C. Like quinine, mepacrine in water is fluorescent. Christophers (1937) found that the base is soluble in water to the extent of $10^{-4·08}$ (0·000084), the undissociated base to the extent of $10^{-4·8}$ (0·000016) : the solubility product is $10^{-8 \cdot 68}$. Magidson and Grigorowsky (1936) showed that watery solutions of mepacrine will not keep indefinitely but will decompose by slow hydrolysis with the formation of the sparingly soluble 3-methoxy-6-chloro-acridone and the very soluble α-diethylamino-δ-aminopentane dihydrochloride. Mietzsch *et al.* (1936) found, however, that a 1 per cent. solution of mepacrine hydrochloride could be kept for three weeks at a temperature of 37° C, without any formation of 2-methoxy-6-chloro-acridone, but after heating for a quarter of an hour at 105° C. decomposition began after a few days. Neither of these decomposition products showed any toxic action in animals.

Mepacrine dimethanesulphonate, or mepacrine musonate, in which two molecules of methanesulphonic acid (CH_3SO_3H) replace two molecules of hydrochloride, has been used for parenteral injection owing to its extreme solubility in water : even with mepacrine musonate it is better to employ only freshly prepared solutions and not to submit these solutions to prolonged boiling.

While mepacrine dihydrochloride and the base can be readily obtained, the monohydrochloride cannot be obtained in an isolated form, owing to the low solubility of the base and the close proximity of the two dissociation constants ($pK_2 - pK_1 = 2 \cdot 59$).

According to Christophers (1937) mepacrine possesses two dissociation constants, both probably connected with the amine portion of the molecule, one very strong, $pK_1 = 3 \cdot 88$, the other weaker, $pK_2 = 6 \cdot 47$. There is a possibility of a third constant, probably in relation to the acridine ring, but if a third constant exists it is weaker than $pK_3 = 11 \cdot 0$. Irwin and Irwin (1946, 1947) believe that mepacrine has two proton-accepting groups, with one dissociation constant, $pK_1 = 7 \cdot 67$ involving the aromatic nucleus and $pK_2 = 10 \cdot 16$ involving the diethylamino side-chain.

A resolution into optical antimers was obtained by Bacher *et al.* (1947) using D-α-brom-camphor-π-sulphonic acid : $[\alpha]_D - 334°$, $+ 335°$ for the hydrochloride in water. Brown and Hammick (1948) prefer to use D-4 : 6 : 4'-6'-tetranitrodiphenic acid when they obtain $[\alpha]_D - 197°$, and 205° for the free base in ethyl alcohol, and $[\alpha]_D - 334°$, $+ 335°$ for the hydrochloride in water.

Mepacrine is readily absorbed from the intestinal tract (Chopra *et al.*, 1937 ; Shannon *et al.*, 1944 ; Shannon and Earle, 1945).

Absorption is only slightly affected by the presence or absence of food in the stomach, hypoacidity in the stomach or inflammation of the intestinal mucosa. Chopra *et al.* (1937) showed that if mepacrine is given with pamaquin in dragees its absorption is greatly reduced. Considerable differences in the rate of absorption have been noted : Yudkin (1946) reported one case of non-absorption of mepacrine from the intestinal canal as demonstrated by non-appearance of the drug in the urine and by lack of response to therapy. Recovery took place immediately after the intramuscular injection of mepacrine musonate. After intramuscular or intravenous injection the blood mepacrine level rises very rapidly but after an intravenous injection the drug disappears rapidly from the circulation and as in the case of quinine 95 per cent. has left the circulation within three minutes of injection. Patients with dysentery absorb both mepacrine and quinine readily and no impairment of absorptive power is seen (Maier, 1948b).

The concentration in the blood varies of course with the dose and with the time at which the observations are made in relation to the time of administration. In addition there is considerable individual variation (Smith *et al.*, 1946). Moderate amounts of ethyl alcohol do not affect the levels. Shannon *et al.* (1944) showed that the greater part of the mepacrine in the blood is located in the white cells ; only about 20 per cent. of the blood mepacrine is partitioned between plasma and the red cells in the ratio of 1 : 1·6 (Army Malaria Research Unit, 1946c). If 10 per cent of carbon dioxide in oxygen is breathed over a two-hour period the concentration of mepacrine in the blood plasma and red cells is doubled. The breathing of CO_2 under these conditions causes an acidosis corresponding to a drop in blood pH from 7·4 to 6·9. Under the same conditions the concentration of mepacrine in muscle tissue and in leucocytes is unchanged (Jailer *et al.*, 1948).

Mepacrine would thus seem to be bound to the white cells in two ways : (i) lightly bound mepacrine increases and decreases rapidly after a dose is given ; (ii) firmly bound mepacrine increases more slowly and reaches a constant value for a given plasma level about the fifth day, when the dosage is 800 mgm. for

MEPACRINE CONCENTRATION IN PLASMA AND BLOOD CORPUSCLES
DURING A THERAPEUTIC COURSE OF MEPACRINE
(Brown and Rennie, 1945)

	Mepacrine concentration, mgm./1,000 ml.			Hæmato-crit.	Mepacrine content of leucocytes per litre of blood.	Leucocytes per c.mm.
	Plasma.	Whole blood.	Red cells.			
Case 1						
½ hour	9	32	48	46	5	5,750
8 hours	65	268	144	44	168	10,350
12 ,,	42	208	144	44	87	9,950
24 ,,	29	132	—	—	—	—
3rd day	63	212	200	44	89	7,650
5th ,,	46	220	208	43	104	6,850
6th ,,	66	268	224	45	131	8,950
8th ,,	56	284	152	47	185	8,900
Case 2						
½ hour	10	28	32	47	8	10,100
8 hours	18	176	72	48	131	10,950
12 ,,	16	176	88	47	122	11,350
24 ,,	32	128	88	47	65	10,250
3rd day	38	232	—	—	—	—
5th ,,	51	420	160	45	152	11,250
6th ,,	45	268	120	45	192	9,050
8th ,,	53	234	108	46	132	5,600
9th ,,	37	256	140	44	158	9,250

two days and then 300 mgm. a day. Parmer (1948) found that
the concentration of mepacrine in rabbits and hens four hours
after a single intramuscular injection of 8 mgm. per kgm. was
1·87 mgm. per kgm. in leucocytes, 0·08 and 0·27 mgm. per kgm. in
plasma and red cells. In two human subjects with leukæmia, bone-
marrow contained twenty times the amount in plasma. Brown and
Rennie (1945) also suggest that the rate of destruction in the tissues
varies with different individuals, thus accounting for the low plasma
levels in certain patients with relapsing vivax malaria. The plasma
level of mepacrine given to patients with infective hepatitis does
not differ from that in normal persons (Maier, 1948a).

Chopra, Ganguly and Roy (1936), and Chen and Geiling (1944),
showed that mepacrine is retained in the tissue for considerable

periods. After a single intravenous injection 80 to 90 per cent. remains in the lung two hours after injection. Dearborn *et al.* (1943) found that a constant level of mepacrine in fæces and urine was reached after seven days, when less than 4 per cent. of the daily intake was excreted. Since the concentration of the drug in the tissues reaches a saturation point it would seem that most of the absorbed mepacrine is destroyed in the body. They also determined the concentration of mepacrine in various tissues after doses of 5 or 50 mgm. per kgm. for periods of one to twenty-four days and found that the greatest concentration was in the liver. Slightly lower concentrations were found in the adrenals, pancreas, bile, spleen, and lung, whilst in the remaining tissues descending concentrations were found in the following order : bone-marrow, kidney, heart, skin, muscles, brain, and blood. Similar results were obtained by the Army Malaria Research Unit (1946b) and Dearborn (1947).

MEPACRINE CONCENTRATIONS (MGM./KGM.) IN TISSUES OF RABBITS AFTER AN INTRAMUSCULAR INJECTION OF 8 MGM. PER KGM. OF BODY WEIGHT OF MEPACRINE DIHYDROCHLORIDE. (Parmer, 1948)

	Time after injection.			
	4 hours.	4 days.	7 days.	11 days.
Rib marrow . . .	5·08	0·89	0·37	Trace
Proximal femoral marrow	4·38	1·02	0·33	Trace
Distal femoral marrow .	3·11	0·69	0·21	Trace
Plasma	0·08	Trace	0	0
Red cells . . .	0·27	Trace	0	0
Leucocytes . . .	1·87	Trace	0	0
Lymph nodes . . .	3·70	1·35	1·05	0·41
Thymus . . .	2·70	0·57	0·10	0
Liver	7·78	1·25	0·46	0·05
Spleen	40·62	1·96	0·44	0·11

Annegers *et al.* (1943) gave 5 mgm. of mepacrine dihydrochloride daily for seven days to rats of 200 gm. body weight and recovered the following amounts from the whole body :—

Days after the last dose.	Average amount recovered in mgm.
1	7·37
3	6·53
7	2·35
12	1·33
17	2·31
28	0·58
40–42	Trace

Five dogs were given thrice daily oral doses of 33 to 50 mgm. of mepacrine for seven days, then killed at intervals and the mepacrine content of the liver determined, with the following results :—

Days after last dose.	Total dose in mgm.	Recovery of mepacrine from liver.	
		Mgm.	Per cent. dose.
1	1,050	63·3	6·0
3	700	34·0	4·8
10	850	14·6	1·4
17	850	17·2	2·2
52	700	3·58	0·51

Foy *et al.* (1936) had already emphasised the high concentrations of mepacrine in liver and spleen.

The distribution of mepacrine was further investigated by Jailer (1945) by a direct fluorescence method, and by Shannon *et al.* (1944), who showed by chemical determinations that mepacrine is localised chiefly in the leucocytes, liver, spleen, and kidney ; frozen sections of tissues were examined by the fluorescence microscope in an aqueous medium buffered at pH 5. In the liver the fluorescence is diffusely distributed throughout the parenchymal cells while the Kupffer cells contain very little. In the kidney the highest degree of fluorescence is seen in the convoluted tubules, less in the collecting tubules, and little or none in the glomeruli. Other organs exhibit very little fluorescence. This method of course makes no distinction between mepacrine and its degradation products. Human hair, however, contains 85 μgm. per gm. ; dark hair usually contains more than light (Army Malaria Research Unit, 1946b).

Storage is greater in the organs of the rabbit, with the exception of the liver, than in those of the hen. Very little mepacrine was stored in the hen's lungs whereas one hour after an intravenous injection of 5 mgm. per kgm. in rabbits the lung contained 72 mgm. per kgm., the kidney 66, spleen 46, adrenal 32, liver 20, brain 15 and muscle 3 mgm. per kgm. As the liver is the largest organ, the absolute amount of mepacrine is largest in the liver. Lymph nodes retain the drug for more than twenty-six days, whereas liver and spleen under the same conditions were free on the eighteenth day (Parmer, 1948). In pregnant rabbits mepacrine passes through the placenta and may be stored in the fœtus. The liver of the mother contained 23 mgm. per kgm. of body weight when that of the fœtus was about 3 mgm. per kgm. (Oldham and Kelsey, 1945). Dikshit (1939) also found that mepacrine will pass through the placenta. In the dog the concentrations in fœtal organs are from one-third to one-half those in maternal organs.

The concentration of mepacrine in the cerebrospinal fluid is much less than in the plasma, ratios varying from 1 : 20 to 1 in 132. When plasma concentrations of mepacrine varied from 18 to 135 μgm. per litre, cerebrospinal fluid concentrations were from 18 to 135 μgm. per litre (Lippincott *et al.*, 1946). Dearborn *et al.* (1943) found that when mepacrine and sulphonamides were administered concurrently the concentration of mepacrine in the tissues was lowered ; blood-levels of mepacrine and sulphonamides were unaffected.

The high concentrations of mepacrine which are found in the tissues are undoubtedly due to the character of the basic side-chain and possibly, as suggested by Henry and Grindley (1945), to the strong tendency towards adsorption at colloid surfaces.

The effects of mepacrine on the cardio-vascular system have also been studied. Ganguli (1933) noted an occasional slight lowering of blood pressure in man, and de Langen and Storm (1934) and Storm (1935) recorded a fall in both diastolic and systolic blood pressure in monkeys after intravenous injections of mepacrine. Hecht (1933, 1935, 1936) obtained similar effects in cats after the intravenous injection of 2 mgm. per kgm. of body weight : intramuscular injection of 20 mgm. per kgm. of body weight was without effect. Smith and Stoeckle (1946) showed that a fall in blood pressure can be regularly obtained in cats, dogs, and rabbits provided the doses administered are large enough. In man, intravenous injection of mepacrine in therapeutic doses has no appreciable effect on blood pressure, but the blood sugar may fall. Meythaler (1942), however, reported that the blood pressure may fall by 15 to 20 mm. of mercury after intravenous injection of mepacrine musonate. Any temporary fall in blood pressure can be counteracted by injection of adrenaline. Russian investigators first showed that mepacrine when injected intravenously diminished the inhibitory action of the vagus on the heart as do quinine and proguanil. Studies on the isolated heart of the frog (Suffolk and Berkshire, 1939) and dog (Smith and Stoeckle, 1946) further suggest that mepacrine has a negative inotropic action on the isolated heart. With dogs this negative inotropic action may sometimes be demonstrated at concentrations of 1 mgm. per litre of blood and is constantly observed with concentrations of 1·5 mgm. per litre and above. Whether this negative inotropic action may occur in man under certain conditions when mepacrine is given intravenously in large doses is still uncertain. Irregularities in cardiac rhythm and in the working capacity of the heart are seen in dogs only with large doses. It is doubtful whether intravenous infusions at the rate of 0·5 mgm. per minute would reach a toxic level. If a severe myocardial failure has been produced it is not easily reversible. Injections of adrenaline cause a slight and transient improvement, but cardiac glycosides such as " strophosid " are said to produce prompt and long-lasting improvement in the working capacity of the failing heart in doses which neither change the heart rate nor cause irregularities in cardiac rhythm. Whereas quinine and quinidine have long been known to arrest auricular fibrillation, mepacrine also has a similar effect (Gertler and Yohalem, 1947, 1949). When mepacrine fails to cure auricular fibrillation, digitalis or quinidine, or both, also fail. In three of six cases of arrhythmia due to causes other than auricular fibrillation, mepacrine caused improvement. Melville (1946) suggests that mepacrine acts as a coronary dilator. Intravenous injections of mepacrine prevent the development of ventricular fibrillation following adrenaline injection during chloroform administration to dogs anæsthetised with pentobarbitol. The same protective action is noted after atropinisation or vagotomy. Unna (1945), on somewhat slender evidence, thinks that circulatory disturbances associated with mepacrine are due to an action on the central nervous system. According to Chin (1937), the excised heart of the rabbit can be rapidly paralysed by direct toxic action on the heart muscle. The effect of adenosine triphosphate on sinus rhythm is inhibited by mepacrine and heart block does not occur (Wayne *et al.*, 1949).

Small doses of mepacrine stimulate the uterus of both pregnant and non-pregnant rabbits and guinea-pigs. Large doses stimulate and later paralyse the uterus. In women there is no evidence that therapeutic doses are liable to cause an interruption of pregnancy, and daily doses of 0·1 gm. do not interfere with menstruation in women living in the tropics.

In nerve-muscle preparations mepacrine depresses the excitability of motor nerve endings (Chin, 1937). Suffolk and Berkshire (1939) found that mepacrine antagonises acetylcholine and depresses the vagal response of the heart but not of the gut. Waelsch and Nachmansohn (1943), on the other hand, believed that mepacrine inhibits cholinesterase, which would be equivalent to stimulation of the vagus. The Army Malaria Research Unit (1946a) studied the gastro-intestinal action of mepacrine radiologically. Single doses of 0·6 to 1·0 gm. in man caused some hypersecretion, increased peristalsis, and increase of tone of the pyloric antrum, followed by atony and pylorospasm. On a suppressive regime of 0·1 gm. daily no effect was noted except for slight hyperæmia of that portion of the gastric mucosa immediately in contact with the tablet. In dogs, according to Babkin and Karp (1947), mepacrine in a dose of 10 mgm. per kgm. of body weight strongly inhibits gastric secretion, but in man doses of 400 mgm. intravenously caused no inhibition (Petch, 1947). Whereas intravenous administration of mepacrine decreases gastric secretion produced by rhythmic vagal stimulation, small doses do not affect gastric secretion evoked by the subcutaneous administration of histamine. The amount of pepsin discharged from peptic cells under the influence of vagal stimulation is decreased by intravenous injection of mepacrine. Mepacrine has an inhibitory action on the secretory response of the gastric glands to sham feeding (Karp, 1948). The fear that mepacrine may possibly cause a tendency to hæmorrhage in patients with gastric ulcer owing to its vasodilatory action was not borne out in persons taking suppressive mepacrine. Hawking (1944) showed that intramuscular or subcutaneous injection of mepacrine caused necrosis less than but similar to that found after injection of quinine.

The action of mepacrine on enzymes is discussed on p. 534. At one period during the war it was feared that mepacrine might decrease the ceiling for oxygen of aeroplane pilots. Such is not the case, nor is there any suggestion that mepacrine affects the eyesight of pilots (Abbey and Lawrence, 1946).

Pick and Hunter (1944), by measuring electro-cortical potentials in cats, came to the conclusion that mepacrine has a depressant action on the brain, the action being related to the concentration of mepacrine present in the brain.

Excretion of Mepacrine

Metabolic degradation products of mepacrine have been isolated in the blood and urine as the result of analytical processes involving differences in solubilities (Brodie and Udenfriend, 1943b ; Craig, 1943).

The main method of excretion both in man and animals is probably by the fæces, but some is found in the urine (Tropp and Weise, 1933 ; Farinaud *et al.*, 1939 ; Dearborn *et al.*, 1943). Tropp and Weise (1933) believed that 50 to 70 per cent. of the drug administered appeared in the urine, but Kehar (1935a and b) suggested that the substances found in the urine were largely disintegration products. Scudi and Jelinek (1944) isolated four separate fractions from the urines of dogs receiving mepacrine. One of these, Fraction A, consisted of unchanged mepacrine dihydrochloride and a non-fluorescent material ; Fraction B contained a compound resembling mepacrine but possessing a phenolic —OH group, which may have replaced the methoxy radical ; Fraction B contained another derivative, possibly representing a partial side-chain degeneration product ; Fraction C contained yet another acridine derivative probably with a phenolic group. From the urine of human beings given the commercial DL-form of mepacrine, only the L-isomer has been isolated (Hammick and Chambers, 1945). This L-isomer is accompanied by degradation products believed to be identical with those in dog urine. King *et al.* (1946a) found that by extraction of alkalinised human urine with ethylene dichloride and subsequent purification and chromatographic distribution seven fractions could be characterised spectrophotometrically. Fractions 2 and 4 are unchanged mepacrine, the other fractions are diphenylamine derivatives. Scudi and Jelinck's Fraction B1 is 2-chloro-5-amino-7-hydroxy-acridine (Hammick and Mason, 1945 ; King *et al.*, 1946a) Other products have been identified by polarographic comparison with known samples of these compounds as 2-chloro-5-(4′-diethylamino-1′-methylbutylamino)-7-hydroxyacridine,   2-chloro-5-amino-7-methoxyacridine and 2 - chloro - 5 - amino - 7 - hydroxyacridine (Hammick and Firth, 1944 ; Hammick and Mason, 1945). Acridanes unsubstituted in the 5 : 10 positions are not excretion products of mepacrine (Tárnoky, 1950).

Jailer *et al.* (1947) studied the effects of giving alkalis, sodium bicarbonate, acid salts and ammonium chloride on the urinary excretion of mepacrine. The amount excreted when the acid salt was given was from fourteen to twenty-five times that excreted in the " alkali period." Acid and alkali made relatively little difference to the plasma mepacrine level. Similar experimental results were obtained with chloroquine and sontoquine. These results are thought to indicate that while some of the drug is excreted by the glomerulus, more is excreted by the proximal convoluted tubules. Some water is absorbed both in the convoluted tubules and in the loop of Henle, while in the distal convoluted tubules the concentration of the drug becomes equal to that in the fluid surrounding the tubules, varying, however, according to the respective pH's of the two fluids. With rapidly excreted drugs like chloroquine or sontoquine it should be possible to increase the rate of excretion by giving ammonium chloride if toxic symptoms occur. As the rate of mepacrine excretion is slow the administration of ammonium chloride would not be effective in cases of mepacrine intoxication. The length of time during which mepacrine or its fluorescent degradation products can be detected in the urine is subject to considerable individual variation, as is shown by the results reported from Malaya by Field, Niven and Hodgkin (1937).

EXCRETION OF MEPACRINE IN THE URINE AFTER CESSATION OF SUPPRESSIVE TREATMENT IN MAN. FLUORESCENCE DUE TO MEPACRINE AND ITS PRODUCTS IN THE URINE.
(Field, Niven, and Hodgkin, 1937)

Period after cessation of suppressive treatment.	Number of samples examined.	Strong.	Moderate.	Weak.	Absent.
1 week	50	17	23	10	0
2 weeks	47	4	24	16	3
3 ,,	46	2	7	26	11
4 ,,	41	0	2	26	13
5 ,,	41	1	0	3	37
6 ,,	48	0	0	3	45
7 ,,	20	0	0	0	20

The rate of excretion of mepacrine appears to vary in different species. In the fowl the rate is more rapid than in the rabbit, a fact which may be correlated with the finding that mepacrine is three times more toxic for the rabbit than for the hen.

Mepacrine is also excreted in the bile. Annegers *et al.* (1943) gave mepacrine to dogs with biliary fistulæ and recovered 4·8 per cent. of the dose administered from the bile when the latter was not returned to the intestine and 8·0 per cent. when it was returned to the intestine. The urinary excretion in these animals was 4·0 per cent. without the return of the bile to the intestine and 5·2 per cent. when bile was returned to the intestine. Mepacrine did not appear in the fæces of intact dogs. There is very slight circulation from bile to intestine, thence to liver and then to bile again. In two patients with biliary fistulæ the concentration was two to three times that in whole blood (Army Malaria Research Unit, 1946b). In individual dogs considerable variations were found in the output of cholic acid during the administration of mepacrine, but on the average the depression in output was only 2 per cent. De Langen and Storm (1935) believed that in persons with depleted glycogen in the liver mepacrine could produce urobilinuria. This has not been confirmed.

In man, the Army Malaria Research Unit (1946d) found that only small amounts of mepacrine were excreted in the fæces after intramuscular injection ; when, however, a daily dose of 100 mgm. was given by mouth nearly 30 per cent. of the dose was excreted in the fæces by some subjects though in others the fæcal output was much smaller. Since mepacrine can be found in the fæces after intramuscular or intravenous injection, fæcal output is not directly related to non-absorption of the orally administered drug. No close relationship exists between fæcal output and either the concentrations in whole blood and plasma or the urinary excretion.

The concentration of mepacrine in the sweat is about the same as that in whole blood, but it is doubtful whether any significant amount is thus excreted, even in the tropics. The saliva also contains concentrations approximately the same as that in whole blood but the concentration in the semen (400 to 1,100 μgm. per litre) is two to four times that in whole blood (Army Malaria Research Unit, 1946b).

Taggart (1946) has shown in a series of 9-aminoacridines closely related to mepacrine that variations in the length and character of the side-chain produce marked differences in plasma drug concentrations, in the extent of plasma binding and tissue localisation, and in the rate of degradation by the tissues. Plasma binding and tissue localisation are greatest when a butyl group separates the nitrogens of the side-chain : these properties are still further enhanced by branching of the alkyl group. The chloro nuclear substituent exerts its greatest effect in promoting tissue localisation, whereas the methoxy substituent seems only to increase the rate of degradation.

Taggart suggests that within this series antimalarial activity depends not on one factor but on the cumulative effects of plasma concentration, plasma binding, tissue localisation, and rate of metabolic degradation.

Estimation of Mepacrine in the Blood, Tissues and Urine

Before 1939 a considerable number of methods had been elaborated for estimating mepacrine in the urine, blood or tissues (Green, 1932 ; Tropp and Weise, 1933 ; Hecht, 1933, 1936 ; Wats and Ghosh, 1934 ; Hicks, 1935 ; Schechter and Taylor, 1936 ; Chopra and Roy, 1935 ; Chopra, Sen and Roy, 1937 ; Chopra and Roy, 1936 ; Weise, 1937, and Gentzkow, 1938). In general these methods consist in extraction with an immiscible solvent, evaporation of the solvent by an acid, and comparison of the colour or of the fluorescence of the resulting solution with appropriate standards.

These techniques are open to serious objections and further methods were elaborated by Masen (1943), Brodie and Udenfriend (1943b) and Brodie *et al.* (1947a, b), Auerbach and Eckert (1944), Lewis (1944) and Lange and Matzner (1946) ; only the method of Brodie and Udenfriend attempts to differentiate between mepacrine and the fluorescent metabolic products which may be present in blood and certainly occur in urine. Masen (1943) extracts the material with an alkaline mixture of *iso*propyl and *iso*butyl alcohol, extracts with sodium hydroxide and finally takes up the residue with acidified *iso*propyl alcohol : the fluorescence of the sample is then compared with that of prepared standards in a suitable photofluorimeter. Brodie and Udenfriend (1943b) extract with ethylene dichloride, and after washing with sodium hydroxide the residue is taken up by lactic acid. Fluorescence is then estimated as before. When plasma estimations are to be made ammonium oxalate or any salt mixture containing ammonia must not be used as an anticoagulant for ammonia displaces mepacrine from leucocytes, thus increasing the apparent plasma concentration (Army Malaria Research Unit, 1945a). Heparin, sodium citrate or potassium oxalate are suitable anticoagulants.

Methods for field examinations were elaborated by Yudkin (1945a and b) and King and Gilchrist (1945a and b). Yudkin adsorbs mepacrine and its metabolites from the urine by means of silica gel. The method is non-specific. King and Gilchrist modified Masen's method, the coloured solution being compared with a coloured disc in the Lovibond comparator. Mepacrine clearance from plasma is directly proportional to the rate of ammonia excretion in the urine (Army Malaria Research Unit, 1945c). This fact has been made the basis of a field method for plasma mepacrine concentrations (Brown and Rennie, 1945 ; Army Malaria Research Unit, 1945a). If the urinary mepacrine and urinary ammonia are known, the plasma mepacrine can be calculated from the formula $PM = K \times \dfrac{UM}{UNH_3}$. Where K is a constant; PM is the plasma mepacrine concentration in microgrammes per litre, UM is the urinary mepacrine concentration in microgrammes per litre, UNH_3 is mgm. of nitrogen per 100 ml. of urine. Brown and Rennie (1945) find that the constant K varies slightly with different dosage regimes of mepacrine. K should be calculated afresh for each course of mepacrine by first carrying out a few plasma mepacrine determinations.

Lange and Matzner (1946) used an ultra-violet light of main wavelength 3,600 Å to detect mepacrine in the skin and nails, since mepacrine in these tissues gives rise to a green fluorescence which can be determined photometrically. The concentration in the skin increases slowly during treatment and is independent of plasma concentrations. It continues as a rule to rise for two to five days after treatment. Deposition in the nails also occurs during treatment and a series of courses of mepacrine given at intervals produces bands of fluorescence in the nails. By examining the nails under ultra-violet light it should therefore be possible to determine whether suppressive mepacrine therapy has been evaded.

Chloroquine and other 4-Aminoquinolines

As the result of Russian (Galperin, 1944), French, and German observations on the antimalarial activity of 4-aminoquinolines, intensive pharmacological and chemotherapeutic tests were carried out in America. Including chloroquine (SN 7,618), the 4-aminoquinolines shown in the table on the opposite page have been studied pharmacologically (Berliner *et al.*, 1948).

Absorption from the gastro-intestinal tract is complete or almost complete, as is indicated by the small amount of drug which can be obtained from the stools.

Survey No.	Nuclear substituents.	Substituent on 4-amino group.
SN 3,294	6-methoxy	diethylamino-1'-methylbutyl
SN 6,911	3-methyl-7-chloro	diethylamino-1'-methylbutyl
SN 7,135	2-methyl-7-chloro	diethylamino-1'-methylbutyl
SN 7,373	7-bromo	diethylamino-1'-methylbutyl
SN 7,618	7-chloro	diethylamino-1'-methylbutyl
SN 8,137	7-chloro	diethylamino-2'-hydroxypropyl
SN 9,584	7-chloro	diethylamino propyl
SN 10,751	7-chloro	α-diethylamino-*o*-cresol
SN 10,960	7-chloro	diethylamino-3-hydroxybutyl
SN 13,425	7-chloro	1'-ethyl-4'-piperidyl

Plasma concentrations of chloroquine on a given dosage are ten to twenty times higher than in the case of mepacrine, but plasma concentrations of chloroquine tend to be higher than those of other 4-aminoquinolines. Concentrations of SN 10,751 are low and even lower than those indicated in the table (Berliner *et al.*, 1948), since the measurement includes a fluorescent metabolic product :—

RELATIONSHIP BETWEEN PLASMA DRUG CONCENTRATION AND DAILY ORAL DOSES OF 4-AMINOQUINOLINES (Berliner *et al.*, 1948)

Drug.	Daily dose (mgm.). [Mean plasma drug concentration μgm./litre].			
	50.	100.	200.	300.
SN 3,294	—	—	—	112
SN 6,911 (sontoquine)	—	—	107	179
SN 7,135	—	—	—	176
SN 7,618 (chloroquine)	22	49	110	176
SN 8,137	16	37	73	98
SN 9,584	19	37	68	126
SN 10,751	3·6	9·3	19	34

SN 3,294 is 6-methoxy-4(4'-diethylamino-1'-methylbutylamino)-quinoline.

The 4-aminoquinolines in the plasma are bound to a considerable extent to the non-diffusible constituents of the plasma although SN 10,751 alone is bound to as great a degree as mepacrine. *In vitro* the percentage of drug bound varies widely. Breathing 10 per cent. carbon dioxide over a two-hour period, thereby causing the blood pH to fall from 7·4 to 6·9, produces a two-fold increase in the concentration of chloroquine in red cells and plasma but no change in the concentration in leucocytes or muscle (Jailer *et al.*, 1948). The amounts of the 4-aminoquinolines found in the tissues follow the dose administered and are similar to the general pattern produced by mepacrine though variations occur between individual aminoquinolines. The smallest amounts of chloroquine are found in plasma ; next come red cells and nervous tissues with ten to twenty-five times the amount in plasma, followed in ascending order by heart, kidney, lung, and liver. The relative concentrations of mepacrine, chloroquine, and SN 3,294 are shown in the table :—

DISTRIBUTION OF 4-AMINOQUINOLINES IN PLASMA AND TISSUES OF RATS COMPARED WITH MEPACRINE (Berliner *et al.*, 1948)

	Mepacrine.	SN 3,294.	Chloroquine.
Days of drug administration . .	10	10	10
Plasma drug concentration, μgm./l .	134	170	157
Tissue/plasma concentration ratio :			
Red cells	2·9	2·9	1·9
Whole blood	7·0	4·1	3·7
Brain	27·6	5·9	31·0
Muscle	194	77	44
Heart	1,420	93	150
Kidney	3,000	100	670
Lung	4,070	150	640
Liver	6,380	130	420

The relative concentrations in plasma, red cells, and whole blood of the rat demonstrate a limited localisation in red cells and a greater localisation in leucocytes. In man, plasma drug levels indicate that the distribution is qualitatively similar though the metabolic rate may differ. SN 9,584 has a concentration in the central nervous system two to three times that of the other 4-aminoquinolines.

All 4-aminoquinolines are rapidly eliminated but, like mepacrine, chloroquine is degraded so that only from 10 to 25 per cent. of the daily oral dose is excreted in the urine. Excretion is increased by acidification and decreased by alkalinisation of the urine though the changes are not as marked as with mepacrine (Jailer *et al.*, 1947). Craig *et al.* (1948), by various fractionation procedures mainly involving the " counter-current " distribution method, found that 4-aminoquinolines yield substances in the urine in which an ethyl group is missing. Deethylation of SN 9,584 and of chloroquine produces compounds which are active in avian malarias. In addition to the formation of the corresponding secondary amines other structural changes may occur (Wiselogle, 1946). Chloroquine probably undergoes a different metabolic breakdown in the monkey, dog, and rat. No data are available on the rates of degradation of individual 4-aminoquinolines. The rates of metabolic degradation and excretion, together with the degree of prior tissue localisation, determine the rate at which plasma drug concentrations fall following the termination of therapy. As seen from the table, chloroquine has a greater persistence in the body than the other 4-aminoquinolines.

RATE OF DISAPPEARANCE OF 4-AMINOQUINOLINES FROM PLASMA DURING A FIVE-DAY PERIOD (Berliner *et al.*, 1948)

Drug.	Number of patients.	Plasma concentrations.		Percentage remaining at 5 days.
		3 hours after the last dose, μgm./l.	5 days after the last dose, μgm./l.	
SN 3,294 . . .	5	214	51	24
SN 6,911 (sontoquine)	4	220	50	23
SN 7,135 . . .	4	201	56	27
SN 7,618 (chloroquine)	6	28	15	53
SN 8,137 . .	10	31	9	29
SN 9,584 . . .	6	25	10	40

The greater persistence of chloroquine is of importance in relation to suppressive dosage.

The method of counter-current distribution appears of particular value for the study of 4-aminoquinolines as well as other antimalarials (Craig *et al.*, 1948 ; Titus *et al.*, 1947).

There is no evidence that chloroquine causes abortion or miscarriage in the pregnant female and, unlike mepacrine, none of the 4-aminoquinolines stains the skin.

Apparent acid dissociation exponents ($\mu = 0\cdot1$; $30°$) for a series of 4-aminoquinolines with identical side-chains (1-methyl-4-diethylamino-butyl) attached to the amino group have been worked out by Irvin and Irvin (1946, 1947). The distinctive substituents and the corresponding values of pK_1 (aromatic nuclei) are :—

$$\begin{aligned}
&\text{6-methyl} &&= 8\cdot75 \\
&\text{6-chloro} &&= 8\cdot06 \\
&\text{2-methyl-7-chloro} &&= 8\cdot51 \\
&\text{3-methyl-7-chloro} &&= 7\cdot28
\end{aligned}$$

pK_2 (diethylamino group) is $10\cdot0$ in each case.

Pamaquin and other 8-Aminoquinoline Derivatives

Pamaquin and other water-soluble 8-aminoquinolines are rapidly absorbed from the gastro-intestinal tract, 85 to 95 per cent. being absorbed within two hours of administration, as shown by the rise in the plasma concentration of the drug after a single oral dose.

Pamaquin is rapidly destroyed when incubated at $37°$ C. in a suspension of fæces, but differences in solubility between various salts of pamaquin do not seem to condition the rate of absorption.

After oral ingestion of pamaquin in monkeys there is a rapid rise in plasma concentration, the peak being reached within one to two hours, after which an equally rapid fall occurs. In man also there is a rapid disappearance from the blood stream, for Zubrod *et al.* (1948) found that upon termination of a fifteen-minute infusion of 20 mgm. of pamaquin only 5 to 6 per cent. could be accounted for in the circulating blood.

Such a rapid disappearance must represent localisation in the tissues rather than metabolism and excretion. In man, considerable variations in plasma concentrations are found in different

PLASMA PAMAQUIN LEVELS THREE HOURS AFTER ADMINISTRATION
OF 20 MGM. (BASE) OF THE DRUG (Zubrod *et al.*, 1948)

Patient.	Plasma pamaquin level after oral dose μgm./litre.	Plasma pamaquin level after intramuscular dose μgm./l.
I	64	84
	69	84
	78	
	75	
II	112	105
	112	77
III	94	91
	120	131
	121	
IV	191	157
	198	170

persons, but in general plasma concentrations are proportional to the oral dose ingested. Thus doses of 3 mgm. per kgm. yield plasma levels of from 20 to 360 μgm. per litre, doses of 6 mgm. per kgm. levels of 20 to 570 μgm. per litre, and doses of 24 mgm. per kgm. levels of 640 to 3,240 μgm. per litre. With small and relatively non-toxic doses the peak plasma level tends to decrease as the period of treatment is prolonged. At the end of eight hours, after a daily dose of 30 mgm., minimal plasma concentrations are negligible, and after a dose of 60 mgm. very small. Such rapid fluctuations can be minimised by giving divided doses at intervals of not more than four hours. In the case of other 8-aminoquinolines plasma levels appear to be related to the side-chain structures of these substances. Compounds with side-chains ending in a primary amino group give lower levels than those with secondary amino groups and these, in turn, yield lower levels than compounds with tertiary amino groupings. Exceptionally high plasma levels are obtained with compounds having terminal 2-piperidyl groups. Both peak and trough plasma levels are greater with these compounds than with the corresponding alkyl or dialkylamino derivatives. Nuclear substitution also affects plasma levels. Compounds without nuclear substituents give as high peak plasma levels as the 6-methoxy compounds and considerably greater trough levels. Compounds with a 6-hydroxy substituent yield very low levels.

Hecht (1935) noted that concentrations of 8-aminoquinolines in the tissues are greater than in the plasma. The concentrations in the dog after a single dose of 10 mgm. per kgm. of pamaquin hydroiodide were found by Zubrod *et al.* (1948) to be as follows :—

Tissue.	Tissue pamaquin concentration. μgm./kgm.	Ratio : tissue pamaquin concentration to plasma pamaquin concentration.
Plasma　.　.　.	610	—
Whole blood.　.　.	814	1·3
Liver　.　.　.　.	22,900	37·6
Muscle　.　.　.	1,360	2·2
Brain　.　.　.　.	6,460	10·6
Spleen　.　.　.	725	1·2
Lung　.　.　.　.	15,830	26·0
Heart　.　.　.　.	3,690	6·0

It is of interest that with comparable dosage the concentrations of pamaquin and plasmocid in the brain are practically the same, though the latter drug is far more toxic for the central nervous system.

Archibald and Weisiger (1948) suggest that the rapid disappearance of pamaquin from the blood may be due to the fact that it reacts rapidly with naturally occurring aldehydes or ketones in the host and parasite. Pamaquin undoubtedly reacts in aqueous solution with one molecule of formaldehyde and one equivalent of acid. A strongly fluorescent quaternary salt is formed which is twenty times more toxic than pamaquin and cannot couple with diazo-reagents.

Excretion occurs in the urine, but on serial oral dosage of 60 mgm. daily only about 1 per cent. of administered pamaquin is found in the urine. Similar data are available for plasmocid, 8-(diethylaminopropylamino)-6-methoxy quinoline (SN 3,115).

The pathway of metabolism of pamaquin is not known, but there is evidence for the presence of two metabolic intermediates. Metabolic alteration appears to occur very quickly.

After intramuscular injection of 20 mgm. doses of pamaquin

the maximum concentration in plasma is reached earlier than after oral administration, usually in from thirty to sixty minutes ; the concentrations also are greater, being from 200 to 400 μgm. per litre. At the end of three hours and thereafter the plasma drug concentration is approximately the same as when the oral route is used. Variability in plasma concentration from patient to patient is noted after intramuscular as well as after oral administration, but the same individual always reproduces the same time of plasma curve (Zubrod *et al.*, 1948). Mepacrine increases the plasma concentration of pamaquin, the maximal concentrations being many times higher than when pamaquin is given alone : in addition the rate of disappearance is greatly reduced. Doses as small as 20 mgm. of mepacrine are capable of producing this phenomenon. Quinine does not produce any similar increase, and it is very doubtful whether chloroquine does so.

Nandi (1940) believes that pamaquin increases the oxygen uptake of the tissues. Jones (1949) has shown that pamaquin and pentaquine in a concentration of 5×10^{-5} M inhibit acid production under anaerobic conditions from glucose by rat-brain extract. Quinine, mepacrine, chloroquine, and proguanil cause no such inhibition even in a concentration of 2×10^{-3} M. The same inhibition takes place when hexose diphosphate is the substrate, when fluoride is present in a concentration of 0·02 M, and when arsenate is substituted for phosphate in the system. Thus these compounds interfere with the conversion of hexose diphosphate to phosphoglyceric acid by animal tissues. Attempts to correlate the power to inhibit acid production under anaerobic conditions with antimalarial activity among the 8-aminoquinolines give no consistent results. De Langen and Storm (1934) found that when injected intravenously in monkeys as a 0·1 per cent. solution a fall in blood pressure occurs. Cardiac arrhythmia was produced by Eichholtz (1935). Tsikimanauri (1931) reported that in dogs and rabbits therapeutic doses cause tachycardia, slight elevation of blood pressure and increased rate and depth of respiration. In animals with the vagi sectioned bradycardia follows pamaquin administration. Pamaquin probably acts directly on the vagal centre. Heimann and Shapiro (1943) found that pamaquin could cause electro-cardiographic changes. The amplitude of all, but especially the T wave, is increased. In concentrations of 1 in 300,000 to 1 in 500,000 pamaquin contracts the isolated uterus of the dog, cat, and guinea-pig : in concentrations of 1 in 100,000 it relaxes the uterine muscle. *In vitro*, pamaquin produces methæmoglobin more readily in hæmolysed than in non-hæmolysed blood. In a concentration of 0·01 per cent. pamaquin causes methæmoglobin formation and slight hæmolysis (Le Heux and de Lind van Wijngaarden, 1929).

Pentaquine, 6-methoxy-8-(5′-*iso*propylamino-amylamino)-quinoline is generally used as the diphosphate, containing 75 per cent. of the base. The drug is rapidly and completely absorbed from the gastro-intestinal tract of the experimental animal. In the dog and monkey, absorption of from 80 to 90 per cent. of the dose administered occurs in two hours. After a single dose the maximal concentration in the plasma occurs in from 90 to 120 minutes ; thereafter the concentration steadily declines ; after six to eight hours traces only are found in the plasma.

After a single dose of 20 mgm. pentaquine, or after three to four doses at eight-hourly intervals, a stable plasma level is reached only after a minimum of six hours and probably more often not till eight hours after the last dose. At such times the level is frequently too low to be estimated accurately by the method employed. The peak plasma level, usually about 120 μgm. per litre, is found about two and a half hours after a single dose. The average pentaquine plasma level is usually higher when quinine and pentaquine are given concurrently than when pentaquine is given alone. A stable plasma pentaquine level is reached approximately on the third or fourth day of treatment ; a stable pamaquin level is not reached till the eighth day of treatment. After the last dose of pentaquine detectable amounts are still present in the plasma forty-eight hours after the last dose, and in one case (Monk, 1948) traces were present four days after the last dose. When pamaquin is given the plasma rarely shows significant amounts longer than thirty-six hours after discontinuing treatment with quinine and pamaquin.

If a stable level of drug in the plasma indicates a stable level in the tissues, and if this is of importance in obtaining a radical cure of benign tertian malaria, then pentaquine would seem to have an

obvious advantage over pamaquin when the drugs are administered at eight-hourly intervals.

The apparent dissociation exponents for pamaquin were first
investigated by Christophers and Fulton (1940), Christophers
(1937) having previously obtained apparent dissociation exponents
for quinine. Kolthoff (1925) had previously obtained similar
figures for quinine. Further investigations were carried out by
Irvin and Irvin (1946, 1948).

Data for pamaquin, its structural isomer, 6-methoxy-4-(4'-
diethylamino-1'-methylbutylamino)-quinoline, quinine, and 4-(6'-
methoxyquinolyl)-α-piperidylcarbinol are shown in the table, the
spectrophotometric absorption data for pamaquin and for
SN 3,294 in aqueous solutions of sulphuric acid being formulated
in terms of the acidity function scale of Hammett and the extended
pH scale of Michaelis.

ACID/DISSOCIATION EXPONENTS (30° C.) OF VARIOUS DERIVATIVES
OF QUINOLINE (Irvin and Irvin, 1948)

Compound.	Ionic strength 0·1.			
	pK'_s.	pK'_1.	pK'_2.	$pK_{(H_2SO)}$.
Quinine	4·33	4·32	8·4	(scale of Michaelis)
Pamaquin	3·49	3·48	10·2	— 1·33
6-Methoxy-4-(4'-diethylamino-1'-methyl-butylamino)-quinoline (SN 3,294) .	8·73	8·68	10·2	— 7·83
4-(6'-Methoxyquinolyl)-α-piperidylcarbinol (SN 2,157)	4·34	4·36	9·3	

These values for pK'_1 and pK'_2 for quinine are in agreement with
Christophers (1937), who reported 4·21 for pK'_1 and 8·36 for pK'_2
at 20° C. Kolthoff (1925) obtained values of 4·50 and 8·23 respectively at 15° C. The value for pK_s, the spectrophotometrically
determined dissociation exponent for the proton exchange concerned with the aromatic nucleus of quinine, is practically identical
with the corresponding value of pK_1 determined potentiometrically. The proton acceptor involved in the equilibrium evaluated
by pK_s (= pK'_1) is almost certainly the nitrogen atom of the

quinoline ring : the proton acceptor in quinine involved in the proton exchange evaluated potentiometrically as pK'_2 is the quinuclidine nitrogen atom.

The values reported by Christophers and Fulton (1940) for the apparent dissociation exponents of pamaquin were 3·55 for pK'_1 and 10·13 for pK'_2 at 20° C., and the ionic strength was about 0·009 in evaluating pK'_1 and 0·0002 in determining pK'_2. These figures agree closely with those given by Irvin and Irvin (1948). With pamaquin the proton acceptor corresponding to pK'_s ($= pK'_1$) is uncertain as both the nitrogen of the quinoline ring and the 8-amino nitrogen are possible acceptors.

Figures for the 4-aminoquinoline derivative 6-methoxy-4(4′-diethylamino-1′-methylbutylamino)-quinoline (SN 3,294) are given by Irvin and Irvin (1947, 1948). The marked strengthening of the acceptance of the first proton by the aromatic nucleus of SN 3,294 and the great weakness of the second proton, as contrasted with the proton exchange of pamaquin, is attributable to the powerful resonance of the monopolar cation of the aromatic nucleus of SN 3,294. The resonance hybrid of this species probably receives contributions both from Kekulé and quinonoid structures, as first suggested by Albert and Goldacre (1944) for the parent 4-amino-quinoline and emphasised by Irvin and Irvin (1947).

Estimation of Pamaquin and Related Compounds

The method of estimating pamaquin based on coupling with diazonium salts, as proposed by Brodie *et al.* (1947b), has been modified by Jones *et al.* (1948) :—

Twenty ml. of heptane and 0·5 ml. of *iso*butyl alcohol are placed in a 60-ml. glass-stoppered bottle : 10 ml. of plasma and 10 ml. of 0·1 N NaOH are added and the mixture shaken for ten minutes. The mixture is then transferred to a 50-ml. centrifuge tube and centrifuged for five minutes. The water phase is aspirated and 15 ml. of the heptane phase is transferred to a 40-ml. glass-stoppered pointed centrifuge tube containing 0·5 ml. of coupling reagent (diazotised sulphanilic acid). The mixture is then shaken for five minutes and centrifuged. The heptane layer is removed by aspiration. Not less than 0·3 ml. of the water layer is transferred to a special microcuvette and the transmission read in a Coleman spectrophotometer at a wave-length of 480 millimicra. This method can be used for all 8-amino-quinolines.

Irvin and Irvin (1948) describe a fluorimetric method of estimating pamaquin : it has also been applied to SN 3,294, 6-methoxy-4-(4'-diethylamino-1'-methylbutylamino)quinoline and SN 13,276, 6 - methoxy - 8 - (5' - *iso*propylaminoamylamino) - quinoline. The method is based on the fluorescence of these compounds in concentrated sulphuric acid and is of interest as it can be applied to mixtures of any one of the above compounds with quinine. The changes in fluorescence of quinine and pamaquin in concentrated aqueous solutions of sulphuric acid are in opposite directions.

Proguanil (Paludrine)

Proguanil (chloriguane, diguanyl, bigumal, 4888) is N_1-*p*-chlorophenyl-N_5-*iso*propylbiguanide, but the term was originally applied to *p*-chlorophenyl-N_5-methyl-N-*iso*propylbiguanide (4430): for such change of nomenclature there is no scientific excuse. The compound is often also referred to as paludrine and chlorguanide (American medical Association, 1948). The monoacetate was originally employed but the monohydrochloride is now generally used. The monoacetate contains 81 per cent. of the base and is soluble in water to the extent of about 2 per cent. : the monohydrochloride contains 87·4 per cent. of the base and is about half as soluble as the monoacetate. Solutions of both salts are stable when boiled. The acetate contains 79·5 per cent. by weight of the base, the hydrochloride 86·5 per cent. Proguanil salts are white crystalline powders, odourless, and slightly bitter in taste. The anhydrous monohydrochloride has its melting point at 240° C. ; it is stable under normal conditions but is somewhat hygroscopic, and if exposed under moist tropical conditions the tablets are liable to disintegrate : hence they are best stored in a dry place in a closed container.

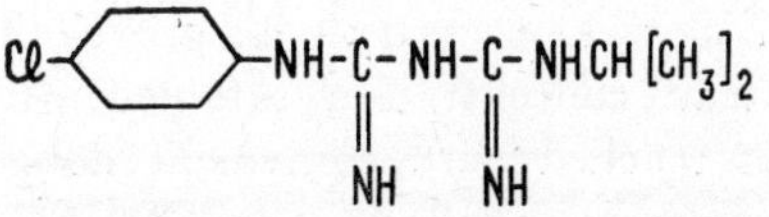

N_1-p-Chlorophenyl-N_5-isopropylbiguanide :
Proguanil (Paludrine : 4888)

The pharmacology of proguanil has been studied in man and in animals. Preliminary studies in man were published by Adams *et al.* (1945) and Maegraith *et al.* (1945, 1946a). More detailed results are provided by Maegraith *et al.* (1946b). After single oral doses of from 100 to 500 mgm. the maximum concentration is reached four hours after administration, the height of the maximum depending largely on the size of the dose. At each dose level there is some individual variation both in the maximum concentration and in the rate of disappearance of the drug. The plasma concentration after twenty-four hours is also related to the oral dose. This persistence of drug in the plasma following the higher single dose is probably of therapeutic importance (Maegraith *et al.*, 1946a). After single oral doses of 5 and 10 mgm. it is possible to detect proguanil in the plasma four hours later, the concentration being 6 μgm. per litre and from 17 to 22 μgm. per litre respectively. For corresponding dosages the plasma concentrations of proguanil are higher than those reached with mepacrine or 3349 (Spinks and Tottey, 1945b). When patients are given therapeutic doses of 50 or 500 mgm. twice daily at twelve-hourly intervals for fourteen days an irregular " plateau concentration " is reached at about the third day. This plateau concentration is between 300 and 500 μgm. per litre during a course of 500 μgm. twice daily and between 50 and 150 μgm. per litre on a course of 50 mgm. twice daily although individual variation occurs outside these limits. After the end of the course the reduction in plasma concentration is rapid, the concentration being below the limits of analysis within three to seven days. The disappearance of the drug from the plasma is more rapid on the lower dose schedule. The plateau concentration of proguanil is reached more rapidly than in the case of mepacrine, so that in view of the very low concentration of proguanil in the plasma which is effective therapeutically it is probable that a " loading dose " or " build up " is not as necessary with proguanil as with mepacrine. The plateau concentration attained with proguanil is higher than that reached with equivalent doses of mepacrine. On 100 mgm. mepacrine the plasma concentration averages after four to six weeks 25 μgm. per litre, compared with 50 to 150 μmg. of proguanil per litre. The existence of a plateau concentration in the plasma as a result of a therapeutic course does not affect the absorption and subsequent plasma concentration reached by further dosage. In other words, the tissues can in no sense be " saturated " with the drug even on the relatively high dosage of 500 mgm. twice daily, while the degradation and excretion of the drug apparently continues normally under such conditions.

PLASMA CONCENTRATIONS OF PROGUANIL (0·97 GM. OF BASE DAILY OR 13·6 GM. FOR FOURTEEN DAYS) AND CONCURRENTLY ADMINISTERED DRUGS (QUININE 23 GM. AND PENTAQUINE 0·84 GM. IN FOURTEEN DAYS). (Jones *et al.*, 1948)

Drug regime.	Range of mean concentration of proguanil in plasma. μgm./litre.	Range of mean concentration of concurrent drug in plasma. μgm./litre.
Proguanil alone . .	630–1,300	—
Proguanil and quinine .	770–1,200	6–13
Quinine alone . . .	—	3–10
Proguanil and pentaquine .	650–1,400	140–450
Pentaquine alone . .	—	29–49

Adams *et al.* (1945) noted the rapid disappearance of proguanil from the body within a week of the cessation of dosage although the drug is often detectable in the urine for a day or so later than in the blood. This rapid disappearance contrasts with the fate of mepacrine. Intravenous doses of 5 to 50 mgm. in physiological saline are followed by a very rapid fall in plasma concentration following injection. This rapid disappearance from the plasma of man has also been noted in the rat and mouse. It is probably indicative, in part at least, of a very rapid fixation in the tissues, but it is also associated with a rapid removal of the drug through the kidneys. When 50 mgm. proguanil is injected intravenously 6·65 mgm. is excreted in the urine in the first ninety minutes.

The ratio of whole blood concentration to plasma concentration remains constant at between 2 : 1 and 3 : 1 during the course of an experiment.

The distribution of proguanil in the tissues of man was investigated in two cases by Maegraith *et al.* (1946b). The drug is most

concentrated in the kidney and thereafter in the liver. Proguanil
thus differs from mepacrine and 3349, which are most concentrated
in the liver. The distribution of proguanil in the red cells and
leucocytes, as compared with plasma concentrations, is shown in
the table.

The administration of proguanil with other drugs such as mepacrine does not modify the plasma concentration of proguanil, as is
shown in the table.

THE DISTRIBUTION OF PROGUANIL AND MEPACRINE IN THE
BLOOD OF MAN (Maegraith *et al.*, 1946b)

	Proguanil.		Proguanil and Mepacrine.		Mepacrine.	
	μgm./l. of blood.	Percentage of blood content.	μgm/l. of blood.	Percentage of blood content.	μgm/l. of blood.	Percentage of blood content.
Red cells .	831	73	820	79·4	28	13·5
Plasma .	154	13·6	147	14·2	21	10
Leucocytes	152	13·4	66	6·4	159	76·5

In a case of lymphatic leukæmia with a white cell count of
70,000 (over 80 per cent. lymphocytes) per c.mm. and an erythrocyte count of 2·8 million per c.mm., each white cell contained
seventy-three times the amount of drug held by an erythrocyte.
With mepacrine the individual white cell concentration is of the
order of 3,000 times that in the red cell. At 23° C. or 37° C. in
normal plasma about 70 to 80 per cent. of the proguanil in solution
is bound, presumably to the protein. This is the same degree of
binding as is found with mepacrine.

Adams *et al.* (1945), in preliminary investigations, found that
on a dosage of 50 to 500 mgm. proguanil daily for fourteen days
between 30 and 50 per cent. of the drug is excreted in the urine.
The substance isolated from human urine is unchanged proguanil
(Spinks and Tottey, 1946a). Further investigations by Maegraith
et al. (1946b) show that after a single oral dose of 50 to 500 mgm.,
urinary excretion amounts to 40 to 60 per cent. of the oral dose :
the amount of the drug falls to less than 1 per cent. of the admini-

stered dose in from three to five days after dosage, the period decreasing with the dose. After full therapeutic doses of 50 mgm. and 500 mgm. twice daily for fourteen days, the drug disappears from the urine in four to six days and six to nine days respectively. The drug stored in the tissues is probably not very firmly fixed and is degraded rapidly. In comparison with mepacrine and 3349, proguanil is more rapidly and more completely eliminated by the kidneys, but the excretion in the urine is very similar to that of quinine ; with quinine 25 to 66 per cent. of the intake is eliminated in the urine and all excretion is over two days after a single dose and in about one week after repeated dosing.

Whereas in the case of mepacrine the urinary excretion is a direct function of the urinary ammonia content and of the plasma mepacrine, no such relationship occurs with proguanil and no close correlation between plasma concentration and urinary concentration could be found. The use of ammonium oxalate as an anticoagulant does not interfere with the distribution of proguanil between plasma and cellular elements as it does in the case of mepacrine. The percentage of the total oral dosage of proguanil excreted in the fæces is of the same order after single doses of 100 and 500 mgm. as it is after repeated dosage : it accounts for about 10 per cent. of the ingested drug. It would therefore seem that as the percentage loss does not increase with the dosage the drug after oral administration is almost completely absorbed from the gut. The drug recovered from the fæces has probably been absorbed from the intestine and excreted into the intestine. Such excretion in the bile occurs with certain other antimalarial drugs, such as mepacrine (Hecht, 1933 ; Annegers *et al.*, 1943), quinine (Bernardbeig and Caujolle, 1935), and 3349 (Spinks and Tottey, 1946a). In the case of mepacrine and 3349, the fæcal excretion accounts for a higher proportion of the total excretion than does urinary excretion, but in the case of proguanil this state of affairs is reversed. Proguanil in plasma is present almost entirely as a singly-charged positive ion with a first pK about 10·9 : it thus differs very considerably from sulphaguanidine, which is unionised with a first pK about 2·5 (Bell and Roblin, 1942).

The pharmacology of proguanil in laboratory animals has been studied by Spinks (1946, 1947), Spinks *et al.* (1946), Butler *et al.*

(1947), Hughes and Schmidt (1947), and Schmidt *et al.* (1947). The results of all these investigations agree closely but differ to a certain extent from those obtained in man.

Proguanil is rapidly and completely absorbed from the gastro-intestinal tract of laboratory animals but somewhat more slowly than quinine, mepacrine, and chloroquine (Spinks, 1946 ; Hughes and Schmidt, 1947).

In the rat, after an oral dose of 80 mgm. per kgm. of body weight, the concentrations in whole blood and in plasma are low and are of the order of 2 and 0·75 mgm. per litre. In rats killed within twelve hours of a single oral dose the concentrations in the tissues are low but the amounts found in the lung, liver, spleen, and kidney are from ten to fifty times as high as those in the plasma. Somewhat higher concentrations in blood and plasma are noted than with 4430. In the mouse, after oral ingestion of 80 mgm. per kgm. of body weight, somewhat higher concentrations are found in the blood while the distribution in the tissues is similar to that in the rat. The oral administration of 80 mgm. per kgm. causes a certain number of deaths two to seven hours after ingestion, the acute lethal blood concentration being of the order of 10 mgm. per litre (Spinks, 1947). In the rabbit the concentration in the red cells is four to six times that in the plasma, whereas in the white cells it is ten to 100 times that in the plasma. Low concentrations in the brain suggest that proguanil does not pass the blood-brain barrier to any extent. Dogs and monkeys store considerably larger amounts in the organs than rats when given comparable doses. Proguanil disappears with extreme rapidity from the tissues after the end of treatment, and at the end of forty-eight hours only traces, if any, can be found. From experiments in mice and rabbits it is doubtful whether proguanil can pass the blood-brain barrier and gain access to the cerebrospinal fluid : in the chick it would appear to reach the brain more easily. After prolonged oral administration there is no tendency for proguanil to accumulate in the plasma, as in the case with mepacrine or chloroquine. Rats given 50 mgm. per kgm. daily for sixty days show levels in the liver, spleen, kidney, and lung of from 2·5 to 50 μgm. per kgm. With similar doses of chloroquine the figures are from 1,100 to 3,700 mgm. per kgm., and of mepacrine from

6,000 to 17,000 mgm. per kgm. In rats and rabbits proguanil is mainly excreted in the urine, though some may reach the small intestine by the bile : very little is excreted by the large intestines in the fæces. Not more than between 30 and 40 per cent. of proguanil ingested can be found in the excreta of laboratory animals. In the rabbit, following 80 mgm. per kgm. by mouth, 8·4 and 13·1 per cent. of the dose was found in urine and fæces : following 8 mgm. per kgm. intravenously, 22·6 and 3·1 per cent. Both in the rat and rabbit a considerable amount of proguanil must be metabolised. The pharmacological properties of proguanil are very similar to those of 4430.

The effects of intramuscular injections of proguanil in animals in doses comparable with those given to man have been examined by Innes (1947). Focal myonecrosis with an inflammatory reaction associated later with fibrosis was seen in sheep, calves, dogs and rabbits, the lesions being very similar to those produced by mepacrine (Hawking, 1943). As proguanil need be given intramuscularly only on those very rare occasions when oral or intravenous administration is impossible, the question of necrosis by proguanil hardly arises (Peeters, 1949).

Proguanil, like mepacrine and quinine, diminishes the action of the vagus on the heart. Burn and Vane (1949) showed that if isolated rabbits' auricles were exposed to proguanil the inhibitory effect of acetylcholine is gradually changed to a stimulation. This change is accompanied by a reduction in the rate and amplitude of the beat. Within seven to thirty-eight minutes after proguanil has been added the auricles cease to beat for periods up to one hour : during this period acetylcholine restarted the beat (Burn and Vane, 1949). Vane (1949) found that in addition to acetylcholine the following drugs restarted the contraction of the auricles : choline, carbaminoylcholine, acetyl-β-methyl-choline, Bovet's acetal compound, and adrenaline. Nicotine and benzoylcholine did not start the beat after treatment. Bülbring *et al.* (1949) have pointed out that whereas *P. gallinaceum* does not synthesise acetylcholine, *Trypanosoma rhodesiense*, which is unaffected by proguanil, does. In large doses in cats proguanil reduces or inhibits the secretion of acid in the stomach produced by histamine.

Burn and Vane (1948) have found that proguanil exerts an inhibitory action on the volume and acidity of gastric juice evoked by histamine. Replacing the *iso*propyl group of proguanil by a methyl group had no effect in abolishing this action in cats. Biguanide, *iso*propylbiguanide and di*iso*propylbiguanide were inactive but N_1-*p*-chlorophenyl-biguanide, N_1-*p*-methoxyphenyl-biguanide, and N_1-*p*-chlorophenyl-N_3-methyl-guanide were all active.

Vane *et al.* (1948) have shown that when 0·9 to 1·0 gm. of proguanil is given by mouth to men two hours before a test meal a significant reduction in the acidity of the gastric juice occurs. Similarly, Doll and Schneider (1948) found that when 1 gm. of proguanil hydrochloride was given two hours before the start of a gruel test meal there was a significant depression of more than 33 per cent. in the concentration of free acid during the first one and a half hours of the meal. No consistent effect was observed with doses up to 400 mgm. of proguanil acetate given intravenously on the gastric secretion in response to histamine.

These observations possibly explain why dogs fed on a diet containing proguanil become disinclined to eat (Hughes *et al.*, 1947), and why on very rare occasions some people, after a large dose or after taking the drug as a suppressive, suffer from loss of appetite or gastro-intestinal symptoms.

Proguanil, according to Vane (1949), antagonises the action of adrenaline on the perfused hind leg of the dog and on the blood pressure of the cat. The refractory period of the auricle is lengthened but the activity of proguanil is only about one-eighth that of quinidine. On the isolated perfused heart of the cat (Langendorff preparation) proguanil reduces the amplitude and rate of contraction as well as causing coronary dilatation. Proguanil abolishes the contraction of the isolated frog rectus muscle and the isolated guinea-pig ileum : in addition it inhibits the normal action of acetylcholine on the isolated rabbit auricle. Blaschko *et al.* (1947) found that the activity of certain cholinesterases, such as the pseudocholinesterase and benzoylcholinesterase of guinea-pig liver, is inhibited by proguanil.

The effects of vagal stimulation on the cat intestine and rabbit respiration were reduced as was the natural tonus of the intestine.

It had a curariform action on the cat sciatic-gastrocnemius, the rat phrenic nerve-diaphragm, and the perfused cervical ganglion preparations.

Proguanil causes vasodilatation of the perfused dog hind leg and in the cat. The dilatation is reduced by antihistamine agents, which suggests that proguanil may release histamine from the tissues. If this is so then the relationship between proguanil and histamine is not easy to understand. Proguanil potentiates the constrictor effect of histamine on the guinea-pig lungs but inhibits histamine-induced gastric secretion in cats. It also inhibits contraction of isolated guinea-pig ileum evoked by histamine.

MacIntosh and Paton (1947) found that certain biguanides and amidines also release histamine from the tissues.

Intravenous injection of proguanil 2·5 mgm. per kgm. of body weight in decerebrate and chloralosed cats causes, according to Davey (1946) :

(i) A transient fall in blood pressure roughly equivalent to that produced by the injection of 1 mgm. per kgm. of mepacrine.

(ii) An increase in the depth of respiration in the inspiratory phase.

(iii) A temporary increase in the intestinal movements, followed by inhibition.

Chen and Anderson (1947) contribute a few further facts to the pharmacology of proguanil. In anæsthetised cats it lowers the blood pressure and increases the respiratory rate. It relaxes the isolated uterus and intestine of the rabbit and also the isolated guinea-pig's intestine : the isolated guinea-pig's uterus, however, responds by contraction. Wiseman (1949) finds that proguanil hydrochloride in a concentration of 200 mgm. per 100 ml. will hæmolyse blood : the rate of hæmolysis depends on the area of glass with which the blood is in contact. Massart (1949) believes that proguanil interferes with cation exchange since it causes a progressive inhibition of the respiration of yeast cells. The inhibition is reversed by metallic ions such as magnesium and by non-toxic basic organic compounds such as spermine.

The Estimation of Proguanil

A method for the estimation of proguanil in biological fluids and tissues was first described by Spinks and Tottey (1945a and c) : the biguanidine molecule is converted by hydrolytic fission to p-chloroaniline which is then estimated colorimetrically by diazotisation and coupling with a dyestuffs end component to give an azo dye.   Later Spinks and Tottey (1946a) modified the method, the duration of hydrolysis being reduced from twelve to four hours.

A 1 per cent. solution of N-β-sulphatoethyl-m-toluidine is employed as coupling component : the solution becomes discoloured in daylight and must be kept in the dark.   A fresh solution must be prepared weekly and must be kept in an amber-coloured, glass-stoppered container : it should be colourless when used.   Proguanil standard solutions are prepared from pure anhydrous base and must be prepared freshly every two weeks, being stored in the refrigerator.

Plasma (5 to 10 ml.) is pipetted into a 30-ml. glass-stoppered bottle and treated with one-quarter of its volume of 40 per cent. sodium hydroxide.   The bottle is warmed at 50° C. for thirty minutes, cooled to room temperature and benzene ethanol (10 ml.) is added, shaken, then centrifuged at 4,000 r.p.m. for ten minutes. As large an aliquot as possible of the upper layer is withdrawn, suction being by vacuum.   The final solution should be colourless or pink.   The volume is noted and the benzene delivered into a glass-stoppered centrifuge-tube.   N/4 Hydrochloric acid (1·2 ml.) is added to the benzene and the tube stoppered and shaken vigorously for two minutes.   The stopper is removed, and the tube centrifuged for five minutes at 1,000 r.p.m.   The lower layer is removed, transferred to an ampoule which is sealed, autoclaved for four hours at 20 to 25 lb. pressure, and allowed to cool.   A 1-ml. aliquot is withdrawn into a tube graduated at 2 ml., and 0·1 per cent. sodium nitrite (0·1 ml.) is added and the tube is shaken. After ten minutes 1 per cent. N-β-sulphatoethyl-m-toluidine (0·2 ml.) is added, followed by 30 per cent. sodium acetate (0·4 ml.), the tube being shaken after each addition.   The yellow colour of the azo dye is changed to red after ten minutes by making up to volume with concentrated hydrochloric acid.   The colour obtained may be matched in either a photoelectric or a visual colorimeter.   If a photoelectric colorimeter is available a standard curve is constructed, using a filter with maximum transmission from 500 to 510 mμ. From such a curve of galvanometer readings against concentration of proguanil in μgm. per ml. the concentration in the final unknown aliquot is read off as y μgm. per ml. Then the concentration in the original plasma sample (c) is given by the formula

$$ c = \frac{y \times 1 \cdot 2 \times 10}{z \times v} \ \mu\text{gm./ml. (mgm./litre)} $$

where z is the aliquot of benzene, and v the volume of the plasma in ml. If a visual colorimeter is used, the standard most closely matching the unknown is chosen and the unknown read against it. The concentration, y μgm./ml. in the final acid aliquot, is then given by the formula

$$ y = \frac{\text{Reading of standard}}{\text{Reading of unknown}} \times s $$

where s is the concentration of the standard in μgm./ml. Samples should be read within one hour of preparation since a yellow colour, probably due to nitroso derivatives, slowly develops.

This method is highly sensitive and of very considerable accuracy, but it is essentially a laboratory procedure, especially as the hydrolysis is most effectively carried out under autoclave conditions.

Gage and Rose (1946) evolved a somewhat simpler method based on the fact that biguanidines are known to form co-ordination complexes with metals such as copper. Proguanil is capable of forming a complex with copper which is insoluble in water but soluble in hydrocarbon solvents such as benzene. When isolated and characterised the complex is found to consist of two molecules of proguanil associated with one atom of metal and one molecule of water. The complex is a dull purple, unstable under acid conditions but more stable in alkali. When a solution of the complex in an organic solvent is shaken with an aqueous solution of diethyldithiocarbamate the characteristic colour of this reagent with copper is produced. The intensity of the colour is dependent on the amount of copper and hence of proguanil present in the test solution. The method is satisfactory for amounts from 5 to

100 mgm. of proguanil per litre in urine. If more than this is present the urine must be diluted. Acid-washed 6 × ⅝ in. test tubes fitted with rubber stoppers are used for extraction of the copper-complex into an organic solvent. The rubber stoppers are well washed and boiled in distilled water before use.

The test is as follows :—

Reagents. (i) Copper sulphate AR (0·5 gm.) and ammonium chloride (1·33 gm.) dissolved in 100 ml. distilled water.

(ii) Sodium diethyldithiocarbamate : 0·1 per cent. aqueous solution. This solution does not keep more than a fortnight.

(iii) Normal caustic soda solution.

(iv) Benzene : the commercial grade redistilled is adequate.

Urine (2 ml.), copper reagent (1 ml.), and caustic soda solution (1 ml.) are pipetted into a tube, mixed and allowed to stand for a few minutes. Benzene (5 ml.) is added ; the tube is stoppered and shaken for two minutes. After separation of the layers the benzene is decanted or pipetted into a second tube, washed with 1 ml. water, transferred to a third tube, and shaken with sodium diethyldithiocarbamate solution (1 ml.) for one minute. The intensity of the golden-yellow colour developing in the benzene layer is estimated in a Spekker absorptiometer using Ilford violet 601 filters and the amount of proguanil present is read from a standard curve constructed from samples of urine containing known amounts of the drug. Small separating funnels may conveniently be used for the estimation. Xylene or chloroform may replace benzene ; the commercial grade of the former may contain a volatile substance which gives a high blank reading, it should be distilled over soda ash before use.

Emulsions have not been encountered with human urines but have been observed when rat's urine has been used. Such emulsions may be broken by sucking up into a capillary pipette and ejecting several times.

Samples of urine from normal human subjects give blank values not exceeding 5 mgm. proguanil per litre. Rat urine gives higher blanks, not exceeding 12 mgm. per litre due, to the extraction of a urinary pigment.

This method has been still further simplified for use in the field by Tottey and Maegraith (1948). The concentration of the various reagents is immaterial to the final colour and the only accurate measurements required are the urine, the standard solution, and the extracting solvent. The volume of the last need not be known provided it is the same for all estimations ; about 10 ml. is required. A graduated test-tube will suffice for the measurements and a pipette is required for the urine and standard solutions. In the absence of a balance, solutions may be prepared as follows :—

Proguanil Standard. A 100-mgm. tablet is dissolved in a small volume of dilute hydrochloric acid and made up to 1 litre with water.

Copper Reagent. One volume saturated copper sulphate solution, 2 volumes saturated ammonium chloride, 40 volumes water.

Caustic Soda. Five volumes saturated sodium hydroxide solution, 95 volumes water.

Sodium diethyldithiocarbamate. Saturated solution.

The procedure is as described by Gage and Rose (1946) and the colours obtained are compared visually with those in a series of standards similarly prepared containing in place of urine :—

0	0·3	0·6	1·0	1·5 ml.	standard solution
i.e., 0	30	60	100	150 μgm.	drug.

Derivatives of *p*-chlorophenylbiguanidine with the following alkyl groups R, and R_2 on the terminal atom

	Proguanil.	4430	5093	4567
R_1	$C_3H_7\beta$	$C_3H_7\beta$	CH_3	$C_4H_9\beta$
R_2	—	CH_3	—	—

gave the same colour reaction with slight variations in intensity : the introduction of methyl groups into one or both of the imino-groups in the proguanil molecule did not interfere. No colour was obtained with biguanidine nor with *p*-chlorophenylbiguanide, the copper complexes of these substances being apparently insoluble in benzene. Alkyl-substituted guanidine derivatives do not produce colour nor does the antimalarial 3349 (Curd *et al.*, 1945). The method is thus rather more specific than that based on the estimation of p-chloroaniline after hydrolysis. It therefore gives lower readings with urine, since it does not include metabolites of the drug which give rise to p-chloroaniline on hydrolysis.

Human Urine.	Proguanil content in mgm./litr e.	
	Copper method.	Hydrolysis method.
1	202	296
2	22·7	15·4
3	412	530
4	421	531
5	17	14·25
6	190	299

The method evolved by King, Wootton, and Gilchrist (1946b) for the estimation of proguanil in blood also involves colorimetric and preferably photo-electric methods. The results obtained agree very closely with those obtained by the diazo methods of Spinks and his colleagues. Schulz (1949) employs hydrogenolysis in acid solution with zinc amalgam to yield a primary aromatic amine. This is then estimated colorimetrically by a modified Bratton-Marshall reaction.

2-p-Chlorophenylguanidino-4-β-diethylaminoethyl-amino-6-methylpyrimidine (3349)

Although this compound is of little value therapeutically in man, its pharmacology is not without interest. It is a colourless substance which crystallises from petroleum ether in needles with a melting point at 154°–155° C. It is insoluble in water but readily soluble in hot ethanol, acetone, and toluene and somewhat less soluble in these solvents in the cold. It forms three series of salts, mono-, di-, and tri-acid salts, with inorganic acids and also with organic acids like acetic acid. The salts are also colourless, like the parent base. The dihydrochloride is readily soluble in water, the monohydrochloride only sparingly soluble, the trihydrochloride hygroscopic.

In the rat, after oral administration, 3349 is rather slowly absorbed and reaches only low concentrations in whole blood and plasma. The maximum concentrations in whole blood and plasma from oral administration of 100 mgm. per kgm. are of the order of 0·8 and 0·2 mgm. per litre respectively. The higher concentration in whole blood is associated with localisation in red and white cells ; although concentrations in the latter are variable both in rabbit and rat, they are higher than in red cells (Spinks and Tottey, 1946b). 3349 is rather persistent in blood. The concentrations in tissues are about 100 to 300 times those in plasma ; the highest concentration after oral administration is in the liver, but after intravenous administration it is found first of all in the lung though later redisposition occurs to give a distribution somewhat similar to that following oral administration. Tissue concentrations from 25 mgm. per kgm. intravenously and 100 mgm. per kgm. orally are similar, suggesting that 3349 may be poorly absorbed when given by the latter route. 3349 persists strongly in the body, being still detectable in considerable amounts six days after administration. In mice and rats, the distribution and rates of absorption are similar in the two species, but blood concentrations in the mouse are two to three times as high as in the rat.

In both the rat and the mouse only a small percentage of 3349 is excreted in the urine. Much larger amounts are found in fæces, giving total recoveries of 63 and 43 per cent. after oral and intravenous administration respectively. If allowance is made for losses during the feeding periods and for drug still remaining in the tissues it is probable that little or none is metabolised. 3349 is very rapidly excreted into the small intestine, about half through the bile and half through the intestinal wall or in secretions other than bile. The drug found in the large intestine is mainly passed on from the small intestine. The excretion of 3349 in the urine in man has been studied by Spinks and Tottey (1945b).

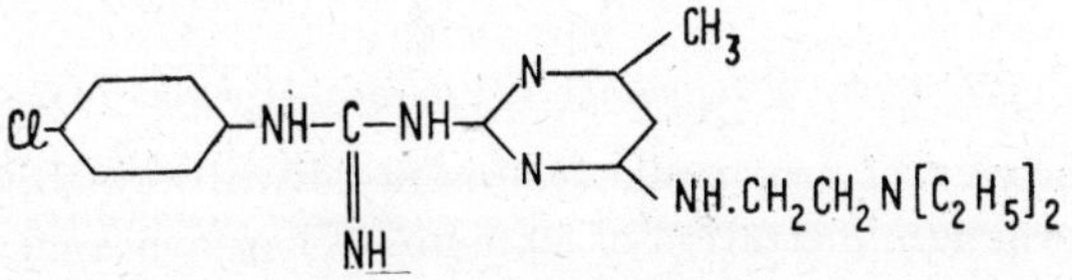

2-p-Chlorophenylguanidino-4-β-diethylaminoethyl-amino-6-methylpyrimidine (3349)

It was found that in man only about 4 per cent. of that administered by mouth can be obtained in the urine. As might be expected from the behaviour of 3349 in animals, excretion in the urine continues long after administration has ceased. In volunteers given 3349 an increase occurs in aromatic amine, the mean increase being equivalent to 2·95 mgm. of p-chloroaniline and its plus or minus limit of error (for $p = 0·05$) 1·54. But this increase is equivalent only to a 0·1 per cent. conversion of 3349 to p-chloroaniline, assuming complete excretion of the latter in the urine. There is no evidence of breakdown of the pyrimidine ring of 3349 to acetone nor is proof of conjugation of the drug or of a phenolic derivative with sulphuric acid obtained. No significant increase in the excretion of ester sulphate occurs, but this is probably to be attributed to a reduction in the activity of the intestinal flora. No metabolite can be detected during isolation experiments.

Methods for the determination of 3349 by a turbidimetric technique and for colorimetric determination have been worked out by Spinks (1945) and Spinks and Tottey (1945a). 3349 and mepacrine both exhibit considerable similarities in their absorption, distribution, and excretion ; the ease with which they are localised in tissues at the expense of plasma and their slow excretion in urine show that these compounds have a strong affinity for tissue cells, thus partially explaining their activity on malarial parasites. Their strong affinity for tissue cells is probably due to the possession of a basic side-chain.

N_1-p-Chlorophenyl-N_5-methyl-N_5-*iso*propyl-biguanide (4430)

The pharmacology of 4430 was studied by Spinks (1946)

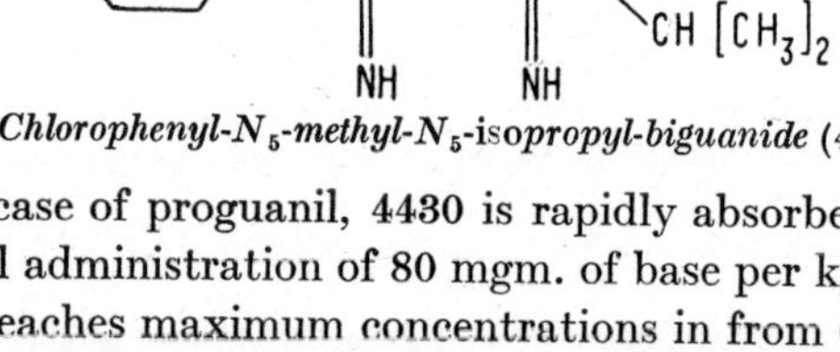

N_1-p-Chlorophenyl-N_5-methyl-N_5-isopropyl-biguanide (4430)

As in the case of proguanil, 4430 is rapidly absorbed in the rat after the oral administration of 80 mgm. of base per kgm. of body weight ; it reaches maximum concentrations in from 0·3 hours of 1·5 mgm. per litre in whole blood and in 1·3 hours of 0·45 mgm.

per litre in plasma. The drug is rather persistent at lower concentrations : the concentrations in tissue are higher than those in plasma, the ratios being from 10 to 50. After intravenous injection 4430 is rapidly distributed through the tissues, initial concentrations being high, especially in the kidney. The high concentration in the kidneys may be associated with the fact that 4430 is more rapidly excreted in the urine than either mepacrine or quinine. It is rapidly cleared from the tissues, the concentrations after twenty-four hours usually being less than 5 mgm. per kgm. However, it can be detected in the urine at least five days after administration. In comparison with mepacrine and 3349, 4430 is more rapidly absorbed and more rapidly eliminated and its maximum concentration is about twice as high in blood and plasma (Spinks and Tottey, 1945c). The most marked point of difference is the low concentration ratio between tissue and plasma. Mepacrine, 3349, and quinine, when given under the same conditions, show tissue/plasma concentrations ratios of 300 : 1,000, 100 : 300 and 50 : 200 respectively.

BLOOD, PLASMA, AND TISSUE CONCENTRATIONS OF 4430 FOLLOWING THE INTRAVENOUS ADMINISTRATION OF 20 MGM. OF BASE PER KGM. OF BODY WEIGHT IN THE RAT (Spinks, 1946)

Time (hours).	Concentrations in mgm. of base per litre or kgm. in					
	Blood.	Plasma.	Liver.	Lung.	Spleen.	Kidney.
0·3	1·95	0·55	36·8	48·9	18·7	119·4
1·0	0·75	0·30	15·5	41·2	21·3	50·4
2·3	0·56	0·19	2·31	23·8	8·3	34·3
7·0	0·52	0·15	1·9	8·5	4·0	5·5
19·0	0·35	0·17	2·9	6·4	3·3	2·8

In the mouse 4430 gives higher blood concentrations than in the rat following the administration of the same doses, and in the mouse the ratios between tissue concentration and blood concentration are also somewhat higher. As in the rat, 4430 is more rapidly absorbed and gives higher concentrations in the blood than 3349.

Concentrations in rabbit blood after a dose of 80 mgm. of base per kgm. of body weight given by stomach tube are between those in mouse and rat ; absorption is slower in the rabbit than in the other two species.

In the rat the percentage of 4430 excreted in the urine is low following both oral and intravenous administration, and as with 3349 considerable amounts are found in the fæces. The ratios between fæcal and urinary excretion differed considerably according to the route of administration, suggesting that a considerable amount of the drug passes through the gut unabsorbed. After intravenous injection 4430 still appears in the intestine, largely as a result of excretion by the bile into the small and thence into the large intestine ; some of the drug, however, is excreted through the walls of the intestine and in secretions other than the bile. Such excretory mechanisms are of a non-specific nature (Spinks and Tottey, 1946b). In the rabbit also 4430 is excreted both in the fæces and the urine, though the excretion in the fæces is more irregular than in the rat. The total excretion in urine and fæces is low, about half and a third of the administered drug being recovered after oral and intravenous administration respectively. As compared with 3349 in the rabbit, a greater percentage of drug is excreted in the urine and less in the fæces. 4430 is almost certainly metabolised both by the rat and rabbit.

Absorption and Excretion of 4430 in Man. In man after the oral administration of single doses of 200 and 400 mgm. of the acetate the drug is rapidly absorbed and blood concentrations of 0·44 and 0·8 mgm. per litre of base result, the concentrations being higher than those attained by mepacrine when given in similar amounts. After repeated doses the maximum concentrations were about 1 mgm. per litre with doses of 400 mgm. three times a day and 0·6 mgm. per litre with doses of 200 mgm. three times a day.

The excretion of 4430 in human urine in twenty-four hours accounted for 24·5 and 24·2 per cent. in two volunteers when the oral dose was 100 mgm. of the acetate. These are higher figures than those obtained with mepacrine or 3349 (Spinks and Tottey, 1945c).

Spinks (1946) suggests that mepacrine, 3349, quinine, and 4430 orm a series with decreasing affinities for cells, the reason for these differences resting mainly on variation of the basic dissociation constant and the length of the alkyl groups in the basic side-chain. It is probable that the alkylbiguanidine side-chain displays the conductophoric function postulated by Magidson *et al.* (1934) and Magidson and Grigorowsky (1936) for the dialkylamino-alkylamino side-chain of mepacrine and pamaquin. As a nitrogen-carbon system capable of displaying tautomeric and mesomeric effects (Curd *et al.*, 1945 ; Curd and Rose, 1946), it also displays the parasiticidal function postulated by Magidson for the heterocyclic nuclei of mepacrine and pamaquin.

In cercopithecus monkeys doses of 5·0 gm. per kgm. by mouth caused vomiting and weakness : with intramuscular injections of 0·2 gm. per kgm. of body weight there was weakness and listlessness: doses of 0·5 gm. per kgm. caused weakness and death in from five to forty-four hours from heart failure, with fatty degeneration of the heart muscle and liver cells. At the site of intramuscular injection there is considerable necrosis and œdema.

The blood concentrations and tissue distributions of some further homologues of proguanil have been studied by Spinks (1948). The relationship of these homologues to proguanil and to one another are as follows :—

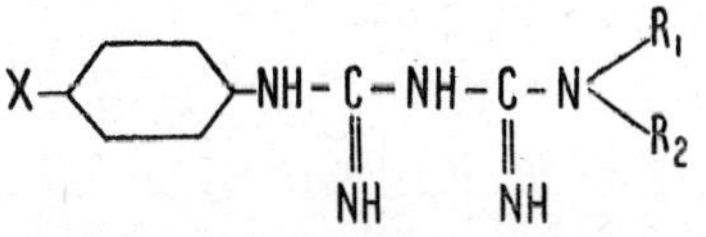

$$X-\langle\bigcirc\rangle-NH-\underset{\underset{NH}{\|}}{C}-NH-\underset{\underset{NH}{\|}}{C}-N\begin{smallmatrix}R_1\\\\R_2\end{smallmatrix}$$

Compound.	X.	R_1.	R_2.
5093 . . .	Cl	H	CH_3
4134 . . .	Cl	CH_3	CH_3
Proguanil . .	Cl	H	$iso\text{-}C_3H_7$
4430 . . .	Cl	CH_3	$iso\text{-}C_3H_7$
3936 . . .	Cl	C_2H_5	C_2H_5
4565 . . .	Cl	H	$n\text{-}C_4H_9$

After oral doses of 80 mgm. per kgm. of the above compounds the blood and plasma concentrations were as follows :—

Compound.	Tissue.	Concentrations in mgm. per litre after					
		½ hour.	1½ hours.	2½ hours.	5 hours.	16 hours.	24 hours.
5093 .	Blood	2·79	3·60	4·36	3·94	—	2·21
	Plasma	0·79	1·11	1·25	0·96	—	0·62
4134 .	Blood	1·44	1·78	2·20	1·23	—	0·86
	Plasma	0·82	0·80	1·42	0·62	—	0·52
Proguanil.	Blood	1·20	1·58	1·26	—	—	0·58
	Plasma	0·29	0·73	0·59	—	—	0·12
4430 .	Blood	1·52	0·77	0·53	—	—	0·15 *
	Plasma	0·18	0·46	0·23	0·11	—	0·07 *
3936 .	Blood	1·22	1·49	0·82	0·62	0·61	—
	Plasma	0·30	0·30	0·25	0·25	0·18	—
4565 .	Blood	0·36	0·66	0·53	0·39	0·37	—
	Plasma	0·13	0·19	0·14	0·10	0·12	—

* After thirty hours.

In the chick proguanil showed the lowest concentrations after an oral dose of 40 mgm. per kgm. The concentration in blood was 0·47 and in plasma 0·24 mgm. per litre after twenty-four hours ; the highest readings were with 4565, where the blood and plasma concentrations were 1·48 and 0·70 mgm. per kgm. Although doses in the chick were only half those in the rat, all compounds except 5093 gave higher concentrations in the former. Similar differences were noted by Butler *et al.* (1947). Both in rat and chick the homologues tend to give increasing blood concentrations with decreasing molecular weight.

In general, the biguanides appear to be distributed similarly with highest concentrations in liver, lung or spleen after eighteen to twenty-four hours.

The ratios between mean tissue and plasma concentrations are shown in the table on p. 175.

These findings show that the inactivity of 5093 is not correlated with difficulty in absorption. Malarial inactivity must therefore be due to faulty metabolism or to low intrinsic activity. The inactivity of 4134 may by analogy be ascribed to one of these two possibilities. However, therapeutic activity rises along the series 5093 to 4635 till proguanil is reached and then falls. As blood

MEAN TISSUE : PLASMA CONCENTRATION RATIOS OF BIGUANIDES IN RAT, CHICK AND RABBIT (Spinks, 1948)

Compound.	Animal.	Route.	Dose. (mgm./kgm.).	Mean ratio for					
				Brain.	Muscle.	Liver.	Lung.	Spleen.	Kidney.
Proguanil	Rat	Oral	80	—	—	49	14	15	20
4430	,,	,,	80	—	—	56	34	22	33
5093	,,	,,	80	—	5	38	31	8	12
Proguanil	Chick	,,	40	6	—	84	29	—	—
5093	,,	,,	80	5	—	30	31	—	—
Proguanil	Rabbit	Intravenous	8	5	21	57	155	97	188
4967	,,	,,	8	8	8	10	53	23	49
5093	,,	,,	8	5	9	15	61	38	42

and plasma concentrations fall continuously along the series the results are not at variance with the hypothesis that the observed therapeutic effects are due to interrelation between this continuous fall and a concomitant continuous increase in intrinsic activity.

Similarity of Pharmacological Effects of Antimalarial Drugs

Despite the differences in chemical constitution between anti-malarial drugs there is a very curious measure of agreement in their pharmacological action which may possibly throw some light on their chemotherapeutic action. The main similarities are shown in the table. Late deaths in rats and mice but not in chicks have been reported by Butler *et al.* (1947) with proguanil, and by Köhlschütter *et al.* (1943) with mepacrine, pamaquin, and certuna in fowls ; the nervous symptoms which accompany the delayed deaths prevent the ingestion of food and thereby hasten death. Proguanil in sublethal doses given to rats, mice, dogs, and monkeys diminishes the intake of food (Hughes *et al.*, 1947). Thus delayed deaths and loss of appetite are apparently symptoms produced by at least four antimalarial drugs, proguanil, pamaquin, certuna, and mepacrine.

Proguanil antagonises the effects of vagal stimulation and of acetylcholine. In smooth muscle the natural tonus is reduced by proguanil (Vane, 1949). Quinine, quinidine, cinchonine, pamaquin, and mepacrine first stimulate and then relax the isolated rat's intestine (Keogh and Shaw, 1943, 1944). Quinine also reduces the depressor response of the cat's blood pressure to acetylcholine. Hiatt *et al.* (1945) similarly showed that quinine, quinidine, and cinchonine all inhibit the action of the vagus on the heart. Proguanil lengthens the refractory period and impairs the contractility of isolated rabbit auricles (Vane, 1949). Quinine, mepacrine, and pamaquin decrease the heart rate and lengthen the conduction time as shown by the electrocardiogram in man and dogs (Molitor, 1941). The lengthening of the refractory period by quinidine and to a lesser extent by quinine is well known. Mepacrine impairs the contractility of the heart (Smith and Stoeckle, 1946).

Vane (1949) demonstrated the curariform action of proguanil on the perfused superior cervical ganglion, on the cat sciatic-gastrocnemius preparation, and on the rat phrenic nerve-diaphragm preparation. Harvey (1939) similarly described a curariform action of quinine on the neuromuscular junction.

Proguanil in large doses antagonises the vasoconstriction caused by adrenaline in the dog's perfused hind leg and on the cat's blood pressure (Vane, 1949). Quinine in large doses similarly reverses the action of adrenaline on the cat's blood pressure (Keogh and Shaw, 1943, 1944). Molitor (1941) demonstrated that mepacrine and pamaquin cause vasodilatation, as does quinine : similarly Vane (1949) showed that proguanil produces vasodilatation in the dog's perfused hind leg and in the cat.

Finally, Madinaveitia and Raventós (1949) showed that antimalarial compounds antagonise the action of adenosine on the guinea-pig heart and on the hen's cæcum, the parallelism between antimalarial activity and the power to antagonise adenosine being demonstrated in most series of antimalarial compounds investigated. There is also some evidence that cinchona alkaloids and mepacrine antagonise the effects of Ca ions on the isolated intestine thus leading to a condition which simulates calcium deficiency.

It may, however, be noted that another group of alkaloids, conessine, *iso*conessine and *nor*conessine, have very little if any antimalarial action even in repeated doses of 40 mgm. per kgm. of body weight in chicks infected with *P. gallinaceum* despite the fact that their pharmacological action is very similar to that of the cinchona alkaloids (Stephenson, 1948).

Similarity in the Pharmacology of Antimalarial Drugs in Animals

	Mepacrine.	Pamaquin.	Quinine and cinchona alkaloids.	Proguanil.	Observers.
Delayed deaths . .	+	+		+	Butler *et al.* (1947). Vane (1949). Köhlschütter *et al.* (1943).
Inhibition of gastric secretion.	+		+	+	Karp (1948). Burn and Vane (1948).
Loss of appetite .	+	+		+	Vane (1949). Schmidt *et al.* (1947). Hughes *et al.* (1947).
Inhibition of acetylcholine.	+	+	+	+	Keogh and Shaw (1943, 1944). Hiatt *et al.* (1945). Vane (1949). Burn and Vane (1949).
Antagonism of adrenaline.			+	+	Keogh and Shaw (1943, 1944). Vane (1949).
Vasodilatation . .	+	+		+	Molitor (1941). Vane (1949).
Curare-like action .			+	+	Harvey (1939). Vane (1949).
Lengthening of refractory period of heart.	+	+	+	+	Molitor (1941). Smith and Stoeckle (1946). Vane (1949).
Relaxation of intestinal muscle.	+	+	+	+	Keogh and Shaw (1943, 1944). Vane (1949).
Inhibition of adenosine action on guinea-pig heart and hen cæcum.	+	+	+	+	Madinaveitia and Raventós (1949).

References

ABBEY, E. A., and LAWRENCE, E. A., 1946, The effect of atabrine suppressive therapy on eyesight in pilots. *J. Amer. Med. Ass.*, **130**, 786.

ACTON, H. W., and CHOPRA, R. N., 1924, The local effects produced in the tissues by intramuscular injections. *Indian J. med. Res.*, **12**, 251.

ACTON, H. W., and CHOPRA, R. N., 1925, The concentration of quinine in the circulating blood. *Indian J. med. Res.*, **13**, 197.

ADAMS, A. R. D., MAEGRAITH, B. G., KING, J. D., TOWNSHEND, R. H., DAVEY, T. H., and HAVARD, R. E., 1945, Studies on synthetic antimalarial drugs. XIII. Results of a preliminary investigation of the therapeutic action of 4888 (paludrine) on acute attacks of benign tertian malaria. *Ann. trop. Med. Parasit.*, **39**, 225.

ALBERT, A., and GOLDACRE, R., 1944, Basicities of the aminoquinolines : comparison with aminoacridines and aminopyridines. *Nature, Lond.*, **153**, 467.

AMERICAN MEDICAL ASSOCIATION, Council on Pharmacy and Chemistry, 1948, Chloroguanide hydrochloride generic term for chlorophenyl *iso*-propyl biguanide hydrochloride. *J. Amer. med. Ass.*, 136, 251.

ANDREWS, J. C., and CORNATZER, W. E., 1947, The metabolism of cinchonine in dogs and in man. *J. nat. Mal. Soc.*, 6, 246.

ANDREWS, J. C., and WEBB, B. D., 1942, The effect of hookworm damage on levels of quinine attained in blood and urine of dogs following single doses of quinine sulphate. *J. Pharmacol.*, 75, 191.

ANNEGERS, J. H., SNAPP, F. E., PASKIND, L., IVY, A. C., and ATKINSON, A. J., 1943, Retention of atabrine in animal body ; excretion in bile and urine and effect on cholic acid output. *War Med.*, 4, 176.

ARCHIBALD, R. M., and WEISIGER, J. R., 1948, Reaction of plasmochin with formaldehyde. *Fed. Proc.*, 7, 143.

ARMY MALARIA RESEARCH UNIT, 1945a, Indirect determination of plasma mepacrine in subjects on a suppressive regime. Method suitable for a field laboratory. *Lancet, i*, 687.

ARMY MALARIA RESEARCH UNIT, 1945b, Prolonged oral administration of mepacrine. I. The effects of tests on organ function. II. Hæmatological effect. *Ann. trop. Med. Parasit.*, 39, 128, 133.

ARMY MALARIA RESEARCH UNIT, 1945c, Factors effecting the excretion of mepacrine in the urine. *Ann. trop. Med. Parasit.*, 39, 53.

ARMY MALARIA RESEARCH UNIT, 1946a, The effect of mepacrine on the gastro-intestinal tract of man. *Ann. trop. Med. Parasit.*, 40, 80.

ARMY MALARIA RESEARCH UNIT, 1946b, Mepacrine in animal tissues. *Ann. trop. Med. Parasit.*, 40, 173.

ARMY MALARIA RESEARCH UNIT, 1946c, Distribution of mepacrine in blood. *Ann. trop. Med. Parasit.*, 40, 181.

ARMY MALARIA RESEARCH UNIT, 1946d, The excretion of mepacrine in fæces. *Ann. trop. Med. Parasit.*, 40, 372.

AUERBACH, M. E., and ECKERT, H. W., 1944, The photofluorometric determination of atabrine. *J. biol. Chem.*, 154, 597.

BABKIN, B. P., and KARP, D., 1947, Effect of quinine and atabrine on gastric secretion (a preliminary communication). *Canad. med. Ass. J.*, 56, 137.

BABKIN, B. P., and RITCHIE, T. W., 1945, Effect of quinine on the para-sympathetic innervation of the heart in the dog. *Rev. canad. Biol.*, 11, 346.

BACHER, F. A., BUHS, R. P., HETRICK, J. C., REISS, W., and TRENNER, N. R., 1947, The resolution of atabrine dihydrochloride. *J. Amer. chem. Soc.*, 69, 1534.

BASU, U. P., MUKHERJEE, S., and BANERJEE, R. P., 1947, Influence of bile salts on absorption of quinine. *J. Amer. pharm. Ass.* (Sci. Edit.), 36, 266.

BELL, P. H., and ROBLIN, R. O., Jr., 1942, Studies in chemotherapy. VII. A theory of the relation of structure to activity of sulfanilamide-type compounds. *J. Amer. chem. Soc.*, 64, 2905.

BERLINER, R. W., EARLE, D. P., Jr., TAGGART, J. V., ZUBROD, C. G., WELCH, W. J., CONAN, N. J., BAUMAN, E., SCUDDER, S. T., and SHANNON, J. A., 1948, Studies on the chemotherapy of the human malarias. VI. The physiological disposition, antimalarial activity and toxicity of several derivatives of 4-amino-quinolines. *J. clin. Invest.*, 27, Suppl., p. 98.

BERNARDBEIG, J., and CAUJOLLE, F., 1935, Sur l'élimination de la quinine par la bile. *Bull. Acad. Méd., Paris*, 113, 147.

BLASCHKO, H., CHOU, T. C., and WAJDA, I., 1947, The inhibition of esterases by paludrine. *Brit. J. Pharmacol.*, 2, 116.

BRODIE, B. B., BAER, J. E., and CRAIG, L. C., 1946, Cinchona alkaloids. 4. Metabolic products in human urine. *Fed. Proc.*, 5, 168.

BRODIE, B. B., and UDENFRIEND, S., 1943a, The estimation of quinine in human plasma with a note on the estimation of quinidine. *J. Pharmacol.*, 78, 154.

BRODIE, B. B., and UDENFRIEND, S., 1943b, The estimation of atabrine in biological fluids and tissues. *J. biol. Chem.*, **151**, 299.

BRODIE, B. B., and UDENFRIEND, S., 1945, The estimation of basic organic compounds and a technique for the appraisal of specificity. Application to the cinchona alkaloids. *J. biol. Chem.*, **158**, 705.

BRODIE, B. B., UDENFRIEND, S., DILL, W., and CHENKIN, T., 1947a, The estimation of basic organic compounds in biological material. III. Estimation by conversion to fluorescent compounds. *J. biol. Chem.*, **168**, 319.

BRODIE, B. B., UDENFRIEND, S., and TAGGART, J. V., 1947b, The estimation of basic organic compounds in biological material. IV. Estimation by coupling with diazonium salts. *J. biol. Chem.*, **168**, 327.

BROWN, B. R., and HAMMICK, D. L., 1948, A resolution of mepacrine [2-chloro-5-(δ-diethylamino-α-methylbutyl)amino-7-methoxyacridine]. *J. chem. Soc.*, 99.

BROWN, M., and RENNIE, J. L., 1945, Indirect determination of plasma-mepacrine during a therapeutic course. *Lancet*, i, 686.

BÜLBRING, E., LOURIE, E. M., and PARDOE, V., 1949, The presence of acetylcholine in *Trypanosoma rhodesiense* and its absence from *Plasmodium gallinaceum*. *Brit. J. Pharmacol.*, **4**, 290.

BURN, J. H., and DUTTA, N. K., 1948, Acetylcholine and body temperature. *Nature, Lond.*, **161**, 18.

BURN, J. H., and VANE, J. R., 1948, The inhibitory action of paludrine on the secretion of gastric juice. *Brit. J. Pharmacol.*, **3**, 346.

BURN, J. H., and VANE, J. R., 1949, The relation between the motor and inhibitor actions of acetylcholine. *J. Physiol.*, **108**, 104.

BURTON, A. F., and KELSEY, F. E., 1943, Studies on antimalarial drugs. The metabolism of quinine in pregnant animals. *J. Pharmacol.*, **79**, 70.

BUTLER, R., DAVEY, D. G., and SPINKS, A., 1947, A preliminary report of the toxicity and the associated blood concentrations of paludrine in laboratory animals. *Brit. J. Pharmacol.*, **2**, 181.

CHEN, G., 1947, Influence of pamaquine and atabrine on the enzymatic degradation of quinine. *Proc. Soc. exp. Biol., N.Y.*, **66**, 313.

CHEN, G., and GEILING, E. M. K., 1944, Observations bearing on the mechanism of the elimination of quinine and atabrine from the circulation and tissues. *J. Pharmacol.*, **82**, 120.

CHEN, K. K., and ANDERSON, R. C., 1947, The toxicity and general pharmacology of N₁-p-chlorophenyl-N₅-isopropyl biguanide. *J. Pharmacol.*, **91**, 157.

CHIN, K., 1937, Ueber die pharmakologische Wirkung des Atebrins. *J. med. Ass. Formosa*, **36**, 159.

CHOPRA, R. N., GANGULY, S. K., and ROY, A. C., 1936, Studies on the action of antimalarial remedies on monkey malaria. The relationship between the concentration of atebrin in the circulating blood and parasite count. *Indian med. Gaz.*, **71**, 443.

CHOPRA, R. N., and ROY, A. C., 1935, On the estimation of minute quantities of atebrin in the blood. *Indian med. Gaz.*, **70**, 504.

CHOPRA, R. N., and ROY, A. C., 1936, On the determination of small quantities of atebrin in the blood. *Indian J. med. Res.*, **24**, 487.

CHOPRA, R. N., SEN, B., and ROY, A. C., 1937, Individual variations in the effectiveness of synthetic antimalarial drugs (a preliminary note). *Indian med. Gaz.*, **72**, 131.

CHRISTOPHERS, S. R., 1937, Dissociation constants and solubilities of bases of antimalarial compounds. I. Quinine. II. Atebrin. *Ann. trop. Med. Parasit.*, **31**, 43.

CHRISTOPHERS, S. R., and FULTON, J. D., 1940, The dissociation constants of plasmoquine. *Ann. trop. Med. Parasit.*, **34**, 1.

CLARK, A. J., 1937, " Applied Pharmacology," 6th edition. London : J. & A. Churchill.

CORNATZER, W. E., and ANDREWS, J. C., 1944, The relative rates of absorption of quinine and some other cinchona salts from isolated intestinal loops of dogs. *J. Pharmacol.*, **82**, 3.

CRAIG, L. C., 1943, Identification of small amounts of organic compounds by distribution studies. Application to atabrine. *J. biol. Chem.*, **150**, 33.

CRAIG, L. C., 1944, Identification of small amounts of organic compounds by distribution studies. II. Separation by counter-current distribution. *J. biol. Chem.*, **155**, 519.

CRAIG, L. C., MIGHTON, H. R., TITUS, E., and GOLUMBIC, C., 1948, Identification of small amounts of organic compounds by distribution studies. Purity of synthetic antimalarials. *Analytical Chem.*, **20**, 134.

CURD, F. H. S., DAVEY, D. G., and ROSE, F. L., 1945, Studies on synthetic antimalaria drugs. II. General chemical considerations. *Ann. trop. Med. Parasit.*, **39**, 157.

CURD, F. H. S., and ROSE, F. L., 1946, Synthetic antimalarials. Part X. Some aryl-diguanide ("biguanide ") derivatives. *J. chem. Soc.*, 729.

DÄHNE, G., 1943, Verhalten der Retikulozyten bei einer für Malaria spezifischen Therapie. *Dtsch. tropenmed. Zischr.*, **47**, 129.

DAVEY, D. G., 1946, Paludrine : a summary of information to February 1946. Report BT 1116. Imperial Chemicals (Pharmaceuticals) Ltd.

DEARBORN, E. H., 1947, The distribution of quinacrine in dogs and in rabbits. *J. Pharmacol.*, **91**, 174.

DEARBORN, E. H., KELSEY, F. E., OLDHAM, F. K., and GEILING, E. M. K., 1943, Studies on antimalarials ; the accumulation and excretion of atabrine. *J. Pharmacol.*, **78**, 120.

DIKSHIT, B. B., 1939, Effect of plasmoquine and atebrin on the fœtus. *Rep. Haffkine Inst.*, 1938, p. 46.

DOLL, R., and SCHNEIDER, R., 1948, The effect of paludrine on human gastric secretion. *Brit. J. Pharmacol.*, **3**, 352.

DRIESBACH, R. H., 1949, Antagonists for fatal and non-fatal doses of quinine intravenously in depressed circulatory states and in hyperthermia. *J. Pharmacol.*, **95**, 347.

DRIESBACH, R. H., and HANZLIK, P. J., 1945, Antagonists for the circulatory depression of quinine injected intravenously and the implied cholinergic action, and nature and importance of the vasodilation, in the depression. *J. Pharmacol.*, **83**, 167.

EARLE, D. P., Jr., WELCH, W. J., and SHANNON, J. A., 1948, Studies on the chemotherapy of the human malarias. IV. The metabolism of cinchonine in relation to its antimalarial activity. *J. clin. Invest.*, **27**, Suppl., p. 87.

EICHHOLTZ, F., 1935, Bemerkungen zur Arbeit von de Langen und Storm. *Klin. Wschr.*, **14i**, 716.

FARINAUD, E., LATASTE, C., BACCIALONE, L., and CANET, J., 1939, Rapports entre la concentration sanguine et l'élimination urinaire de la quinacrine. *C.R. Soc. Biol. Paris*, **130**, 623.

FIELD, J. W., NIVEN, J. C., and HODGKIN, E. P., 1937, The prevention of malaria in the field by the use of quinine and atebrin. Experiments in clinical prophylaxis. *Quart. Bull. Hlth. Org. L.o.N.*, **6**, 236.

FOY, H., KONDI, A., and PERISTERIS, M., 1936, Studies on atebrin. A controlled field experiment to test the relapse value of atebrin. *Trans. R. Soc. trop. Med. Hyg.*, **30**, 109.

GAGE, J. C., and ROSE, F. L., 1946, The estimation of paludrine in urine. *Ann. trop. Med. Parasit.*, **40**, 333.

GALPERIN, E. P., 1944, Quinoline compounds with side-chain in position 4. *Amer. Rev. Soviet Med.*, **1**, 220.

GANGULI, P., 1933, Treatment of malaria with atebrin with records of blood pressure and electrocardiogram. *Arch. Schiffs-u. Tropenhyg.*, **37**, 413.

GENTZKOW, C. J., 1938, A method for the determination of atabrine in the blood. *Amer. J. trop. Med.*, **18**, 149.

PHARMACOLOGY 181

GERTLER, M. M., and KARP, D., 1947, Effect of atabrine on the parasympathetic innervation of the dog heart *in situ*. *Rev. canad. Biol.*, **6**, 229.

GERTLER, M. M., and YOHALEM, S. B., 1947, The effect of atabrine on auricular fibrillation in man. *Canad. med. Ass. J.*, **57**, 249.

GERTLER, M. M., and YOHALEM, S. B., 1949, The effect of atabrine (quinacrine hydrochloride) on cardiac arrhythmias. *Amer. Heart J.*, **37**, 79.

GOLJACHOWSKI, N. W., 1934, Ueber die Bedeutung der aktuellen Reaktion des milleus für die Wirkung der Gifte. (Der Einfluss der Wasserstoffonenkonzentration auf die Giftigkeit des Chinins und die Salicylsäure fur das Froschherz.) *Arch. int. Pharmacodyn.*, **48**, 271.

GREEN, R., 1932, A report on fifty cases of malaria treated with atebrin. A new synthetic drug. *Lancet*, *i*, 826.

HAAG, H. B., LARSON, P. S., and SCHWARTZ, J. J., 1943, Effect of urinary pH on elimination of quinine in man. *J. Pharmacol.*, **79**, 136.

HAMMICK, D. L., and CHAMBERS, W. E., 1945, Optical activity of excreted mepacrine. *Nature, Lond.*, **155**, 141.

HAMMICK, D. L., and FIRTH, D., 1944, Mepacrine derivatives in urine. *Nature, Lond.*, **154**, 461.

HAMMICK, D. L., and MASON, S. F., 1945, Primary degradation products of mepacrine in human urine. *Nature, Lond.*, **156**, 718.

HARVEY, A. M., 1939, The actions of quinine on skeletal muscle. *J. Physiol.*, **95**, 45.

HAWKING, F., 1943, Intramuscular injection of mepacrine (atebrin) : histological effect. *Brit. med. J.*, *ii*, 198.

HAWKING, F., 1944, Histological effect of injection of mepacrine (atebrin) dihydrochloride. *Brit. med. J.*, *ii*, 209.

HECHT, G., 1933, Pharmakologisches über Atebrin. *Arch. exp. Path. Pharmak.*, **170**, 328.

HECHT, G., 1935, Experimentelle Untersuchung von Zirkulations-störungen durch Plasmochin und Atebrin. Erwinderung auf die Arbeit von de Langen und Storm. *Klin. Wschr.*, 14i, 714.

HECHT, G., 1936, Die Verteilung des Atebrins in Organismus. *Arch. exp. Path. Pharmak.*, **183**, 87.

HEIMANN, H. L., and SHAPIRO, B. G , 1943, Effects of plasmoquin, atebrin and quinine on the electrocardiogram, *Brit. Heart J.*, **5**, 131.

HENRY, A. J., and GRINDLEY, D. N., 1945, The adsorption-fluorescence estimation of mepacrine and stilbamidine. *Ann. trop. med. Parasit.*, **39**, 1.

HIATT, E. P., 1944, Plasma concentrations following the oral administration of single doses of the principal alkaloids of cinchona bark. *J. Pharmacol.*, **1**, 160.

HIATT, E. P., 1949, The antagonism of cinchona alkaloids to the circulatory effects of intravenous epinephrin. *Fed. Proc.*, **8**, 74.

HIATT, E. P., BROWN, D., QUINN, G., and MACDUFFIE, K., 1945, The blocking action of the cinchona alkaloids and certain related compounds on the cardio-inhibitory vagus endings of the dog. *J. Pharmacol.*, **85**, 55.

HIATT, E. P., and QUINN, G. P., 1945, The distribution of quinine, quinidine, cinchonine and cinchonidine in fluids and tissues of dogs. *J. Pharmacol.*, **83**, 101.

HICKS, E. P., 1935, Atebrin musonate : a note on the rate of absorption and on the local effects of intramuscular injection. *Rec. Malar. Surv. India*, **5**, 203.

HUGHES, H. B., and SCHMIDT, L. H., 1947, On the metabolism of paludrine in the rat. *Fed. Proc.*, **6**, 339.

HUGHES, H. B., SCHMIDT, L. H., and SMITH, C. C., 1947, On the pharmacology of paludrine. *Fed. Proc.*, **6**, 368.

INNES, J. R. M., 1947, The effect of intramuscular injection of paludrine and mepacrine in experimental animals. *Ann. trop. Med. Parasit.*, **41**, 46.

IRVIN, J. L., and IRVIN, E. M., 1946, Acid-base reactions of quinoline and acridine derivatives. *Fed. Proc.*, **5**, 139.

IRVIN, J. L., and IRVIN, E. M., 1947, Spectrophotometric and potentiometric evaluation of apparent acid dissociation exponents of various 4-aminoquinolines. *J. Amer. chem. Soc.*, **69**, 1091.

IRVIN, J. L., and IRVIN, E. M., 1948, A fluorometric method for the determination of pamaquine, SN 13,276, and SN 32,941. *J. biol. Chem.*, **174**, 589.

JAILER, J. W., 1945, Fluorescent microscopic study of the physiological distribution of atabrine. *Science*, **102**, 258.

JAILER, J. W., ROSENFELD, M., and SHANNON, J. A., 1947, The influence of orally administered alkali and acid on the renal excretion of quinacrine, chloroquine and santoquine. *J. clin. Invest.*, **26**, 1168.

JAILER, J. W., ZUBROD, C. G., ROSENFELD, M., and SHANNON, J. A., 1948, Effect of acidosis and anoxia on the concentration of quinacrine and chloroquine in blood. *J. Pharmacol.*, **92**, 345.

JONES, R., Jr., 1949, Effect of antimalarial drugs an anaerobic glycolysis (acid production) in tissue extracts. *Fed. Proc.*, **8**, 304.

JONES, R., Jr., CRAIGE, B., Jr., ALVING, A. S., WHORTON, C. M., PULLMAN, T. N., and EICHELBERGER, L., 1948, A study of the prophylactic effectiveness of several 8-aminoquinolines in sporozoite-induced *vivax* malaria (Chesson strain). *J. clin. Invest.*, **27**, Suppl., p. 6.

KARP, D., 1948, The effect of quinine and atabrine on gastric secretory function in the dog. *Rev. Canad. Biol.*, **7**, 508.

KEHAR, N. D., 1935a, Observations on the absorption and excretion of atebrin. *Rec. Malar. Surv. India*, **5**, 393.

KEHAR, N. D., 1935b, The influence of food in the stomach on the absorption and excretion of atebrin. *Rec. Malar. Surv. India*, **5**, 405.

KELSEY, F. E., and BRUNSCHWIG, A., 1947, Concentration of quinine in gastrointestinal cancers (preliminary report). *J. Nat. Cancer Inst.*, **7**, 355.

KELSEY, F. E., and GEILING, E. M. K., 1942, Micro determination of quinine in blood and tissues. *J. Pharmacol.*, **75**, 183.

KELSEY, F. E., GEILING, E. M. K., OLDHAM, F. K., and DEARBORN, E. H., 1944, Studies on antimalarial drugs. The preparation and properties of a metabolic derivative of quinine. *J. Pharmacol.*, **80**, 391.

KELSEY, F. E., and OLDHAM, F. K., 1943, Studies on antimalarial drugs. The distribution of quinine oxidase in animal tissues. *J. Pharmacol.*, **79**, 77.

KELSEY, F. E., OLDHAM, F. K., and GEILING, E. M. K., 1943, Studies on antimalarial drugs. The distribution of quinine in the tissue of the fowl. *J. Pharmacol.*, **78**, 314.

KELSEY, F. E., OLDHAM, F. K., and GEILING, E. M. K., 1945, Studies on antimalarial drugs. The metabolism of quinine and quinidine in birds and mammals. *J. Pharmacol.*, **85**, 170.

KELSEY, F. E., OLDHAM, F. K., CANTRELL, W., and GEILING, E. M. K., 1946, Antimalarial activity and toxicity of a metabolic derivative of quinine. *Nature, Lond.*, **157**, 440.

KEOGH, P., and SHAW, F. H., 1943, The pharmacology and toxicity of Alstonia alkaloids. *Aust. J. exp. Biol. med. Sci.*, **21**, 183.

KEOGH, P. P., and SHAW, F. H., 1944, The mode of action of quinine alkaloids and other antimalarials. *Aust. J. exp. Biol. med. Sci.*, **22**, 139.

KING, E. J., and GILCHRIST, M., 1945a, Field method for estimating mepacrine in urine. *Lancet*, *i*, 686.

KING, E. J., and GILCHRIST, M., 1945b, Field method for direct estimation of mepacrine in plasma and blood. *Lancet*, *i*, 814.

KING, E. J., GILCHRIST, M., and TÁRNOKY, A. L., 1946a, Spectrophotometric study of the excretion products of mepacrine compared with synthetic acridine and diphenylamine derivatives. *Biochem. J.*, **40**, 706.

KING, E. J., WOOTTON, I. D. P., and GILCHRIST, M., 1946b, Estimation of paludrine in blood., *Lancet*, *i*, 886.

KNOX, W. E., 1946, The quinine-oxidizing enzyme and liver aldehyde oxidase. *J. biol. Chem.*, **163**, 699.

PHARMACOLOGY 183

KÖHLSCHÜTTER, E., ZIPF, H. F., and TRILLER, G., 1943, Zur Toxikologie der Malariamittel Plasmochin, Atebrin, Certuna und Chinin. *Arch. exp. Path. Pharmak.*, **201**, 402.

KOLTHOFF, J. M., 1925, Die Dissoziationskonstante, das Löslichkeitsprodukt und die Titrierbarkeit von Alkaloiden. *Biochem. Z.*, **62**, 289.

KYKER, G. C., McEWEN, M., HEDGPETH, E. M., and YOUNG, V., 1946, Quinine, avitaminosis, and motility. *Fed. Proc.*, **5**, 142.

LANGE, K., and MATZNER, M. J., 1946, The distribution of atabrine in the blood, the skin and its appendages. Methods for the rapid and simple detection of the presence of atabrine in blood, skin and nails. *J. Lab. clin. Med.*, **31**, 742.

LANGEN, C. D. DE, and STORM, C. J., 1934, Experimenteel onderzoek van circulatiestoornissen door plasmochine en atebrine. *Geneesk. Tijdschr. Ned.-Ind.*, **74**, 1646.

LANGEN, C. D. DE, and STORM, C. J., 1935, Observations on the modern medical treatment of malaria : a clinical and experimental study. *Trans. Far-East. Ass. trop. Med. 9th Congr.*, **2**, 233.

LE HEUX, J. W., and DE LIND VAN WIJNGAARDEN, C., 1929, Über die pharmakologische Wirkung des Plasmochins. *Arch. exp. Path. Pharmak.*, **144**, 341.

LEWIS, R. A., 1944, A simple method for estimating serum atabrine concentration. *J. Lab. clin. Med.*, **29**, 1303.

LIPPINCOTT, S. W., ELLERBROOK, L. D., HESSELBROCK, W. B., CARRICO, C. C., and MARBLE, A., 1946, The relationship of spinal fluid to plasma concentrations of quinacrine and quinine. *J. Nat. Mal. Soc.*, **5**, 85.

MacINTOSH, F. C., and PATON, W. D. M., 1947, The release of histamine by amidines and other compounds. XVII. *Int. physiol. Congr.*, p. 240.

McLAY, K., 1922, Malaria in Macedonia, 1915–1919. Part III. Hæmatological investigations on malaria in Macedonia. *J.R. Army med. Cps.*, **38**, 93.

MADINAVEITIA, J., and RAVENTÓS, J., 1949, Antimalarial compounds as antagonists of adenosine. *Brit. J. Pharmacol.*, **4**, 81.

MAEGRAITH, B. G., ADAMS, A. R. D., KING, J. D., TOWNSHEND, R. H., DAVEY, T. H., and HAVARD, R. E., 1945, Studies on synthetic antimalarial drugs. XIV. Results of a preliminary investigation of the therapeutic action of 4888 (paludrine) on acute attacks of malignant tertian malaria. *Ann. trop. Med. Parasit.*, **39**, 232.

MAEGRAITH, B. G., ADAMS, A. R. D., KING, J. D., TOTTEY, M. M., RIGBY, D. J., and SLADDEN, R. A., 1946a. Paludrine in the treatment of malaria. *Brit. med. J.*, i, 903.

MAEGRAITH, B. G., TOTTEY, M. M., ADAMS, A. R. D., ANDREWS, W. H. H., and KING, J. D., 1946b, The absorption and excretion of paludrine in the human subject. *Ann. trop. Med. Parasit.*, **40**, 493.

MAGIDSON, O. Y., DELEKTORSKAYA, N. M., and LIPOWITCH, I. M., 1934, Die Derivate des 8-Aminochinolins als Antimalariapräparate. Mitt. III. Der Einfluss der Verzweigung der Kette in Stellung 8. *Arch. Pharm. Berl.*, **272**, 74.

MAGIDSON, O. Y., and GRIGOROWSKY, A. M., 1936, Acridin-Verbindungen und ihre Antimalaria-Wirkung (I. Mitteil). *Ber. dtsch. chem. Ges.*, **69**, 396.

MAIER, J., 1948a, Quinacrine levels in plasma of persons with infectious jaundice during and after suppressive malaria therapy. *Amer. J. trop. Med.*, **28**, 395.

MAIER, J., 1948b, The absorption of quinine and quinacrine in dysentery patients. *Amer. J. trop. Med.*, **28**, 397.

MARIANI, F., 1903, L'assorbimento e l'eliminazione della chinina e de 'suoi sali : deduzioni per la terapia e la profilassi del l'infezione malariea. *Boll. Soc. lancis. Osp.*, **23**, 1.

MARSHALL, P. B., 1945a, Loss of antimalarial properties in quinine degradation products. *Nature, Lond.*, **156**, 505.

MARSHALL, P. B., 1945b, The absorption of cinchona alkaloids in the chick and its relationship to antimalarial activity. *J. Pharmacol.*, 85, 299.

MARSHALL, P. B., and ROGERS, E. W., 1945, A colorimetric method for the determination of cinchona alkaloids. *Biochem. J.*, 39, 258.

MARSHALL, P. B., and ROGERS, E. W., 1948, The determination of quinine degradation product in blood and its absorption in the chick. *Biochem. J.*, 43, 414.

MASEN, J. M., 1943, The quantitative determination of atabrine in blood and urine. *J. biol. Chem.*, 148, 529.

MASSART, L., 1949, Paludrine and cation exchange. *Arch. int. Pharmacodyn.*, 80, 470.

MEAD, J., and KOEPFLI, J. B., 1944, The structure of a new metabolic derivative of quinine. *J. biol. Chem.*, 154, 507.

MEAD, J. F., RAPPORT, M. M., and KOEPFLI, J. B., 1946, The synthesis of potential antimalarials. The reaction of organic lithium compounds with quinolinemethanols. *J. Amer. chem. Soc.*, 68, 2704

MELVILLE, K. I., 1946, The protective action of atabrine against chloroform-adrenaline ventricular fibrillation. *J. Pharmacol.*, 87, 350.

MEYTHALER, F., 1942, Die therapie der Malaria. *Münch. med. Wschr.*, 89, 812.

MIETZSCH, F., MAUSS, H., and HECHT, G., 1936, Experimental studies on atebrin. *Indian med. Gaz.*, 71, 521.

MONK, J. F., 1948, Results of an investigation of the therapeutic action of pentaquin on acute attacks of benign tertian malaria. *Trans. R. Soc. trop. Med. Hyg.*, 41, 663.

NANDI, B. K., 1940, Observations on the respiratory metabolism of tissues in the presence of plasmoquine. *J. Mal. Inst. India*, 3, 475.

OLDHAM, F. K., and KELSEY, F. E., 1943, Studies on antimalarial drugs. The influence of pregnancy on the quinine oxidase of rabbit liver. *J. Pharmacol.*, 79, 81.

OLDHAM, F. K., and KELSEY, F. E., 1945, Studies on antimalarial drugs. The distribution of atabrine in the tissues of the fowl and the rabbit. *J. Pharmacol.*, 83, 288.

OVERMAN, R. R., 1948, Reversible cellular permeability alterations in disease. *In vivo* studies on sodium, potassium and chloride concentrations in erythrocytes of the malarious monkeys. *Amer. J. Physiol.*, 152, 113.

PARMER, L. G., 1948, Blood and bone marrow concentration of atabrine and and its rôle in aplastic anemia. *J. Lab. clin. Med.*, 33, 827.

PEETERS, E. M. E., 1949, Essai thérapeutique de la malaria par un anti-paludique de synthése injectable (lactate de paludrine). *Ann. Soc. belge. Méd. trop.*, 29, 225.

PETCH, C. P., 1947, Action of mepacrine on gastric secretion. *Lancet, ii*, 561.

PLOYÉ, M., 1950, Un medicament trop peu employé : la quinidine. *Rev. Palud.*, 8, 123.

PICK, E. P., and HUNTER, J., 1944, Action of atabrine on electro cortico-potentials. *J. Pharmacol.*, 80, 354.

PIRK, L. A., and ENGELBERG, R., 1945, Hypothrombinemic action of quinine sulfate. *J. Amer. med. Ass.*, 128, 1093.

QUEVAUVILLER, A., 1946, L'elimination de la quinine injectée au lapin est ralentie par un " véhicule-retard," le subtosan. *Rev. Palud.*, 4, 225.

RAMSDEN, W., LIPKIN, I. J., and WHITLEY, E., 1918, On quinine in animal tissues and liquids, with methods for its estimation. *Ann. trop. Med. Parasit.*, 12, 223.

ROGERS, L., 1918, The advantages of intramuscular injections of soluble cinchonine salts in severe malarial infections. *Brit. med. J., ii*, 459.

SCHECHTER, A. J., and TAYLOR, H. M., 1936, Atabrine pigmentation. *Amer. J. med. Sci.*, 192, 645.

PHARMACOLOGY 185

SCHMIDT, L. H., HUGHES, H. B., and SMITH, C. C., 1947, On the pharmacology
of N_1-para-chlorophenyl-N_5-isopropyl-biguanide (paludrine). *J. Phar-
macol.*, **90**, 233.
SCHULZ, R., 1949, Hydrogenolysis as a method for determining chloroguanide
(paludrine). *J. Amer. pharm. Ass.*, **38**, 84.
SCUDI, J. V., and JELINEK, V. C., 1944, Urinary excretion products of atabrine.
J. biol. Chem., **152**, 27.
SHANNON, J. A., and EARLE, D. P., Jr., 1945, Recent advances in the treatment
of malaria. *Bull. N.Y. Acad. Med.*, **21**, 467.
SHANNON, J. A., EARLE, D. P., Jr., BRODIE, B. B., TAGGART, J. V., and
BERLINER, R. W., 1944, The pharmacological basis for the rational
use of atabrine in the treatment of malaria. *J. Pharmacol.*, **81**, 307.
SILVESTRI, S., 1923, Assorbimento, eliminazione, tossicita della cinconina.
Policlinico, sez. med., **30**, 601.
SMITH, L. H., and STOECKLE, J. D., 1946, Effect of quinacrine hydrochloride
(atabrine) on isolated mammalian heart. *Proc.Soc.exp.Biol.,N.Y.*,**62**,179.
SMITH, P. K., GALLUP, B. N., and CAIN, L. J., 1946, Blood plasma atabrine
levels obtained with suppressive and therapeutic doses of atabrine
dihydrochloride. *J. Pharmacol.*, **87**, 360.
SPINKS, A., 1945, Studies on synthetic antimalarial drugs. VII. Turbidimetric determination of 2-*p*-chlorophenylguanidino-4-β-diethylamino-
ethylamino-6-methylpyrimidine (3349). *Ann. trop. Med. Parasit.*,**39**,182.
SPINKS, A., 1946, The pharmacology of paludrine in animals. *Trans. R. Soc.
trop. Med. Hyg.*, **40**, 3.
SPINKS, A., 1947, Studies on synthetic antimalarial drugs. XVIII The
absorption, distribution and excretion of paludrine in experimental
animals. *Ann. trop. Med. Parasit.*, **41**, 30.
SPINKS, A., 1948, Studies on synthetic antimalarial drugs. XX. The blood
concentrations and physiological distribution of some homologues of
paludrine in relation to their antimalarial activities. *Ann. trop. Med.
Parasit.*, **42**, 190.
SPINKS, A., and TOTTEY, M. M., 1945a, Studies on synthetic antimalarial
drugs. VIII. Colorimetric determination of 2-*p*-chlorophenylguanidino-
4-β-diethylaminoethylamino-6-methylpyrimidine (3349). *Ann. trop.
Med. Parasit.*, **39**, 190.
SPINKS, A., and TOTTEY, M. M., 1945b, Studies on synthetic antimalarial
drugs. IX. The excretion of 2-*p*-chlorophenylguanidino-4-β-diethyl-
aminoethylamino-6-methylpyrimidine (3349) in human urine. *Ann.
trop. Med. Parasit.*, **39**, 197.
SPINKS, A., and TOTTEY, M. M., 1945c, Studies on synthetic antimalarial
drugs. XII. Determination of N_1-*p*-chlorophenyl-N_5-methyl-N_5-iso-
propylbiguanidine (4430) and N_1-*p*-chlorophenyl-N_5-isopropylbiguanide
(paludrine): a preliminary report. *Ann. trop. Med. Parasit.*, **39**, 220.
SPINKS, A., and TOTTEY, M. M., 1946a, Studies on synthetic antimalarial
drugs. XV. Hydrolytic determination of paludrine. *Ann. trop. Med.
Parasit.*, **40**, 101.
SPINKS, A., and TOTTEY, M. M., 1946b, Studies on synthetic antimalarial
drugs. XVI. The absorption, distribution and excretion of 2-*p*-chloro-
phenylguanidino-4-β-diethylaminoethylamino-6-methylpyrimidine (3349)
in experimental animals. *Ann. trop. Med. Parasit.*, **40**, 145.
SPINKS, A., TOTTEY, M. M., and MAEGRAITH, B. G., 1946, The pharmacology
of paludrine and some other new antimalarials. *Biochem. J.*, **40**, Procs. i.
STEPHENSON, R. P., 1948, The pharmacological properties of conessine,
isoconessine and neoconessine. *Brit. J. Pharmacol.*, **3**, 237.
STORM, C. J., 1935, Über die Anwendung des Suprarenins bei intravenöser
Injektion von Atebrin im Affenversuch. *Klin. Wschr.* 14i, 756.
SUFFOLK and BERKSHIRE, Earl of, 1939, Pharmacological actions of acridine
derivatives, with especial reference to those of acriflavine and atebrin.
Quart. J. exp. Physiol., **29**, 1.

TAGGART, J. V., 1946, The physiological disposition of a series of 9-amino acridines. *Fed. Proc.*, 5, 206.

TAGGART, J. V., BERLINER, R. W., ZUBROD, C. G., WELCH, W. J., EARLE, D. P., Jr., and SHANNON, J. A., 1946, Cinchona alkaloids. 3. Physiological disposition in man. *Fed. Proc.*, 5, 206.

TAGGART, J. V., EARLE, D. P., Jr., BERLINER, R. W., ZUBROD, C. G., WELCH, W. J., WISE, N. B., SCHROEDER, E. F., LONDON, I. M., and SHANNON, J. A., 1948, Studies on the chemotherapy of the human malarias. III. The physiological disposition and antimalarial activity of the cinchona alkaloids. *J. clin. Invest.*, 27, Suppl., p. 80.

TÁRNOKY, A. L., 1950, Some properties of acridane and 2-chloro-7-methoxyacridane : their possible relationship to excretion products of mepacrine. *Biochem. J.*, 46, 297.

TEN CATE, J., and BOELES, J. T. F., 1948, The effect of quinine on the nervous system. *Arch. int. Pharmacodyn.*, 77, 468.

TITUS, E. O., CRAIG, L. C., GOLUMBIC, C., MIGHTON, H. R., WEMPEN, I. M., and ELDERFIELD, R. C., 1947, Identification by distribution studies. IX. Application to metabolic studies of 4-amino-quinoline antimalarials. *J. organ. Chem.*, 13, 39.

TOTTEY, M. M., and MAEGRAITH, B. G., 1948, Field method of estimating paludrine in urine. *Trans. R. Soc. trop. Med. Hyg.*, 41, 348.

TROPP, C., and WEISE, W., 1933, Untersuchungen über die Ausscheidung von Atebrin durch Harn und Fäzes. *Arch. exp. Path. Pharmak.*, 170, 339.

TSIKIMANAURI, G., 1931, Zur Pharmakologie des Plasmochins. *Arch. Schiffs-u. Tropenhyg.*, 35, 89.

UNNA, K., 1945, Toxic effects of atabrine following intravenous injection. *J. Amer. pharm. Ass.*, 34, 20.

VANE, J. R., 1949, Some pharmacological actions of paludrine. *Brit. J. Pharmacol.*, 4, 14.

VANE, J. R., WALKER, J. M., and WYNN PARRY, C. B., 1948, The effect of paludrine on gastric secretion in man. *Brit. J. Pharmacol.*, 3, 350.

WAELSCH, H., and NACHMANSOHN, D., 1943, On the toxicity of atabrine, *Proc. Soc. exp. Biol.*, *N.Y.*, 54, 336.

WAHI, P. N., 1947, Action of certain antimalarial drugs on plasma prothrombin level in normal and malarial subjects. *Indian Physician*, 6, 1.

WALETSKY, E., and BROWN, H. W., 1943, Studies on the mode of action of quinine in avian malaria. *J. nat. Mal. Soc.*, 2, 53.

WATS, R. C., and GHOSH, B. N., 1934, Quantitative and qualitative methods for detection of atebrin in urine. *Rec. Malar. Surv. India*, 4, 367.

WAYNE, E. J., GOODWIN, J. F., and STONER, H. B., 1949, The effect of adenosine triphosphate on the electrocardiogram of man and animals. *Brit. Heart J.*, 11, 55.

WEISE, W., 1937, Untersuchungen über die Resorption und Ausscheidung des Atebrins. 1. Methoden zur Bestimmung des Atebrins in Harn, Stuhl und Blut. *Arch. Schiffs-u. Tropenhyg.*, 41, 715.

WINCKEL, C. W. F., KOK, K., DE JONGH, D. K., and KNOPPERS, A. T., 1950, Plasma concentration and excretion of quinine carbonate and ethylcarbonate in man, as compared with quinine sulphate. *Doc. neerl. indon. Morb. trop.*, 2, 90.

WISEMAN, G., 1949, Hæmolysis with paludrine and its acceleration in the hæmocytometer chamber. *J. Physiol.*, 108, 23P.

YUDKIN, J., 1945b, Simple methods for the estimation of mepacrine in urine. *J. trop. Med. Hyg.*, 48, 1.

YUDKIN, J., 1946, Non-absorption of mepacrine—description of a case. *Brit. med. J.*, i, 271.

ZUBROD, C. G., KENNEDY, T. J., and SHANNON, J. A., 1948, Studies on the chemotherapy of the human malarias. VIII. The physiological disposition of pamaquin. *J. clin. Invest.*, 27, Suppl., p. 114.

CHAPTER VI

TOXIC REACTIONS TO ANTIMALARIAL DRUGS

(1) Cinchona Alkaloids

ALTHOUGH it is improbable that quinine will ever again be employed in malaria to the same extent as it was before 1940, yet as cinchona febrifuge is cheap its further use among certain poverty-stricken communities may possibly continue and toxic reactions may therefore still be seen. In addition, in the treatment of relapsing vivax malaria, quinine in association with pamaquin or some other 8-aminoquinoline is still the most useful medicament, as it is also in the immediate treatment of certain complications of falciparum malaria. Although one of the advantages of quinine has always been its low toxicity, it must be remembered that quinine is a general cytoplasmic poison. Its toxic effects may be classified as due to :—

(1) Hypersensitivity : the patient displays the symptoms of cinchonism after therapeutic doses which do not affect the normal person.

(2) Idiosyncrasy : the patient displays signs and symptoms such as skin rashes which never occur in the normal person.

(4) Acute poisoning : Raven (1927) has described death after 18·0 gm., but Kobert (1906) reported a patient who recovered after 19·8 gm. There was depression of all rather than of one particular system. Heathcote (1941) described a fatal case where 1 gm. of quinine was given intravenously in error.

(4) Acute hæmolysis associated with hæmoglobinuria.

(5) Cardiac changes.

The commonest reactions to the administration of quinine are those due to hypersensitivity, buzzing in the ears, slight deafness, and some degree of mental depression. Tinnitus and impairment of hearing rarely occur when the quinine plasma concentrations are less than 10 mgm. per litre. There is no evidence that it causes sterility in the male nor that it is responsible for dental caries, two widely held beliefs in the British Army. In fact, solutions of quinine inhibit spermatozoa less strongly than do solutions of mepacrine (Beck and Frommel, 1947). The great majority of persons can take 5 gr. (0·3 gm.) of quinine daily without any inconvenience, but 10 gr. (0·6 gm.) per day causes mild symptoms of cinchonism in a considerable proportion.

Severe toxic reactions are, however, rare. A child aged twenty months took between 50 and 100 gr. (3·2 and 6·6 gm.) and died two hours later after collapse, with muscular twitchings and cyanosed lips (Lynch and Brandt, 1940). Agranulocytosis has been seen once by the writer. Franks and Davis (1943) could find only four recorded cases to which they added one of their own, a patient who was given 15 gr. (1·0 gm.) a day : leucopenia was followed five days later by a sore throat. Anti-histamines are of value.

The most alarming reaction is undoubtedly amblyopia. The first instance of amblyopia after quinine was reported by Giacomini (1841, 1842). At this time enormous doses of quinine sulphate were the vogue. Anderson (1856) speaks of 100 to 150 gr. (6·6 to 10 gm.) being given in two days, so that it is hardly surprising that indistinct vision was not unheard of. In just over one hundred years under 250 cases have been reported, so that when the many millions who have taken quinine are considered the proportion affected is infinitesimal. Amblyopia does not necessarily follow large doses for the condition was rare in the 1914–18 war, when large doses were still often given. Bishay (1946), in Egypt, found that of seven patients only two had taken large doses though all had taken quinine on an empty stomach. One case in an Australian soldier is reported after 40 gr. (2·6 gm.) of quinine in two days (Hertzberg, 1946), but others have followed doses of 0·6 and 0·75 gm. Smith (1934) records a case after 1·0 gm. The blindness not infrequently comes on suddenly within a few minutes or up to one hour after taking quinine. The main signs and symptoms are blanching of the conjunctiva and anæsthesia of the cornea, though this is not invariably present. The pupil is dilated, the iris immobile, the optic discs pale, and the retinal blood vessels contracted. There is diminution of colour perception, particularly of reds and greens, while the field of vision is contracted. This contraction of the field of vision is seen in patients without complete blindness : it may also persist during recovery when a form of tubal vision continues. Œdema of the retina and pallor and haziness of the optic discs have also been reported but are inconstant. Changes in the retina may however be so profound as to resemble the changes produced by occlusion of the central artery of the retina. Elliot (1918) believed that the important signs of quinine amblyopia were (1) the completeness of the loss of vision and the suddenness of onset ; (2) the possibility of recovery ; (3) the fact that central vision is first regained, peripheral vision more slowly and often incompletely ; (4) the frequent damage to colour sense ; (5) the diminution in the sense of light, and not infrequently night blindness.

The cause of quinine amblyopia has been attributed to (1) the toxic action of quinine on the retinal cells ; (2) contraction of the retinal blood vessels.

Although it was at first thought that quinine acts on the vasomotor centres, later studies have demonstrated conclusively that the primary lesion is in the ganglion cells of the retina, vasoconstriction of the retinal vessels being a secondary effect. Richardson (1936) believes that the administration of quinine to the expectant mother may cause blindness in the fœtus, Nicloux (1909) having shown that quinine passes from the maternal to the fœtal circulation. Mosher (1938) gave quinine to pregnant guineapigs and found hæmorrhages in the cochlear vessels of both mothers and fœtuses. Swab (1932) and Sawyer (1933) have seen amblyopia developing after ethylhydrocupreine medication.

Although most cases of quinine amblyopia recover spontaneously, improvement may be very slow. The administration of strychnine in large doses and of vasodilators such as amyl nitrite or sodium nitrite intravenously has been recommended (Pelner and Saskin, 1942) : Bishay (1946) claims excellent results from paracentesis. Sympathectomy, as used in retinitis pigmentosa, is indicated in patients in whom contraction of the visual fields and reduced vision persist. McGregor and Loewenstein (1944) believe that in addition purgation, copious drinks, and thecal drainage are indicated. Alagna (1948) recommends riboflavin. Taylor (1934, 1935) suggested that prenatal medication of the mother is a causative factor in deafness in the newborn, since quinine produces degenerative changes in the ganglion cells of the spiral ganglion of the internal ear. Forbes (1940) especially has brought forward evidence that cases of so-called congenital deafness can be correlated with the ingestion of large amounts of quinine by the mother during pregnancy. Of 234 patients with nerve deafness, ninety-two gave a history of having themselves taken quinine over considerable periods of time and eighteen of these attributed their deafness to quinine. Of 832 cases of deafness, other than nerve deafness, only eighty-two had taken quinine and none of these associated the taking of quinine with their deafness. Winckel (1948) draws attention to the fact that only fifteen cases of congenital deafness and two of congenital blindness have been ascribed to the ingestion of quinine by the mother either during pregnancy or just before labour. All these cases come from the United States, yet the world consumption of quinine is 600,000 to 800,000 kgm. a year. If quinine were an important cause of congenital deafness or blindness, it is strange that cases have not been reported more frequently and from all parts of the world. In addition in the United States of America there is no correlation between the endemic incidence of malaria in the various States and the proportion of the inhabitants who are deaf, mute or blind. The effects of rubella on the fœtus were not appreciated at the time Taylor made his original suggestion. Ezes (1949) described a case of Turner's syndrome in a girl of seventeen. Her height was only 1·29 metres and the secondary sexual characteristics were absent and coarctation of the aorta was present. The mother of the child had been given large doses of quinine during pregnancy for malaria.

Skin rashes are occasionally seen as the result of sensitivity to quinine. A European soldier in West Africa who had never previously taken quinine developed a maculo-papular rash after two doses of 0·3 gm. of quinine sulphate on two successive days. The rash covered the face, trunk, arms, and legs and was associated with œdema of the face, hands, forearms, and prepuce. Patch tests with quinine hydrochloride produced wheals 6 cm. in diameter. This patient was sensitive also to mepacrine.

As quinine salts are known to produce contractions of the

uterine muscle, they have obtained a reputation as abortifacients, which is probably quite undeserved. In hyperendemic malarial zones premature termination of pregnancy is more likely to occur from malaria than from the administration of quinine. Evidence suggests that quinine may interfere with the action of calcium. Keogh and Shaw (1944) reported that the addition of Ca^{++} to isolated intestine previously treated with quinine induces contraction rather than the usual response of relaxation, an effect seen when calcium deficiency is induced by other means.

There is considerable evidence to show that in patients infected with certain strains of *P. falciparum* small doses of quinine will precipitate attacks of hæmoglobinuria (blackwater fever), but only so long as the malarial infection is uncontrolled (Fairley and Murgatroyd, 1940). The relationship of quinine to the onset of blackwater fever is discussed by Stephens (1937) and Findlay (1949). In addition, a series of cases has been recorded in which patients who have never had malaria and have never been exposed to infection have developed hæmoglobinuria after taking quinine. Two factors are common to all these cases. All have occurred in women in early pregnancy and all have ended fatally with two exceptions. Seitz (1927) reported three cases. The patients had taken only from 1·2 to 1·5 gm. of quinine. In one instance there was a rapid onset within five hours from the last of three doses. The urine was dark red and contained oxyhæmoglobin and other hæmoglobin derivatives : the blood urea rose to 250 mgm. per ml. Death took place on the twelfth day. The other cases were similar. Kutz and Traugott (1925) described two cases, but the necropsy notes are poor. Frommolt (1932) also reported two cases which at necropsy were diagnosed as hæmorrhagic nephritis. Petri (1930) recorded the case of a patient who had been given 1 gm. of quinine and 1 gm. of barbitone for three days. Hæmoglobin derivatives were found in the renal tubules.

The patient reported by Terplan and Javert (1936) had taken twenty tablets of 5 gr., a total of 6 gm., but the exact delay before arrival in hospital was unknown. On admission the patient was anæmic and had albuminuria but no hæmoglobinuria. The blood urea was raised and later hæmoglobinuria developed. The urinary secretion was reduced, red cells appeared in the urine,

and the patient died in coma after six days in hospital. At the
necropsy the kidneys showed blocking of the tubules, œdema of
the liver with hæmosiderosis, and uræmic gastritis with a purple
rash on the back and over the sacrum. Vartan and Discombe
(1940) described the case of a woman of thirty-four years of age
who took 6·08 gm. of quinine sulphate (= 5·04 gm. of the pure
alkaloid). There was fever, vomiting, a vaginal hæmorrhage,
urticaria, methæmalbumin in the plasma, and hæmoglobinuria.
The leucocytes rose to 26,800 cells per c.mm. and the blood urea
to 325 mgm. The pathological changes at necropsy were similar
to those found in blackwater fever.

In some of these patients the dose of quinine was high, 6 to
6·6 gm., but in others not more than 45 gr. (3·0 gm.) was taken in
three days. The patient described by Licciardello and Stanbury
(1948) was a woman aged forty-two, who was said to have taken
an unknown amount of quinine fourteen days before the sudden
appearance of hæmoglobinuria and profuse vaginal bleeding :
the red-cell count was 2,800,000 per c.mm. with 50,700 leucocytes
per c.mm., 86 per cent. being polymorphonuclear leucocytes.
Complete hæmolysis of the red cells occurred in 0·55 per cent.
saline solution and partial hæmolysis with 0·6 per cent. saline, as
compared with normal controls of 0·38 per cent. and 0·42 per
cent. Urine on the day of admission contained 1·3 mgm. of
quinine per litre. The patient recovered. Tests for cold agglutinins,
hæmolysins, and acid hæmolysis were negative, as was the Donath-
Landsteiner test. Wakeman *et al.* (1932) also reported the case
of a twenty-year-old girl who, having taken an unknown amount
of quinine, developed jaundice, hæmoglobinæmia, oliguria, and
uræmia. Another patient, three months pregnant, took 12·9 gm. :
she failed to abort and her only complaint was slight amaurosis
(Lewis, 1950).

The mechanism of the hæmolytic process is obscure. Acute
intravascular hæmolysis following quinine has been reported in
man apparently only in the presence of malaria and pregnancy.
Ponder and Abels (1936) found that in rabbits after large
doses of quinine there was a fall in red-cell concentration
and the erythrocytes became more susceptible to saponin and
sodium taurocholate hæmolysis. The quantity of quinine required

to produce this effect was far in excess of that known to have caused severe hæmolytic anæmia in man. These experiments might well be repeated in pregnant animals. Possibly quinine renders the red cells more susceptible to hæmolysins that may be present in pregnancy and malaria. Findlay and Markson (1947) have brought forward evidence that blackwater fever may be associated with an antigen-antibody reaction, while in animal experiments Nocht and Kikuth (1929) showed that very small amounts of quinine may facilitate amboceptor hæmolysis.

Quinine in therapeutic doses in man was not found by Rosenfeld *et al.* (1948) to produce methæmalbumin in the plasma although the administration of pamaquin and quinine together invariably did so. Blake (1948) believes that the presence of methæmalbuminæmia in the presence of both drugs is due to two phenomena, an increase in the catabolism of hæmoglobin and an interference with its subsequent degradation. Whereas the first of these two phenomena probably results from the synergistic action of pamaquin and quinine, the second is probably due to quinine itself. Increased hæmoglobin catabolism as evidenced by increased fæcal urobilinogen excretion is seen during combined drug administration but not when either drug is given in the same dosage alone. When moderate hæmolysis is simulated by small intravenous injections of hæmoglobin, no measurable methæmalbumin is formed. During quinine administration such an injection of hæmoglobin leads to the definite formation of serum methæmalbumin, the methæmalbumin formation being of the same order of magnitude as when similar injections of hæmoglobin are given to patients on a combined drug regimen. When pamaquin is given alone simulated hæmolysis may lead to traces of methæmalbumin and, when added to quinine, pamaquin may slightly increase the methæmalbuminæmia resulting from the intravenous injection of hæmoglobin. This effect of pamaquin would seem to be due to a retardation of the removal of serum methæmalbumin rather than to an increase in its formation, as is the case with quinine. Pamaquin retards methæmalbumin disappearance by about 11 per cent per day, an effect not increased by quinine.

The detection of methæmalbumin, first described by Fairley and Bromfield (1934), has been further particularised by Foy and

Kondi (1938), who used the absorption band at 623 mμ for its identification and estimation. Rosenfeld *et al.* (1948) have found that a band at 405 mμ is of greater intensity, thus permitting greater accuracy in measurement. The molar extinction coefficient is probably $\sum \dfrac{\text{mol.}}{405 \text{ m}\mu} = 7{\cdot}5 \times 10{\cdot}4$, calculated per mol. of hæmatin iron, while blackwater fever may be an allergic manifestation to infection with certain strains of *P. falciparum* the commonest sensitivity reaction to quinine is a skin rash. Other allergic manifestations are, however, seen.

Mamou (1947) records a case where after 1 gm. of quinine given intramuscularly there developed a petechial purpura with profuse hæmorrhages from the mucous membranes, epistaxis, gingival bleeding, hæmaturia and melæna. The number of red cells fell below two million per c.mm. For eight days blood transfusions of 300 ml. were given every two or three days but without stopping the hæmorrhage. Then on the eighth day, after a transfusion of 500 ml., hæmorrhage ceased suddenly. Some eleven years later the patient was again given 0·3 gm. of quinine by mouth : a generalised purpura again developed. This patient, it may be noted, was intolerant also to aspirin. Thrombocytopenic purpura following the administration of quinine has been reported on a number of occasions (Peshkin and Miller, 1934 ; Fasal and Wachner, 1933 ; Maritschek and Markowicz, 1933 ; Beiglböck, 1937, and Bais, 1941). Condorelli (1941) and Siegenbeek van Heukelom and Wahab (1941) also have recorded similar cases in a European and a Chinese. Hæmorrhage may occur at the site of an intramuscular injection and is not always closely correlated with the number of platelets present in the blood. In some cases there has been no hæmorrhage when the platelets are below 10,000 per c.mm., while in others it may begin when their number is above 50,000 per c.mm.

Similar instances of thrombocytopenic purpura have been reported after the administration of quinidine (Broch, 1941 ; Nudelman, Leff and Howe, 1948). Another manifestation of hypersensitivity is extreme flushing which may or may not be associated with intense generalised pruritus. There is some evidence that sensitivity to quinine may be transmitted hereditarily, possibly as a Mendelian dominant. Hauer (1939) records a family where a father, two daughters, and a grand-daughter were all sensitive to quinine.

Contact dermatitis through handling quinine is comparatively rare among nurses and others giving the drug therapeutically : nevertheless it is by no means uncommon in factories where quinine tablets are prepared. Werz (1949) found in Holland that about 10 per cent. of the workers in a quinine factory had skin lesions. With one exception all had been working for less than three months in the factory. Clinically there was dermatitis with œdema of the hands, forearms, face, and sometimes the genitals : in others the same areas showed chronic eczema. Nineteen of the twenty-two patients affected had to carry pans of boiling hot acid solutions of quinine as part of their duties. Patch tests with quinine salts were positive in sixteen of twenty-two patients but in some cases it took from three to fourteen days before the positive reaction could be detected.

Cinchonine also may cause blurring of vision, dizziness, drowsiness, dryness of the mouth and constipation. In addition, with doses of 3·0 to 4·0 gm. daily, Taggart *et al.* (1948) observed urinary retention necessitating catheterisation. Daily doses of 2·0 gm. cinchonine produced none of the unpleasant effects, nor did 2·0 gm. of cinchonidine or 1·0 gm. of quinidine daily.

Intramuscular injection of quinine inevitably leads to muscle necrosis and occasionally to abscess formation, while cases of tetanus and gas gangrene have been recorded. In African children injections of quinine into the buttocks have precipitated polio-myelitis, affecting especially the legs. Brown (1945) has recorded calcification in soft tissues as a sequela to therapeutic injections. The fall in blood pressure associated with intravenous administration of quinine, the duration of the cardiac depression and the necessity to control the injections by blood pressure readings whenever the general condition is poor, have long been recognised (McCarrison and Cornwall, 1919). In fourteen of twenty-four malaria patients given 2·66 gm. of quinine by a daily intravenous injection in 10 ml. of distilled water in a period of five days, myo-cardial impairment as indicated by electrocardiogram readings appeared after the fifth injection (Heilig and Visveswar, 1944).

Depression of the R-T segment and the reduction or abolition of the T wave is also recorded (Hughes, 1931). The mechanism of the circulatory depression is not fully understood, but Dreisbach and Hanzlik (1945) show that in serious cases of collapse in man the cardiac damage may be irreversible and no treatment is then of any avail. Divry (1948) found that ventricular fibrillation occurred in a pregnant woman who took a large but unknown dose of quinine between the second and third month. Pregnancy was not brought to an end. Aneurin may have an effect in counteracting this depressing action of quinine. It is perhaps the lack of aneurin in the food which explains the dangerous effects of intravenous quinine recorded from the General Hospital, Colombo, during the great epidemic of 1935 (de Silva, 1935).

Starvation and malaria were associated in this epidemic, where intravenous quinine appeared to be contraindicated whenever the systolic pressure was below 90 mm. Hg. (Fernando and Sandarasagara, 1935). Similarly Strahan (1948), in giving intravenous quinine to badly nourished prisoners of war in Singapore, records four fatal cases of collapse with *P. falciparum* infections and one with *P. vivax*. Details of these cases are as follows :—

Species of plasmodium.	Intensity of infection.	Notes.
Falciparum	Heavy	Intravenous injection of 0·5 gm. : immediate epileptiform convulsions and death.
Falciparum	Very heavy.	Intramuscular quinine 0·66 gm., followed one hour later by intravenous quinine 0·2 gm. : twenty minutes later collapse and death.
Falciparum	Moderate	Death during an intravenous injection.
Falciparum	Heavy	Intravenous quinine, 1·0 gm. in 5 ml. water. Immediate epileptiform convulsions. Death.
Vivax	—	Epileptiform convulsion during mepacrine therapy : 0·26 gm. quinine intravenously : immediate death.

It would appear advisable, though at present on empirical grounds, to administer aneurin to all patients with intense malarial infections whenever it is proposed to give quinine intravenously.

Rigdon (1949), in rhesus monkeys infected with *P. knowlesi*, found that electrocardiographic changes were induced by quinine when the monkeys were anæmic. If the red cell count varied from

1·9 to 3·24 million per c.mm. the lethal dose of quinine was from 28 to 47 mgm. per kgm. (Average for six monkeys, 33·2 mgm. per kgm.) For normal monkeys the lethal dose was 56 to 77 mgm. per kgm.

The so-called " paradoxical fever " sometimes, but very rarely, seen when quinine is given over long periods is as yet unexplained. As soon as quinine is withdrawn the fever ends (Reed, 1940).

Acute delirium after quinine administration has been recorded (Mishra, 1947). Some concern followed a report by Pirk and Engelberg (1945) that quinine in therapeutic doses caused hypo-thrombinæmia. These results have not been confirmed, for large doses failed to influence the prothrombin level in rabbits, and in guinea-pigs the effects were very doubtful (Fantl, *et al.*, 1947).

(2) Mepacrine

The pharmacology and therapeutics of mepacrine are now largely of historical interest, but its toxic effects still require some attention, since they may involve claims for compensation or pension. The toxic conditions produced are discussed by Findlay (1947b). Single doses of 1·0 to 1·5 gm. have repeatedly been given without untoward effect, while larger doses have occasionally been taken either in error or with suicidal intent (Barbosa, 1934 ; Foy *et al.*, 1936). Burnham (1946) recorded a case where a man took 90 gr. (6·0 gm.) in an attempt at suicide : recovery was complete and no apparent signs of liver damage remained. Markson and Dawson (1945) also reported the case of a patient who, after taking 0·7 gm. of mepacrine weekly as a suppressive for sixteen months, swallowed 250 tablets (25 gm.) with suicidal intention. Ten minutes later he began to vomit and suffered from diarrhœa ; he then became weak and drowsy. When found three hours later he was collapsed and stuporose : his skin was cold and clammy, the pulse barely perceptible, the pupils contracted and all tendon reflexes were highly active. The plasma mepacrine concentration was 906 μgm. per litre. On the second day the plasma mepacrine was 183 μgm. per litre, and on the third day it had fallen to 90 μgm. per litre. At no time was mepacrine found in the cerebro-spinal fluid. The urine contained no albumin, bile, sugar or acetone. The patient was given adrenaline, 2 pints of 30 per cent. glucose in saline, and 5 mgm. of riboflavin intravenously ; in twenty-four hours he had recovered. Wright and Lillie (1943), however, found that in rats given 80 mgm. of mepacrine per kgm. of body weight the toxic effects were not reduced by a daily dosage of riboflavin, 5 to 10 mgm. per kgm. of body weight. Williamson *et al.* (1946) believed that the toxic effects of mepacrine in rats were enhanced by a high calcium dietary : such a diet resulted in higher concentrations of mepacrine in the livers and spleens.

Occasionally in patients given therapeutic doses of mepacrine there are symptoms of nausea associated with abdominal discomfort (Green, 1932 ; Chopra *et al.*, 1933 ; Schulemann, 1935 ; Hoops, 1935 ; Banerjee, 1936a, b). Among 49,681 cases which were treated with either prophylactic or therapeutic doses of mepacrine Bispham (1941), however, found only thirty-eight in which there were severe symptoms : vomiting, diarrhœa, anorexia, epigastric or precordial pain and restlessness. Kahlstorf (1947) described jaundice and liver damage in a soldier who had taken at least 5·2 gm. in three weeks. It is not clear whether the jaundice was due to mepacrine or to an intercurrent infective hepatitis.

The unpleasant gastro-intestinal effects may be due, it has been suggested, to inactivation of choline esterase, an enzyme-destroying acetylcholine. Inhibition of choline esterase would produce symptoms similar to those resulting from stimulation of the vagus. Waelsch and Nachmansohn (1943) showed that mepacrine in a concentration of 4 μgm. of free base per ml. reduces by more than half the activity of choline esterase. In a concentration of 0·25 μgm. per ml. it inhibits the contraction caused by barium chloride and histamine on the guinea-pig ileum (Beck, 1949). Quinine was some 200 times less effective than mepacrine, while physostigmine was from 100 to 200 times more effective. If vagus stimulation were the cause of the symptoms it is curious that bradycardia is not prominent as a symptom in those who suffer from gastro-intestinal symptoms and are taking mepacrine.

Cellulose-acetate-phthalate is a satisfactory enteric coating for mepacrine if vomiting occurs ; it does not interfere with the ultimate absorption of the drug.

During the war of 1939–45, when mepacrine was taken as a suppressive by large numbers of troops, mild symptoms referable to the abdomen were common during the first ten to fifteen days of suppressive therapy when nausea, eructations, diarrhœa and a feeling of fullness in the abdomen occurred. These symptoms usually disappeared completely, but in about 2 per cent. of cases they continued and necessitated the withdrawal of mepacrine. Headache, insomnia, temporary giddiness and faintness were less common. Slight mental depression has been noted, but this is less than that associated with the prolonged taking of suppressive quinine (Findlay and Stevenson, 1944). During the war years a number of surveys were made of the effects of mepacrine on volunteers in a cool climate, on troops who had returned to a cool climate after taking mepacrine for from twelve to eighteen months and on troops still serving in the tropics who had taken 0·1 gm. mepacrine for periods of one to three years. No evidence could be found of damage to the respiratory, cardio-vascular, hæmatopoietic or nervous systems or to the functional activity of the liver or kidneys. Any abnormalities observed in the electrocardiogram could be attributed to other causes (Levine and Erlanger, 1946). Mepacrine is not demonstrably more toxic at 18,000 ft. than at ground level, so that its use by flying personnel is not contraindicated (Van Liere and Emerson, 1942 ; Smith, 1943). Observations on nursing officers serving in West Africa showed that there was no interference with their menstrual periods. Similar observations were made in England by the Army Malaria Research Unit (1946).

Severe toxic reactions to mepacrine have involved the skin, the central nervous system, hæmatopoietic system, and the eyes.

(1) **Skin Lesions.** Even before the Second World War there had been occasional reports of skin lesions due to mepacrine. Nayadu (1937), for instance, described two patients with giant urticaria which was believed to be due to mepacrine, and Storey (1938) observed a patient with round or oval macules on a diffuse erythematous background, a rash closely resembling that of endemic typhus : two days after the drug was discontinued the rash faded. Loewenthal (1947) mentions a case seen by him in 1935 in Uganda which he believes to have been due to mepacrine. In doctors and nurses handling mepacrine, skin lesions had also been seen, while in those exposed to an atmosphere containing mepacrine dust, lacrimation, photophobia and eczematous patches

had been known to occur. Whitehill (1945) described the case of a nurse who as a result of handling mepacrine developed a contact dermatitis on both eyelids and behind the right ear. The yellow pigmentation of the skin was also well known (Soni, 1935 ; Schechter and Taylor, 1936). Its intensity varies greatly in different persons. It is most clearly seen on the dorsal surface of the fingers and on the forehead and face, but only very rarely on the scleræ. When the conjunctivæ are tinted the yellow colour is seen most distinctly on the parts not exposed to light. If mepacrine is applied to the conjunctiva it merely causes irritation, but West African troops, by adding mepacrine to an alkaline base, found that it was possible to stain the conjunctivæ deeply, thus simulating jaundice. The yellow tint in the skin may last for from two to four months after ceasing to take mepacrine. It appears to be due to the staining of the tissues by an acridine dye which renders the tissues fluorescent when exposed to ultra-violet light. Ginsberg and Shallenberger (1946) find that fluorescence on exposure to Wood's light disappears from the finger nails in from three to six months, but in the toe nails fluorescence is detectable up to twelve months after administration of mepacrine. Apart from the æsthetic discomfort which is specially felt by women, the yellow discoloration is of no significance. A far less striking finding is a bluish-grey or slate-coloured pigmentation of the nail beds, either a diffuse pigmentation involving the entire nail bed or a transverse band near the middle of the nail. Such bluish pigmentation may also involve the skin of the nose, the hard palate, the epiglottis and the tracheal rings, and the skin at the sides of the nails. On the hard palate it is usually first seen near the midline, whence it extends to the gum margins. It may vary in colour from slate-grey to blue-black. Biopsy specimens show that the pigment contains iron. It was by no means uncommon in Europeans in West Africa in those who had been taking mepacrine for more than a year, while it was also noted in the Pacific area (Lippard and Kauer, 1945 ; Lutterloh and Shallenberger, 1946). In American troops this type of pigmentation was present in 27·3 per cent. of those taking mepacrine for from seven to twelve months, in 54·8 per cent. of those taking mepacrine for from thirteen to eighteen months, and in 63·8 per cent. of those taking mepacrine for from nineteen to twenty-four months. The blue pigmentary changes also fade in from two to three months.

During the latter part of 1943 reports began to appear of a curious lichenoid skin disease which was becoming not uncommon among Australian and American troops fighting in the Pacific area. At first, as in the report by Ambler (1944) and Myers (1944), the large number of patients suffering from lichen planus hypertrophicus was noted. Hellier (1944) described two patients, one from North, the other from West Africa : Roxburgh (1944) saw a soldier from Libya. Later the suspicion arose that these cases were in some way associated with the prolonged administration of mepacrine (Harvey *et al.*, 1944 ; Schmitt *et al.*, 1945 ; Mitchell, 1945, and others). For security reasons much information was suppressed during the actual continuance of hostilities, but with the coming of peace it became possible to give a full account of the subject.

The " mepacrine dermatitis complex," as it has been called, was seen in all theatres of war where, owing to the presence of malaria, mepacrine suppression was necessary. It was most prevalent in the Pacific zone, though cases were reported from Australia, Burma, India (Livingood and Dieuaide, 1945 ; Agress, 1946), Assam, North Africa and Italy (Nelson, 1945 ; Grant-Peterkin and Hair, 1946 ; Grant-Peterkin, 1947, and Loewenthal, 1947), and West Africa. Its incidence, however, in different areas varied greatly. Even in the Pacific and South-east Asia the incidence was higher in some localities than in others, suggesting that climatic and geographical factors may have played a contributory *rôle*. No race appears to have been exempt, since cases were seen in Americans, British, South Africans, Australians, New Zealanders, Maoris, Mexicans, Negroes, Filipinos, American Indians, Indians, Chinese and Japanese. Judging from the clinical reports which have appeared, the disease seems to have been far more common among Americans, Australians and New Zealanders than among other nations ; more than 1,000 cases have been reported by American observers : Butler (1947) 247 cases ; Bazemore *et al.*, (1946) over 400 cases ; Bereston (1946) 200 cases ; Epstein (1945) sixty-five cases ; Bagby (1945) twenty-five cases ; Dantzig and Marshall (1946), twenty-four cases ; Kierland (1946) forty-nine cases ; Rosenthal (1946) five cases. Grant-Peterkin (1947) mentions only fifty-three British cases seen by him in the Mediterranean zone. Loewenthal (1947) mentions some fifty cases in South African military hospitals in Italy, and Singh (1948) eighty-three cases among Indian troops in Burma. In West Africa the incidence of lichen planus and lichenoid conditions was no higher among British troops after March, 1943, when mepacrine suppression was begun, than it had been in 1941 and 1942, when British troops were taking quinine : in addition the incidence of lichen planus and, incidentally, exfoliative dermatitis was no higher among British troops in West Africa, who were taking mepacrine, than among African troops who were not taking any suppressive (Findlay, 1946) ; only three cases of exfoliative dermatitis occurred in two years among 15,000 British troops. Russell (1947) describes one patient who had never left the British Isles, while Wallace (1947) reports one case from West Africa. Agress (1946), in Chinese, estimated the incidence of exfoliative dermatitis as one among 2,000 to 3,000 of those given mepacrine ; Singh (1948), among Indians, one in 3,000. There is a suggestion from American sources that women, in proportion to their numbers, were more frequently affected than men in the South-West Pacific area, while brunettes were more often affected than blondes. Of 259 patients 82 per cent. were brunettes (Bazemore *et al.*, 1946). Temperamental differences were not significantly associated with the diseases, but Kierland (1946) believes that the age distribution was higher than the average age in the area. In Burma, fifty-six of eighty-three occurred during the monsoon with a humidity of 80 to 100 per cent., and twenty-one in September, October and November. The disease, which at first was termed " atypical lichen planus," is characterised by various combinations of the following lesions : violaceous and erythematous, hypertrophic, lichenoid papules and plaques, often with a rough verrucous surface ; violaceous and erythematous, oozing or scaling ezcematoid plaques, well demarcated in some cases, ill-defined in others ; flat, squamous, geographic plaques on the trunk, axillæ and groins, similar to tinea lesions ; white, sometimes violet-tinged, slightly raised mucous membrane lesions identical with those seen in typical lichen planus ; oozing intertriginous dermatitis in the groins, axillæ, and posterior surface of the ears ; ecthymatous lesions ; scaling and superficial fissuring of the lips and scaling erythematous eczematoid dermatitis of the eyelids. In some patients the lesions are predominantly lichenoid, in others most of the plaques are eczematoid. Many patients have at some time both violaceous hypertrophic lichenoid plaques and some form of cutaneous eczematoid reaction. During the course of the disease a considerable number of these patients suffer from acute " explosive " generalised exacerbations, manifested by oozing eczematoid dermatitis, especially on the flexor surfaces of the limbs, the groins, axillæ, extremities, and neck. Such exacerbations merge into a true secondary exfoliative dermatitis, quite as severe as that seen in primary exfoliative dermatitis. As Nisbet (1945) has emphasised, the condition thus superficially resembles almost every known dermatosis.

At the onset the first appearance is usually that of localised violaccous or erythematous eczematoid plaques on the dorsal surface of the hands or feet, upper part of the back, or on the sides of the neck, ears, nose and around the mouth. The plaques often appear first as tiny follicular papules 1 to 2 mm. in diameter, later coalescing to form the violaceous plaques 2 to 5 mm. in diameter. These plaques in turn fuse to form thick plates of violct-grey, desquamating skin up to 30 cm. in diameter and sometimes as much as 1 cm. in thickness. The tops of the lesions are flat and Wickham's striæ are frequently seen ; later the tops are covered with fine adherent silvery scales (Bazemore *et al.*, 1946). New lesions continue to develop in fresh parts of the body. The soles and palms are often solid plaques which crack and bleed on motion. Barker (1947) has noted hyperkeratosis of the palms and soles as the sole symptom. The lesions were symmetrical and disappeared slowly as the yellow colour of the skin decreased. On the face there was often a typical spectacle frame dermatitis. A variable degree of horny follicular plugging on the back and shoulders was not uncommon (Williams, 1947). Reticulation is seen in almost every case. Bagby (1945) has described five cases in which pustules were replaced in healing by lesions of atypical lichen planus. The polygonal shiny lesions characteristic of true lichen planus did not occur.　After the appearance of the initial lesions there was usually a generalisation over the whole body, though not infrequently the middle zone of the trunk was exempt. The parts most severely affected were the legs, forearms, dorsal surface of the hands and feet, face and eyelids, buttocks, over the sternum and neck and the genitalia.　Lesions were particularly liable to develop at the sites of trauma and on areas recently affected by tinea or scabies.　Early and destructive lesions of the nails were common but not permanent.　Sometimes in addition to discoloration there was a heaping up of the nail substance, the so-called " Beau-line."　Wallace (1947) observed one case where a prickly-heat type of eruption first developed round the ankles followed after a few days by a widespread eruption all over the body, œdema of the ankles and ulceration of the mouth.　The site of the initial lesions in 302 patients is shown in the table.　In addition to the lichenoid plaques some cases more rarely showed lesions resembling psoriasis or even pityriasis rosacea.

THE SITE OF THE INITIAL LESION IN LICHENOID DERMATITIS
(Bazemore *et al.*, 1946)

Location.	Number of cases.	Percentage of cases.
Hands and wrists	103	33·7
Feet and ankles	72	23·8
Legs	49	16·2
Groin	12	4·0
Arms	11	3·6
Thighs	9	3·0
Eyelids	8	2·3
Ears	5	1·6
Lips	5	1·6
Face and scalp	5	1·6
Chest	4	1·3
Axillæ	4	1·3
Mouth	3	1·0
Abdomen	3	1·0
Neck	3	1·0
Scrotum	3	1·0
Other sites	3	1·0

Mucous membrane lesions also appeared with blisters and ulcers in the mouth, fissures on the lips and at the corners of the mouth, and rawness on the edges of the tongue. Involvement of the lips, buccal mucosa, and tongue may suggest syphilitic mucous patches. The mucosa of the colon or rectum was rarely involved, but Butler (1947) has described lesions resembling condylomata on the genitalia and in the perianal region. The glans penis, however, was scarcely ever affected. Œdema of the ankles was very common. Burning irritation of the hands and feet has been noted in a patient who also developed mental symptoms (Clarke, 1949).

Pathological Changes. The histological changes present in the skin have been very fully investigated by Rosenthal (1946) and Kierland (1946). Three stages which merge into one another may be distinguished, the earliest lesions resembling those of ordinary lichen planus. The main features are the hyperkeratinisation and plugging of the openings of the hair follicles, degenerative and liquefactive changes in the basal layer, and the presence of infiltrating cells in the papillary and subpapillary connective tissue around the hair shafts, hair follicles and some of the dermal glands. The number of the invading cells, histiocytes, lymphocytes and eosinophils, with very few polymorphonuclear leucocytes and plasma cells, depends on the severity of the disease. The changes in the basal layer are somewhat patchy and vary in different regions. They are best seen in the acute stage, but even then they may not be distinguishable from those of other dermatoses. There is no vascular or collagenous change other than that accompanying acute inflammation. Œdema is frequently seen in the acute and subacute stages, both extracellularly and intracellularly, in the prickle cell and basal layers as well as in the upper layers of the corium. Atrophy of sebaceous glands and infiltration around sweat glands are frequent ; sweat glands may in fact be destroyed by the infiltration. Of all the changes noted, the one that is common to all stages is the lesion in the basal layer, and this layer of the epidermis is the last to return to normal when the disease has subsided. An outstanding feature is the aggregation of pigment in the papillary and subpapillary connective tissue. These collections of pigment are specially seen in the acute stages, most characteristically at the tips of the papillæ and around the sweat glands, but frequently also in the sub-papillary connective tissue : the pigment is found either within macrophages or scattered in the connective tissue. It gives negative reactions for hæmosiderin or hæmofuscin but positive tests for melanin. The pigmentation is not limited to the acute stage but is found in appreciable amounts even in the papillary or subpapillary connective tissue. The normal pigment of the basal layer is generally increased. The increase in pigmentation is extreme unless acanthosis is severe. The acanthosis may be so extreme that the change may suggest an epithelioma. Elastic tissue is not changed.

In addition to the lichenoid lesions, a condition of eczematoid dermatitis has been seen in persons taking suppressive mepacrine. Bilateral, symmetrical, violet-tinged, vesicular, eczematoid or oozing plaques occur involving more especially the hands, arms, feet, legs and less commonly other parts of the body. The nail bed and skin of the nail folds are frequently affected, resulting in exfoliation of the nails without true suppurative paronychia. The lesions usually begin as patches of closely set, deep-seated miliary vesicles, which clear up and relapse to form erythematous, eczematoid patches. The term symmetrical eczematoid dermatitis has been applied to this condition (Medical Consultants Division Rept., U.S.A., 1945). The lichenoid and the eczematous conditions may frequently be combined in the same patient. While a broad division may be made into those lesions that are raised above the skin surface and those that are not it is possible to distinguish the following types which together make up the mepacrine-dermatitis complex :—

(1) A non-weeping form with the primary characteristics of a lichenoid dermatitis.

(2) Eczematous dermatitis.

(3) Combined lichenoid and eczematous dermatitis.

(4) Pustules replaced in healing by lichenoid lesions.

(5) Exfoliative dermatitis secondary to (1) to (4) or (8).

(6) Primary exfoliative dermatitis.

(7) Hyperkeratosis of the palms of the hands and soles of the feet.

(8) Discrete maculo-papular or scarlatiniform rashes.

A number of secondary complications have been described. There is usually loss of body hair, while the scalp hair shows lesions recalling those of alopecia areata. When the hair returns it is often darker. Bazemore *et al.* (1946) describe one case where the hair was at first white but later returned to normal. Total alopecia has occurred. When no hair is lost groups of follicular papules may be seen on the hair scalp. Itching is sometimes severe and is not necessarily related to the severity of the lesions. In some instances a prodromal stage was noted in which intense itching was present in the absence of lesions. Pruritus, also, did not correspond with the severity of the condition. Nervous phenomena occasionally occurred ; sharp shooting pains were present in the legs, patches of anæsthesia and paræsthesia in the skin, and in rare instances disturbance of vision with contraction of the visual fields. Polyneuritis has also been seen. Mental depression was not infrequent, while Butler (1947), among 247 cases, describes three in which there were hallucinations and delusions. Secondary bacterial infection with pustules or abscesses, sometimes with the formation of septic ulcers, was seen in about 10 per cent. of cases, and the lymph nodes, more especially those in the inguinal region, often exhibited a non-suppurative adenitis : lymphangitis has occurred. Staphylococci and streptococci, diphtheroids, and coliform organisms have been isolated. Infection of hair follicles, both superficial and furuncular, was common, the usual organism being *Staphylococcus pyogenes.*

Interference with sweating in the affected areas was very common. Some patients were sensitive to light. Venous stasis with œdema in the lower limbs was occasionally seen. Anorexia and diarrhœa were sometimes present ; in one patient blood was passed per rectum. Most patients lost weight, decreases of 10 to 30 lbs. (4·5 to 13·5 kgm.) being not infrequent. A low-grade fever was often present. Depigmentation or hyperpigmentation with deposits of melanin and atrophy of the skin were also encountered. In a negro, patches of vitiligo developed. Diffuse follicular accentuation in the skin over the upper part of the back, shoulders and extremities and loss of or changes in the nails were sometimes seen. Telangiectasia also occasionally developed.

Simple anæmia was not uncommon, and in a few patients aplastic anæmia occurred, while Bereston and Saslaw (1946) described one patient who in the course of an exfoliative dermatitis showed symptoms of glomerulo-nephritis with albumin, red blood corpuscles, and granular and pus casts in the urine. The skin became a dark coffee colour and a profound anæmia developed. (Hæmoglobin percentage 58, erythrocytes 2,810,000 per c.mm.) A high eosinophil count, up to 54 per cent., was sometimes encountered in the absence of helminthic infection or Löffler's syndrome. Liver function tests as a rule revealed no abnormality. A number of other complications have also been seen in association with the mepacrine dermatitis complex, but it is doubtful whether there was any causal relationship. Pericarditis, hepatitis, atypical pneumonia, ascites and œdema have all been recorded. Occasional deaths have occurred. Butler (1947) records one which took place three months after the last dose of mepacrine. In this instance degenerative changes were found in the myocardium. Agress (1946) saw three deaths among five Chinese suffering from exfoliative dermatitis due to mepacrine : all these patients had some degree of hepatitis. Lum (1946) also describes a fatal acute hepatitis associated with lichenoid dermatitis.

During convalescence recurrent attacks of pyoderma super-imposed on the flattening lichenoid lesions may develop, and thrombophlebitis has sometimes been seen. Wallace (1947) observed a patient who four years after onset had recurrent attacks of soreness of the tongue with gross lichenoid changes in the mouth and tongue, suggestive of early leukoplakia. In addition, atrophic lichenoid changes were present on the body and scalp, while warty growths were present on the forehead : these growths recurred after cauterisation. In view of the chronicity of some lesions and the sensitivity to ultra-violet light, Scoltern (1946) has given a warning of the possible development of ultra-violet light carcinomata. Recurrence of eczematous lesions has also been recorded months or even years after ceasing to take mepacrine. The recurrent lesions are less commonly symmetrical. Some patients have complained that since their original attack they have become far more sensitive to a large number of other substances, an example of a specific eczema becoming non-specific as a result of a broadening of the allergic base (Schmitt, 1949).

The relationship of the skin lesions to mepacrine was suggested at an early stage. Senear *et al.* (1945) had reported skin lesions of a lichenoid type in a husband and wife who had used mepacrine as a suppressive for a considerable period, and Noojin and Callaway (1942) had incriminated mepacrine as the cause of an exfoliative dermatitis in a diabetic patient. Duemling (1945) also suggested that mepacrine was a causal factor in three cases of exfoliative dermatitis seen by him in the South-West Pacific area. The arguments which have been put forward in favour of the view that mepacrine is the primary causal factor in this symptom complex are as follows :—

(1) The syndrome has been seen in all areas where large bodies of troops have taken mepacrine as a malarial suppressive and in one man who had never left the British Isles (Russell, 1947).

(2) Those persons who have taken more than 0·7 gm. of mepacrine a week appear to be more liable to develop the syndrome than those who have not exceeded this dosage.

(3) When in 1943 in the South-West Pacific area the dose was increased to 0·7 gm. weekly and discipline was enforced to see that this dose was taken the incidence of the disease increased.

(4) Only 20 per cent. of the cases developed lesions within three months of beginning mepacrine therapy, whereas in 80 per cent. they had developed in seven months.

(5) Some, but by no means all, patients failed to improve till mepacrine was stopped.

(6) Readministration of mepacrine caused a late chronic lichenoid reaction identical with the original lesions in 19·3 per cent. of cases (Bazemore *et al.*, 1946).

(7) On experimental readministration of mepacrine to forty-six patients with lichenoid eruptions, exacerbations occurred in nine ; in six the reinvolvement was extensive, and in three only a few lesions were seen. The earliest relapse of lichenoid lesions occurred in twenty-three days and the longest in ninety-seven days. In the majority of cases the time of relapse was between forty and sixty-three days. The exacerbations of atypical lichen planus on experimental readministration occurred in the same

frequency within three months as they had on initial ingestion of the drug (Bazemore *et al.*, 1946).

(8) Lichen planus has occasionally been recorded after the long-continued administration of gold, bismuth, mercury or arsenical preparations (Bigham, 1949).

The evidence which suggests that mepacrine itself is not the primary factor in the production of the lichenoid eruption is as follows :—

(1) The far greater prevalence of atypical lichen planus in the South-West Pacific area among American, Australian, and New Zealand troops.

(2) Many patients, despite lichenoid eruptions, continued to take 0·1 gm. mepacrine daily but nevertheless improved ; others failed to improve long after mepacrine medication was terminated.

(3) Improvement occurred when the patients were sent to Australia or the United States of America, but relapse occurred when they returned to the South-West Pacific area.

(4) In 80·7 per cent. of patients readministration of mepacrine failed to produce a recurrence of lichenoid lesions.

(5) In thirty-seven out of forty-six patients with lichenoid lesions readministration of mepacrine caused no exacerbation and the majority of the relapses occurred between forty and sixty-three days after again taking mepacrine. Mepacrine hydrochloride, 0·3 gm. daily for four days, given to five men who were convalescent, failed to cause any relapse (Bagby, 1945).

(6) The application of mepacrine as a wet dressing did not increase the severity of the lichenoid lesions (Epstein, 1945).

(7) The statement by Butler (1947), but otherwise unconfirmed, that a similar disease was known to Filipinos before the war. Bagby (1945) records that in 1943 several men were seen in the western part of the Solomon Islands with simple lichen planus but none with the atypical form till 1944, though mepacrine suppression was in force in both years.

(8) The failure to demonstrate sensitivity either by patch tests or by passive transfer tests in the majority of patients with lichenoid eruptions (Grant-Peterkin and Hair, 1946 ; Kierland, 1946 ; Nelson, 1947). Holbrook (1948) describes two cases from

the South Pacific area, where typical signs and symptoms were present but mepacrine had never been taken.

It must therefore be confessed that the ætiology of the lichenoid eruption is still obscure. No fungi, spirochætes or bacteria of ætiological significance have been isolated and attempts to demonstrate a virus by inoculation of biopsy material into embryonated eggs have yielded negative results. It is possible, however, that a virus may have been the cause of the lichen planus, infection occurring only in patients whose tissues have been prepared by administration of mepacrine, bismuth, gold or arsenic. Slight physical trauma, such as irritation from a wrist-watch strap, may precipitate the lesions. Individual idiosyn-crasy appears to play an important *rôle*, but the greater prevalence in the Pacific area suggests that the condition may be due to degradation products which are formed more readily from some brands of mepacrine than from others. As a rule the lesions were not seen until mepacrine had been taken for some months : Bigham (1949) saw a few Europeans affected in India who had been on suppressive mepacrine only a few weeks.

The cause of the eczematous dermatitis, on the other hand, is simply a drug sensitivity similar to that described before the Second World War among those who had to handle mepacrine. Patch tests are, as a rule, positive in cases of this nature, and readministration of mepacrine is followed by the reappearance of symptoms after a short interval. Becker (1946), for instance, saw two patients who had recovered from eczematous dermatitis due to mepacrine in the Pacific area. When on leave in the United States of America they developed attacks of malaria and were given therapeutic courses of mepacrine. Within twenty-four hours both patients had developed skin lesions, in one instance urticarial, in the other of the vesicular-bullous, eczematoid type. Harvey *et al.* (1944), working in New Guinea, reported an exacerba-tion of lesions in from twenty-four to seventy-two hours in seven of nine patients after administration of the drug. In each patient the exacerbation was described as oozing or crusted and not of a lichenoid nature. Agress (1946) produced exfoliative dermatitis in a Chinese with only 0·1 gm. of mepacrine.

Thus the mepacrine dermatitis complex contains at least two

separate conditions : the eczematous dermatitis is due to drug sensitivity ; in the ætiology of the lichenoid condition mepacrine probably plays an important part but its exact *rôle* is still uncertain. The eczematous dermatitis can occur and become extremely severe with small doses of mepacrine and with a very low plasma concentration. In this group positive reactions to patch tests with mepacrine are to be expected. The second type is localised and morphologically resembles lichen planus. Prolonged administration of the drug is apparently necessary to elicit this reaction. In this connection it may be of interest to note that Forman (1947) has recently emphasised the frequency with which lichenification of the skin is associated with anxiety states and hysterical traits or with depression.

Treatment. The treatment of the lesions associated with the mepacrine dermatitis complex is unsatisfactory. Mepacrine must be stopped, although in some patients no improvement may occur until they have ceased taking the drug for from two to three months. Some patients who ceased to take mepacrine failed to improve till penicillin had been administered. Systemic penicillin is of particular value in the generalised eczematous cases to guard against secondary bacterial infection (Nisbet, 1945). Ferreira-Marques (1949) recommends nicotinamide 0·2 gm. in association with penicillin injections. Neither thiobismol, arsenical preparations nor large doses of vitamin A caused any improvement (Bazemore *et al.*, 1946). Wilson (1946) believed that deficiency of vitamin A was a predisposing cause. Intravenous sodium thiosulphate is of no value (Schmitt *et al.*, 1945). In view of the fact that lesions similar to those of riboflavin deficiency may be seen and that mepacrine may possibly interfere with the metabolism of riboflavin, large doses of vitamins of the B complex, as recommended by Hellier (1944) and Bereston and Cheney (1946), and more especially of riboflavin, may be of value. Many of the patients who suffered from skin lesions due to mepacrine in the Pacific area are said by Butler (1947) to have been living on a diet deficient in fresh vegetables, milk, and meat. The Indians reported by Singh (1948) were living on a diet of rice or atta (whole wheat flour) ; and pulses fresh vegetables, fish and meat were only rarely eaten. Other observers, however, state that the diet was excellent (Rosenthal,

1946). Russell (1947) noted that his patient who contracted the disease in England was malnourished. On the other hand, in West Africa, British troops lived on an excellent diet. It may be noted that in rats Scudi and Hamlin (1944) and FitzHugh *et al.* (1945) have pointed out that a high-protein, low-fat diet reduces the toxicity of mepacrine, especially in relation to the extent of the liver lesions. Hegsted *et al.* (1944a) believe, also, that on a low dietary intake mepacrine impairs utilisation of food. No lipotropic action was noted by Hegsted *et al.* (1944b). Ershoff (1948) found that in addition to vitamins of the B group there are other protective factors in yeast and liver, particularly in the water-soluble fraction of whole liver.

Bland, non-irritating solutions such as 1 : 9,000 potassium permanganate solution soaks may be of value. Sulphonamide ointments, tincture of iodine, and mercurial ointments should be avoided. As some patients are light-sensitive, exposure to sunlight must be avoided. In patients with exfoliative dermatitis intravenous glucose or plasma may be necessary, especially if œdema is present (Feder, 1949).

It would be interesting to know whether persons who have developed lichenoid lesions while taking mepacrine subsequently show a recrudescence of the lesions after prolonged therapy with either bismuth or arsenical preparations.

(2) **Toxic Psychoses.** Very shortly after mepacrine had been introduced reports began to appear of toxic psychoses and other nervous phenomena which were attributed to its use. In some cases, as in those described by Chopra and Abdul Wahed (1934), Decherd (1937), Choremis and Spiliopoulos (1938), and Ayala and Bravo (1942), mepacrine had been combined with pamaquin and there was some uncertainty whether the nervous symptoms were due to one or other of these drugs or to their combination. Kingsbury (1934), however, with two years' experience in Malaya, was able to collect twelve cases ; others were added by Green (1934a and b). One case was reported from India by Govindaswamy (1936), while from China, Kang and Garvis (1936) recorded one case and Wilkinson (1939) three others. The malarial epidemic in Ceylon, when soluble mepacrine (atebrin musonate) was extensively used intramuscularly, in addition to

mepacrine by mouth, provided a considerable number of cases (Briercliffe, 1935 ; Udalagama, 1935 ; Hay *et al.*, 1935). Reports before 1939 had rather suggested that mepacrine psychoses were more common among members of Eastern races than among those of European extraction. Allen *et al.* (1937), however, reported nine cases among persons given therapeutic malaria in America ;

THE INCIDENCE OF NERVOUS REACTIONS FOLLOWING ADMINISTRATION OF MEPACRINE

Number of persons given mepacrine.	Number with nervous involvement.	Incidence per 1,000 cases.	Observers.
30,000	35	1·16	Lidz and Kahn (1946).
20,000	2	0·1	Nieto-Caicedo and Guerrero (1946).
13,649	0	0	Noyan (1949).
11,584	3	0·25	Findlay (1947a).
9,000	4	0·44	Hoops and Barrowman (1938).
7,604	35	4·6	Gaskill and FitzHugh (1945).
4,876	19	3·9	Sheppeck and Wexberg (1946).
4,112	0	0	Coda (1949).
1,628	6	3·6	Field (1939).
1,207	1	0·82	Hoops (1935).
750	2	2·66	Green (1934a).
†644	7	10·8	Udalagama (1935).
500	0	0	Field (1939).
493	1	2·0?	Einhorn and Tomlinson (1946).
422	1	2·3	Bispham (1936).
450	4	8·8	Vollmer and Liebig (1944).
450	16	35·3	Nandi (1947).
*300	5	16·6	Read *et al.* (1946).
†203	2	9·8	Field (1939).
110	6	5·4	Bang *et al.* (1947).
99	6	6·06	Maier *et al.* (1948).
65	0	0	Cooper *et al.* (1949).
Totals 108,146	155	1·43	

* Therapeutic malaria for neurosyphilis.
† Soluble mepacrine and mepacrine *per os*.

Bispham (1936 and 1941) observed one case, while Lerro (1941), in Panama, also recorded a case. Sheppeck and Wexberg (1946) subsequently described nineteen cases seen between 1935 and 1943 in the Gorgas Hospital, Panama. Since the war there have been reports of cases in white troops. Greiber (1947) described thirty-four, Perk (1947) twenty-three cases.

The incidence of psychoses due to mepacrine is extremely low, as is shown in the table opposite. It will be seen that the numbers tend to be highest among those given malaria for cerebral syphilis and subsequently treated with mepacrine as well as among those groups where soluble mepacrine was given intramuscularly. No explanation is forthcoming for the high percentage recorded by Nandi (1947) among Indians after an average dose of 2·8 gm. Possibly dietary factors may predispose to the onset of psychosis. Among specially selected persons, such as European troops in West Africa, the incidence was extremely low among those treated with therapeutic courses of mepacrine, and among approximately 30,000 Europeans taking 0·1 gm. mepacrine from March, 1943, to March, 1946, there were no cases of toxic psychoses. Perk (1947) found only one patient in the Middle East who developed a psychosis as a result of suppressive mepacrine : this attack was precipitated by an emotional crisis. The high incidence reported by Udalagama (1935) in Ceylon, in those treated therapeutically, may be due to the fact that he included all states of depression following mepacrine administration : these may or may not have been due to the drug. Guija Morales (1945a and b) finds that of thirty-six cases studied by him only two occurred between the ages of twenty-three and forty-five years. It is possible that a high initial dose may predispose to involvement of the nervous system. Maier *et al.* (1948) gave 1·2 gm. in the first twenty-four hours of treatment with a total of 3·6 gm. in six days : six of ninety-nine patients had nervous symptoms.

As an experiment Hoobler (1947) gave thirty-one normal officers a fairly high dosage schedule, 0·1 gm. daily for one to two weeks, 0·1 gm. twice daily for one week, 0·4 gm. three times daily for one day, 0·3 gm. three times on the next day, and 0·1 gm. thrice daily for the remaining four days. After this excessive dosage, which would never be given in practice, it is not surprising that twenty-four officers suffered from mental disturbances. Increased dreaming and insomnia were common, minor psychotic changes such as increased tension, restlessness, tremor, over-activity, over-talkativeness, headache, chilly sensations and increased sweating were also seen. Nine were depressed, five elated. Three developed frank psychoses with delusions, hallucinations and profound changes in mood.

Mepacrine psychoses related to therapeutic dosage usually, though not invariably, begin after the fever has subsided and parasites have disappeared from the blood stream. Bang *et al.* (1947) regard the fifth or sixth day of treatment as the most critical. Symptoms have been noted before the third day of treatment or as long as twenty-one days after cessation of mepacrine therapy, but the interval is usually shorter. Gaskill and FitzHugh (1945) found the onset most common six days after completion of treatment, though some patients developed symptoms on the third day after having taken 0·9 gm. by mouth. Kingsbury (1934), with Asiatics, had an average of five and a half days after commencement of treatment, the shortest interval being one and a half days. Sheppeck and Wexberg (1946), in their series of nineteen cases, found that the average interval between the disappearance of fever and the onset of psychosis was 2·2 days, the median two days ; the average interval between the disappearance of parasites and the onset of psychosis was 2·6 days, the median two days. Briercliffe (1935) noted that when mepacrine was given by mouth mental symptoms usually began at the end of five days ; with intramuscular injections the onset would be shortly after the first or within twenty-four hours of the second injection.

Psychoses may also develop in association with mepacrine suppression. Greiber (1947) showed that psychoses were most likely to develop in those whose previous history suggested that they would fall an easy prey to mental disease if the proper " trigger " mechanism were applied. Thus of thirty-four patients with mepacrine psychoses twenty-seven had a previous history of mental trouble (twelve emotionally unstable, seven cyclothymic, five schizoid, three psychopathic). These patients developed mepacrine psychoses as early as the seventeenth day or as late as the 170th day of suppressive therapy, whereas those with no previous mental trouble developed psychoses from the forty-fourth to the eighty-fourth day of suppressive therapy. Those who fall into the " primary " group appear to be sensitive to the drug for, on retesting with mepacrine, five patients in the primary group relapsed. Guija Morales (1945a, b) found that of thirty-four patients with mepacrine psychoses eighteen gave a family history of psychotic trouble. Perk (1947) reported that of twenty-three

patients only one had been on mepacrine suppression, 0·2 gm. daily
for nine months. Of those developing nervous symptoms while
under treatment ten had been under emotional stress and two were
alcoholics. In the Middle East the proportion of officers to other
ranks who developed mepacrine psychoses during the war was
very high. The symptoms associated with mepacrine psychosis
vary. States of manic or hypomanic excitement with euphoria
are most common. Probably those cases labelled " cerebral "
excitation by some of the earlier observers fall into this group.
Some patients become filled with original ideas which enable
them to write poems, compose music or paint pictures; others
have profound depression for which they can offer no explanation
(Nistico, 1948). There are two main types of symptoms :
(1) manic, (2) schizophrenic-like. The symptomatology varies
widely, being coloured, at least in part, by the prepsychotic
personality of the individual. Delirium, visual or auditory
hallucinations combined with an otherwise catatonic condition,
schizophrenic-like symptoms, paranoid syndromes and acute
confusional states have all been reported, while depression is less
common and in only one instance has prolonged coma been noted
(Beckman, 1942). Sometimes it is not easy to differentiate the
symptoms from those of alcoholic delirium, as in the patient
described by Lourdenadin (1949) who was persecuted by a room
full of snakes. Women suffer from sexual excitement and
delusions of having been raped. Disorientation as to time, place,
and person is not uncommon, while a fine tremor has been
observed (Mergener, 1945). Delusions are usually of an exalted
character. Two possible instances of fugue have been reported
by MacDonald (1947). The deep reflexes are often impaired
(Burack, 1946). The mental integration of the patient would
seem to be of importance in determining the type of psychotic
reaction, though it may not have anything to do with initiating
the condition.

The onset is usually sudden, but in a few cases it may be
preceded by a short period, a day or less of nervousness, malaise,
restlessness and especially insomnia. When the onset is insidious,
loss of recent memory may be well marked, the patient becoming
withdrawn and secretive. After an outburst of noisy, talkative

insomnia the psychosis develops rapidly to a climax within a day or even less and remains at its height for from one day to five weeks. During the climax insight may be totally lost, but many patients have an exceedingly clear memory of events preceding and during the psychotic episode. As a rule there is rapid subsidence of symptoms. Sheppeck and Wexberg (1946) found the average duration of symptoms to be 8·5 days, the median 2·5 days. The outcome is very generally complete recovery but there may be difficulty in concentrating or in remembering for some time, while the speech is rather slow. Gaskill and FitzHugh (1945) found that thirty-three of thirty-five patients completely recovered in from eight to eighty-five days, the average being twenty-three days. Two patients who developed schizophrenia did not recover. Perk (1947), however, believes that about 20 per cent. of cases go on to a chronic psychosis. Some fatal cases have been recorded. One patient, while in a state of profound depression committed suicide (Nieto-Caicedo and Guerrero, 1946). In another instance a fatal psychosis developed after 2·4 gm. mepacrine had been given to a patient who was apparently suffering from undiagnosed dementia paralytica. A third patient, after receiving 3 gm. of mepacrine, developed two days later a subacute toxic delirium, associated with fever ; death took place thirteen days later with hyperpyrexia.

No correlation appears to exist between the type of malarial parasite and the incidence of psychosis.

There is no regular relationship between the dose of mepacrine and the liability to develop symptoms, since toxic psychoses have been seen after as little as 0·5 gm. There is no relation between skin sensitivity and the tendency to develop mepacrine psychoses. Shiers (1946), for instance, reported a case of marked cerebral excitement after very small doses, the attacks returning whenever mepacrine was given. Newell and Lidz (1946) believe that mepacrine psychoses were rare when not more than 2·8 gm. was given as treatment in seven days. When, later, massive dose schedules became popular the incidence of toxic psychoses increased and Newell and Lidz (1946) found that psychoses were not uncommon when 3·8 to 4·8 gm. were given in seven days, or 1·4 gm. in twenty-four hours. Perk (1947), in the Middle East, observed symptoms only when 3·4 gm. in six days replaced the previous standard treatment of quinine, mepacrine, and pamaquin.   This is in agreement with the finding of the Malaria Commission of the League of Nations (1937), who believed that the incidence of psychoses increased with large doses, with the length of the period over which mepacrine was given, and with the use of atebrin musonate.   Allen *et al.* (1937) suggested that a relationship existed between the dose of mepacrine per kgm. of body weight and the duration of symptoms.   The correlation, however, is not very exact, for while four patients who took more than 25 mgm. per kgm. of body weight had symptoms of over ten days' duration, two patients who had symptoms lasting more than ten days had taken only 19·1 and 24·1 mgm. per kgm. of body weight.   Gaskill and FitzHugh (1945) gave mepacrine to sixteen patients who had recovered without untoward result in fifteen days ; one patient became mildly excited.   In the case reported by Shiers (1946) the symptoms returned when mepacrine was readministered, while Agress (1946) noted a return of symptoms in a Chinese after 0·7 gm. in three days.

Very rarely, and particularly in small children, acute forms of polyneuritis or myelo-radiculoneuritis have been ascribed to the taking of mepacrine.   Two cases have been described in Italians (Moschini, 1935, and Valentini, 1937) and six in Greek children by Choremis and Spiliopoulos (1938), associated with polyneuritis and paralyses of the lower limbs.   It must be remembered that a very similar neurological picture has been recorded in malarial patients treated with quinine ; the question therefore arises whether mepacrine is the main factor in the ætiology of the polyneuritis.   Lerro (1941), in an adult treated with mepacrine, observed paræsthesia over the whole body, nausea, vomiting and a choking sensation.   Epileptiform fits are reported by Vardy (1935), Field and Niven (1936), and Siegenbeck van Heukelom and Overbeck (1936), a matter of some interest, as according to Molitor (1941) clonic convulsions are produced in animals by large doses of mepacrine.   Van Slype (1936) observed three cases of convulsions in children and one case of bulbar paralysis with flaccid paralysis of the lower extremities.   Some observers, such as Welch *et al.* (1948), believe that in advanced syphilis of the central nervous system treated by malaria, mepacrine is much more likely than quinine to bring on convulsions. With lesser degrees of organic deterioration the convulsion rates for mepacrine and quinine are the same.

Not all psychoses occurring in patients with malaria treated with mepacrine are necessarily suffering from mepacrine psychoses. The psychosis may have been present before the attack of malaria or it may have been precipitated by malaria alone. In most cases the attack probably has a multifactorial causation. Mohanty (1945), in India, regards deficiency of the vitamin B complex as the predisposing factor. However, riboflavin deficiency is not usually associated with psychotic phenomena so that a sudden interference with riboflavin metabolism by mepacrine is not a probable cause. As the African diet is very often deficient in riboflavin, the administration of mepacrine to Africans should, if this theory were correct, result in a high incidence of psychotic reactions : this certainly was not noticeable among African soldiers treated with mepacrine.

The symptoms are not those of cerebral malaria nor do they bear any relationship to a Jarisch-Herxheimer reaction which might equally be due to destruction of malarial parasites by other antimalarial drugs. It seems probable therefore that the psychosis is due to a direct interference with the metabolism of the nerve cell by mepacrine. In animals, Hecht (1933) found evidence of cerebral stimulation after lethal doses. Molitor (1941) states that occasionally high concentrations of mepacrine are found in the cerebrospinal fluid, but no mepacrine was present in the cerebrospinal fluid of the patient with acute poisoning described by Markson and Dawson (1945). Certain experiments by Manifold (1941) are of interest in this connection. Various acridine dyes, not however mepacrine, were tested for their action on the carbohydrate and pyruvate oxidation systems of brain tissue *in vitro*. Acriflavine was found to inhibit oxidation in high concentrations, the action suggesting a breakdown in carbohydrate metabolism similar to that found in the absence of aneurin, a possible explanation for a certain similarity between the psychiatric pictures caused by mepacrine and by a deficiency of aneurin. Lidz and Kahn (1946) have suggested that mepacrine, without giving rise to actual psychoses, may produce mental impairment as judged by scores on the Kohs-Block test, in which the mental age is assessed by forming standard patterns with coloured cubes, whenever the serum levels are above 18 μgm. per 100 ml. Thus doses of 2·1 gm. of mepacrine in seven days were without action in causing impairment of the mental faculties, but 4·5 gm. in six days caused a very definite impairment. It would thus seem that mepacrine psychoses are likely to develop only if the plasma or serum levels are allowed to remain at a consistently high level.

Gaskill and FitzHugh (1945) suggest that these toxic psychoses represent either an unusual sensitivity reaction to mepacrine or a complex-conditioned sensitivity in which mepacrine is one of several factors which must be combined in a given individual. The diagnosis of mepacrine psychosis usually presents little difficulty, but the possibility of functional psychosis must always be considered. Allen (1944), however, has drawn attention to a case where the euphoria and delusions of grandeur caused a diagnosis of general paralysis to be made. It should be remembered in this connection that a recent attack of malaria may cause a false positive Kahn or Wassermann reaction : differentiation is necessary from cerebral malaria and from endogenous or biogenic psychosis. With cerebral malaria there is confusion only, whereas mepacrine causes delirium or coma. In mepacrine psychosis it is rare to find malaria parasites in the blood. Differentiation from a biogenic psychosis is not always easy for administration of the drug may obviously be one of the precipitating causes of a chronic psychosis. In the early stages it is not possible to distinguish between the acute reaction to mepacrine and a chronic psychosis associated with it. Psychoses caused by malaria alone are usually depressive in type (Turner, 1936). Delirium tremens may possibly be confused with a mepacrine psychosis in alcoholics.

The value of any particular treatment in mepacrine psychoses is difficult to assess, since in so many patients the symptoms subside spontaneously. Treatment similar to that used in alcoholic psychoses has been suggested by Sheppeck and Wexberg (1946) : this consists of aneurin hydrochloride 50 mgm. intravenously four times a day, aneurin hydrochloride tablets 10 mgm.

and nicotinic acid 50 mgm. three times a day and two compound vitamin B capsules three times a day, each capsule containing 5 mgm. aneurin hydrochloride, 25 mgm. riboflavin, and 25 mgm. nicotinamide. It should, however, be noted that in rats Hegsted *et al.* (1945) found that mepacrine retarded the onset of vitamin B_1 deficiency. In addition, fluids are given in large quantities and the bowels are kept open. The effects of large doses of riboflavin alone would be of interest and glucose intravenously might be of value since it is known that soluble mepacrine given intravenously reduces the blood sugar. Convulsive treatment has been tried by Perk (1947), but the results are not impressive. Colette and Porot (1949) recommend insulin shock in mania.

(3) **Hæmatopoietic Lesions.** In rare instances, aplastic anæmia, agranulocytosis, and acute hepatitis have been seen in association with either the lichenoid-eczematoid syndrome or with exfoliative dermatitis (Drake and Moon, 1946). Similar blood changes have also occurred in those taking mepacrine in the absence of skin lesions (Livingood and Dieuaide, 1945 ; Fishman and Kinsman, 1949). Custer (1946) found that in the United States Army the case incidence of aplastic anæmia in areas where mepacrine suppression was in force rose during the years 1943 and 1944 from 0·66 to 2·84 per 100,000 compared with a case incidence of 0·04 to 0·18 in other theatres of war. In forty-seven cases of aplastic anæmia occurring in those who had taken mepacrine, the period of mepacrine suppression varied from one to thirty-four months. The mepacrine dermatitis complex preceded the aplastic anæmia in twenty cases but the dermatological therapy employed was not a significant causal factor. The pathological findings were typical of those found in aplastic anæmia. Liver lesions were found in ten patients at necropsy but in five these hepatic lesions were indistinguishable from those seen in infective hepatitis. The hæmatological features were essentially those of normocytic, normochromic anæmia with leucopenia and thrombocytopenia. Reticulocytes were usually very scanty. A hæmorrhagic tendency was frequently noted early and the subsequent course was almost invariably marked by fever and hæmorrhagic phenomena. Four out of forty-seven patients survived for from two to seven months. Rosenthal (1946) also has described two cases of aplastic

anæmia in association with the lichenoid dermatitis. One patient recovered but the other died. At necropsy, apart from widespread petechial hæmorrhages there was chronic focal myocarditis ; the liver showed œdema, periportal degeneration of liver parenchyma, and infiltration by lymphocytes, and fibroblasts with localised masses of pigment, mostly within macrophages in the periportal regions. The pigment gave a reaction for melanin with Becker's stain. A few cases of agranulocytosis have also been recorded. Treatment is unsatisfactory.

When large doses of mepacrine of the order of 50 to 200 mgm. per kgm. of body weight daily were given to rats, mice, rabbits, hamsters, guinea-pigs, dogs, monkeys, chickens, and ducks, peculiar basophilic inclusions, usually associated with vacuoles, appeared in the cytoplasm of lymphocytes. Inclusions of a similar nature occurred in the erythrocytes of the rat, mouse and hamster and rarely in the monocytes of rat. Anæmia, " polynucleosis," lymphopenia, and monocytosis occurred in the rat, while " polynucleosis " and lymphopenia developed in other species. The nature of these inclusions is unknown but they do not appear to be parasitic in nature (Mushett and Siegel, 1946), and nothing like them has been seen in man. They differ from Pappenheimer's bodies in that they do not stain with iron (McFadzean and Davis, 1947). Russell (1945) has described an eosinophilia in man as a result of prolonged mepacrine administration. This finding has not been confirmed and was probably due to other causes.

(4) **Ophthalmological Changes.** A new industrial hazard has been found to occur among those engaged in handling mepacrine in large quantities. Reference has already been made to the occurrence of skin eruptions on exposed parts of the body, puffiness of the eyelids, lacrimation, and pain over the frontal sinuses. Mann (1947) has now described a curious corneal condition in six male workers handling mepacrine ; all had a pigmented yellow skin. The patients worked in an atmosphere which contained clouds of very fine mepacrine dust for short periods without goggles, masks or protective clothing. They had no dermatitis, but the conjunctivæ also were yellow. After working for some weeks they all noticed that at night a point source of light had a

blue halo round it. One yard (0·9 m.) away the halo began 2 in. (5 cm.) from the source and was about 3 in. (7·5 cm.) wide. It was dark blue at the inner edge and pale blue at the outer edge. At a distance of 6 yds. (5·4 m.) faint yellow, green and reddish-brown bands appeared outside the blue ring. All the men had normal visual acuity.

On slit-lamp examination the condition of all patients was similar. There was yellow discoloration of the conjunctiva in the interpalpebral space, and a slight dulling and yellowing of the cornea which was barely visible macroscopically. Under magnification there appeared to be an actual deposit of minute dark-brown dots at the exposed margins of the limbus. The whole surface of the cornea was peppered with very fine dust-like particles, which appeared dark yellowish-brown by direct illumination and opaque by transmitted light. The size of the particles was estimated as between 5μ and 10μ in diameter—that is, about the size of the nucleus of a corneal epithelial cell. The corneal surface was perfectly smooth and bright, and the change was present only in the surface layer of cells. In the lower part of each cornea there was a series of wavy yellow lines which were composed of closely aggregated dots similar to those peppered over the cornea but closer together and of a bright yellow colour. One patient noticed the haloes after being employed for less than a year ; they disappeared within two months of a transfer to a different job. Later he returned to work with mepacrine, and the phenomenon reappeared in six months although it did not reach its previous intensity. There was no evidence of glaucoma in any of the patients, and it seems reasonable to attribute the condition to a diffraction effect.

Two male volunteers, who had both taken 100 mgm. of mepacrine by mouth for seven months, showed a pale-yellow staining of the skin generally, but their eyes were normal and they had never seen blue haloes. Mepacrine dust blown directly on to the eyes of rabbits produced in six days an appearance on slit-lamp examination similar to that of human subjects. These observations suggest that the corneal condition is caused by direct contamination with mepacrine dust. The particles seen may not be mepacrine itself, since this is soluble in the tears, and the exact

nature of the precipitates is doubtful, although they are probably
an insoluble breakdown product of mepacrine. Histological
examination of an affected rabbit's eye was carried out, and the
yellow granules in the cytoplasm could be seen in unfixed specimens : they were very small and amorphous. The opaque yellow
dots seen with the slit-lamp are the whole aggregation of these
amorphous particles within the cell containing them. It was
suggested that they might be composed of 2-chloro-7-methoxy-
acridone, an insoluble substance which is formed by hydrolysis of
mepacrine. Among West African troops a self-inflicted ocular
injury was caused by putting mepacrine in the conjunctival sac.
A mild conjunctivitis was seen in the early stages and in some a
striate keratitis was observed. The most usual finding was staining
of the bulbar conjunctiva in an area surrounding the limbus and
extending laterally in an area corresponding with the palpebral
fissure. The bulbar conjunctiva above and below was devoid of
staining and the lines of demarcation above and below were sharp.
Thus exposure, possibly associated with oxygen uptake, may play
an essential part in the ability of cells to take up staining granules.
The cornea was hazy and had a yellow green coloration. A
biopsy specimen of the conjunctiva showed the presence of
mepacrine. The condition took some weeks to clear up (Somerville-
Large, 1947). Roper-Hall (1950) observed similar lesions in
Mauritian troops.

An additional toxic effect on the eyes has been noted by Reese
(1946), who saw three patients suffering from œdema of the
corneal cells as a result of taking large doses of mepacrine.
Blurring of vision was noted in both eyes, and examination with
a slit-lamp showed " bedewing " of the cornea due to isolated
points of œdema. One patient had taken 0·2 gm. daily for twenty-
seven days, but others had had large therapeutic doses, in
addition to suppressive mepacrine. On stopping mepacrine the
œdema disappeared but recurred when mepacrine was readministered. Chamberlain and Boles (1946) similarly recorded four
cases ; three of their patients had taken mepacrine for only four
to six weeks in doses of 0·1 gm. daily. In one instance the visual
acuity was as low as 1 : 200 in each eye, and in all some degree of
hepatic dysfunction was noted. The corneal opacities were for

the most part located near the level of Bowman's membrane. It is estimated that at least twenty-five cases of this type occurred in the Pacific theatre.

Observations made during the war showed that suppressive doses of 0·1 gm. daily did not interfere with the vision of flying personnel in the Air Force ; after high blood-mepacrine levels suddenly attained the only visual changes noted were minor and temporary scotomas and blind-spot enlargement (Dame, 1946).

Mepacrine and Blackwater Fever

The question whether mepacrine therapy precipitates an attack of blackwater fever is of some interest. It has long been recognised that quinine may be a precipitating factor, while pamaquin is also known to give rise to methæmalbumin in the blood, and, if this compound is formed in sufficient amounts, to the escape of hæmo-globin derivatives through the kidney into the urine. Many cases have been recorded where the administration of a combina-tion of pamaquin and mepacrine has been followed by hæmo-globinuria (Banerjee and Brahmachari, 1933 ; Amy, 1934 ; Naumann, 1933 ; Moir, 1934 ; Murray, 1934, and Chopra and Chaudhuri, 1935). Nagelsbach (1933), however, recorded the case of a woman in labour who developed blackwater fever while taking mepacrine ; some of the cases recorded by Naumann (1934) had mepacrine only ; Foy and Kondi (1937) reported three cases of blackwater fever where mepacrine had been given but quinine had not been taken for at least three months ; Gunther (1938) also described one case where blackwater fever appeared to be precipitated by the administration of mepacrine, and Lucherini (1938) and Abbott (1946) one each. It is noticeable that the blackwater fever developed as a rule either after very small doses of mepacrine, in one instance 0·4 gm. in forty-eight hours, or after the completion of what would now be regarded as an inadequate dosage (1·5 gm. in five days) for the treatment of an attack of malaria.

Hoops (1935) found that the use of mepacrine in a labour force in Malaya reduced the incidence of blackwater fever. The experi-ence of Findlay and Stevenson (1944) and Findlay (1949) in West Africa was similar : among European troops the introduction of mepacrine as a suppressive, 0·6 or 0·7 gm. weekly, with mepacrine only in the treatment of malarial attacks, 0·8 gm. being given in the first twenty-four hours, completely abolished blackwater fever.

Fairley (1945) came to similar conclusions as to the correlation between the reduction of blackwater fever and mepacrine suppression among Australian troops in the South West Pacific area, and Foy and his colleagues (1948) made similar observations in Greece.

Siegel and Mushett (1944) showed that a massive hæmoglobinuria could be produced in young rats only by giving large doses far in excess of those ever given to man therapeutically. It thus seems that mepacrine is far less likely to precipitate blackwater fever than is quinine.

Patrono (1942), on very slender evidence, suggests that the administration of mepacrine, and in fact of quinine also, precipitates a state of hypovitaminosis C.

To concentrate on its toxic reactions is obviously to give an entirely false picture of the results obtained with mepacrine in the treatment and prevention of malaria. Mepacrine, it should be emphasised, was given without the least ill-effect to hundreds of thousands of Service personnel during the war of 1939–45, and it must therefore be looked on as a drug of very low toxicity. While it would be an exaggeration to say that mepacrine won the war in the East, there is no doubt that without its aid the sickness rates would have been much higher, the deaths would have been far more numerous, and ultimate victory would have been longer delayed.

(3) Chloroquine and 4-Aminoquinolines

As part of the extensive survey of antimalarial drugs described by Wiselogle (1946), considerable attention was paid to the toxicity of the 4-aminoquinolines in experimental animals while the toxicity of chloroquine was also studied in man.

In the dog there are two types of reaction due to these compounds. One, in its acute phase, is characterised by vomiting, extreme irritability and tonic convulsions continuing for six to eight hours. In its chronic phase this syndrome consists of great nervousness and hyperirritability, accompanied by profuse and almost continuous salivation and a few convulsions of short duration, occurring when the animals are specially excited.

The second type of reaction in its acute phase is characterised by the prancing horse appearance, the " levade " of the Spanish riding school. The dog moves stiff-legged with neck arched and jaw pointed down. Respiratory difficulties are present and death may occur from respiratory failure. In its chronic phase there are muscular tremors, weakness, and depression. With both types of reaction loss of weight and anorexia are seen and intestinal movements are slowed down.

The same two types of reaction are also noted in the monkey, one reaction being associated with hyperirritability, the other with great depression. The latter is accompanied by blurred vision, but the prancing horse response is not observed.

There are no blood changes, but the germinal centres in the spleen are enlarged and hyperactive : the pancreas is brown and microscopically the cells contain masses of secreting granules. Similar changes are seen in the rat. In animals chronically intoxicated the liver exhibits fatty degeneration, while in the rat at least one 4-aminoquinoline produced extensive liver necrosis. The most active compound in causing liver necrosis is SN 6,911, 7-chloro - 4 - (4'- diethylamino-1'- methyl 1-butylamino)-3-methyl-quinoline. Chloroquine shows considerable variations in toxicity for different species of laboratory animals : thus :—

In the mouse a daily dose by mouth of 400 mgm. per kgm. constituted an LD 100.

In the dog a daily dose by mouth of 20 mgm. per kgm. constituted an LD 100 ; 10 mgm. per kgm. caused severe toxæmia.

In the monkey a daily dose by mouth of 50 mgm. per kgm. constituted an LD 100 ; 25 mgm. per kgm. caused slight toxæmia.

In the rat a daily dose by mouth of 150 mgm. per kgm. constituted an LD 100 ; 50 mgm. per kgm. depressed the growth rate by 50 per cent.

By oral administration the toxicity of chloroquine is nearly the same as that of mepacrine, but acute intravenous toxicity in the dog is greater than for mepacrine.

Toxicity in the 4-aminoquinolines increases with length of side-chain : partial oxidation of the methylene chain separating the two nitrogens reduces toxicity. Increasing the size of the substituent increases toxicity, while the introduction of a methyl group into the nucleus increases toxicity when the methyl group is located at position 3. SN 10,751, 4-(7'-chloro-4'-quinolylamino)-α-diethylamino-*o*-cresol differs from other 4-aminoquinolines in that toxic symptoms may develop and deaths occur in the first two weeks after the end of treatment. SN 10,751 appears to produce irreversible toxic changes, but these are not associated with definite pathological changes.

Chloroquine has much less action on the gastro-intestinal tract of animals than other 4-aminoquinolines and, unlike mepacrine, it does not cause vomiting and diarrhœa either in the monkey or the dog. Chloroquine also has a steeper dose-response curve than other 4-aminoquinolines : in other words, doses below the lethal dose have little or no effect on the well-being of the animals. This is a point of considerable importance, for it is the sublethal toxicity of a drug which often precludes its routine administration in man. The development of tolerance to the toxic action of the 4-aminoquinolines is said to be an important characteristic of the 4-aminoquinolines. In tests extending for not more than thirty days chloroquine appeared a little more toxic for rat and monkey than mepacrine but for periods from 30 to 120 days mepacrine was the more toxic. Slow absorption is probably the reason why water-soluble salts of 4-aminoquinolines are less toxic than the corresponding water-insoluble salts. The toxicity of some 4-aminoquinolines in terms of chloroquine for different animals is shown in the table on page 230.

When rats have fed on a stock diet containing 1,000 parts per million of chloroquine they survived for from thirteen to twenty-one weeks. At death there was replacement of cardiac muscle by fibrous tissue, similar but less extensive replacement of voluntary muscles and moderate centrolobular necrosis and fibrosis of the liver. Other lesions found at necropsy were hunched back, paleness of the viscera, cardiac atrial thrombosis, testicular atrophy, and generalised cytoplasmic basophilia. With 400 parts per million or less in the diet some rats survived for two years without showing any pathological lesions (FitzHugh and Nelson, 1947, and Nelson and FitzHugh, 1947). The degree of damage is

The Toxicity of 4-Aminoquinolines
(Wiselogle, 1946)

Compound.	Chloroquine equivalent.				Type of reaction.
	Mouse.	Rat.	Dog.	Monkey.	
SN 7,618 : 7-Chloro-4-(4-diethylamino-1-methylbutylamino) quinoline (chloroquine).	1·0	1·0	1·0	1·0	Chronic: depression acute, " levade " phenomenon.
SN 6,911 : 7-Chloro-4-(4'-diethylamino-1'-methyl 1-butylamino)-3-methylquinoline (sontoquine, nivaquine).	1·0	0·8	0·25	0·6	Chronic: hyperirritability, acute convulsions.
SN 8,137 : 1-(7-Chloro-4-quinolylamino)-3-diethylamino-2-propanol.	0·3	0·5	0·12	0·5	,, ,, ,,
SN 9,584 : 7-Chloro-4-(3-diethylamino-propylamino) quinoline.	0·6	0·8	0·50	1·0	,, ,, ,,
SN 10,751 : 4-(7'-Chloro-4'-quinolylamino)-α-diethylamino-o-cresol.	0·6	0·5	0·25	1·0	,, ,, ,,
SN 7,135 : 7-Chloro-4-(4-diethylamino-1-methylbutylamino) quinoline.	1·2	1·2	1·0	1·5	Chronic: depression acute, " levade " phenomenon.
SN 14,079	—	1·0	—	1·0	,, ,, ,,
SN 15,062	—	2·0	—	1·5	,, ,, ,,
SN 13,425	—	1·0	0·25	1·0	Atypical.

proportional to the dose of chloroquine. Further observations on the chronic oral toxicity of chloroquine have been recorded by FitzHugh *et al.* (1948) and Nelson and FitzHugh (1948).

Groups of weanling rats were fed over a two-year period on diets containing up to 1,000 parts per million (p.p.m.) ; at 400 p.p.m. there was a significant inhibition of growth during the first three months of the experiment though this retardation was made up later. At 800 p.p.m. growth was greatly retarded and all rats receiving these higher concentrations died within a year. The lesions at necropsy included testicular atrophy, the presence of foamy macrophages in several locations, pigment in uterine muscle and renal convoluted tubular cells, and degenerative changes in the pancreatic acinar cells. The really serious lesions were (*a*) a slowly developing focal necrosis of striated muscle, particularly cardiac, (*b*) a moderate degree of centrolobular hepatic necrosis and fibrosis.

The lowest dosage of chloroquine in relation to body weight of rats was 4 mgm. per kgm. per day for two years. The recommended dose in human malaria is 300 mgm. on the same day each week for suppression and for the treatment of an acute attack of vivax malaria—600 mgm. as an initial dose, followed by 300 mgm.

after six to eight hours and a single dose of 300 mgm. on each of the next two days. These doses approach the toxic levels in rats and render it doubtful whether chloroquine is a suitable suppressive to administer for long periods to indigenous populations in the tropics.

The toxic reactions to therapeutic doses in man are usually of a minor character, but Gordon *et al.* (1947) found that they were rather more numerous than with mepacrine. Their nature and frequency are seen in the table :—

MINOR TOXIC REACTIONS IN PATIENTS TREATED WITH THERAPEUTIC COURSES OF CHLOROQUINE AND OF MEPACRINE

	Chloroquine (SN 7,618).	Mepacrine.
Number of patients	236	137
Number with toxic reactions	54 (22·9 per cent.)	12 (8·7 per cent.)
Nausea	8	2
Vomiting	2	2
Anorexia	10	2
Diarrhœa	8	6
Abdominal cramps	4	0
Dizziness	2	0
Pruritus	17	0
Urticaria	2	0
Rash	1	0

Most *et al.* (1946) also observed few toxic reactions. Some dizziness and light-headedness were not uncommon and fifty-six, or 20 per cent., of 284 patients complained of pruritus ; this was usually localised and generally confined to the first two days of treatment : in seven patients (2·4 per cent.) erythema, urticaria or a mild papular rash was noted. In no case were the symptoms severe enough to interrupt symptoms. Slight visual disturbances have also been noted.

U.S. Army Medical Department (1947) reported the following reactions among 1,277 patients with *P. vivax* and forty-four with *P. malariæ* :—

Pruritus	.	.	.	124	Diarrhœa	.	.	.	33
Anorexia	.	.	.	86	Malaise	.	.	.	3
Vertigo and/or tinnitus	.			76	Urticaria	.	.	.	4

These reactions were generally mild, and only in rare instances required discontinuance of the drug.

Alving *et al.* (1948b) carried out extensive toxicity tests on groups of volunteers given either 0·5 gm. of chloroquine base by mouth once a week for one year or a total daily dosage of 0·3 gm. of the base in two daily doses (0·1 gm. and 0·2 gm.) for seventy-seven days. On the higher daily dosage schedule the main toxic symptoms were visual disturbances, headache, bleaching of the hair, electrocardiographic changes and slight loss of weight. These changes caused no incapacity and diminished or disappeared when the dosage was decreased. The second group, receiving 0·5 gm. of chloroquine base weekly, had occasionally headaches, with slight loss of weight : in two out of the thirty volunteers a lichen planus eruption similar to that seen with mepacrine developed (Craige *et al.*, 1948). Maier (1948) gave 0·3 gm. of the base weekly for periods up to twenty weeks to approximately 400 men. Three men were forced to discontinue the drug because of gastrointestinal reactions, four had milder gastro-intestinal reactions, and twelve had headaches. Chaudhuri (1948) noted five patients with insomnia, pruritus or gastro-intestinal irritation among fifty treated in India.

The electrocardiographic changes were noted in twelve out of twenty men ; they consisted of a concordant diminution of the height of the T waves in some or all of the leads, similar to that recorded with antimony, arsenic, emetine, and histamine. The visual symptoms consisted of a difficulty in changing focus quickly from a near to a far object. Tests for visual acuity, power of monocular accommodation, and diplopia failed to demonstrate objective abnormality. Bleaching of the hair occurred only in blond subjects. The lichen planus-like eruptions appeared only during the last few months of drug administration : they were limited to the flexor surfaces of the extremities and to the trunk. Reddish violaceous papules and annular reddish macules with a ring of papules about a paler centre were noted. The skin symptoms disappeared rapidly after stopping the drug. Alving *et al.* (1948b) did not note any cutaneous eruptions in twenty men who took 0·5 gm. daily for eleven weeks, or seven times the usual suppressive dose. Hayman *et al.* (1946), among 284 patients noted only six with erythema, urticaria or mild papular eruptions ; fifty-six, however, had pruritus. Loeb *et al.* (1946) gave chloroquine to more than 5,000 patients without seeing any case of lichen planus. Persons with lichen planus-like eruptions due to mepacrine have successfully taken chloroquine, but in one instance a mepacrine-induced dermatitis has been exacerbated by taking chloroquine (Craige *et al.*, 1948).

Berliner *et al.* (1948) gave thirty-two volunteers graded doses of from 50 to 400 mgm. daily for a week, the first dose being preceded by a loading dose of from 200 to 600 mgm. Twenty men developed symptoms : one had generalised itching when on 400 mgm. daily, one when on 300 mgm. daily developed dizziness, weakness and spells of lightheadedness, and eighteen had eye symptoms when on 400 mgm. a day. Blurring of vision on looking from a near to a distant object was seen in one subject, the others complained of feeling heavy about the eyes or having something wrong with them.

Although chloroquine thus seems to be a safe suppressive its effect on the eyes requires more careful investigation before it can be safely given to those who may have to drive motor cars or pilot aeroplanes.

FitzHugh *et al.* (1948) have compared the toxicity of chloroquine and mepacrine. Short-term chronic experiments in rats, as well as monkeys, extending up to 180 days showed that chloroquine is slightly less toxic than mepacrine (Wiselogle, 1946). In the dog chloroquine is more toxic than mepacrine when the acute toxicity is compared, but in experiments to test the chronic toxicity there was no significant difference. In a two-year test in rats chronic toxicity tests showed that when 100 parts per million were added to the diet there was little or no effect, but effects became progressively more severe with each increase in dosage (FitzHugh *et al.*, 1948). The lowest concentration producing a significant retardation of growth was 400 p.p.m. At dosage levels of 200 p.p.m. or more, mortality increased progressively till 800 and 1,000 p.p.m. caused early death of all animals. The most striking finding was a leucocytosis, predominantly neutrophilic. This was scarcely noticeable with 200 p.p.m. but very marked with 800 p.p.m. Histological changes similarly were negligible on 100 p.p.m. but marked at 800 p.p.m. The two most prominent changes were focal necrosis of striated muscle, especially cardiac muscle, and some degree of central lobular necrosis and fibrosis in the liver. In relation to body weight in rats, the lowest doses of chloroquine which produced slight toxic effects in some animals correspond to approximately 4 mgm. per kgm. per day for two years. When compared with similar tests made on rats by FitzHugh *et al.* (1945), the anatomical changes produced by chloroquine and mepacrine are seen to be very similar although the toxicity of chloroquine is on the whole rather less than that of mepacrine. At the dosage level of 4 mgm. per kgm. of body weight per day there is no noticeable difference between the toxicities of the two compounds.

The toxic actions of other 4-aminoquinolines also have been studied in man.

The results obtained by Gordon *et al.* (1947) on 7-chloro-4-(4'-diethylamino-1'-methyl 1-butylamino)-3-methylquinoline (sontoquine, SN 6,911) and 1-(7-chloro-4-quinolylamino)-3-diethylamino-2-propanol (SN 8,137) are shown in the table :—

Toxicity in Man of Sontoquine and SN 8,137

	Sontoquine.	SN 8,137.
Number of patients .	82	63
Number with toxic reactions . . .	16 (19·5 per cent.)	21 (33·3 per cent.)
Nausea . . .	5	1
Vomiting . . .	3	1
Anorexia . . .	0	1
Diarrhœa . . .	6	5
Abdominal cramps .	0	1
Dizziness . . .	0	4
Tinnitus . . .	2	2
Blurring of vision . .	0	2
Pruritus . . .	0	2
Urticaria . . .	0	1
Rash	0	1

The incidence of toxic reactions was thus slightly greater than with chloroquine or mepacrine.

Hering *et al.* (1948) compared the effects of sontoquine, chloroquine, SN 8,137, mepacrine, and metanilamide when given as suppressives for six weeks to men who were unaware what drug they were taking : a placebo was given to a control group.

THE COMPARATIVE TOXICITY OF SONTOQUINE, CHLOROQUINE, SN 8,137, MEPACRINE, METANILAMIDE AND A PLACEBO
(Hering *et al.*, 1948)

	Sonto-quine.	Chloro-quine.	SN. 8,137.	Mepa-crine.	Metanil-amide.	Placebo.
Number of men .	170	152	165	172	154	142
Weekly dose . .	0·6 gm.	0·3 gm.	0·6 gm.	0·24 gm.	2·0 gm.	—
Anorexia . .	—	—	—	—	1	—
Chest pains .	—	—	—	—	—	2
Chills . . .	1	3	2	2	4	4
Constipation. .	—	—	—	4	1	—
Cramps (abdominal)	3	1	7	5	4	3
Diarrhœa . .	4	9	7	11	4	5
Dizziness . .	—	—	1	5	2	—
Drowsiness . .	4	2	4	1	1	1
Exhaustion . .	1	1	2	—	—	2
Flatulence . .	—	1	—	1	2	—
Flush . . .	6	8	8	16	7	6
Headache . .	12	6	4	13	7	5
Nausea . .	9	2	6	20	1	—
Rash . .	2	—	2	—	—	—
Stomach pains .	6	—	2	4	2	2
Syncope . .	—	—	1	—	—	—
Vomiting . .	4	1	3	4	26	2
Itch . .	—	—	1	—	—	—
Back pains . .	1	—	—	—	—	—
Miscellaneous .	3	1	—	1	1	—
Refusal, non-specific	—	1	1	—	5	1
Totals . .	56	36	51	41	114	34

Mepacrine and sontoquine showed an increase in refusals from week to week, though after the fourth week there was a general stabilisation with all suppressives. Chloroquine gave rise to as few complaints as the placebo.

Motor co-ordination, as reflected by firing scores, was not affected by any of these suppressive drugs.

Berliner *et al.* (1948) did not find any symptoms attributable to

SN 8,137 in sixteen volunteers receiving up to 600 mgm. of the drug daily. The toxicities of the following 4-aminoquinolines were also studied in man :—

U.S.A. Survey No.	Nuclear substituents.	Substituent on 4-amino group.
SN 9,584 . .	7-chloro	diethylamino propyl
SN 10,751 . .	7-chloro	α-diethylamino-o-cresol
SN 13,425 . .	7-chloro	1'-ethyl-4'-piperidyl

SN 9,584 caused severe itching, most severe at night, in nine of sixteen volunteers ; nausea, vomiting, nervousness, anxiety and tremor were also seen in those taking 400 mgm. a day.

SN 10,751 produced lassitude, lack of energy and insomnia in twelve of sixteen men on 300 mgm. daily. Feelings of abdominal uneasiness, anorexia and nausea and vomiting developed, in some cases when only 200 mgm. daily was being taken.

SN 13,425 caused symptoms in twelve of sixteen volunteers. Itching accompanied in four of seven subjects by a papular rash was the most common complaint. Nervousness, and in one man also an acute anxiety state, developed with insomnia and sleeplessness. Camoquin in field experiments is even less toxic than chloroquine (Hoekenga, 1950).

Thus of the 4-aminoquinolines which have been investigated in man the least toxic are chloroquine, camoquin, SN 8,137, and sontoquine (SN 6,911). All have advantages over mepacrine in their lower toxicity and in the smaller dosage required to produce a given effect. Chloroquine from experiments in the field would appear to have a considerable margin of safety, but in view of its effect on the eyes its use in those in charge of aeroplanes and mechanically driven transport requires further study.

(4) Pamaquin and other 8-Aminoquinolines

Very soon after the introduction of pamaquin, when large doses of from 0·10 to 0·15 gm. were given daily, toxic reactions began to be noticed (Fischer and Rheindorf, 1928, and Le Heux and de Lind van Wijdgaarden, 1929). Even with small daily doses of from 0·04 to 0·06 gm., or 0·02 gm. if prolonged for ten days or more, toxic reactions were not uncommon (Missiroli and Marino, 1934). Bastianelli, Mosna and Canalis (1937), at an early stage, found that as small a dose as 0·02 gm. for five days caused a reaction in nearly 50 per cent. of people, the chief signs and symptoms being cyanosis, vomiting, gastralgia, and asthenia. The cyanosis is specially noticeable in the lips, tongue, and finger nails, and occasionally in the lobules of the ear. It is due to the formation of methæmalbumin.

The three main effects of pamaquin in man are :—
(1) The formation of methæmalbumin ;
(2) Acute hæmolytic anæmia, sometimes associated with hæmoglobinuria ;
(3) Granulocytopenia.

Methæmalbumin Formation. In 1934 Tate and Vincent showed that *in vitro* pamaquin, even in a dilution of 1 in 50,000, when mixed with blood is capable of producing what was at first thought to be methæmoglobin but is now known to be methæmalbumin. Blake *et al.* (1946), Rosenfeld *et al.* (1948), and Blake (1948) have brought forward evidence to suggest that methæmalbumin is more readily formed in the blood when quinine is given together with pamaquin. In addition, while a daily dose of 30 mgm. for fourteen days may or may not produce methæmalbumin it almost invariably does so if mepacrine has also been previously administered for varying periods of time (Earle *et al.*, 1948). Thus among fifty negroes given pamaquin who had previously received mepacrine five had hæmolytic anæmia : of twenty-six who had not had mepacrine only one developed hæmolytic anæmia. The amount of methæmalbumin, calculated as hæmatin, which follows 90 mgm. of pamaquin and 2 gm. of quinine varies from 6 to 45 mgm. per litre of serum, the average value being 30 mgm. per litre. Dixon (1933) noted that cyanosis is more likely to occur in patients who are constipated ; it would seem also to be more common in non-Caucasians than in those of white race.

In addition to the spectroscopic test for absorption bands at either 623 or 405 mμ, Schumm's test is said by most authorities to be specific for methæmalbumin, although Schumm himself says that it is specific for hæmatin. The test is as follows : fresh concentrated ammonium sulphide solution is added to plasma, and if methæmalbumin is present the α-band of ammonium hæmochromogen is sharply defined at 558 mμ. It should be noted that Weise (1941) believes that methæmalbumin is in fact hæmatin in a solution of plasma. The degree of methæmalbuminæmia is not necessarily correlated with that of hæmolytic anæmia.

Acute Hæmolysis. In patients who have taken pamaquin, anæmia may develop slowly or as the result of an acute hæmolysis. Anæmia is undoubtedly common both in Indians and negroes, and some 5 to 10 per cent. of such patients will develop it after from three to five days of medication with therapeutic doses. The incidence of hæmolytic anæmia among white patients on comparable doses is very low. Dimson and McMartin (1946) described eighteen cases among 8,000 Indians given quinine, mepacrine, and pamaquin. Mann and Smith (1943) drew attention to the curious racial incidence of pamaquin hæmoglobinuria among troops in the Middle East theatre of war. In eighteen months there were fifteen cases in military personnel distributed racially as follows :—

Indian	. .	7	Polish Jew	. 1	Mauritian	. 1
Basuto	. .	2	Palestinian Jew	1	Rhodesian	
Greek	. .	1	East African	. 1	(white)	. 1

Not a single British soldier developed hæmoglobinuria, and it is noteworthy that all those who suffered from hæmoglobinuria had lived for long in endemic areas. The hæmoglobinuria developed in every case while pamaquin was being given as part of the standard quinine, mepacrine, pamaquin course then in vogue in Army hospitals. In four patients the infection was due to *P. falciparum*, in two to *P. vivax*, and in the remainder uncertain. Six of the fifteen died. The question is whether pamaquin is directly the cause of the hæmolysis and hæmoglobinuria or whether it acts as a " trigger," as does quinine, to precipitate classical blackwater fever.

Earle *et al.* (1946, 1948) found that of seventy-four coloured patients given 30 mgm. or more of pamaquin a day six developed acute hæmolytic anæmia, while of seventy-three white patients given the same doses only one developed a gradual hæmolytic anæmia. The occurrence of anæmia is not causally related to the plasma drug level, to the occurrence of fever or to chronic malarial infection ; nor can it be correlated with the presence of isoagglutinins, isohæmolysins, autoagglutinins, cold agglutinins, changes in the resistance of the red cells to hypotonic saline or to mechanical trauma. The absence of correlation between the degree of methæmalbuminæmia and hæmolytic anæmia has already been mentioned. In some instances the degree of hæmolysis may be so great that hæmoglobin products pass the kidney threshold and appear in the urine, the signs and symptoms being identical with those in blackwater fever. Amy and Boyd (1936) drew attention to the fact that in some parts of India the widespread use of pamaquin was associated with an increased admission rate for hæmoglobinuria. In association with the hæmoglobinuria there are seen such symptoms as epigastric pain, anorexia, vomiting, slight fever, weakness, giddiness, dyspnœa, palpitation, and thirst. Anuria may also occur, such anuria being unassociated with blockage of the urinary tubules. Even in the absence of frank hæmoglobinuria there may be hyperbilirubinæmia, increased urobilinogen in urine and fæces, and an increase in urinary and fæcal coproporphyrins.

While race and individual idiosyncrasy play an important part in inducing these toxic changes, allergy may have some *rôle*, for a previous history of pamaquin administration is by no means rare (Banerjee and Brahmachari, 1933).

Granulocytopenia. Granulocytopenia has not been noted as a consistent manifestation of pamaquin therapy : however, Hasselmann and Hasselmann-Kahlert (1929) noted only one death due to agranulocytosis and " toxic hepatitis " among 103 subjects given 60 to 120 mgm. pamaquin hydroiodide daily. Schmidt (1948) observed granulocytopenia in monkeys given large doses, while Zubrod *et al.* (1946) and Earle *et al.* (1948) found that in volunteers infected with the Chesson strain of vivax malaria the daily administration of 90 mgm. of pamaquin base for fourteen days, together with quinine sulphate, caused a polymorphonuclear leucocytosis on the sixth or seventh day, followed by a gradual fall which reached a minimum sixteen to seventeen days after beginning pamaquin. Five days after stopping the drug the count began to rise again. Mature polymorphonuclear leucocytes were chiefly destroyed.

In addition to these rather dramatic reactions there have been noted dizziness, drowsiness, headache, fever and generalised urticaria (Paladino-Blandini and Marino-Assereto, 1934). Icterus has occasionally been described apart from hæmolytic anæmia.

In some of the earlier deaths from pamaquin poisoning the exact cause was not ascertained, but even as early as 1936 six fatal cases had been described (Nocht and Mayer, 1936). Some of these deaths may have been due to blackwater fever.

In one case reported by Blackie (1935) death was preceded by a gripping sensation in the throat with tightness of breath. The kidneys at necropsy showed evidence of an acute nephritis with hæmorrhages, and the liver exhibited a parenchymatous necrosis. Similar lesions can be produced experimentally in rhesus monkeys by the daily administration of from 0·0005 to 0·001 gm. per kgm. of body weight.

In fatal cases the dose of pamaquin has shown considerable variation. The patient described by Blackie (1935) is said to have received therapeutic doses only : Löken and Haymaker (1949) saw a fatal result in a patient who had taken 1·2 gm. in one day, twenty times the therapeutic dose if this be taken as 0·06 gm. Cordes (1928) describes two fatal cases where one and a half times the therapeutic dose had been taken for three days. Simcons (1936) had two fatal cases after only 0·03 gm. daily for three days, among 5,600 patients.

According to Heimann and Shapiro (1943), pamaquin has an effect on the electrocardiogram of convalescent malarial patients. The amplitude of the various deflections, especially the T wave, is increased and the S–T segment appears such as to simulate the cardiogram of a coronary thrombosis. Mepacrine, on the other hand, decreases the amplitude of the various deflections and restores the S–T segment to the isoelectric level after it has been elevated by pamaquin. In addition, with large doses of pamaquin, Moe and Seevers (1946) have obtained evidence of central impairment of sympathetic reflexes. It has long been recognised that pamaquin and mepacrine, if given together or with only a short interval between them, are liable to cause severe toxic reactions. Hardgrove and Applebaum (1946), for instance, gave ambulatory suppressive treatment to 4,361 labourers in Panama : 0·1 gm. of mepacrine was given three times a day for five days followed by an interval for two days and then 0·01 gm. of pamaquin dihydrochloride three times a day for five days. No less than 489, or 10·13 per cent., of the labourers developed symptoms, the toxic reactions in decreasing order of frequency being abdominal pain, dark urine, anorexia, jaundice, headache, nausea, vomiting, fever, weakness, and backache. Among the rarer findings were enlarged liver and spleen, cyanosis, and pallor. The urine was not infrequently concentrated and gave positive reactions for oxyhæmoglobin and methæmoglobin. Three-quarters of the patients had red cell counts below 4 million per c.mm. and 21 per cent. below 2 million per c.mm. West and Henderson (1944) observed toxic symptoms in twenty-four of 846 patients given 0·01 gm. three times daily for three days. Pamaquin treatment began two days after a course of quinine and mepacrine. The symptoms were headache, nausea, vomiting, dizziness, abdominal pains, jaundice, and fever. Two patients were psychotic and one passed into coma. Bile and albumin were constantly present in the urine, and hæmoglobin was frequent. In fatal cases late symptoms include numbness of the face, difficulty in speaking, dyspnœa, and palatal paralysis.

A possible explanation of the toxicity of combined pamaquin and mepacrine has been given by Kennedy *et al.* (1946). In man the oral administration or intramuscular injection of 20 mgm. of pamaquin base causes a maximal plasma concentration one to two hours later with negligible concentrations in eight hours. When pamaquin is given to patients who have recently taken mepacrine the plasma pamaquin level is raised from two to ten times and the rate of disappearance is slower. When 30 mgm. of mepacrine is given daily the rate of disappearance of pamaquin from the plasma is practically nil, and after a single dose of 500 mgm. mepacrine the resulting retardation of pamaquin excretion lasts for as long as six weeks.

Very much less is known of the toxic reactions due to other 8-aminoquinolines. Some produce reactions similar in type to those of pamaquin, but others give rise to an entirely different type of reaction.

Wiselogle (1946) classifies the toxic actions caused by 8-amino-quinolines into those affecting :—

(1) The hæmatopoietic organs and the formed elements of the blood ;

(2) The central nervous system ;

(3) The heart and circulation.

When the hæmatopoietic system is particularly affected the reaction is termed " the pamaquin reaction " ; when the central nervous system is chiefly involved the reaction is classified as of the " plasmocid " type, plasmocid being 8-(diethylamino-1-methyl propylamino)-6-methoxyquinoline (SN 3,115). The atypical reaction involving the heart and circulation is seen particularly with SN 10,309, which has an α-piperidyl group, —NH(CH₂)₂CH NH CH₂ CH₂ CH₂ CH₂, in place of terminal

$$-NH(CH_2)_2CH\ NH\ CH_2\ CH_2\ CH_2\ CH_2-$$

alkylamino groups on the side-chain.

The pamaquin reaction in the monkey and dog are very similar, There is depression of physical and mental activities, extreme weakness, cramps in the abdomen, tenesmus, loss of appetite, cachexia, cyanosis and circulatory and respiratory impairment. Eye lesions were seen in the dog but not in the monkey. Cyanosis was less intense in the monkey and most marked in the second week of treatment : thereafter it decreased in intensity, being scarcely detectable between the fourteenth and twenty-first days.

In monkeys there was frequent leucopenia with a considerable fall in the polymorphonuclear leucocytes. This neutropenia, with loss of two-thirds of the normal number of leucocytes, was associated with ulcerative lesions on the gums, surface of the tongue and on the buccal mucosa. Vincent's organisms (fusiforms, spirochætes and Gram-positive cocci with Gram-negative bacilli) were found in the lesions.

The red cells showed poikilocytosis, anisocytosis, polychromato-philia ; erythroblasts and normoblasts were present. Methæm-albuminæmia was less marked in monkeys than in dogs. Bili-rubinæmia was present. The bone marrow showed suppression of myeloid activity, enlargement of the spleen, which was engorged with red cells, while the liver exhibited necrosis in the central zone of the lobules. In the brain there was slight shrinkage of the neurones of the III, IV and VI cranial nerves with concentration of Nissl substance (Schmidt *et al.*, 1947a).

The plasmocid reaction is associated with severe abdominal cramps, hyperæsthesia, nystagmus, loss of pupillary reflexes, loss of vision, vertigo, inability to co-ordinate bodily movements, and spastic paralysis of the lower limbs, with dysbasia, dysergia and dysmetria. There is destruction of cells in the cochlear, vestibular, cerebellar, abducens, trochlear and oculomotor nuclei (Richter, 1949). The reactions due to plasmocid are irreversible, those due to pamaquin reversible (Schmidt and Schmidt, 1947, 1948). In a fatal case in man examined by Löken and Haymaker (1949) the most pronounced lesions were in the lower part of the pons, a somewhat curious distribution if anoxia be the cause of the lesions. Although the ischæmic changes in the cerebral cortex were consistent with anoxia, the globus pallidus, commonly involved in such conditions as carbon monoxide poisoning, was unaffected. The nuclei specially attacked were the oculo-motor, trochlear, abducent and vestibular, so that the same localisation is seen both in man and monkey.

In rhesus monkeys with large doses of plasmocid there is death within eighteen to forty-eight hours, associated with complete obliteration of all cells in the cochlear, vestibular, cerebellar, abducens, trochlear, and oculomotor nuclei. There is also drastic destruction of cell groups associated with these nuclei in ascending and descending pathways. The perineuronal spaces are empty or contain shrunken remnants of neurones. In severe chronic intoxications of from two to four weeks the lesions involved the same areas and practically all pathways in the brain stem and striatum. In the cord, the column of Clarke and at least some of the anterior horn cells are involved. The medium-sized pyramidal cells of the motor areas of the cerebral cortex show only slight changes. In low-grade chronic intoxication more restricted lesions are found, limited to the nuclei of cranial nerves, III, IV, VI and VIII, the cerebellar nuclei, the lateral cuneate nucleus, the column of Clarke and a very few anterior horn cells. Most cell groups associated with these nuclei remain normal. Plasmocid thus appears to have a specific toxic effect on nuclei in the proprioceptive and some reflex paths, as well as on extrapyramidal nuclei. Proprioceptive nuclei of the cord and medulla are first affected, later the vestibular nuclei and finally cochlear and visual reflex nuclei.

The atypical reaction is associated with cardiac failure and sudden death.

The type of toxicity exhibited by 8-aminoquinoline derivatives depends primarily on the side-chain : the degree of toxicity on the other band depends chiefly on the nuclear structure. Smith and Schmidt (1947) concluded that all compounds in which the terminal nitrogen of the side-chain was unsubstituted produced effects on the hæmatopoietic system. Compounds with one or two alkyl groups on the terminal nitrogen produced reactions which depended on the number of methylene groups separating the nitrogen atoms in the side-chain. With four exceptions the central nervous system was involved when compounds had two or three methylene groups. With derivatives having hexyl or longer methylene chains hæmatopoietic reactions developed but with side-chains containing four or five methylene groups the reactions were mixed. Atypical reactions on the heart and circulation were associated with compounds in which 2-piperidyl groupings replaced the terminal alkylamino groups.

The toxicity of pentaquine in animals may be compared with that of pamaquin. Pentaquine is considerably less toxic than pamaquin in animals : in the rat its toxicity is only one third, in the dog one-half and in the monkey one-half to one-fourth that of pamaquin. In the rat the toxic symptoms due to pentaquine and pamaquin are essentially similar, but in the dog there are differences. Both cause the formation of methæmalbumin, though pentaquine is less active : both cause abdominal pain and discomfort, pentaquine again being less active. Pentaquine has little effect on appetite, while with pamaquin dogs show loss of appetite and extreme emaciation. Pamaquin causes lesions in the third cranial nerve, paralysis of the nictitating membrane and divergent strabismus. These reactions are not met with in dogs given pentaquine. When a toxic level is present in the blood stream both pamaquin and pentaquine cause ill-defined effects on the heart and circulation, more marked in the case of pentaquine.

In the monkey the toxic action of pentaquine is chiefly on the cardiovascular system. Anæmia, leucopenia, methæmalbuminæmia, hyperbilirubinæmia, emaciation, depression and liver necrosis are not seen as they are with toxic doses of pamaquin. In normal men postural hypotension is caused by large doses of pentaquine (Freis and Wilkins, 1947). Doses of 120 to 240 mgm. of the base per day produce a significant fall in blood pressure after some days of therapy. Pentaquine depresses sympathetic nervous reflexes and causes a prolonged fall in pressure unassociated with a quickening of the pulse.

Both in the monkey and rat the toxicity of both compounds is increased two to four times by concurrent administration of quinine. The toxic manifestations are unaltered qualitatively. In man the toxicity of pentaquine for adults is one-half to three-quarters that of pamaquin. Thus, according to Loeb (1946), 15 to 45 mgm. of pentaquine base is equivalent to 15 mgm. pamaquin base per day. Sixty mgm. of pentaquine base with 2 gm. of quinine per day in divided doses for fourteen days equals in toxicity 30 to 45 mgm. of pamaquin base combined with the same dose of quinine. At this latter dosage there is invariably anorexia, abdominal discomfort and a slight degree of methæmalbuminæmia (average for forty-four patients 4·5 mgm. per 100 ml.). When methæmalbuminæmia exceeds 6 per cent. of the total hæmoglobin, cyanosis is noticeable.

A rise in leucocyte count above 12,000 per c.mm. is common, and occasionally a leucopenia below 3,600 per c.mm. The differential leucocyte count, however, remains normal. With doses of 120 to 180 mgm. daily of pentaquine base the toxic symptoms are naturally more severe. Of twenty volunteers studied by Craige *et al.* (1948) the majority suffered from severe abdominal and chest pain, nausea, anorexia and methæmalbuminæmia (5 to 13 per cent.) similar to that produced by toxic doses of pamaquin : in addition there was considerable loss of hæmoglobin. It is uncertain whether malaria tends to aggravate the toxicity of pentaquine. Straus and Gennis (1948) found toxic reactions in thirty-six of forty-nine patients but in none was it so severe as to necessitate discontinuance of the drug. Nausea, anorexia and occasional vomiting in the first four days, and mild abdominal pain after the first week, were not uncommon. Six patients showed a decrease of one million red cells or less per c.mm., but no frank hæmolysis occurred. Fever (99·6–103·4° F.) lasting for one day occurred in seven patients from the seventh to the ninth day. Alving *et al.* (1948a) noted that the concomitant administration of quinine lessened toxicity in man, contrary to its effect in experimental animals (Loeb *et al.*, 1946). Three subjects developed long-persistent postural hypotension and syncope somewhat similar to that produced by sodium nitrite. Whereas, however, the effects of nitrites are transient the tendency to postural hypotension in two of these subjects persisted for a month. In addition, the venous tone was reduced and adrenalin was ineffective in preventing the postural hypotension and syncope. Severe anoxia also developed ; this can be explained only by changes in the peripheral circulatory bed, a concept supported by the finding of a decreased venous tone. Doses of 120 to 180 mgm. daily are, of course, two to three times those used in ordinary antimalarial chemotherapy. Leucopenia and agranulocytosis have not been seen when pentaquine has been given to man, but a moderate leucocytosis has been noted. Whether or not an acute hæmolytic anæmia or hæmoglobinuria may occur is as yet unknown. Urinary abnormalities have not so far been observed and the urinary output remains normal. Alving *et al.* (1948c), among ninety-nine white subjects given from 15 to 60 mgm. per day for fourteen days found that abdominal discomfort was the main complaint. Occasionally the pain radiated from the epigastrium to the retrosternal area ; it was unrelieved by food. A small decrease of hæmoglobin is common, and in eleven of seventeen subjects it exceeded 1 gm. per 100 ml. of blood. It seems probable that the toxicity of pentaquine is too great to allow it to be used as a suppressive for prolonged periods, but in the treatment of relapsing vivax malaria, in association with quinine, it may well prove of greater value than pamaquin, since plasma concentrations are sustained for longer periods with pentaquine. Electrocardiograms revealed a diminution in the height of the T waves in some or all of the leads. T_3 sometimes became inverted ; in other patients an inverted T_3 became upright. In only a few instances was the T wave amplitude reduced below normal height. Serial electrocardiograms showed a return to normal after the course of treatment had been completed. Very occasionally unexplained attacks of fever occurred from the fourth to the tenth day of treatment. The comparative toxicity of pamaquin and pentaquine is shown in the table :—

Toxic Reactions after Therapeutic Administration of Pamaquin (60 mgm. for Twelve Days) and Pentaquine (60 mgm. for Fourteen Days) to Twenty-two Patients (Spicknall and Terry, 1948)

Symptom.	Pamaquin (number of cases).	Pentaquine (number of cases).
Abdominal pain . .	7	14
Cyanosis . . .	5	5
Anorexia . . .	—	4
Headache . . .	3	3
Dizziness . . .	—	1
Nausea . . .	1	—
No signs or symptoms .	9	6

Toxic reactions after pentaquine are rather numerous. Monk (1948) found that among twenty-five patients given 20 mgm. eight-hourly for ten days eleven had toxic reactions, seven suffering from cyanosis, seven from gastric disturbances ; among twenty-six patients given the same dose of pentaquine and 10 gr. of quinine eight-hourly for ten days thirteen had toxic reactions, twelve with cyanosis and eight with gastric disturbances. Cyanosis usually appeared about the third or fourth day and outlasted treatment by three or four days. It became apparent as a dusky grey colour most marked in the lips and conjunctivæ mucosa and accompanied in many cases by anorexia and nausea, sometimes epigastric pain and flatulence. One patient on a course of quinine and pentaquine developed cyanosis on the fourth day of treatment and by the sixth day there was marked tenderness under right costal margin, nausea, anorexia and central abdominal pain of a sharp and continuous nature. The liver was not palpable and the urine showed no abnormality, but the temperature rose above 102° F., although the patient had been apyrexial for the previous five days. The peripheral blood remained free from parasites. These signs and symptoms, except for the cyanosis, had disappeared within forty-eight hours of discontinuing treatment and did not reappear during the subsequent administration of a six-day course of pamaquin and quinine. The cyanosis gradually faded during administration of the latter course. This case suggests that some hepatic disturbance had occurred from the administration of pentaquine.

THE INCIDENCE OF TOXIC REACTIONS IN PATIENTS INFECTED WITH *Plasmodium vivax* (INDIAN, BURMESE AND FAR-EASTERN STRAINS) (Monk, 1948)

Number of cases.	Course.	Number with toxic signs.		Total number with toxic signs.
		Cyanosis.	Gastric disturbances.	
25	Pentaquine 20 mgm. : eight hourly for ten days	7 (28%)	7 (28%)	11 (44%)
26	Pentaquine 20 mgm. and quinine 10 gr. : eight hourly for ten days . .	12 (46%)	8 (30%)	13 (50%)
168	Quinine 10 gr. and pamaquin 10 mgm. : eight hourly for ten days . . .	11 (7%)	8 (5%)	18 (11%)
179	Proguanil 250 mgm. and pamaquin 10 mgm.: eight hourly for ten days . . .	30 (18%)	43 (25%)	63 (37%)
22	Pamaquin 10 mgm. eight hourly for ten days	Nil	1 (3·5%)	1 (3·5%)
24	Proguanil 250 mgm. twelve hourly for ten days	Nil	1 (4%)	1 (4%)

The toxic reactions following proguanil are very low when compared with those occurring with other courses. Monk (1948) has compared the incidence following six different courses. Pamaquin and proguanil, when given alone, showed very low toxicity, but curiously enough proguanil and pamaquin given together caused toxic reactions in just over a third of the patients. The reason for this increased toxicity requires further investigation. It is possible that the toxicity of pamaquin and other 8-aminoquinolines may be due, as suggested by Archibald and Weisiger (1948), to interaction with a naturally occurring aldehyde or ketone. Pamaquin reacts in aqueous formaldehyde solution binding irreversibly one equivalent of acid and one molecule of formaldehyde. The resulting compound, which cannot couple with diazo reagents, is twenty times more toxic than pamaquin ; it decomposes irreversibly in alkaline solution to give at least two new compounds neither of which is soluble in non-polar solvents, thus suggesting the persistence of the quaternary structure.

The toxicity of other 8-aminoquinolines has been studied in man by Jones *et al.* (1948) and Alving *et al.* (1948c). Methæmalbumin was present, and when the methæmalbumin exceeded 5 to 6 per cent. of the total hæmoglobin, cyanosis also was noted. The average total hæmoglobin values fell slowly and gradually. White counts were erratic, both mild leucopenia and slight leucocytosis being observed. Electrocardiograms in many cases showed a slight and transient diminution in the height of the T waves. The T waves changes were not attended by other evidence of cardiovascular abnormality. Drug fever appeared on the fourth to sixth day of treatment in three subjects receiving SN 1,452 in daily doses of 240 mgm. base. Drug fever or abdominal pain caused termination of treatment in three patients given SN 1,452. Alving *et al.* (1948c) found that SN 191, SN 13,619, SN 13,697 and SN 12,694 were peculiar in that they did not cause significant methæmoglobinæmia : the first three of these compounds have no 6-methoxy radical on the nucleus, while the last has a chloro substituent in the five position as well as a 6-methoxy radical. Pruritic vesicular rashes were seen in two out of five persons treated with SN 13,232.

(5) Proguanil

The toxicity of proguanil in laboratory animals has been studied by Davey (1946), Spinks (1947), Butler *et al.* (1947), and Schmidt *et al.* (1947a). The acute toxicity of proguanil for the mouse, rat, dog and rhesus monkey as recorded by Schmidt and his colleagues following oral and intramuscular injection is recorded in the table on page 250.

The LD 50, according to Schmidt *et al.* (1947b, c), for mice by the oral route is 23 mgm. per kgm. of body weight and by the intramuscular route 20 mgm. per kgm. of body weight.

According to Davey (1946) the minimal lethal dose for mice per kgm. of body weight varies slightly according to the body

THE ACUTE TOXICITY OF PROGUANIL FOR LABORATORY ANIMALS
(Schmidt *et al.*, 1947a)

Species.	Proguanil base dose in mgm. per kgm. of body weight.	Number of deaths per number of animals treated.	Remarks.
	Oral toxicity		
Mouse . .	15	0/20	Survivors exhibit no toxic symptoms.
	20	4/45	
	25	14/20	
	30	42/45	
Rat . .	100	0/4	No toxic effects.
	200	3/6	Survivors lose weight.
	400	6/8	
	800	4/4	
Dog . .	25	0/1	No toxic effects.
	50	0/1	
	100	0/1	Repeated vomiting two to four hours after administration.
	200	0/1	
	400	0/1	
Rhesus monkey	25	0/1	No toxic effects.
	50	0/1	
	100	0/1	
	200	0/1	Repeated vomiting two to four hours after administration.
	400	0/1	
	Intramuscular toxicity		
Mouse . .	15	0/20	No toxic symptoms in survivors.
	20	9/20	
	25	16/20	
	50	19/20	
Dog . .	20	0/1	No toxic symptoms.
	40	0/1	
	80	0/1	Depression of twelve hours' duration.
	160	1/1	
	320	1/1	
Rhesus monkey	20	0/1	No toxic symptoms.
	40	0/1	
	80	0/1	Depression of eight hours' duration.
	160	1/1	
	320	1/1	

weight. The toxicities for rats and mice of different weights were as follows :—

Species.	Route of administration.	Minimal lethal dose in mgm./kgm.
Mice (18–22 gm.)	Acute oral toxicity	50–75
	Acute intravenous toxicity	25
	Acute intraperitoneal toxicity	25
	Chronic oral toxicity (dosed twice daily for five days)	25–30
Mice (14–16 gm.)	Chronic oral toxicity (dosed twice daily for fourteen days)	20
Rats (80–100 gm.)	Acute intravenous toxicity	40
	Chronic oral toxicity (dosed once daily)	50
Rats (40 gm. : newly weaned)	Chronic oral toxicity	50 (growth unaffected at 30)

For chicks of 50 to 80 gm. body weight a dose of 60 mgm. per kgm. of body weight given twice daily caused a few deaths after two or three days' medication. The minimal lethal dose for chicks after intravenous injection was 80 mgm. per kgm.

In the dog and rhesus monkey, proguanil is more toxic intramuscularly than orally, a dose of 160 mgm. per kgm. given intramuscularly being fatal in both species. Death in coma was preceded by slowing of the heart and respiration and by profound lethargy.

In unpublished observations it was found that with baboons and vervet monkeys (*Cercopithecus æthiops centralis*) doses by mouth up to 500 mgm. per kgm. of body weight caused slight nausea and vomiting but were not fatal (Findlay, 1945). Dog and monkey are thus less susceptible in acute toxicity tests than rats and mice, the last being the most susceptible.

The toxicity of proguanil given intravenously or intraperitoneally has been compared with that after oral administration by Butler *et al.* (1947).

After intravenous or intraperitoneal injection of proguanil in rats and mice death may not occur for from one to twenty-four hours later ; a second injection one to forty-eight hours after the first has an additive effect which is probably due to the formation of some metabolite of greater toxicity than proguanil itself.

THE ACUTE TOXICITY OF PROGUANIL IN LABORATORY ANIMALS
(Butler *et al.*, 1947)

Species.	Route of administration.	LD 0 (mgm./kgm.).	LD 50 (mgm./kgm.).	LD 100 (mgm./kgm.).
Chick (wt. 50 gm.)	Oral	200	400–60	—
	Intravenous	40	60–80	100
Mouse (wt. 18–22 gm.)	Oral	50	60–80	100
	Intravenous	10	20–30	40–50
	Intraperitoneal	10	20–30	40–50
Rat (wt. 100 gm.)	Oral	80	100–150	—
	Intravenous	20	40	60
	Intraperitoneal	20	40	60
Rabbit (wt. 1,500 gm.)	Oral	—	150	—
	Intraperitoneal	30	50	—

Chicks do not exhibit delayed deaths with proguanil. It is possible
that late death is due to interference with some enzyme system,
for Vane (1949) showed that when prostigmine is injected in
doses of 90 or 180 μgm. per kgm. the proportion of immediate
deaths is increased and the proportion of delayed deaths correspondingly decreased. In chronic toxicity tests it was found by
Butler *et al.* (1947) that a daily oral dose of 12·5 mgm. per kgm.
for five days produced no deaths and no effect on growth. The
LD 50 for this type of experiment was 25 mgm. per kgm. of body
weight. Rats given 30 mgm. per kgm. by mouth showed a normal
growth curve ; 40 mgm. per kgm. caused a slight deviation in the
weight curve, while 50 mgm. per kgm. caused an immediate effect
on the weight curve, associated with some deaths. The concentration of proguanil in the blood at death was, however, only 1·4 mgm.
per litre. No characteristic pathological changes were found in
animals dying as a result of the chronic toxic action of proguanil.

Schmidt *et al.* (1947a) found that the addition of 0·04 to 0·08
per cent. of proguanil to the diet of mice was sufficient to cause
death. A simple oral dose of 9 mgm. per kgm. of body weight was
sufficient to cause symptoms. If however a dose of 32 mgm. per
kgm. of body weight was divided into four doses and given in the
course of twenty-four hours, no toxic results followed, this being
further evidence that proguanil is not stored in the tissues. In
rats, daily oral doses of 11 to 23 mgm. per kgm. were without

any toxic action, but daily doses of 45 mgm. per kgm. caused loss of appetite and failure of growth. In chronic toxicity tests in dogs doses of more than 10 mgm. per kgm. of body weight were fatal. Bradycardia preceded death. Rhesus monkeys given 10 and 20 mgm. per kgm. of body weight survived up to sixty-three days ; those given 40, 80, and 160 mgm. per kgm. died in twenty-two, eighteen, and seven days respectively. The symptoms of chronic poisoning in dogs and monkeys are salivation, loss of weight, hæmoconcentration, and increase in hæmoglobin and in red cell counts.

In dogs given proguanil by mouth there develops a disinclination to eat (Schmidt *et al.*, 1947b). The loss of appetite and death from starvation are possibly due to some as yet obscure action on the gastro-intestinal tract, but they are possibly related to the inhibitory action of proguanil on the volume and acidity of the gastric juice evoked by histamine (Burn and Vane, 1948). The symptoms of chronic poisoning rapidly disappear once proguanil is withdrawn, a striking difference from the findings with mepacrine and chloroquine.

It thus appears that the mouse and rat are highly susceptible to the toxic action of proguanil : chickens, dogs, and monkeys are far less susceptible. Yet in the highly susceptible rat a toxic dose of 50 mgm. produces a plasma concentration of only 0·23 mgm. per litre and far higher concentrations have been noted in man in the absence of toxic symptoms. In the rat also the persistence of proguanil in the plasma is less than in man. The same is true of the chick, which may have plasma concentrations ten times as high as those found in mice and rats without exhibiting toxic effects. A study of the tissue distribution of proguanil in the susceptible rat and the relatively insusceptible chick does not reveal any important difference. Equivalent doses of proguanil give higher plasma concentrations and the drug is more persistent in chicks than in rats and mice. It would therefore seem that in rats and mice proguanil is changed to a toxic product which persists in the body, whereas in the chicken, monkeys and possibly the dog this product is either not formed to the same degree or is rapidly destroyed or excreted.

As compared with mepacrine and chloroquine, the acute oral

toxicity of proguanil is twenty to forty times greater in the mouse, but in the rat the acute oral toxicity of all three drugs is approximately the same. In the dog the acute intramuscular toxicity of proguanil is one-half that of mepacrine and one-eighth that of chloroquine : in the monkey proguanil has approximately one-half of the acute intramuscular toxicity of mepacrine and chloroquine.

The Toxicity of Proguanil in Man. It was at first assumed that man reacted to proguanil in the same way as one of the more susceptible species. It now appears that the toxicity of proguanil for man is very low. A dose of 700 mgm. of proguanil twice daily was found to produce only very mild toxic effects (Adams *et al.*, 1945), and in the treatment of acute attacks there have been few complaints of toxic reactions. There is no evidence that, as was at first feared, nephritis may be produced. The toxic reactions both in Europeans and non-Europeans treated with proguanil during acute attacks are generally so mild as not to require the cessation of treatment. Gastro-intestinal symptoms are not uncommon, but are rarely seen if the drug is taken after food. Weakness, anorexia, and drowsiness have been complained of on very rare occasions ; pain in the back is rather more common.

Fairley (1946), who found that with doses of 300 mgm. daily for from ten to twenty-one days there were no toxic symptoms, obtained evidence of intolerance when 1,000 mgm. daily was administered. At this dosage the symptoms were gastro-intestinal, and hæmatological, together with changes in the urine.

(1) GASTRO-INTESTINAL. Vomiting was not infrequent in cases of malaria, but in one case it was so severe as to necessitate stopping treatment. Œsophagoscopy on this patient revealed reddening and œdema of the lower end of the œsophagus and a diagnosis of œsophageal spasm appeared consistent with the clinical findings.

In two patients after a single dose of 1,000 mgm. there were abdominal pain, vomiting, and diarrhœa.

(2) URINARY CHANGES. These were associated with overt malaria and high doses. Blood and epithelial cells and a few hyaline or granular casts were present in the urine. One case developed gross hæmaturia after a single dose of 100 mgm. ; another had hæmaturia and albuminuria with granular and blood casts during a course of 1,000 mgm. daily in divided doses ; a

raised blood urea was also present in this second patient, who may have had a previous renal lesion. These renal complications all disappeared when the dose was reduced. Similar observations have not been recorded on patients with smaller doses, but hæmaturia has also been observed in a child of three years given 300 mgm. daily.

(3) Hæmatological. Doses of 1,000 mgm. daily cause a slight increase in myelocytes to an average maximum of slightly more than 1 per cent. between the seventh and tenth days. The highest number recorded was 10 per cent. of the total leucocytes. A single dose of 100 mgm. was associated with a slight increase from the seventh to tenth days referable to the malaria rather than to the proguanil, for similar changes may occur after the use of mepacrine or pamaquin : proguanil in the absence of a malarial attack has no such action. Novoselova (1948), after a course of 600 mgm. on the first day, followed by 300 mgm. daily for four or nine days, found an increase in myelocytes in the blood and a diminution in Stab forms : the Arneth index showed a shift to the left. It would seem that proguanil may have a direct effect on the bone marrow, which is more marked after an attack of malaria. Hæmaturia has been reported in a girl of seven after 0·8 gm. proguanil taken in forty-eight hours (Thiodet and Fabregoule, 1949).

Urticaria has appeared on rare occasions and itching, puffiness of the face and erythema of the face, palms of the hands, and soles of the feet. The areas affected by erythema may subsequently exhibit desquamation. Very rarely blurring of vision has been complained of. There are suggestions of doubtful validity that proguanil may induce a polymorphonuclear leucocytosis, thus simulating a coccal infection, and that proguanil may interfere with the curative action of penicillin and sulphonamides. Among those who have taken proguanil as a suppressive in the tropics there have been complaints of lassitude, gastro-intestinal upset, loss of appetite followed by loss of weight, and sometimes looseness of stools on doses of 100 mgm. daily (Shearer, 1949). Often these symptoms do not appear till proguanil has been taken for at least two or three months. Loss of appetite may be correlated with the reduction in the secretion of acid by the stomach caused by doses of 900 mgm. (Doll and Schneider, 1948 ; Vane *et al.*, 1948). Gastro-intestinal symptoms are prevented if the drug is given on a full stomach. Canet (1948), in Indo-China, noted anorexia, headache and insomnia in from 6 to 10 per cent. of patients given thera-peutic doses of proguanil. Klopper *et al.* (1948), among 602 adults given 100 mgm. as a weekly suppressive, saw general malaise in four, abdominal pain in seven, headache in one and vertigo in one : among 580 children given 50 mgm., four had headache and abdominal pain, nine had headache alone and two had abdominal pain alone. It is not yet known whether proguanil has any relation to the onset of blackwater fever. The patient with blackwater fever described by Best (1949), in the Sudan, had received quinine in doses of 30 gr. (2 gm.) daily for three days as his falciparum infection was not controlled by proguanil. Billington (1950) with 400 mgm. daily noted hypersensitivity of the carotid sinus reflex and peripheral neuritis.

Combined Toxicity of Antimalarial Drugs

In view of the fact that a combination of two or more drugs is often used, especially in the treatment of relapsing vivax infections, data on combined toxicity are of some interest. French workers use a combination of equal parts of rhodoquine and pamaquin under the name rodopréquine or præquine. Rhodoquine and pamaquin (præquine) are both gametocyticidal, but the combination is said to be less toxic for whereas pamaquin causes cyanosis, rhodoquine is apt to cause giddiness and the mixture contains insufficient to cause symptoms. Similarly, a mixture of ten parts of mepacrine and one part of rodopréquine has been largely used under the name prémaline. Here again there is said to be complete absence of toxicity. Chen and Geiling (1947) tested a number of combinations of different drugs in mice. Quinine and mepacrine acted indepen-dently and similarly as regards toxicity ; so also did quinine and hydroxyethylapocupreine. When mepacrine and pamaquin were tested the lethal effect of the latter was not influenced by a sublethal dose of the former, indicating that the two substances act on the host independently but in different ways. When mepacrine was used in the lethal range, however, the addition of pamaquin produced a greater mortality than would be expected. This combination, first used by Mühlens and Fischer (1932), is now regarded as too toxic for general use in man (Banerjee and Brahmachari, 1933). Quinine and pamaquin, or quinine and pentaquine, display a synergistic action as regards toxicity to the host.

References

ABBOTT, P. H., 1946, A case of blackwater fever during mepacrine therapy. *Trans. R. Soc. trop. Med. Hyg.*, **40,** 354.

ADAMS, A. R. D., MAEGRAITH, B. G., KING, J. D., TOWNSHEND, R. H., DAVEY, T. H., and HAVARD, R. E., 1945, Studies on synthetic antimalarial drugs. XIII. Results of a preliminary investigation of the therapeutic action of 4888 (paludrine) on acute attacks of benign tertian malaria. *Ann. trop. Med. Parasit.*, **39,** 225.

AGRESS, C. M., 1946, Atabrine as a cause of fatal exfoliative dermatitis and hepatitis. *J. Amer. med. Ass.*, **131,** 14.

ALAGNA, G., 1948, Intossicazione chininica ed occhio. *Atti 37 Congr. Soc. Oftal. ital.*, **10,** 37.

ALLEN, C., 1944, Diagnosis of psychotic symptoms in atebrin intoxication. *Brit. med. J.*, **ii,** 831.

ALLEN, E. W., ALLEN, H. D., Jr., and FULGHUM, C. B., 1937, Psychosis following the administration of atabrine for malaria. *J. med. Ass. Ga.*, **26,** 62.

ALVING, A. S., CRAIGE, B., Jr., JONES, R., Jr., WHORTON, C. M., PULLMAN, T. N., and EICHELBERGER, L., 1948a, Pentaquine (SN-13,276), a therapeutic agent effective in reducing the relapse rate in vivax malaria. *J. clin. Invest.*, **27,** Suppl. p. 25.

ALVING, A. S., EICHELBERGER, L., CRAIGE, B., Jr., JONES, R., Jr., WHORTON, C. M., and PULLMAN, T. N., 1948b, Studies on the chronic toxicity of chloroquine (SN-7,618). *J. clin. Invest.*, **27,** Suppl. p. 60.

ALVING, A. S., PULLMAN, T. N., CRAIGE, B., Jr., JONES, R., Jr., WHORTON, C. M., and EICHELBERGER, L., 1948c, The clinical trial of eighteen analogues of pamaquin (plasmochin) in vivax malaria (Chesson strain). *J. clin. Invest.*, **27,** Suppl. p. 34.

AMBLER, J. V., 1944, Experience of a dermatologist in the Southern Pacific. *Arch. Derm. Syph.*, Chicago, **49,** 224.

AMY, A. C., 1934, Hæmoglobinuria : a new problem on the Indian Frontier. *J. R. Army Med. Cps*, **62,** 178.

AMY, A. C., and BOYD, J. S. K., 1936, Malaria in India ; the synthetic drugs and the relapse rate. *J. R. Army Med. Cps*, **67,** 83.

ANDERSON, THOMAS, 1856, " Handbook for yellow fever describing its pathology and treatment as observed in unintermitted practice during half a century. . . ." London : John Churchill & Sons.

ARCHIBALD, R. M., and WEISIGER, J. R., 1948, Reaction of plasmochin with formaldehyde. *Fed. Proc.*, **7,** 143.

ARMY MALARIA RESEARCH UNIT, OXFORD, 1946, Prolonged oral administration of mepacrine. *Ann. trop. Med. Parasit.*, **40,** 128.

AYALA, F., and BRAVO, G., 1942, Psicosis obervadas en el tratamiento de la malaria con atepé. *Rev. clin. esp.*, **7,** 70.

BAGBY, J. W., 1945, A tropical lichen planus-like disease. *Arch. Derm. Syph.*, Chicago, **52,** 1.

BAIS, W. J., 1941, Nog een geval van thrombopenische purpura door kinine. *Geneesk. Tijdschr. Ned.-Ind.*, **81,** 2213.

BANERJEE, K., 1936a, Some unnatural phenomena in the course of atebrin treatment. *Calcutta med. J.*, **30,** 515.

BANERJEE, K., 1936b, Two cases of poisoning after injection of atebrin musonate. *Calcutta med. J.*, **31,** 41.

258 TOXIC REACTIONS TO ANTIMALARIAL DRUGS

BANERJEE, N. G., and BRAHMACHARI, P., 1933, The occurrence of hemoglobinuria during treatment of malarial fever with atebrin and plasmoquine. *Indian med. Gaz.*, **68**, 149.
BANG, F. B., HAIRSTON, N. G., TRAGER, W., and MAIER, J., 1947, Treatment
of acute attacks of vivax and falciparum malaria. A comparison of
atabrine and malaria. *Bull. U.S. Army med. Dept.*, **7**, 75.
BARBOSA, A., 1934, Contribucion al tratamiento del paludismo con la atébrina.
Med. Páis. cálidos, **7**, 73, 123 and 157.
BARKER, L. P., 1947, Hyperkeratosis of the palms and soles due to the ingestion of quinacrine hydrochloride. *Arch. Derm. Syph.*, Chicago, **55**, 256.
BASTIANELLI, G., MOSNA, E., and CANALIS, A., 1937, Prevention and treatment
of malaria by synthetic drugs. *Quart. Bull. Hlth Org. L.o.N.*, **6**, 822.
BAZEMORE, J. M., JOHNSON, H. H., SWANSON, E. R., and HAYMAN, J. M., Jr.,
1946, Relation of quinacrine hydrochloride to lichenoid dermatitis
(atypical lichen planus). *Arch. Derm. Syph.*, Chicago, **54**, 308.
BECK, I. T., and FROMMEL, E., 1947, De l'action comparative de la quinine,
de l'atébrine et de la plasmochine sur la survie des spermatozoides du
cobaye. *Compt. rend. Soc. Phy. Hist. nat. Genève*, **64**, 100.
BECKER, F. T., 1946, Dermatitis due to quinacrine hydrochloride. *Arch.
Derm. Syph.*, Chicago, **54**, 338.
BECKMAN, H., 1942, "Treatment in general practice." 4th edit. Philadelphia.
W. B. Saunders Co.
BEIGLBÖCK, W., 1937, Ein Fall von thrombopenischer Purpura bei echter
Chinenüberempfindlichkeit. *Z. klin. Med.*, **131**, 308.
BERESTON, E. S., 1946, Lichenoid dermatitis. *J. invest. Derm.*, **7**, 69.
BERESTON, E. S., and CHENEY, G., 1946, Vitamin B complex in the treatment
of Lichenoid dermatitis. *Arch. Derm. Syph.*, Chicago, **54**, 425.
BERESTON, E. S., and SASLAW, M. S., 1946, Complications of lichenoid derma-
titis. Glomerulonephritis and severe pigmentary changes in the exfoliative
stage of lichenoid dermatitis. *Arch. Derm. Syph.*, Chicago, **54**, 325.
BERLINER, R. W., EARLE, D. P., Jr., TAGGART, J. V., ZUBROD, C. G., WELCH,
W. J., CONAN, N. J., BAUMAN, E., SCUDDER, S. T., and SHANNON, J. A.,
1948, Studies on the chemotherapy of the human malarias. VI. The
physiological disposition, antimalarial activity and toxicity of several
derivatives of 4-aminoquinoline. *J. clin. Invest.*, **27**, Suppl. p. 98.
BEST, A. M., 1949, Proguanil and blackwater fever. *Brit. J. Med.*, **i**, 324.
BIGHAM, A., 1949, Mepacrine dermatitis. *Brit. med. J.*, **ii**, 387.
BILLINGTON, V. L., 1950, Side effects of proguanil therapy. *Brit. med. J.*, **i**,
671.
BISHAY, A., 1946, Quinine amblyopia. *Brit. J. Ophthal.*, **30**, 281.
BISPHAM, W. N., 1936, A report on the use of atabrine in the prophylaxis of
malaria. *Amer. J. trop. Med.*, **16**, 547.
BISPHAM, W. N., 1941, Toxic reactions following the use of atabrine in malaria.
Amer. J. trop. Med., **21**, 455.
BLACKIE, W. K., 1935, A fatal case of plasmoquinine poisoning. *S. Afr. med.
J.*, **9**, 147.
BLAKE, W. D., 1948, Methemalbumin. II. Effect of pamaquine and quinine
on pathways of hemoglobin metabolism. *J. clin. Invest.*, **27**, Suppl.,
p. 144.
BRIERCLIFFE, R., 1935, The Ceylon Malaria epidemic 1934–35. Report by the
Director of Medical and Sanitary Services. Sessional Paper XXII.
Colombo, Ceylon, Government Press.
BROCH, O. J., 1941, Trombopenisk purpura etter kinindin. *Nord. med.*,
10, 1542.
BROWN, J. S., 1945, Soft tissue calcification secondary to therapeutic quinine.
Brit. J. Radiol., **18**, 183.
BURACK, S., 1946, Problems of military neuro-psychiatry. *J. nerv. ment. Dis.*,
104, 284.

BURN, J. H., and VANE, J. R., 1948, The inhibitory action of paludrine on the secretion of gastric juice. *Brit. J. Pharmacol.*, 3, 346.

BURNHAM, R. C., 1946, Acute atabrine intoxication : report of a case. *Nav. med. Bull., Wash.*, 46, 434.

BUTLER, A., DAVEY, D. G., and SPINKS, A., 1947, A preliminary report of the toxicity and the associated blood concentrations of paludrine in laboratory animals. *Brit. J. Pharmacol.*, 2, 181.

BUTLER, M. G., 1947, Atypical lichen planus tropicalis. *Arch. Derm. Syph., Chicago*, 55, 535.

CANET, J., 1948, Essais de traitement curatif du paludisme aigu dans la paludrine en Indochine. *Bull. Soc. Path. exot.*, 41, 690.

CHAMBERLAIN, W. P., and BOLES, D. J., 1946, Edema of cornea precipitated by quinacrine (atabrine). *Arch. Ophthal., Chicago*, 35, 120.

CHAUDHURI, R. N., 1948, Treatment of malaria. *Indian med. Gaz.*, 83, 225.

CHEN, G., and GEILING, E. M. K., 1947, The acute joint toxicity of atabrine, quinine, hydroxyethylapocupreine, pamaquine and pentaquine. *J. Pharmacol.*, 91, 133.

CHOPRA, R. N., and ABDUL WAHED, A. K. M., 1934, Toxic effects produced by combined treatment with atebrin and plasmochin. *Indian med. Gaz.*, 69, 213.

CHOPRA, R. N., and CHAUDHURI, R. N., 1935, Some observations on the toxicity of synthetic antimalarial remedies. *Indian med. Gaz.*, 70, 1.

CHOPRA, R. N., DAS GUPTA, B. M., and SEN, B., 1933, Atebrin in the treatment of Indian strains of malaria. *Indian med. Gaz.*, 68, 425.

CHOREMIS, K., and SPILIOPOULOS, G., 1938, Paralytische Erscheinungen nach Gebrauch von synthetischen Antimalaria-Mitteln. *Dtsch. med. Wschr.*, 64, 1680.

CLARKE, G. H. V., 1949, A case of mepacrine dermatitis. *Brit. med. J.*, ii, 58.

CODA, D., 1949, Expériences sur la chimioprophylaxie du paludisme au Brésil. *Bull. Soc. Path. exot.*, 42, 168.

COLETTE, MLLE, and POROT, M., 1949, Les psychoses quinacriniques. *Algérie méd.*, No. 7, p. 375.

CONDORELLI, L., 1941, Porpora emorragica chininica de malaria. (Considerazioni patogenetiche sulla porpora da malaria). *Riv. Malariol.*, 20, 8.

COOPER, W. C., RUHE, D. S., COATNEY, G. R., JOSEPHSON, E. S., and YOUNG, M. D., 1949, Studies in human malaria. VIII. The protective and therapeutic action of quinacrine against St. Elizabeth strain vivax malaria. *Amer. J. Hyg.*, 49, 25.

CORDES, W., 1928, Zwischenfäke bei der Plasmochin-behandlung. *Arch. Schiffs-u. Tropenhyg.*, 32, 143.

CRAIGE, B., Jr., EICHELBERGER, L., JONES, R., Jr., ALVING, A. S., PULLMAN, T. N., and WHORTON, C M., 1948, The toxicity of large doses of pentaquine (SN 13, 276), a new antimalarial drug. *J. clin. Invest.*, 27, Suppl. p. 17.

CUSTER, R. P., 1946, Aplastic anæmia in soldiers treated with atabrine (quinacrine). *Amer. J. med. Sci.*, 212, 211.

DAME, L. R., 1946, The effects of atabrine on the human visual system. *Amer. J. Ophthal.*, 29, 1432.

DANTZIG, L., and MARSHALL, L. E., 1946, Tropical lichen planus : New Guinea variety ; clinical report on 24 cases. *N.Y. St. J. Med.*, 46, 991.

DAVEY, D. G., 1946, Paludrine : a summary of information to February, 1946. Rept. BT 1116. Imperial Chemicals (Pharmaceuticals) Ltd.

DECHERD, G. M., Jr., 1937, A fatality after atebrin-plasmochin treatment of malaria. *J. trop. Med. Hyg.*, 40, 90.

DIMSON, S. B., and McMARTIN, R. B., 1946, Pamaquin hæmoglobinuria. *Quart. J. Med.*, 15, 25.

DIVRY, A., 1948, Intoxication par la quinine. *Rev. méd. Liege*, 3, 316.

DIXON, H. B. F., 1933, A report on 600 cases of malaria treated with plasmoquine and quinine. *J.R. Army med. Cps.*, 60, 431.

260 TOXIC REACTIONS TO ANTIMALARIAL DRUGS

Doll, R., and Schneider, R., 1948, The effect of paludrine on human gastric secretion. *Brit. J. Pharmacol.*, **3**, 352.

Drake, J. B., and Moon, H. D., 1946, Atabrine dermatitis and associated aplastic anemia. *Calif. med.*, **65**, 154.

Dreisbach, R. H., and Hanzlik, P. J., 1945, Antagonists for the circulatory depression of quinine injected intravenously and the implied cholinergic action, and nature and importance of the vasodilation, in the depression. *J. Pharmacol.*, **83**, 167.

Duemling, W. W., 1945, Cutaneous diseases in the South Pacific. *Arch. Derm. Syph., Chicago*, **52**, 75.

Earle, D. P., Jr., Bigelow, F. S., Zubrod, C. G., and Kane, C. A., 1948, Studies on the chemotherapy of malaria. IX. Effect of pamaquine on the blood cells of man. *J. clin. Invest.*, **27**, Suppl. p. 121.

Earle, D. P., Jr., Knowlton, P., Berliner, R. W., Taggart, J. V., Zubrod, C. G., Welch, W. J., and Shannon, J. A., 1946, Pamaquin. 3. Occurrence of hemolytic anæmias. *Fed. Proc.*, **5**, 176.

Einhorn, N. H., and Tomlinson, W. J., 1946, Estivo-autumnal (*Plasmodium falciparum*) malaria : a survey of 493 cases of infection with *Plasmodium falciparum* in children. *Amer. J. Dis. Child.*, **72**, 137.

Elliot, R. H., 1918, Quinine poisoning : its ocular lesions and visual disturbances. *Amer. J. Ophthal.*, **1**, 547.

Epstein, E., 1945, The lichen planus-eczematoid dermatitis complex of the South-west Pacific : a study of 65 cases. *Bull. U.S. Army med. Dept.*, **4**, 687.

Ershoff, B. H., 1948, The effects of B vitamins, liver and yeast on atabrine toxicity in the rat. *J. Nutrit.*, **35**, 269.

Fairley, N. H., *et al.*, 1945, Chemotherapeutic suppression and prophylaxis in malaria. An experimental investigation undertaken by medical research teams in Australia. *Trans. R. Soc. trop. Med. Hyg.*, **38**, 311.

Fairley, N. H., *et al.*, 1946, Researches on paludrine (M 4888) in malaria. *Trans. R. Soc. trop. Med. Hyg.*, **40**, 105.

Fairley, N. H., and Bromfield, R. J., 1934, Laboratory studies in malaria and blackwater fever. Part III. A new blood pigment in blackwater fever and other biochemical observations. *Trans. R. Soc. trop. Med. Hyg.*, **28**, 307.

Fairley, N. H., and Murgatroyd, F., 1940, Recurrent blackwater fever induced by quinine. *Trans. R. Soc. trop. Med. Hyg.*, **34**, 187.

Fantl, P., Rome, M. N., and Nance, M. H., 1947, The influence of quinine hydrochloride on the plasma coagulation mechanism. *Aust. J. exp. Biol. med. Sci.*, **25**, 183.

Fasal, P., and Wachner, G., 1933, Symptomatische thrombopenische Purpura als Folge einer Chinin Safran Intoxikation. *Wien. klin. Wschr.*, **46**, 747.

Feder, A., 1949, Clinical observations on atypical lichen planus and related dermatoses presumably due to atabrine toxicity. *Ann. inter. Med.*, **31**, 1078.

Fernando, P. B., and Sandarasagara, A. P., 1935, A clinical study of 647 patients treated for malaria during the Ceylon epidemic of 1934–35. *Ceylon J. Sci.*, **3**, 195.

Ferreira-Marques, J., 1949, Contribution à l'étude du traitement du lichen plan par l'association nicotinamide-penicilline. *Acta derm.-venereol. stockh.*, **29**, 1009.

Field, J. W., 1939, Notes on the chemotherapy of malaria. *Bull. Inst. med. Res. F.M.S. No. 2 of 1938.*

Field, J. W., and Niven, J. C., 1936, A clinical comparison of atebrin-musonate with quinine bihydrochloride ; a preliminary report based on the treatment of 286 cases of acute malaria. *Trans. R. Soc. trop. Med. Hyg.*, **29**, 647.

FINDLAY, G. M., 1945, The toxicity of paludrine in monkeys. Unpublished Report.

FINDLAY, G. M., 1946, Mepacrine and lichen planus. *Lancet, i*, 252.

FINDLAY, G. M., 1947a, Unpublished Report.

FINDLAY, G. M., 1947b, The toxicity of mepacrine in man. *Trop. Dis. Bull.*, 44, 763.

FINDLAY, G. M., 1949, Blackwater fever in West Africa 1941–45. I. Blackwater fever in European military personnel. *Ann. trop. Med. Parasit.*, 49, 140.

FINDLAY, G. M., and MARKSON, J. L., 1947, Attempts to induce blackwater fever experimentally. *Ann. trop. Med. Parasit.*, 41, 22.

FINDLAY, G. M., and STEVENSON, A. C., 1944, Investigations into the chemotherapy of malaria in West Africa. II. Malaria suppression—quinine and mepacrine. *Ann. trop. Med. Parasit.*, 38, 168.

FISCHER, O., and RHEINDORF, G., 1928, Zur Frage der Plasmochin-Nebenwirkung. *Arch. Schiffs-u. Tropenhyg.*, 32, 594.

FISHMAN, A. P., and KINSMAN, J. M., 1949, Hypoplastic anemia due to atabrine. *Blood*, 4, 970.

FITZHUGH, O. G., and NELSON, A. A., 1947, The chronic toxicity of chloroquine (SN 7,618). *Fed. Proc.*, 6, 330.

FITZHUGH, O. G., NELSON, A. A., CALVERY, H. O., and GLASSMAN, J. M., 1945, The chronic toxicity of quinacrine (atabrine). *J. Pharmacol.*, 85, 207.

FITZHUGH, O. G., NELSON, A. A., and HOLLAND, O. L., 1948, The chronic oral toxicity of chloroquine. *J. Pharmacol.*, 93, 147.

FORBES, S. B., 1940, The etiology of nerve deafness with particular reference to quinine. *Sth. med. J., Nashville*, 33, 613.

FORMAN, L., 1947, Evipan used in the investigation of some chronic dermatoses. *Brit. J. Derm. Syph.*, 59, 45.

FOY, H., and KONDI, A., 1937, Three cases of blackwater fever following the oral administration of atebrin. *Trans. R. Soc. trop. Med. Hyg.*, 31, 99.

FOY, H., and KONDI, A., 1938, Spectrographic analysis of pigments in serum and urine of blackwater fever. *Trans. R. Soc. trop. Med. Hyg.*, 32, 49.

FOY, H., KONDI, A., DAMKAS, C., DEPANIAN, M., LEFCOPOULOU, T., BACH, L. G., DAX, R., PITCHFORD, J., SHIELE, P., and LANGTON, M., 1948, Malaria and blackwater fever in Macedonia and Thrace in relation to D.D.T. *Ann. trop. Med. Parasit.*, 42, 153.

FOY, H., KONDI, A., and PERISTERIS, M., 1936, Studies on atebrin—a controlled field experiment to test the relapse value of atebrin. *Trans. R. Soc. trop. Med. Hyg.*, 30, 109.

FRANKS, A. G., and DAVIS, M. I. J., 1943, Agranulocytosis: complication following quinine in case of malaria therapy. *Amer. J. Syph.*, 27, 314.

FREIS, D., and WILKINS, R. W., 1947, Effect of pentaquine in patients with hypertension. *Proc. Soc. exp. Biol., N.Y.*, 64, 455.

FROMMOLT, G., 1932, Methämoglobinurie bie Kriminellem. *Z. Geburtsh. Gynäk.*, 101, 454.

GASKILL, H. S., and FITZHUGH, T., Jr., 1945, Toxic psychoses following atabrine. *Bull. U.S. Army Med. Dept.* No. 86 (March), p. 63.

GIACOMINI, G., 1841, Effetti del solfato di chinina sugli animali, ed avvelenamento pel solfato di chinina nell' uomo sano. *Ann. Univ. Med.*, 97, 325.

GIACOMINI, G., 1842, Effets du sulfate de quinine chez la animaux et observation d'empoisonnement par ce sel chez l'homme. *J. Pharm. Chim. Paris. NS.*, 2, 268.

GINSBERG, J. E., and SHALLENBERGER, P. L., 1946, Woods' light fluorescence phenomenon in quinacrine medication. *J. Amer. med. Ass.*, 131, 808.

GORDON, H. H., DIEUAIDE, F. R., MARBLE, A., CHRISTIANSON, H. B., and DAHL, L. K., 1947, Treatment of *Plasmodium vivax* malaria of foreign origin : a comparison of various drugs. *Arch. intern. Med.*, 79, 365.

GOVINDASWAMY, M. V., 1936, Atebrin poisoning. *Lancet, i,* 56.

GRANT-PETERKIN, G. A., 1947, Sequelæ of tropical disease skin conditions. *Edin. med. J.,* 54, 36.

GRANT-PETERKIN, G. A., and HAIR, H. C., 1946, Preliminary report of a dermatosis due possibly to mepacrine. A description of 26 cases seen in Italy. *Brit. J. Derm. Syph.,* 58, 263.

GREEN, R., 1932, A report on fifty cases of malaria treated with atebrin. A new synthetic drug. *Lancet, i,* 826.

GREEN, R., 1934a, Toxic effects associated with the use of atebrin. *Malaya med. J.,* 9, 22.

GREEN, R., 1934b, Lectures on the development and use of the synthetic antimalarial drugs. *Bull. Inst. Med. Res. F.M.S.,* No. 2.

GREIBER, M. F., 1947, Psychoses associated with the administration of atebrine. *Amer. J. Psychiat.,* 104, 306.

GUIJA MORALES, E., 1945, " Psicosis palúdicas y atebrínicas. Trastornos psiquicos en el paludismo espontáneo, en el terapéutico y en los tratamientos con preparados atébrínicosi." Barcelona. J. M. Masso.

GUNTHER, C. E. M., 1938, Blackwater fever following the administration of " atebrin." *Med. J. Aust., ii,* 1119.

HARDGROVE, M., and APPLEBAUM, I. L., 1946, Plasmochin toxicity   analysis of 258 cases. *Ann. intern. Med.,* 25, 103.

HARVEY, A. M., MAIER, J., PAPENHEIMER, A. M., Jr., BANG, F. B., and HAIRSTON, N. G., 1944, Clinical and laboratory studies on atypical lichen planus with particular reference to the *rôle* of atabrine. Rept. to Surgeon-General U.S.A., Dec. 3.

HASSELMANN, C. M., and HASSELMANN-KAHLERT, M., 1929, Erfahrungen und Zwischenfälle bei der Plasmochin-Behandlung autochthoner Malaria in den Tropen. *Dtsch. med. Wschr.,* 55, 1635.

HAUER, A., 1939, Beispiel einer familiären Form von vererbbarer Chinin-überempfindlichkeit. *Arch. Schiffs-u. Tropenhyg.,* 43, 203.

HAY, D. C., SPAAR, A. E., and LUDOVICI, H. L., 1935, Atebrin treatment in malaria. *Indian med. Gaz.,* 70, 678.

HAYMAN, J. R., Jr., MOST, H., LONDON, I. M., KANE, C. A., LAVIETES, P. H., and SCHROEDER, E. F., 1946, Chloroquine (SN 7,618), a new highly effective antimalarial drug for routine use in treatment of acute attacks of vivax malaria. *Trans. Ass. Amer. Phys.,* 59, 82.

HEATHCOTE, R. ST. A., 1941, Toxicology—Quinine. *Med. Ann.,* 59, 380.

HECHT, G., 1933, Pharmakologisches über Atebrin. *Arch. exp. Path. Pharmak.,* 170, 328.

HEGSTED, D. M., McKIBBIN, J. M., and STARE, F. J., 1944a, Nutrition and tolerance to atabrine. *J. Nutrit.,* 27, 141.

HEGSTED, D. M., McKIBBIN, J. M., and STARE, F. J., 1944b, The effect of atabrine on choline deficiency in the young rat. *J. Nutrit.,* 27, 141.

HEGSTED, D. M., McKIBBIN, J. M., and STARE, F. J., 1945, The effect of atabrine on thiamine deficiency in the young rat. *J. Nutrit.,* 29, 361.

HEILIG, R., and VISVESWAR, S. K., 1944, The influence of intravenous injections of quinine on the myocardium. *Indian med. Gaz.,* 79, 514.

HEIMANN, H. L., and SHAPIRO, B. G., 1943, Effects of plasmoquin, atebrin and quinine on the electrocardiogram. *Brit. Heart J.,* 5, 131.

HELLIER, F. F., 1944, in discussion on : Dowling, G. B., 1944, Erythematous lichen planus. *Proc. R. Soc. Med.,* 37, 410.

HERING, E. R., PATT, H M., and LEAVITT, H. J., 1948, Tolerability studies of some new antimalarial drugs. *J. nat. Mal. Soc.,* 7, 322.

HERTZBERG, R., 1946, Quinine amaurosis : a report of a case. *Med. J. Aust., ii,* 92.

HOEKENGA, M. T., 1950, Camoquin treatment of malaria : a preliminary report. *Amer. J. trop Med.,* 30, 63.

HOLBROOK, A. A., 1948, Lichen planus, atypical. A report of ten cases. *Amer. J. Med.*, 4, 525.

HOOBLER, S. W., 1947, Psychotic reactions to the ingestion of large doses of quinacrine in normal subjects. *Amer. J. trop Med.*, 27, 477.

HOOPS, A. L., 1935, The advantages of atebrin in the treatment of malaria amongst controlled labour forces in Malaya. *Trans. R. Soc. trop. Med. Hyg.*, 29, 249.

HUGHES, T. A., 1931, The effect of intravenous injections of quinine on the electrocardiogram in man. *Indian J. med. Res.*, 19, 113.

JONES, R., Jr., CRAIGE, B., Jr., ALVING, A. S., WHORTON, A. C., PULLMAN, T. N., and EICHELBERGER, L., 1948, A study of the prophylactic effectiveness of several 8-aminoquinolines in sporozoite-induced vivax malaria (Chesson strain). *J. clin. Invest.*, 27, Suppl. p. 6.

KAHLSTORF, A., 1947, Ueber eine Leber schädigung durch hohe Atebrindosen. *Klin. Wschr.*, 24–25, 632.

KANG, T., and GARVIS, B. W., 1936, Maniacal symptoms following use of atebrin. Report of a case. *Chin. med. J.*, 50, 976.

KENNEDY, T. J., Jr., ZUBROD, C. G., BIGELOW, F. S., BERLINER, R. W., and SHANNON, J. A., 1946, A mechanism of drug " potentiation " : pamaquin metabolism as influenced by quinacrine. *Fed. Proc.*, 5, 185.

KEOGH, P., and SHAW, F. H., 1944, The mode of action of quinine alkaloids and other antimalarials. *Aust. J. exp. Biol. med. Sci.*, 22, 139.

KIERLAND, R. R., 1946, Drug eruption due to atebrine and resembling lichen planus. *Proc. Mayo Clin.*, 21, 404.

KINGSBURY, A. N., 1934, Psychoses in cases of malaria following exhibition of atebrin. *Lancet, ii*, 979.

KLOPPER, S., SLOP, D., and OP'T LAND, C., 1948, Een onderzoek naar de suppressieve werking van paludrine bij malaria tertiana. *Ned. Tijdschr. Geneesk.*, 92, 3922.

KOBERT, R., 1906, "Lehrbuch des Intoxikationen." 2nd Edit., Vol. 2, p. 1126. Stuttgart, F. Enke.

KUTZ, A., and TRAUGOTT, C., 1925, Ueber einen mit Hämatoporphyrurie unter dem Klinischen Bilde des Schwarzwasserfiebers todlich verlaufenden Fall von gleichzeitiger Idiosynkrasie gegen Chinin und veronal. *Münch. med. Wschr.*, 72i, 154.

LEAGUE OF NATIONS, 1937, The treatment of malaria. Study of synthetic drugs, as compared with quinine in the therapeutics and prophylaxis of malaria. Fourth general report of the malaria commission. *Quart. Bull. Hlth Org. L.o.N.*, 6, 895.

LE HEUX, J. W., and DE LIND VAN WIJNGAARDEN, C., 1929, Über die pharmakologische Wirkung des Plasmochins. *Arch. exp. Path. Pharmak.*, 144, 341.

LERRO, S. J., 1941, Report of two cases of toxicity to atabrine. *Mil. Surg.*, 89, 668.

LEVINE, H. D., and ERLANGER, H., 1946, Atabrine and the electrocardiogram. *Amer. J. med. Sci.*, 212, 538.

LEWIS, B. S., 1950, A case of acute quinine poisoning. *J. R. nav. med. Serv.*, 36, 38.

LICCIARDELLO, A. T., and STANBURY, J. B., 1948, Acute hemolytic anemia from quinine used as an abortifacient. *New Engl. J. Med.*, 238, 120.

LIDZ, T., and KAHN, R. L., 1946, Toxicity of quinacrine (atabrine) for the central nervous system. III. An experimental study on human subjects. *Arch. Neurol. Psychiat., Chicago*, 56, 284.

LIPPARD, V. W., and KAUER, G. L., Jr., 1945, Pigmentation of the palate and subungual tissues associated with suppressive quinacrine hydrochloride therapy. *Amer. J. trop. Med.*, 25, 469.

LIVINGOOD, C. S., and DIEUAIDE, F. R., 1945, Untoward reactions attributable to atabrine. *J. Amer. med. Ass.*, 129, 1091.

264   TOXIC REACTIONS TO ANTIMALARIAL DRUGS

LOEB, R. F., 1946, Activity of a new antimalarial agent, pentaquine (SN 13,276). Statement approved by the Board for Coordination of Malarial Studies. *J. Amer. med. Ass.*, **132**, 321.

LOEB, R. F., CLARK, W. M., COATNEY, G. R., COGGESHALL, L. T., DIEUAIDE, F. R., DOCHEZ, A. R., HAKANSSON, E. G., MARSHALL, E. K., Jr., MARVEL, C. S., McCOY, O. R., SAPERO, J. J., SEBRELL, W. H., SHANNON, J. A., and CARDEN, G. A., Jr., 1946, Activity of a new antimalarial agent, chloroquine (SN 7,618). Statement approved by the Board for Coordination of Malarial Studies. *J. Amer. med. Ass.*, **130**, 1069.

LÖKEN, A. C., and HAYMAKER, W., 1949, Pamaquine poisoning in man, with a clinicopathologic study of one case. *Amer. J. trop. Med.*, **29**, 341.

LOEWENTHAL, L. J. A., 1947, Tropical lichenoid dermatitis. *Arch. Derm. Syph.*, *Chicago*, **56**, 868.

LOURDENADIN, S., 1949, Mepacrine psychosis. *Proc. Alumni Ass. King Edw. VII Coll. Med. Singapore*, **2**, 169.

LUCHERINI, T., 1938, Primo casa in Italia di emoglobinuria da atebrin. *Policlinico, sez. prat.*, **45**, 1849.

LUM, L. C., 1946, Fatal hepatitis associated with tropical lichenoid dermatitis. *Med. J. Aust.*, *ii*, 866.

LUTTERLOH, C. H., and SHALLENBERGER, P. L., 1946, Unusual pigmentation developing after prolonged suppressive therapy with quinacrine hydrochloride. *Arch. Derm. Syph.*, *Chicago*, **53**, 349.

LYNCH, P. P., and BRANDT, C. W., 1940, Quinine poisoning. Report of a fatal case. *N.Z. med. J.*, **39**, 191.

McCARRISON, R., and CORNWALL, J. W., 1919, Pharmaco-dynamics of quinine. *Indian J. med. Res.*, **6**, 248.

MacDONALD, D. R., 1947, Fugue after mepacrine administration. *Brit. med. J.*, *ii*, 959.

McFADZEAN, A. J. S., and DAVIS, L. J., 1947, Iron-staining erythrocytic inclusions with especial reference to acquired hæmolytic anæmia. *Glasg. med. J.*, **28**, 237.

McGREGOR, I. S., and LOEWENSTEIN, A., 1944, Quinine blindness. *Lancet*, *ii*, 566.

MAIER, J., 1948, A field trial of chloroquine (SN 7,618) as a suppressive against malaria in the Philippines. *Amer. J. trop. Med.*, **28**, 407.

MAIER, J., BANG, F. B., and HAIRSTON, N. G., 1948, A comparison of the effectiveness of quinacrine and quinine against falciparum malaria. *Amer. J. trop. Med.*, **28**, 401.

MAMOU, H., 1947, Intolérance grave à la quinine. Guérison par transfusions massives. *Rev. Palud.*, **5**, 273.

MANIFOLD, M. C., 1941, The effect of certain antiseptics on the respiration of brain tissues in vitro. *Brit. J. exp. Path.*, **22**, 111.

MANN, I., 1947, " Blue haloes " in atebrin workers. *Brit. J. Ophthal.*, **31**, 40.

MANN, W. N., and SMITH, S., 1943, Hæmoglobinuria following the administration of plasmoquine. *Trans. R. Soc. trop. Med. Hyg.*, **37**, 151.

MARITSCHEK, M., and MARKOWICZ, H., 1933, Ueber einen Fall von Chinenuberempfindlichkeit mit Purpura, vorwiegend der oberen Luft and Speiseweg. *Mschr. Ohrenheilk.*, **67**, 410.

MARKSON, J. L., and DAWSON, J., 1945, Investigations in the chemotherapy of malaria in West Africa. IV. Report on a case of acute mepacrine poisoning. *Ann. trop. Med. Parasit.*, **39**, 117.

MEDICAL CONSULTANTS' DIVISION, (1945) REPORT TO SURGEON-GENERAL'S OFFICE, U.S.A. Evaluation of the untoward reactions attributable to atabrine. *Bull. U.S. Army Med. Dept.*, **4**, 653.

MERGENER, J. C., 1945, Pychosis following administration of quinacrine hydrochloride for malaria. Neuropsychiatric study of a case. *War Med.*, **8**, 250.

MISHRA, K. C., 1947, Delirium after quinine administration. *Antiseptic*, **44**, 614.

MISSIROLI, A., and MARINO, P., 1934, Anwendung des Chinoplasmin zur Malariasanierung. *Arch. Schiffs-u. Tropenhyg.*, **38**, 1.

MITCHELL, J. H., 1945, in discussion on : Duemling, W. W., Cutaneous diseases in the South Pacific. *Arch. Derm. Syph.*, *Chicago*, **52**, 84.

MOE, G. K., and SEEVERS, M. H., 1946, Central impairment of sympathetic reflexes by plasmochin. *Fed. Proc.*, **5**, 193.

MOHANTY, J. K., 1945, Mepacrine intoxication and vitamin B deficiency. *Indian med. Gaz.*, **80**, 459.

MOIR, K. T., 1934, Blackwater fever following atebrin. *W. Afr. med. J.*, **7**, 121.

MOLITOR, H., 1941, Antimalarials other than quinine : in " A symposium on human malaria with special reference to North America and the Caribbean Region," edited by F. R. Moulton. *American Ass. Advancement Science*, Publ. 15, p. 261.

MONK, J. F., 1948, Results of an investigation of the therapeutic action of pentaquin on acute attacks of benign tertian malaria. *Trans. R. Soc. trop. Med. Hyg.*, **41**, 663.

MOSCHINI, S., 1935, Polineurite cerebrospinale acuta motoria, di natura tossica, ad inizio apoplettiforme in una bambina di due anni. *Riv. Clin. Ped.*, **33**, 823.

MOSHER, H. P., 1938, Does animal experimentation show similar changes in the ear of mother and fetus after ingestion of quinine by the mother ? *Laryngoscope*, *St. Louis*, **48**, 361.

MOST, H., LONDON, I. M., KANE, C. A., LAVIETES, P. H., SCHROEDER, E. F., and HAYMAN, J. M., Jr., 1946, Chloroquine for treatment of acute attacks of vivax malaria. *J. Amer. med. Ass.*, **131**, 963.

MÜHLENS, P., and FISCHER, O., 1932, Über Malariabehandlung mit Atebrin. *Arch. Schiffs-u. Tropenhyg.*, **36**, 196.

MURRAY, A. J., 1934, Blackwater fever following atebrin—a fatal case. *W. Afr. med. J.*, **8**, 17.

MUSHETT, C. W., and SIEGEL, H., 1946, Hematological changes following the administration of large doses of quinacrine hydrochloride. *Blood*, **1**, 537.

MYERS, W. K., 1944, Clinical impressions of skin disease in a tropical operational area. *Med. J. Aust.*, **ii**, 10.

NAGELSBACH, E., 1933, Schwarzwasserfieber und Atebrin. *Arch. Schiffs-u. Tropenhyg.*, **37**, 337.

NANDI, D. K., 1947, Toxic symptoms associated with quinacrine treatment. *Indian med. Gaz.*, **82**, 273.

NAUMANN, H. E., 1933, Betrachtungen zum Schwarzwasserfieber. *Arch. Schiffs-u. Tropenhyg.*, **37**, 299.

NAUMANN, H. E., 1934, Schluss zu Betrachtungen zum Schwarzwasserfieber. *Arch. Schiffs-u. Tropenhyg.*, **38**, 171.

NAYADU, R. V. N., 1937, Malaria and its treatment by the synthetic remedies : atebrin and plasmochin. *Indian med. Gaz.*, **72**, 531.

NELSON, A. A., and FITZHUGH, O. G., 1947, Pathological changes produced by feeding of chloroquine (SN 7,618) to rats. *Fed. Proc.*, **6**, 397.

NELSON, A. A., and FITZHUGH, O. G., 1948, Chloroquine (SN 7,618). Pathologic changes observed in rats which had been fed various proportions for two years. *Arch. Path.*, **45**, 454.

NELSON, L. M., 1945, Dermatitis from atabrine. *Bull. U.S. Army med. Dept.*, **4**, 725.

NELSON, L. M., 1947, Unusual dermatoses simulating lichen planus and lichen corneus hypertrophicus. *Arch. Derm. Syph.*, *Chicago*, **55**, 12.

NEWELL, H. W., and LIDZ, T., 1946, The toxicity of atabrine to the central nervous system. *Amer. J. Psychiat.*, **102**, 805.

NICLOUX, M., 1909, Etude d'ensemble sur le passage des substances chimiques de la mére au fœtus mecanisme de ce passage. *Obstétrique*, 2, 840.

NIETO-CAICEDO, M., and GUERRERO, L., 1946, Psicosis toxica por atebrina y metoquina. *Rev. Med. trop. Parasit.*, 12, 76.

NISBET, T. W., 1945, A new cutaneous syndrome occurring in New Guinea and adjacent islands, preliminary report. *Arch. Derm. Syph.*, *Chicago*, 52, 221.

NISTICO, G., 1948, Sopra un caso di psicosi da ingestione di atebrin. *Clin. nuova*, 6, 219.

NOCHT, B., and KIKUTH, W., 1929, Über hämolytische Chininwirkungen. *Arch. Schiffs-u. Tropenhyg.*, 33, 355.

NOCHT, B., and MAYER, M., 1936, " Die Malaria," 2nd Edit. Berlin. Springer.

NOOJIN, R. O., and CALLAWAY, J. L., 1942, Generalised exfoliative erythroderma following atabrine. Report of a case. *N.C. med. J.*, 3, 239.

NOVOSELOVA, E. I., 1948, [Changes in the white cells in treatment of malaria with proguanil.] *Klin. Med. Mosk.*, 27 (i), 76.

NOYAN, A., 1949, Malaria prophylaxis in Turkey. Unpublished Observations.

NUDELMAN, P. L., LEFF, I. L., and HOWE, C. D., 1948, Thrombopenic purpura following quinidine. *J. Amer. med. Ass.*, 137, 1219.

PALADINO-BLANDINI, A., and MARINO-ASSERETO, P., 1934, La chinoplasmina nella profilassi della malaria a Schiavonea (bonifica di Sibari). *Riv. Malariol.*, 13, 161.

PATRONO, V., 1942, Il chinino e l'atebrina quali possibili fattori di ipovitaminosi C nella malaria. *Policlinico, sez. prat.*, 49, 1685.

PELNER, L., and SASKIN, E., 1942, Amaurosis due to quinine. Treatment with sodium nitrite administered intravenously. *J. Amer. med. Ass.*, 119, 1175.

PERK, D., 1947, Mepacrine psychoses. *J. ment. Sci.*, 93, 756.

PESHKIN, M. M., and MILLER, J. A., 1934, Quinine and ergot allergy and thrombocytopenic purpura. *J. Amer. med. Ass.*, 102, 1737.

PETRI, E., 1930, Pathologische Anatomie und Histologie der Vergiftungen. in : Henke, F., und Lubarsch, O., " Handbuch der Speziellen Pathologischen Anatomie und Histologie," Vol. 10, p. 398. Berlin. J. Springer.

PIRK, L. A., and ENGELBERG, R., 1945, Hypoprothrombinemic action of quinine sulfate. *J. Amer. med. Ass.*, 128, 1093.

PONDER, E., and ABELS, J. C., 1936, Effect of quinine hydrochloride on resistance of rabbit red cells. *Proc. Soc. exp. Biol.*, *N.Y.*, 34, 162.

RAVEN, H. M., 1927, Death from quinine poisoning. *Brit. med. J.*, ii, 59.

READ, H. S., KAPLAN, L. I., BECKER, F. T., and BOYD, M. F., 1946, An analysis of complications encountered during therapeutic malaria. *Ann. intern. Med.*, 24, 444.

REED, A. C., 1940, The treatment of malaria. *J. Amer. med. Ass.*, 115, 602.

REESE, F. M., 1946, Edema of the corneal epithelium caused by atabrine. Observations on three patients. *Bull. Johns Hopk. Hosp.*, 78, 325.

RICHARDSON, S., 1936, The toxic effect of quinine on the eye. *Sth. med. J.*, *Nashville*, 29, 1156.

RICHTER, R., 1949, The effect of certain quinoline compounds upon the nervous system of monkeys. *J. Neuropath. exp. Neurol.*, 8, 155.

RIGDON, R. H., 1949, Lethal and electrocardiographic changes produced by quinine dihydrochloride in monkeys infected with *P. knowlesi*. *Fed. Proc.*, 8, 327.

ROPER-HALL, M. J., 1950, Self-inflicted conjunctivitis. *Brit. J. Ophthal.*, 34, 119.

ROSENFELD, M., ZUBROD, C. G., BLAKE, W. D., and SHANNON, J. A., 1948, Methemalbuminaemia. I. Appearance during administration of pamaquine and quinine. *J. clin. Invest.*, 27, Suppl. p. 138.

ROSENTHAL, J., 1946, Atypical lichen planus. *Amer. J. Path.*, 22, 473.

RUSSELL, B., 1947, Mepacrine eruptions : a case in the British Isles. *Lancet, ii,* 205.

RUSSELL, H. K., 1945, Eosinophilia caused by atabrine. *Nav. med. Bull., Wash.,* 44, 574.

SAWYER, G. M., 1933, Quinine amblyopia or retrobulbar neuritis consequent to giving optochin base. *J. Iowa St. med. Soc.,* 23, 25.

SCHECHTER, A. J., and TAYLOR, H. M., 1936, Atabrine pigmentation. *Amer. J. med. Sci.,* 192, 645.

SCHMIDT, I. G., and SCHMIDT, L. H., 1947, Studies on the 8-aminoquinolines. II. The effects of plasmocid on the central nervous system. *Fed. Proc.,* 6, 368.

SCHMIDT, I. G., and SCHMIDT, L. H., 1948, Neurotoxicity of the 8-amino-quinolines. I. Lesions in the central nervous system of the rhesus monkey induced by administration of plasmocid. *J. Neuropath. exp. Neurol.,* 7, 368.

SCHMIDT, L. H., 1948, quoted by EARLE, D. P., Jr., BIGELOW, F. S., ZUBROD, C. G., and KANE, C. A., 1948, Studies on the chemotherapy of the human malarias. IX. Effect of pamaquine on the blood cells of man. *J. clin. Invest.,* 27, Suppl. p. 121.

SCHMIDT, L. H., HUGHES, H. B.and SMITH, C. C., 1947a, On the pharmacology, of N_1-*para*-chlorophenyl-N_5-*iso*propyl-biguanidine (paludrine). *J. Pharmacol.,* 90, 233.

SCHMIDT, L. H., HUGHES, H. B., and SMITH, C. C., 1947b, On the pharmacology of paludrine, *Fed. Proc.,* 6, 368.

SCHMIDT, L. H., SMITH, C. C., HUGHES, H. B., and CARTER, C., 1947c, Studies on the 8-aminoquinolines. I. The toxicity of pamaquin and plasmocid in different animal species. *Fed. Proc.,* 6, 369.

SCHMITT, C. L., 1949, Present status of quinacrine (atabrine) dermatitis : report of six cases. *Arch. Derm. Syph., Chicago,* 59, 16.

SCHMITT, C. L., ALPINS, O., and CHAMBERS, G., 1945, Clinical investigation of new cutaneous entity. *Arch. Derm. Syph., Chicago,* 52, 226.

SCHULEMANN, W., 1935, The new synthetic drugs. *Indian med. Gaz.,* 70, 83.

SCOLTERN, A. H., 1946, New Guinea lichen planus. *J. Maine med. Ass.,* 37, 96.

SCUDI, J. V., and HAMLIN, M. T., 1944, Biochemical aspects of the toxicity of atabrine. II. The influence of the diet upon the effects produced by repeated doses of the drug. *J. Pharmacol.,* 80, 150.

SEITZ, L., 1927, Die Schwangerschaftshämolyse, Schwangerschafshämoglobinämie und hämoglobinurie. In : Halban, J., and Seitz, L., "Handbuch der Pathologie des Weibes," Vol. 7i, p. 815. Berlin und Wien, Urban und Schwarzenberg.

SENEAR, F. E., CARO, M. R., and STUBENRAUCH, C. H., 1945, Lichen planus in husband and wife. *Arch. Derm. Syph., Chicago,* 51, 353.

SHEARER, G., 1949, Second thoughts on proguanil. *Brit. med. J., i,* 775.

SHEPPECK, M. L., and WEXBERG, L. E., 1946, Toxic psychoses associated with administration of quinacrine. *Arch. Neurol. Psychiat., Chicago,* 55, 489.

SHIERS, D., 1946, Cerebral excitement following mepacrine therapy. *Brit. med. J., i,* 762.

SIEGEL, H., and MUSHETT, C. W., 1944, Structural changes following administration of quinacrine hydrochloride. *Arch. Path.,* 38, 63.

SIEGENBEEK VAN HEUKELOM, A., and OVERBEEK, J. G., 1936, Behandeling van de acute malaria—aanval met atebrine pro injectione. *Geneesk. Tijdschr. Ned.-Ind.,* 76, 2507.

SIEGENBEEK VAN HEUKELOM, A., and WAHAB, —, 1941, Thrombopenische purpura door idiosyncrasie voor kinine. *Geneesk. Tijdschr. Ned.-Ind.,* 81, 906.

SILVA, S. DE, 1935, Observations on some interesting cases occurring during the malaria epidemic in Ceylon. *J. trop Med. Hyg.,* 38, 66.

268 TOXIC REACTIONS TO ANTIMALARIAL DRUGS

SIMEONS, A. T. W., 1936, Mass treatment with injectable atebrin. *Indian med. Gaz.*, **71**, 132.
SINGH, I., 1948, Mepacrine dermatitis. *Brit. J. Derm. Syph.*, **60**, 90.
SMITH, C. C., and SCHMIDT, L. H., 1947, Studies on the 8-aminoquinolines. III. On the relations between structure and pharmacological activities. *Fed. Proc.*, **6**, 372.
SMITH, E. C. T., 1934, Quinine amblyopia. *Med. J. Aust.*, *ii*, 289.
SMITH, P. K., 1943, Atabrine and anoxia tolerance. A.A.F. School of Aviation Medicine Project 112, Rept. 1.
SOMERVILLE-LARGE, L. B., 1947, Mepacrin and the eye. *Brit. J. Ophth.*, **31**, 191.
SONI, R. L., 1935, A note on yellow discoloration in atebrine therapy. *Indian med. Gaz.*, **70**, 211.
SPICKNALL, C. G., and TERRY, L. L., 1948, Combined quinine-plasmochin and quinine-pentaquine treatment of relapsing vivax Malaria. *Sth. med. J., Nashville*, **41**, 338.
SPINKS, A., 1947, Studies on synthetic animal drugs. XVIII. The absorption, distribution and excretion of paludrine in experimental animals. *Ann. trop. Med. Parasit.*, **41**, 30.
STEPHENS, J. W. W., 1937, " Blackwater fever : a historical survey and summary of observations made over a century." Liverpool : University Press. London : Hodder & Stoughton.
STOREY, W. E., 1938, Toxic exanthemata following prolonged atabrine administration and resembling Brill's typhus fever. Report of case. *J. med. Ass. Ga.*, **27**, 317.
STRAHAN, J. H., 1948, Quinine by continuous intravenous drip in the treatment of acute falciparum malaria. *Trans. R. Soc. trop. Med. Hyg.*, **41**, 669.
STRAUS, B., and GENNIS, J., 1948, Evaluation of pentaquine as a cure of relapsing vivax malaria : a controlled study of ninety-five cases. *Bull. N.Y. Acad. Med.*, **24**, 395.
SWAB, C. M., 1932, Amblyopia from ethylhydrocupreine. *Arch. Ophthal., Chicago*, **7**, 285.
TAGGART, J. V., EARLE, D. P., Jr., BERLINER, R. W., ZUBROD, C. G., WELCH, W. J., WISE, N. B., SCHROEDER, E. F., LONDON, I. M., and SHANNON, J. A., 1948, Studies on the chemotherapy of the human malarias. III. The physiological disposition and antimalarial activity of the cinchona alkaloids. *J. clin. Invest.*, **27**, Suppl. p. 80.
TATE, P., and VINCENT, M., 1934, The action of atebrin on bird malaria. *Parasitology*, **26**, 523.
TAYLOR, H. M., 1934, Prenatal medication as a possible etiologic factor of deafness in the newborn. *Arch. Otolaryng., Chicago*, **20**, 790.
TAYLOR, H. M., 1935, Further observations on prenatal medication as possible etiologic factor of deafness in newborn. *Sth. med. J., Nashville*, **28**, 125.
TERPLAN, K. L., and JAVERT, C. T., 1936, Fatal hemoglobinuria with uremia from quinine in early pregnancy. *J. Amer. Med. Ass.*, **106**, 529.
THIODET — and FABREGOULE —, 1949, Hématurie au cours d'accès palustres traités par la chloriquane. *Bull. Mém. Soc. med. Hôp. Paris*, **65**, 1082.
TURNER, C. C., 1936, Neurologic and psychiatric manifestations of malaria. *Sth. med. J., Nashville*, **29**, 578.
UDALAGAMA, L., 1935, Mental derangement in malaria cases treated by atebrin-musonate injections. *Indian med. Gaz.*, **70**, 679.
VALENTINI, P., 1937, A proposito di una grave sindrome mieloradicolneuritica insorta nel corso di terapia atebrinica. *Pediatria*, **45**, 51.
VAN BREUSEGHEM, R., 1949, Sensibilisation à la quinine et à d'autres medicaments. *Ann. Soc. belge Méd. trop.*, **29**, 247.
VANE, J. R., 1949, Some pharmacological actions of paludrine, *Brit. J. Pharmacol.*, **4**, 14.

VANE, J. R., WALKER, J. M., and WYNN PARRY, C. B., 1948, The effect of paludrine on gastric secretion in man. *Brit. J. Pharmacol.*, 3, 350.

VAN LIERE, E. J., and EMERSON, G. A., 1942, The influence of certain anti-malarials and related agents on lethal effects of anoxia. *J. aviat. Med.*, 13, 182.

VAN SLYPE, W., 1936, Atébrine injectable et paludisme aigu. *Ann. Soc. belge Méd. trop.*, 16, 429.

VARDY, E. C., 1935, Notes on a clinical investigation of the treatment of malaria by atebrin musonate injections. *Malaya med. J.*, 10, 67.

VARTAN, C. K., and DISCOMBE, G., 1940, Death from quinine poisoning. *Brit. med. J.*, i, 525.

VOLLMER, H., and LIEBIG, H., 1944, Nebenwirkungen des Atebrins am Zentralnervensystem. *Dtsch. med. Wschr.*, 70, 415.

WAELSCH, H., and NACHMANSOHN, D., 1943, On the toxicity of atabrine. *Proc. Soc. exp. Biol., N.Y.*, 54, 331.

WAKEMAN, A. M., MORRELL, C. A., EISEMAN, A. J., SPRINT, D. L., and PETERS, J. P., 1932, Metabolism and treatment of blackwater fever. *Amer. J. trop. Med.*, 12, 407.

WALLACE, H. J., 1947, Tropical lichenoid dermatitis. *Proc. R. Soc. Med.*, 40, 502.

WEISE, W., 1941, Über das Pseudo-Methämoglobin (Methæmalbumin) N. H. Fairley's. *Dtsch. Tropenmed. Z.*, 45, 218.

WELCH, W. J., BAUMAN, E., KNOWLTON, P., and BERLINER, R. W., 1948, Syphilis of the central nervous system. Effect of quinacrine hydro-chloride on the incidence of convulsions. *Arch. Derm. Syph., Chicago*, 57, 868.

WERZ, J. F. C., 1949, Een onderzoek naar aanleiding van het tijdelijk veel vuldig voorkomen van contact dermatitis bij arbeiders in kininefabrieken. *Ned. Tijdschr. Geneesk.*, 93, 170.

WEST, J. B., and HENDERSON, A. B., 1944, Plasmochin intoxication. *Bull. U.S. Army med. Dept.*, No. 82, p. 87.

WHITEHILL, R., 1945, Skin sensitivity to atabrine. *Bull. U.S. Army med. Dept.*, 4, 724.

WILKINSON, P. B., 1939, Mental disturbance after the exhibition of atebrin. *Caduceus*, 18, 267.

WILLIAMS, W., 1947, Tropical lichen planus syndrome. *Brit. med. J.*, ii, 901.

WILLIAMSON, A., HEGSTED, D. M., McKIBBEN, J. M., and STARE, F. J., 1946, Effect of variations in level of dietary calcium upon growth of young rats receiving atabrine. *J. Nutrit.*, 31, 647.

WILSON, D. J., 1946, Eczematous and pigmentary lichenoid dermatitis, atypical lichen planus. Preliminary Report. *Arch. Derm. Syph., Chicago*, 54, 377.

WINCKEL, C. W. F., 1948, Quinine and congenital injuries of ear and eye in the fœtus. *J. trop. Med. Hyg.*, 51, 2.

WISELOGLE, F. Y., edited by, 1946, "A Survey of Antimalarial Drugs," 1941–45. 2 vols. Ann Arbor, Michigan, J. W. Edwards.

WRIGHT, C. I., and LILLIE, R. D., 1943, Toxic effects of atabrine and sulfa-diazine in growing rats. *Publ. Hlth. Rep., Wash.*, 58, 1242.

ZUBROD, C. G., KNOWLTON, P., WELCH, W. J., BERLINER, R. W., TAGGART, J. V., EARLE, D. P., Jr., and SHANNON, J. A., 1946, Pamaquin: 4. Occurrence of leucopenia. *Fed. Proc.*, 5, 217.

CHAPTER VII

THE CHEMOTHERAPEUTIC TREATMENT OF PLASMODIAL INFECTIONS

I⊤ is now recognised that a number of chemical compounds with very differing constitutions are capable of acting on malarial parasites. It has also become apparent that the same drug does not necessarily act on all species of malarial parasites to the same degree or even in the same way : this difference applies not only to avian and simian plasmodia but also to the four species of plasmodium responsible for producing malaria in man. In addition to interspecific differences in reaction to antimalarial drugs there are also intraspecific differences between certain strains of the same species of plasmodium. These strain differences are probably of as great or even greater importance than the interspecific differences. Finally, the developmental stages of the same species react differently to chemotherapeutic drugs. Those patients who have already acquired some degree of immunity require smaller doses to terminate a clinical attack than those who are not immune. Before discussing in detail the treatment of the human malarias it is proposed to describe the action of the various antimalarial chemotherapeutic drugs on the plasmodia of birds, animals, and man. These drugs include the cinchona alkaloids, mepacrine, pamaquin, chloroquine, proguanil, and the sulphonamides.

The Chemotherapeutic Action of Cinchona Alkaloids

Shortly after the first importation of cinchona bark from South America to Rome in the seventeenth century, it became apparent that if good therapeutic results were to be obtained certain rules of treatment must be observed. Instructions for using the new drug were therefore issued as a broadsheet in 1649 under the ægis of the Society of Jesus by Pietro Paolo Puccerini, apothecary of the Collegio Romano. The information contained in this " Schedula Romana," republished by Sturm in 1659, seems to have been based very largely on the results obtained by the Spaniard Fonseca, physician to Pope Innocent X. One of the first patients to be treated in accordance with the Schedula was the Archduke Leopold of Austria ; although he was cured of his double quartan fever he relapsed one month later. Thereupon his physician, Jean Jacques Chifflet (Chiffletio, 1653) began that bitter and wordy polemic on the merits of cinchona which lasted for nearly two hundred years. As there was then no accurate method of diagnosing which fevers were malarial and which were not, cinchona bark was given indiscriminately to all patients who were febrile. Those who were suffering from malaria were cured, at any rate temporarily ; those who were suffering from typhoid, typhus, pneumonia, erysipelas, yellow fever or relapsing fever were presumably unaffected.

It was in fact only in 1712 that Torti suggested that the bark was specific solely in agues ; by his insistence on the therapeutic test he did much to undermine the then universally held doctrine that all fevers are due to one and the same cause ; this is an early example of the effects of chemotherapeutic investigation on general medical theory. During the seventeenth century, at any rate in Protestant countries, cinchona was, in addition, regarded with suspicion on political grounds as being the Jesuits' bark ; there were not wanting those who were convinced that the bark was being used as an active and deadly poison. The great merit of the English empiric Sir Robert Talbor (Tabor, or finally Talbot) (1672, 1682) was that when others feared he was not afraid to give the bark in large and repeated doses ; for more than one hundred years no one seems to have realised the value of his contribution (Baker, 1785) ; the majority of physicians who prescribed the bark were content to follow Thomas Sydenham, who wrote in a letter in 1677 : " I am sure that an ounce of bark, given between the two fits, cures." Sir Thomas Browne, however, in a letter to a medical student, Henry Power, was greatly concerned over the right use and dosage of Peruvian bark (Keynes, 1946), but it was not till 1768 that Lind demonstrated quite clearly that to obtain the best results the bark must be given in full doses as soon as the disease is diagnosed.

It is now agreed that though quinine may have a slight action on the gametocytes of *P. vivax* and *P. malariæ* (League of Nations, 1933) yet its action is very slow (Parrot *et al.*, 1937) : it is without action on the sexual forms of *P. falciparum* (League of Nations, 1937) and its main action and that of the other cinchona alkaloids is on the young asexual erythrocytic forms, not only of human malaria but of animals and birds. The only exception to this general rule is in the case of *P. rouxi*, which can be radically cured in canaries not only by mepacrine and pamaquin but by quinine as well (Manwell, 1932, 1933, 1934) : presumably these drugs act also on the exo-erythrocytic forms of *P. rouxi*. A clear demonstration that the effects of quinine are restricted to the asexual erythrocytic forms of *P. gallinaceum* is given by the fact that while the parasites can be removed from the blood of chickens by quinine nevertheless the bird will die because the exo-erythrocytic forms distend the cells lining the brain capillaries : the life of the hen can be saved only by sulphonamides, which destroy the exo-erythrocytic forms (Lobato Paraense, 1947). The crucial experiments on man which showed that quinine does not attack sporozoites were recorded in 1943 by Shannon.

The experience in the treatment of malaria of such seventeenth-century physicians as Willis (1659), who found that cinchona bark could cure the acute attack but would not prevent relapses, was fully confirmed during the war of 1914–18, when quinine was given in all practicable and many impracticable doses. It was, however, shown by Yorke and Macfie (1924) that when malaria was transmitted from one person to another by an injection of blood it could be entirely eradicated by quinine, whereas when it was transmitted by the bite of an anopheline mosquito the infection could not be eradicated by quinine. As James (1931) pointed out, this could only mean that when a man was bitten by a mosquito a tissue-inhabiting form of the parasite was injected and this form was not affected by quinine. More recent observations, such as those of Berliner *et al.* (1946), have shown that the cinchona alkaloids have no action on schizonts or exo-erythrocytic forms of human malarial parasites ; their action is limited to the asexual erythrocytic forms.

Some strains of *Plasmodium vivax* are, however, more resistant to quinine than others, and with Italian strains greater concentrations of quinine are necessary than with Indian strains (League of Nations, 1937). This is clearly brought out by results given by James *et al.* (1932) and Shute (1946), from which it is seen that Italian and Sardinian strains require much more quinine than those from India, Africa and Roumania :—

THE AMOUNT OF QUININE REQUIRED TO CONTROL ATTACKS OF VIVAX MALARIA (Shute, 1946)

Origin of strain.	Total quinine in gm. during a primary attack.	Total quinine in gm. during the whole course.	Average amount in gm. per case in primary attack.	Average amount in gm. during whole course.
Roman and Sardinian (13 cases) . .	282·4	1,423·1	21·8	109·2
Other strains (2 Indian, 2 West African, 2 Roumanian and 1 Tanganyikan) (19 cases) . .	50·2	145·1	2·6	7·6

Gordon *et al.* (1947) found little difference in reaction to quinine of Mediterranean and Pacific strains. Zubrod *et al.* (1946) noted that more quinine was necessary to control the Chesson strain than the McCoy strain of *P. vivax.* James (1932) believed that the biological susceptibility of a parasite to the action of drugs is more important than its morphology. Two Roman strains were highly resistant (James *et al.*, 1932), as is the Costa strain of *P. falciparum* (Shannon, 1949).

In addition to the strain differences, in some persons quinine salts are not readily adsorbed from the intestinal tract. Taggart *et al.* (1946) showed that after an oral dose of 300 mgm. of quinine in thirty subjects the plasma levels of quinine varied from 2 to 8·9 mgm. per litre. Chopra *et al.* (1937) reported that this difference is due to defective intestinal absorption. It is perhaps rather more than a coincidence that it was in the war of 1914–18 that cases of non-absorption of liquid quinine first became common : they were also seen in the war of 1939–45 (Howie and Murray-Lyon, 1943) among persons who had particular reasons for not wishing to recover from malaria. Non-absorption must be carefully distinguished from failure to swallow a drug.

The insolubility of certain quinine sulphate tablets in the intestinal tract has of course long been recognised.

There is considerable evidence to show that once a dose of quinine sufficient to remove parasites from the blood stream has been administered, further increase in the oral dose does not increase the therapeutic action (Knoppers, 1948). With the St. Elizabeth strain of vivax malaria Coatney et al. (1948) showed that 2 gm. a day of quinine sulphate does not give better results than 1 gm. a day for six days.

With a blood-induced infection of the McCoy strain of vivax malaria a sustained quinine concentration of 2 mgm. per litre produces an uncertain effect : consistent fall in the temperature within twenty-four hours, and of the parasitæmia to the extent of 50 per cent., can be attained only by a plasma concentration of 3·0 to 4·0 mgm. per litre. A complete interruption of the asexual cycle, what Shannon (1946) terms a Class III effect, is attained by a concentration of 6 mgm. per litre, parasites then being absent from the blood stream for more than fourteen days. The critical level for Class III effects is between 4 and 5 mgm. per litre (Berliner et al., 1946).

Correlations between the oral dose and the therapeutic effect of quinine are poor, but the daily administration of 0·82 gm. of quinine, as quinine sulphate, will give a plasma concentration of 5 to 9 mgm. per litre. The erythrocytic phase of vivax malaria is equally susceptible to quinine whether the parasites are derived from a mosquito-induced or a blood-induced infection.

The relative values of the other cinchona alkaloids for the control of the erythrocytic phases of human malaria parasites as compared with quinine have received considerable attention since the Report of the Madras Cinchona Commission (India) in 1868.

Fletcher (1923) and other early observers were essentially correct in concluding that each of the three other cinchona alkaloids has an antimalarial activity of a suppressive type which compares well with that possessed by quinine : however, the critical plasma concentration of each alkaloid required to produce a Class III effect varies (Shannon, 1946 ; Zubrod et al., 1946 ; Taggart et al., 1948).

PLASMA LEVELS OF CINCHONA ALKALOIDS NECESSARY TO PRODUCE
A CLASS III EFFECT ON BLOOD-INDUCED *P. vivax* INFECTIONS
(McCOY STRAIN). (Shannon, 1946 ; Taggart *et al.*, 1948)

	Plasma concentrations (mgm. per litre).			
	Quinine.	Quinidine.	Cinchonine.	Cinchonidine.
Minimum plasma concentration to produce a Class III effect.	5·0	1·0	less than 0·1	2·5
Concentration obtained by a serial daily dose of 1 gm. .	5·6	(4·6)	0·2	2·4
Ratio of plasma concentration to a Class III effect . .	1·1	(4·6)	2·0	0·8

The quinine equivalent of the three other cinchona alkaloids,
based on total oral dosage against blood-induced *P. vivax* (McCoy
strain), are recorded by Taggart *et al.* (1948) as follows :—

Alkaloid.	Quinine equivalent.
Quinine	1·0
Cinchonidine	0·5
Quinidine	2·0
Cinchonine	0·5

These figures are obviously of considerable significance in relation to the widespread use of totaquina.

From what has been said it will be obvious that if the therapeutic effects of an excessive dose of quinine sulphate such as 2 gm.
daily is compared with the same dose of cinchonine or cinchonidine
there will be little or no difference, but if a minimal dose of quinine
sulphate such as 0·75 gm. of quinine sulphate is compared with
0·75 gm. of either cinchonine or cinchonidine then the last two
will be seen to be therapeutically inferior.

With all the cinchona alkaloids, however, the combined rates
of metabolism and excretion are such that dosage every six hours
is necessary to assure the maintenance of the effective plasma drug
levels. Thus the cinchona alkaloids are at a considerable disadvan-

tage for suppressive purposes when compared with some of the newer synthetic antimalarial drugs which require to be administered only at weekly intervals.

Although in man no obvious sex differences have been noted in the effectiveness of quinine in malarial infections, yet in chickens infected with *P. gallinaceum* Bennison and Coatney (1948) have found that quinine is less effective in reducing the parasitæmia in female than in male chicks.

The lowest oral doses required to produce a Class III effect on blood-induced *P. vivax* (McCoy strain) and *P. falciparum* (McLendon strain) and the corresponding plasma concentrations (Wiselogle, 1946) are as follows :—

	Alkaloid.							
	Quinine.		Cinchonidine.		Quinidine.		Cinchonine.	
	P. falciparum.	*P. vivax.*	*P. falciparum.*	*P. vivax.*	*P. falciparum.*	*P. vivax.*	*P. falciparum.*	*P. vivax.*
Total oral dose in gm.	3·6–4·0	0·95–1·2	2·4	1·7	1·1	0·4	9·0	3·0
Mean plasma concentration (mgm. per litre)	4·5–8·1	4·1–5·1	3·6	1·5	1·1	0·9	0·50	0·10

It will be seen that whereas the oral dosage for all the cinchona alkaloids is of the same order, except in the case of quinidine, the mean plasma concentration varies considerably. Higher concentrations in the plasma are required to control *P. falciparum* than *P. vivax* in the blood. This confirms older observations, such as those of James (1931), that falciparum infections are less readily controlled than those due to *P. vivax*. The McLendon strain in particular is very resistant to cinchonine (Taggart *et al.*, 1948). An entirely different set of values was obtained by Marshall (1945), who correlated antimalarial activity against *P. gallinaceum* in the chick with the rate of absorption and red cell concentration. The results, shown in the table on p. 277, demonstrate that in three optically active pairs of alkaloids the D-isomers all showed higher antimalarial activity than the L-isomers, together with a greater rate of absorption and higher concentrations within the red cells.

ANTIMALARIAL ACTIVITY AND METABOLISM OF
CINCHONA COMPOUNDS (Marshall, 1945)

Alkaloid.	Antimalarial activity (quinine equivalent).	Percentage of alkaloid absorbed from the gut after two hours.	Conc. alkaloid in red cells (area of conc. time graph.).	μgm. Alkaloid destroyed by 0·5 gm. chick liver in two hours.
Quinine (L)	1·0	62	150	77
Quinidine (D)	1·6	92	422	35
Cinchonidine (L)	1·5	40	291	2
Cinchonine (D)	1·9	80	327	0
Niquine (L)	0·3	75	5	38
Niquidine (D)	1·7	57	285	46
Dihydroquinine (L)	2·0	73	68	28
Dihydroquinidine (D)	1·6	50	723	34

Saturation of the double bond in quinine doubles the activity against *P. gallinaceum*, but dihydroquinidine shows no greater activity than niquidine.

The order of effectiveness of the various cinchona alkaloids for bird malarias varies very considerably.

For *P. relictum* the order is quinine = quinidine > cinchonidine > cinchonine.

P. gallinaceum the order is cinchonine > quinidine > cinchonidine > quinine.

P. lophuræ the order is quinine = quinidine = cinchonidine > cinchonine.

Earlier reports suggested that quinine had very little effect on *P. knowlesi* in monkeys. Row *et al.* (1933) found that a dose of 2·5 gr. (0·16 gm.) of quinine checked the blood infection, but a recrudescence occurred which was fatal unless further treatment was given. Chopra *et al.* (1935) were unable to save monkeys with high doses of quinine once the number of parasites had reached one million per c.mm. Nauck (1934) believed that *P. knowlesi* was more refractory to quinine than the human species of plasmodia. In all these experiments the method of drug administration varied as did the time in relation to infection at which treatment was begun. Using a standardised infection of fifty million parasites per kgm. of body weight given intravenously, Richardson *et al.* (1946) showed that a dose of 37·25 mgm. per kgm.

a day for five days produced a variable but significant effect, whereas 75 mgm. per kgm. per day exerted a distinct antimalarial effect in all animals. Daily doses of 150 mgm. per kgm. for five days had a profound effect with survival of all animals for an indefinite time, though a few parasites were still seen in the peripheral blood. Quinine also controls blood infections with *P. cynomolgi* but does not act as a causal prophylactic or bring about a radical cure (Genther *et al.*, 1948 ; Schmidt *et al.*, 1948).

Quinine in blood-induced infections in mice with *P. berghei* has a chemotherapeutic index of 1 in 4 (Schneider *et al.*, 1949).

There are few drugs with which quinine and the other cinchona alkaloids are incompatible. According to Harned and Cole (1942), quinine given to rats at the same time as sulphapyridine increases the amount of the latter drug which is excreted in the acetyl form. Mepacrine in association with sulphapyridine, sulphadiazine or sulphathiazole does not exert a similar action (Bercovitz, 1945).

The action of quinine on saurian parasites, *P. floridense* and *P. mexicanum*, resembles qualitatively the action on avian plasmodia (Thompson, 1946a).

Routes of Administration

Quinine is given by mouth, intravenously or intramuscularly. Even the most enthusiastic advocates of quinine have, however, ceased to claim that a waistcoat padded with cinchona bark was an invaluable remedy (MacBride, 1777). If intramuscular injections are the only available means then, as Winckel (1947) recommends, the relatively soluble quinine hydrochloride rather than the irritating bihydrochloride should be used. Doses of 0·25 or 0·5 gm. can be added to 1 ml. of distilled water to which, to deaden pain, 0·125 gm. of phenazone or 0·25 gm. of urethane is added. The *p*H of these solutions can be raised to 7·2 by the addition of a little quinine base, a method used in the preparation of the German compound " solvochin." For intramuscular injection the solution should be diluted three times with sterile distilled water or physiological saline and for intravenous use ten times ; not more than 0·5 gm. of the quinine salt should be given at one time. Injections, if into a vein, must be given slowly over a period of ten minutes. The depressing effects of quinine on the circulation can be neutralised by the injection of adrenaline or neosynephrine. Calcium chloride also is said to have some effect, as has aneurin (Dreisbach and Hanzlik, 1945) : atropine is of no value. Dreisbach (1949) found that adrenaline was the only drug which would prevent the blood pressure-lowering effect of quinine in cats suffering from hæmorrhage or hyperthermia. For a man of 70 kgm. who has received 10 mgm. of quinine per kgm. of body weight a dose of 1·4 mgm. of epinephrine or 3·5 mgm. of neosynephrine should be given intravenously. As a rule, the seat of the vasodilation is in the peripheral blood vessels, but in severe generalised collapse there is also a toxic action on the myocardium (Dreisbach and Hanzlik, 1945).

One serious drawback to the use of quinine, and possibly to the other cinchona alkaloids in the control of infections caused by *P. falciparum*, lies in the danger of precipitating an attack of blackwater fever. The suggestion that quinine is responsible for the occurrence of hæmoglobinuria in persons infected with some strains of *P. falciparum* was first put forward by Dutroulau (1868). Since then almost all who have studied blackwater fever have been struck by the relation between the administration of quinine and the onset of blackwater fever.

It was not, however, until the war years that by the use of mepacrine it was possible to abandon quinine both in suppression and in treatment of falciparum malaria. When quinine salts were thus abandoned in West Africa in 1943 the incidence of blackwater fever among European troops fell in a most striking manner (Findlay and Stevenson, 1944 ; Findlay, 1949).

The only circumstances under which quinine salts may be legitimately given to persons suffering from *P. falciparum* infections are in cerebral malaria, intractable vomiting when nothing can be given by mouth, hyperpyrexia, and where there is a marked idiosyncrasy to mepacrine, proguanil and chloroquine.

Blood-induced infections due to *P. malariæ* resemble *P. falciparum* in that they are less readily controlled by quinine than those due to *P. vivax* (James, 1931). Winckel (1949) believes that there is no advantage from giving large doses of quinine for infections due to *P. malariæ:* 1 gm. a day is ample.

Treatment by Intravenous Injections of Quinine. In view of the known effects of quinine on the blood pressure and myocardium many workers have given the drug in high dilution in normal saline or glucose saline in the treatment of cerebral malaria or hyperinfection with *P. falciparum* (James, 1913 ; Wright, 1915 ; Thomas and Sydenstricker, 1938 ; Simpson and Sagebiel, 1943 ; FitzHugh *et al.*, 1944). These workers used doses of from 0·32 to 2·0 gm. in 250 to 500 ml. or more given very slowly, and in some cases repeated at intervals of six to eight hours until pernicious symptoms had disappeared and oral therapy could be begun. Lindsay (1943) advocated 0·9 gm. per litre of normal saline in algid cases. The Surgeon-General of the U.S. Army (1943) recommended 0·66 gm. in 300 to 400 ml. saline, repeated if necessary after six to eight hours : for vomiting a continuous drip of dextrose with aneurin added is suggested. Hanzlik and Cutting (1945), after clinical trials with quinine and adrenaline, obtained the best results with 0·5 gm. quinine and 1 mgm. adrenaline in 250 ml. isotonic sodium chloride injected in not less than thirty minutes with not more than two or three injections properly spaced in the twenty-four hours. There is a general belief that the fall in blood pressure due to quinine is less with dilute infusions (Bramachari, 1922), although this belief is not supported (McCarrison and Cornwall, 1919). Intravenous quinine medication was begun in 1831 by Adami (Premuda, 1947).

The use of the continuous intravenous drip method of injecting quinine was employed in West Africa by Don and Meyer (1944), who treated a patient, who after three days had passed into coma, with 35 per cent. of red cells infected by *P. falciparum:* after twenty-four hours on a continuous drip containing 2·0 gm. of quinine the patient recovered despite an attack of blackwater fever. Repeated small injections of 0·5 to 0·8 gm. were given every two to three hours by Perrine (1826) until the symptoms, as judged by the pulse and skin, were subdued. Craig (1909) recommended 0·3 to 0·6 gm. every four to six hours. Beckman and Smith (1944), in avian malarias, preferred a similar regime. Kahn (1945) apparently employed the same method in an Indian hospital during the war. Bratton (1945) also devised a continuous method of drug administration for testing chemotherapeutic drugs against *P. lophurœ* infections in ducks. Marshall (1949) finds quinine three or four times as effective in a single daily dose as when given continuously in lophuræ but not in cynomolgi infections. The most extensive series of human cases is that reported by Strahan (1948), who treated by continuous intravenous drip fifteen patients with heavy *falciparum* infection : all the patients were prisoners of war and all were extremely badly nourished. Patients with counts of from 800,000 to 1,240,000 parasites per c.mm. are reported to have been cured by this method.

The solution used for injection contained 0·06 gm. of quinine bihydrochloride in 2 ml. of sterile saline ; the rate of injection was 2 ml. per minute and the usual dose given at one injection was 0·5 to 0·66 gm. A total dose of 2 gm. was given in twenty-four hours.

The dangers of this method are sudden collapse, mild phlebitis from irritation when the cannula is left *in situ* for two to three days, and the risk of severe septic phlebitis.

Metabolic Derivatives of Quinine

The antimalarial activity of the metabolic products of the cinchona alkaloids is not without interest. The lævorotatory 2′-hydroxy-6′-methoxy-3-vinylruban-9-ol was thought by Marshall (1945) to be inactive against *P. gallinaceum*, but Kelsey *et al.* (1946) showed that this quinine metabolite was capable of suppressive action in fowls if given intravenously in daily doses of 40 to 70 mgm. per kgm. a day, the antiplasmodial effect being equivalent to that of 15 mgm. per kgm. of quinine ; it thus showed one-third to one-fifth the activity of quinine. When the same compound is added to the diet of ducks infected with *P. lophuræ* a definite suppressive action was observable though the activity is only one-twentieth that of quinine. The degradation product is, however, less toxic than quinine. Marshall and Rogers (1948) have shown that the reduction of antimalarial action is not due to decreased absorption. The respiration of chicken red cells parasitised with *P. gallinaceum* is suppressed as effectively as with quinine, but the metabolic product is far less active in inhibiting aerobic and anaerobic glycolysis. This suggests that the metabolic products of other quinoline compounds with substitution in the 2-position might interfere with respiration of the parasites.

2'-Hydroxy-quinine has only one-twentieth and one-quarter the activity of quinine against *P. lophuræ* and *P. gallinaceum* in chicks (Kelsey *et al.*, 1946). Thus it is improbable that the antimalarial activity of quinine is due to conversion into 2'-hydroxy-quinine. 2'-Hydroxy-cinchonine has been shown by Welch *et al.* (1946) to have some action in suppressing blood-induced vivax malaria (McCoy strain). Its quinine equivalent based on total oral dosage is 0·1, and a Class III effect in vivax infections in man is obtained with an oral daily dose of 3 gm. in contrast to 1 gm. of cinchonine (Earle *et al.*, 1948b).

Other Cinchona Alkaloids

In the treatment of acute attacks of vivax malaria cinchonine, cinchonidine, and quinidine have been carefully compared with quinine. MacGilchrist (1915) concluded that judging by the minimum therapeutic doses, quinine, cinchonine, and quinidine sulphates were for all practical purposes of equal value ; cinchonine if anything was slightly the best and quinidine slightly the worst.

Cinchonine. The use of cinchonine was first suggested by Chomel (1821) and Bally (1826). Pepper, in 1853, also wrote on the possibilities of replacing quinine by cinchonine. Since then a number of observers have shown that cinchonine is effective in vivax malaria (Silvestri, 1921 ; Bini, 1921 ; Amantea, 1922 ; Filipella, 1923 ; Baqué *et al.*, 1925 ; Ciuca *et al.*, 1925). Fletcher (1925), in Malaya, found that in doses of 0·1 gm. per kgm. of body weight cinchonine was less effective than this dose of quinine in reducing fever and overcoming parasitæmia : in doses of 0·1 gm. per lb. of body weight cinchonine was as effective as quinine. Ciuca *et al.* (1925) also regarded cinchonine as less effective than quinine. In falciparum infections Cordes (1924) found 0·5 gm. cinchonine hydrochloride per day for three days less efficient than 0·2 gm. quinine hydrochloride.

Quinidine. Somewhat variable results have been obtained with quinidine. The Special Report of the Medical Research Council (1925) failed to show that quinidine was more effective in vivax infections than quinine. Fletcher (1925) believed that quinidine was as good as, or even slightly better than, quinine bisulphate. Kligler *et al.* (1924) also found quinidine as effective as quinine both in adults and children. Ascoli (1926) believed that quinidine was more effective than quinine in falciparum infections, 0·5 to 0·66 gm. of quinidine being equal to 1·0 gm. of quinine. The effective plasma concentration for clinical suppression of strains of *P. vivax* is 1·0 mgm. per litre, a concentration obtained by the daily dose of 0·25 gm. of the base (Taggart *et al.*, 1948). Sanders and Dawson (1932) and Sanders (1935) obtained good results with a short course of quinidine.

Cinchonidine. In treating chronic cases in Algeria the Sergents and Catanei (1925) found cinchonidine equal to cinchonine in overcoming parasitæmia but superior in reducing splenomegaly.

In cases where there is an idiosyncrasy to one cinchona alkaloid another has been successfully substituted. Fletcher and Travers (1923) gave 16 gr. (1·06 gm.) a day of cinchonine to a patient in whom quinine dihydrochloride had caused a dermatitis. Dawson and Garbade (1930) similarly report a patient sensitive to the dextrorotatory but not to the lævorotatory cinchona alkaloids.

Malarial Suppression with Quinine

During the Middle Ages many substances were used to ward off attacks of the ague. By the seventeenth century, however, some scepticism was being expressed as to the value of " chips from the gallows and places of execution " (Sir Thomas Browne, 1652).

Cinchona bark and quinine have now been in use for more than 150 years for the suppression of malaria. When or by whom cinchona bark was first used to ward off attacks of malarial fever as a prophylactic is unknown, but by 1693 Jesuit missionaries, in treating malarial patients in China, including the Emperor, had shown that it was possible to abort an attack by giving cinchona bark on the day before a paroxysm was due (Jesuits, 1743).

Lind (1777) states that since the last edition of his " Essay on the Diseases incidental to Europeans in Hot Climates," which had been published in 1771, " the ships of war on the Guinea station are ordered to be supplied with a large quantity of bark in powder and of wine to be issued occasionally to those who are sent in boats up rivers and on shore." Durand (1806), the French Governor of the Isle de St. Louis in Senegal from 1785 to 1787, mentions that during his period of office it was usual, in order to guard against fever, to drink, fasting, a little brandy in which bark had been infused. Matthews (1788), who resided in Sierra Leone during the. same period, recommends " fires and the bark " as the best preservatives against fever. However, even at the end of the eighteenth century, the prophylactic use of cinchona bark was not widespread. The disastrous attempt to found a colony on the island of Bulama, in 1792, failed because of the excessive death-rate from malaria (Beaver, 1805).

Owing to the pernicious influence of James Johnson (1813) in Calcutta, cinchona in malaria treatment was superseded by mercury. To contradict the prevailing belief in mercury was dangerous, for in Bengal the unfortunate Halliday (1821) was dismissed by the Governor in Council for daring to assert that mercury so far from curing increased the death rate from fever. In Africa a succession of exploring expeditions ended in disaster because of the failure to control malarial infections. On Mungo Park's second expedition, of forty-four Europeans who accompanied him from the Gambia (Park, 1815–16), thirty-nine died from fever and dysentery between Shrouda and Sansandine. Major Peddie and Captain Campbell, who in 1816 tried to reach the Niger from the Atlantic coast, also died (Gray and Dochard, 1825). The expedition to the Congo in 1816 also met with disaster though in this case the mortality was due to yellow fever as well as malaria (Tuckey, 1818). In the MacGregor Laird-Oldfield expedition of 1837 (Laird and Oldfield, 1837) of forty Europeans nine returned alive. Finally, in the expedition to the Niger in 1841, under Captain Trotter, R.N. (McWilliam, 1843 ; Allen and Thomson, 1848), of 143 Europeans forty-three died from fever, and at the return of the expedition only nine retained some semblance of health.

The general attitude to quinine during this period is typified by the advice given in 1829 by Sir John Webb, a recognised authority on tropical medicine, to Richard and John Lander when they set out on their expedition to discover the mouth of the Niger (1832). They were recommended to take with them 4 oz. of quinine sulphate ; this was to be taken in doses of 2 to 4 gr. in the form of pills every six hours, but only as a strengthener after fever and dysentery.

In August, 1826, twenty of the crew of H.M.S. *North Star* were detailed to work ashore or in boats on the Sierra Leone River. They all had wine and bark with the exception of Lieutenant Boultbee, R.N., who declined to take the drug ; he alone suffered from fever (Boyle, 1831). Bryson (1847) records a whole series of occasions from 1833 to 1845 when cinchona bark or quinine played an important part in protecting the crews of H.M. ships from malaria, even though they were working in such malarial spots as the Gambia, the Sherbo, and Old Calabar Rivers. It was noted that quinine should be continued for at least fourteen days after leaving a malarial area. Bryson concluded that " the introduction of quinine wine as a preventive of fever has not only reduced the number of febrile attacks but has lessened the severity of those that do occur and thus the mortality has been reduced to a level which does not materially exceed the death rate from fever on some more healthy stations."

The value of quinine as a suppressive was still further emphasised by the naval surgeons of a later generation. Eames (1861), for instance, in H.M. sloop *Bloodhound*, found that quinine greatly reduced the incidence of malaria although the ship was operating in a highly infected area. Quinine was given daily on parade and in one year 18 gallons of rum were used for the administration of the drug. Eames also recognised that quinine does not lose its suppressive properties by long-continued administration, in other words the parasites do not become quinine resistant.

The most striking indication of the suppressive action of quinine undoubtedly occurred in 1854, when Surgeon W. B. Baikie, R.N., led a scientific expedition up the Niger in the most unhealthy season of the year. The path of the earlier expeditions was followed, but in this one as soon as the bar of the river was crossed each man took 6 to 8 gr. of quinine daily. After four months in the river all the twelve Europeans returned in good health, with the exception of one of the second mates who had declined to take the drug (Hutchinson, 1855 ; Baikie, 1856).

Since then, although it may not always have been followed too closely in practice, the official policy has been that all Europeans resident in hyperendemic areas should take 5 gr. of quinine daily. Even in 1900, however, during the operations incidental to the relief of Kumasi, many British officers, not conversant with health conditions in West Africa, were sceptical of the suppressive value of the daily 5 gr. of quinine. When they had had an attack of malaria they were willing to take it regularly (Armitage and Montanaro, 1901).

It was only in the war of 1939–45 that the value of drugs other than quinine became apparent. The results of chemoprophylaxis with mepacrine are discussed on pp. 345–50, and with proguanil and chloroquine on pp. 327 and 485. It is now recognised that as quinine has no action on the sporozoites of any form of human malaria, nor has it a destructive action on the exo-erythrocytic forms, it is not therefore a true causal prophylactic. Nevertheless quinine has value as a suppressive agent. Findlay and Stevenson (1944) showed that with West African strains of *P. falciparum* under field conditions failure to take 5 gr. (0·3 gm.) of quinine was abruptly followed by a rise in the malaria incidence. Of 600 British officers and men who ceased taking quinine ninety-three developed malaria in the ensuing three weeks, usually in from ten to fourteen days : of 648 officers and men in the same units who continued on quinine only forty-two developed malaria, percentage rates of 15·5 and 6·4 respectively. Fairley (1945a), working with New Guinea strains of *P. falciparum* under laboratory conditions with European volunteers, found that 10 gr. (0·6 gm.) daily failed to prevent overt attacks of malaria. With New Guinea strains of *P. vivax* 5 gr. (0·3 gm.) daily was incapable of preventing attacks of overt benign tertian malaria : when the dosage was increased to 10 gr. (0·6 gm.) daily complete suppression was afforded in some instances. In mixed infections volunteers taking quinine all developed splenomegaly, hepatomegaly, anæmia, and parasitæmia.

The taking of daily doses of quinine may sometimes delay the onset of a primary malarial attack. Murgatroyd *et al.* (1939) recorded a case where *P. ovale* infection developed nine months after infection. There is still some uncertainty whether a single dose of quinine once a day is as effective as small doses repeated at intervals throughout the day. Dearborn (1948) found that in lophuræ malaria in the duck a single daily dose of 8 mgm. per kgm. was as effective as 24 mgm. per kgm. a day divided into six equal doses.

Totaquina

The fact that the alkaloids of cinchona, other than quinine, possess therapeutic activities suggested the possibility of using the crude total alkaloids of cinchona bark or of the alkaloids still remaining in the bark after the removal, in whole or in part, of quinine. Such extracts, known as quinetum, or cinchona febrifuge, which are obviously less expensive than the total alkaloids, were first prepared in Madras by John Broughton (1871) at the instance of Dr. J. E. de Vrij (1874), who suggested the manufacture of a powder containing all the cinchona alkaloids, including quinamine discovered by Hesse in 1872, derived from the red bark of *Cinchona succirubra* in which quinine constitutes about one-third of the alkaloids present. This powder was at first termed quinetum or febrifuge. By 1903 trees of *Cinchona succirubra* had become very rare in India since, from the idea that quinine was the only cinchona alkaloid of value in malaria, attention had been focussed almost entirely on the cultivation of *C. calisaya* and *C. ledgeriana* and their hybrids, species yielding a yellow bark in which quinine constitutes some 70 per cent. of the alkaloid present. *C. calisaya* and *C. ledgeriana,* though they can be raised with extreme care in the eastern Himalayas, grow with ease only in their natural habitat in Bolivia and, as the result of careful acclimatisation, in Java. Cinchona febrifuge was therefore usually made from the alkaloids which remain after the extraction of quinine from yellow bark, some quinine being added to make it more or less similar in composition to the original febrifuge made from red bark. It is, therefore, not surprising that somewhat variable results were obtained in the treatment of malaria with this practically un-standardised febrifuge. In order to overcome these difficulties the Malaria Commission of the League of Nations (1933) introduced an improved and standardised mixture known as " totaquina." This mixture must consist of 70 per cent. of crystallisable alkaloids of which not less than 15 per cent. is quinine : on the other hand, it should contain not more than 20 per cent. of water, while the mineral ash must not exceed 5 per cent., and if possible, 3 per cent.

Two types of totaquina have been suggested. Type I is prepared from the total alkaloids of *C. succirubra.* Its large-scale production requires the existence of a large number of trees of this species. Type II, in which there is as a rule more cinchonine than in Type I, is prepared from *C. ledgeriana* residues with the addition of enough quinine to bring it up to specification. All totaquina differs from the salts of the cinchona alkaloids in that it contains only free bases : to be absorbed it must be transformed into a salt by the free acid in the stomach. It must therefore dissolve readily in the stomach. Although there have been complaints that totaquina is not completely soluble in an acid mixture, and undoubtedly complete standardisation of composition cannot be obtained, nevertheless there is general agreement (Pampana, 1934, and Fletcher, 1934) that totaquina acts like quinine as a potent remedy in all forms of malaria. Hicks and Chand (1935), in India, found that both types of quinine were equally efficacious, provided daily doses of 0·6 gm. per 70 kgm. of body weight were given in vivax infections and 1·2 gm. per 70 kgm. of body weight in falciparum infections. In Roumania, Parvulescu *et al.* (1934) and Slatineanu *et al.* (1934) found Type II less effective than Type I, and in Malaya, Field (1934) showed that with Type II totaquina parasites disappeared more slowly than with quinine.

In the Philippines, Maranon *et al.* (1935) found a locally prepared Type II totaquina almost as efficient as quinine sulphate. Some specimens of totaquina were undoubtedly very low in quinine content. Totaquina possesses no advantage therapeutically over quinine and, as Knoppers (1948) has pointed out, since quinine is generally agreed to be more effective than the other cinchona alkaloids against all forms of human malaria it could hardly be as effective as quinine, weight for weight, unless it could be shown that the action of the other cinchona alkaloids combined with quinine is of a synergistic nature : actually there is no evidence of synergism but only of an additive action between cinchona and the other cinchona alkaloids. Despite its reduced efficiency, the cost of totaquina is so much lower than that of quinine and also of that of the newer synthetic compounds such as mepacrine, sontoquine and proguanil that its use will probably continue for some time to come in countries such as India where, as Russell (1937) points out, at least 100 million persons a year contract malarial infections. In countries where *P. vivax* is the prevailing parasite, and the risk of inducing blackwater fever is therefore very low, totaquina allows those who are in process of acquiring immunity to tide over the more acute symptoms of periodic clinical attacks without interfering with the acquirement of immunity. In areas such as Africa south of the Sahara, where *P. falciparum* is the prevailing parasite, the indiscriminate use of totaquina, as of quinine, undoubtedly entails the danger of inducing blackwater fever in those indigenous inhabitants who have not yet acquired or have lost their immunity to the local strains of plasmodia.

Since the adoption of totaquina by the British Pharmacopœia (1932), its use has become widespread in malarious countries. In the Philippines, as in India, totaquina of Type I has been prepared from the total alkaloids extracted from the bark of either *C. succirubra* or *C. robusta* (Ejercito and Santos, 1937). Totaquina has also been prepared in Tanganyika, whence increasing amounts are being exported to other East African countries (Raymond, 1946).

In Colombia (Figueroa, 1942), where the barks of *C. lancifolia* and *C. cordifolia* have been used as the crude source, totaquina has the following composition :—

	Per cent.
Quinine .	45·55
Cinchonidine .	10·79
Quinidine	4·59
Cinchonine	3·31
Amorphous alkaloids	10·76
Resin	5·12
Inert excipient	8·00
Moisture.	11·88

In Ecuador the bark of *C. pitayensis* is specially rich in alkaloids (Chevalier, 1946).

In South Carolina, Yeager *et al.* (1946) tested a totaquina of unspecified composition. In a negro population largely infected with *P. falciparum*, totaquina appeared as effective in treatment as quinine ; it did not cause any severe reactions.

Green (1945) compared the effects of totaquina with those of

quinine and mepacrine in the treatment of the acute attack in a
series of American soldiers, 268 of whom were suffering from
P. vivax, fifteen from *P. falciparum,* and twenty-one from mixed
infections. The totaquina employed contained 9·6 per cent. of
anhydrous quinine and 73·0 per cent. of total anhydrous crystallisable cinchona alkaloids. Quinine and totaquina were given in
doses of 1 gm. three times daily for five days ; mepacrine was
given in a dose of 0·2 gm. every six hours for five doses, followed
by 0·1 gm. three times a day after meals for six days. The results
are shown in the table :—

Drug.	Time in days till bloods were negative.	Time in days till temperature was normal.	Time in days till disappearance of all symptoms.
Totaquina .	2·73	2·2	3·68
Quinine .	2·53	2·25	3·7
Mepacrine .	2·25	2·7	3·53

The relapse rate for both types of infection, which were not
distinguished, was about the same for patients treated with
totaquina and quinine : of eighty cases treated with totaquina
fifty-two relapsed over an observation period of twelve weeks ;
of eighty cases treated with quinine fifty-six relapsed, while of
eighty cases treated with mepacrine thirty-one relapsed. The

Toxic Symptoms after Treatment of Eighty Cases with
Totaquina and Eighty Cases with Quinine (Green, 1945)

Symptom.	Drug.	
	Totaquina.	Quinine.
Nausea	70	16
Vomiting	32	6
Tinnitus	7	75
Deafness	0	50
Blurring of vision . . .	8	0
Vertigo	24	8
Urticaria	1	1
Headache after each dose .	1	0

intervals between attacks were with totaquina 13·2 days, quinine 15·2 days, and mepacrine 37·4 days.

While only seven of the eighty cases treated with mepacrine complained of symptoms, nausea, vomiting and nervousness, seventy of those given totaquina and seventy-nine of those given quinine had symptoms. A difference in the incidence of symptoms was, however, noted, as shown in the table at the foot of page 290.

The high incidence of nausea and vomiting and of giddiness with totaquina is specially noteworthy.

Chloroquine

Chloroquine (resorchin, résoquine, résochin, nivaquine B, nivaquine, aralen, SN 7,618) is 7-chloro-4-(α-methylbutylamino-δ-diethylamino) quinoline. As the diphosphate, prepared by Surrey and Hammer (1946), it was extensively studied during the war by American investigators, having originally been synthesised as early as 1934 by German workers.

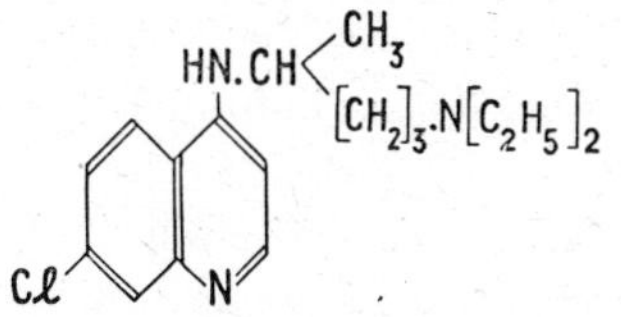

Chloroquine.

Chloroquine is more active than mepacrine in all the avian malarias in which it has been tested. If the activity of mepacrine be taken as 1, then the mepacrine equivalent of chloroquine is in

P. cathemerium infection in the duck and canary . 3·5
P. lophuræ infection in the duck . . . . 5 to 13.

Chloroquine controls trophozoite-induced infections of *P. cynomolgi* in monkeys in doses of 2·5 mgm. per kgm. of body weight as compared with 80 mgm. per kgm. of quinine (Genther *et al.*, 1948). It does not eradicate sporozoite-induced infections due to *P. cynomolgi* (Schmidt *et al.*, 1948). Chloroquine has a quinine equivalent of thirteen against *P. berghei* in mice, this being equal to its quinine equivalent against *P. gallinaceum*, as determined by Goodwin (1949).

The resolution of chloroquine was obtained with D-bromo-camphor sulphonic acid by Kiegel and Sherwood (1949). Neither of the optically active forms showed any marked difference in antimalarial activity in birds from the racemate.

Like mepacrine, chloroquine does not eradicate infection nor is it a causal prophylactic against sporozoite-induced cathemerium malaria in the canary, gallinaceum malaria in the chick or cyno-molgi malaria in the monkey. The quinine equivalent of chloro-quine varies with the host in which a particular avian parasite is present : thus it has a quinine equivalent against *P. cathemerium* of fifteen in the canary but sixty in the duck, against *P. lophuræ* of thirty in the chick but fifteen in the duck, while against *P. gallina-ceum* its quinine equivalent is fifteen.

The earliest report by Loeb *et al.* (1946b) suggested that in the treatment of an acute attack of malaria in man, due either to *P. falciparum* or to *P. vivax*, an initial dose of 0·6 gm. of the base followed six to eight hours later by 0·3 gm. and by a single dose of 0·3 gm. on each of two consecutive days, is enough to remove symptoms in from twenty-four to forty-eight hours, while parasites disappear from the blood stream in from forty-eight to seventy-two hours. This *régime* will also eradicate infections due to *P. falci-parum.* In the case of vivax infections, a single weekly suppressive dose of 0·3 gm. following this dose schedule will control relapses, though not invariably.

Most *et al.* (1946) used three treatment schedules for vivax infections : (1) 1·0 gm. of the diphosphate in twenty-four hours, (2) 1·5 gm. in four days, (3) 2·0 gm. in seven days. The initial dose was 0·3 to 0·4 gm. at the time of diagnosis and 0·3 gm. four hours later. Chloroquine produced rapid disappearance of symp-toms and of parasites from the blood. Slight toxic symptoms were seen among the 365 patients treated by these observers, but in no case was it necessary to interrupt symptoms. Dizziness or light headedness was not uncommon. In fifty-six, or 20 per cent., of 284 patients pruritus was seen : pruritus was generally localised and was most common during the first two days of treatment ; in seven patients there was erythema, urticaria or mild papular eruptions.

Gordon *et al.* (1947) treated vivax infections with the following doses of the base : either 2·0 gm. in six days, 1·2 gm. in three days,

or 0·8 gm. being given in three days. Chloroquine appeared equal
to mepacrine in controlling acute attacks, at the end of twenty-four
hours 48 per cent. of those given chloroquine and 53 per cent. of
those given mepacrine were free from parasites, but fifty-four of
236 patients given chloroquine had minor toxic reactions, whereas
only twelve of 137 patients given mepacrine had minor toxic
complaints.

Tablets containing 0·3 gm. of the base were at first manufactured : those now produced contain 0·15 gm. of the base or
0·25 gm. of the diphosphate. Warthin *et al.* (1948) gave 1·0 gm.
of the diphosphate followed in eight hours by 0·5 gm. A single
dose of the diphosphate was then given on the second and third
days and thereafter the patient took 0·5 gm. of the diphosphate
every Sunday for five weeks. All patients were suffering from
P. vivax infections contracted in the Pacific. In acute attacks
chloroquine was as effective as mepacrine and was better tolerated
in acute relapses. It did not reduce the relapse rate to any greater
degree than does mepacrine.

Young and Eyles (1948) treated nineteen patients infected with
the Chesson strain and one with the Pait strain, which also origi-
nated in the Pacific : the total dose was 1·5 gm. on the first day,
0·9 gm. was given in two doses at an interval of from six to eight
hours and on the two following days one dose of 0·3 gm. was
administered. At the end of twenty-four hours 74 per cent. of
parasites were removed from the peripheral blood stream and at
the end of five days all patients were free.

Hayman *et al.* (1946) found that for the control of acute attacks
due to *P. vivax* a concentration of 10 μgm. of chloroquine per litre
of blood was essential. Doses of 1·0 gm. in a day, 1·5 gm. in 4 days
and 2·0 gm. in seven days all controlled fever and parasitæmia
about equally. Within twenty-four hours 38 per cent. of patients
were parasite-free, and in seventy-two hours 96 per cent. Of
244 patients with recurrent attacks only five had fever for more
than twenty-four hours.

In the United States Army (1947a and b) the routine treatment
is 0·5 gm. on admission immediately after a blood film has been
taken and 0·5 gm. four hours later. At 9 a.m. the next morning,
and on two additional days at the same time, the patient is given

0·5 gm. Thus the total dose is 2·5 gm. or 1·5 gm. of the base in four days. This dosage should not be exceeded. Among 1,077 cases where figures are available the disappearance of fever was as follows :—

> 55 (5 per cent.) afebrile on admission.
> 255 (64·6 per cent.) afebrile within twenty-four hours.
> 71 (6·6 per cent.) afebrile within forty-eight hours.

The disappearance of parasites among 700 patients was as follows :—

418 (59·7 per cent.) were free from parasites within twenty-four hours.

205 (29 per cent.) were free from parasites within forty-eight hours.

19 (2·7 per cent.) were free from parasites within seventy-two hours.

Of a total of 1,321 patients, 1,277 had vivax infections and forty-four malariæ infections.

The reactions of the St. Elizabeth strain of vivax malaria to chloroquine were studied by Coatney *et al.* (1949b). In early attacks parasitæmia was rapidly controlled by 0·8 gm. on the first day (0·2 gm. every six hours), followed by 0·4 gm. per day (0·1 gm. every six hours) for 1·5 to five days. Relapses occurred in from 164 to 293 days after the last day of treatment. Very similar results were obtained with late attacks. In a total of twenty-three early and late attacks parasites were cleared from the blood stream in from one to four days (mean 2·3 days) and fever was terminated in one to two days (mean 1·2 days). Mean plasma concentrations ranged from 84 to 362 μgm. per litre, but peak levels were not attained until near the end of therapy. The peak levels varied from 229 to 705 μgm. per litre. After the end of therapy approximately four weeks were required for concentrations to fall to 10 μgm. per litre.

In Spain, Morales (1949) treated twenty-one patients with vivax infections with chloroquine ; 900 mgm. was given in the first twenty-four hours, 600 mgm. in the second twenty-four hours and 300 mgm. in the third twenty-four hours, a total of 1·8 gm. During an observation period of four to eleven months no relapses were seen.

Chloroquine was given by Halawani *et al.* (1948) in Egypt to six cases of falciparum and thirty-six of vivax infection in a dose of 2·5 gm. in forty-eight hours. All patients were symptom- and parasite-free within three days, but four patients with vivax infections relapsed in from 204 to 308 days after treatment. In French West Africa, Delahousse (1947) treated forty-six patients with *P. falciparum*. The daily dose for adults was 0·3 gm., with children in proportion. The temperature fell to normal in from thirty to thirty-six hours : parasitæmia also disappeared rapidly, but one patient continued to show parasites for five days. One child is known to have relapsed four weeks later.

In North Africa, Schneider and Méchali (1948) treated nineteen patients with *P. falciparum* and nine with *P. vivax* infections. The dosage was 0·6 gm. on the first day, 0·5 gm. on the second, and 0·3 gm. on the next three days. Children from five to twelve years of age had half the above dose. In the infections due to *P. falciparum* fever lasted 1·7 days and schizonts remained in the blood stream for 2·76 days. In *P. vivax* infections the corresponding figures were 1·62 and 2·2 days. In India, Chaudhuri *et al.* (1948) treated eighteen patients with *P. falciparum* and twenty-seven with *P. vivax* infections : two *régimes* were used, a single dose of 1·5 gm. of the base and alternatively 0·5 gm. followed after six hours by 0·25 gm., the latter dose being repeated on each of the next two days, so that 1·25 gm. was given in three days. With *P. falciparum* fever fell in an average of twenty-three hours and parasitæmia had gone in 34·6 hours ; with *P. vivax* the figures were twenty-five and 33·2 hours. Two patients with *P. falciparum* relapsed in thirty and forty-five days, and two with vivax infections in forty-five and 210 days. Chaudhuri (1948) records similar results, chloroquine being less effective against *P. falciparum* than against *P. vivax*. In Panama, Lucena (1948) gave adults total doses of 1·5 to 2·5 gm. in divided doses for from one to three days. *P. vivax* was removed from the blood stream more rapidly than *P. malariæ*, and *P. malariæ* more rapidly than *P. falciparum*.

Chloroquine is effective also in controlling acute attacks due to *P. malariæ*, but its action in a dose of 1·5 gm. in three days is rather slower than in the case of *P. vivax* (Young and Eyles, 1948). Larger doses of chloroquine are of no advantage.

The suppressive action of chloroquine was tested by Goldsmith (1946) on a tea estate in Assam, where malaria is hyperendemic. One tablet containing 0·48 gm. (0·3 gm. of the base) was given once weekly to seventy-three labourers while seventy-four were given 0·1 gm. of mepacrine daily : seventy-six controls took no suppressive. After eight weeks the controls were also given one tablet of chloroquine a week : the administration of this drug to the two groups was continued till the fourteenth week. The mepacrine group ceased taking the drug in the eighth week. A similar experiment was made with three groups of twelve children from six to fourteen years of age : here the dosage was halved. From the fourth week there was a sharp rise in the parasite rate of the controls and a significant fall in the parasite rates of the mepacrine- and chloroquine-protected groups, amounting in the latter to a complete disappearance of parasitæmia. The few cases of " break-through " in the mepacrine group were possibly due to irregularities in taking the drug. There were a few cases of intolerance to mepacrine, none to chloroquine. Pregnant women tolerated chloroquine quite easily, and even on an empty stomach it did not produce any reactions, while some intolerance to mepacrine was seen. The large bulk of the chloroquine tablets appears to be their main disadvantage.

Doucet (1948), in the Belgian Congo, gave one tablet of 0·25 gm. of the base once a week for six months to thirty Europeans. All were free from malaria during that period and in no case was there any evidence of toxicity. Twenty-five children, aged from six to seven years, were left as controls ; 80 to 96 per cent. were infected during that period. Twenty-five children, of whom 84 per cent. were infected with *P. falciparum*, were given 0·125 gm. once a week. In six days all schizonts had disappeared, but at first the number of gametocytes was increased, though, after two months, no gametocytes were present. In Panama, Boldt and Goodwine (1949) found weekly prophylaxis very effective, but in Nigeria Bruce-Chwatt and Bruce-Chwatt (1950) record a failure rate of 23·5 per cent.

The effect of various doses on the suppression of the St. Elizabeth strain of *P. vivax* was studied by Coatney *et al.* (1949b). In one series of five volunteers 0·8 gm. of the base was given on the fourth

day before exposure, on the day of exposure and for six days afterwards. All volunteers developed malaria in from 254 to 308 days
after exposure. Another five volunteers were given 0·4 gm. of
base for four days before, on the day of infection and for twenty
days after exposure, 10 gm. in twenty-five days. Infections
developed in from 256 to 309 days after exposure. Chloroquine
does not therefore prevent the development of infections due to
P. vivax. In those given the prolonged suppressive course dizziness
and blurring of vision occurred in all. With the smaller suppressive and therapeutic courses slight dizziness, nervousness, and
blurring of vision were not uncommon, but in only one patient
was it necessary to reduce the dose.

Berberian (1948), in Syria, used curative followed by suppressive
therapy in two villages. Of thirty cases of falciparum malaria
treated and then given 0·5 or 1 gm. weekly none relapsed, but three
of twenty-three vivax infections relapsed.

Chloroquine has also been used by Smith *et al.* (1948) and
Packer (1947) in field trials, where it has been compared in efficiency
with proguanil.

Chloroquine was employed by Kierland and McCreight (1948)
to control fever in twenty-five cases of therapeutic malaria induced
by injections of blood containing *P. vivax*. The total dosage in
twenty-three cases was 2·5 gm. and in two cases 3·0 gm. The
course was 1 gm. followed in six hours by 0·5 gm.; 0·5 gm. was then
given twenty-four hours and forty-eight hours later. In twenty-
one cases there was no further fever, but four had an additional
paroxysm. There was less likelihood of an additional paroxysm
when the drug was given during defervescence. Chloroquine has
now been used with success in controlling clinical symptoms in
many parts of the world (Kamal and Abdel Messih, 1947 ; Aparicio
Garrido and Benitez Calvo, 1949 ; Pachecho *et al.*, 1946 ; Mein
and Rosado, 1948 ; Enriquez-Navarro and Rognoni, 1948 ; Smith
et al., 1949). Intramuscularly in doses of 200 mgm. of the base
it causes little or no local reaction (Culwell *et al.*, 1948).

There is evidence that, as in the case of mepacrine, infections
due to *P. falciparum* are radically cured by the prolonged use of
suppressive chloroquine.

Chloroquine thus has an action in human malarias very similar to but even more rapid than that of mepacrine. It does not stain the skin yellow like mepacrine, and in addition it can be taken as a suppressive once a week instead of every day, as in the case of mepacrine. Only very occasionally have severe toxic symptoms been seen (Reimann, 1947). Chaudhuri (1948) noted only five patients with insomnia, pruritus, and gastro-intestinal upset among fifty treated. Chloroquine can be given to those who are sensitive to mepacrine.

In vivax infections chloroquine does not prevent relapses, but there is some evidence, not entirely convincing, that the period before a relapse occurs is longer than in patients treated with mepacrine.

Chloroquine has now been adopted by the United States Army Medical Department (1947b) as a routine drug : the diphosphate is commonly used, 1 gm. corresponding to 0·6 gm. of the base.

Oxychloroquine

Oxychloroquine, SN 8,137, is 7-chloro-4-(3-diethylamino-2-hydroxypropylamino)quinoline : it resembles chloroquine in many ways but is thought to be less toxic to man and at the same time rather less active against experimentally induced malarias (Berliner et al., 1948b). The diphosphate contains 62 per cent. of the base.

Small-scale trials in experimental and naturally acquired malaria by Gordon et al. (1947) and Packer (1947) failed to show any advantage over chloroquine. In India, however, it has been suggested that oxychloroquine is rather more effective than chloroquine. It does not appear to have been given any effective trial as a suppressive (Elmendorf, 1948).

In monkeys infected with trophozoites of *P. cynomolgi*, daily doses of 5 mgm. per kgm. for seven days were required to keep

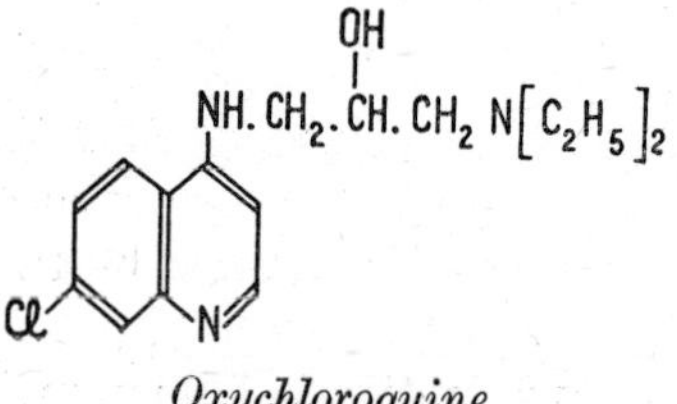

Oxychloroquine.

the blood stream free from parasites for twelve consecutive weeks. Under the same conditions 10 mgm. of mepacrine and 0·25 mgm. of chloroquine were effective (Genther *et al.*, 1948). Sporozoite-induced infections of *P. cynomolgi* were controlled by the same doses but radical cure was not produced by doses sixty times greater (Schmidt *et al.*, 1948).

Sontoquine

3 - Methyl - 4 - diethylamino*iso*amylamino - 7 - chloroquinoline ; 7 - Chloro -4' - (4' - diethylamino -1' - methylbutylamino) - 3 - methyl quinoline) (SN 6,911)

Sontoquin, santoquine, santochin, sontochin, nivaquine, SN 6,911, R.P. 3,308, was originally studied by Kikuth (1945) in bird malaria under the name of sontochin. It was originally synthesised by Andersag *et al.* (1941). The dichlorhydrate has been termed nivaquine C in France, where nivaquine M and nivaquine R refer to methylene dioxynaphthol and resorcin carbonate derivatives ; nivaquine B, however, is chloroquine. All nivaquine now produced in France is chloroquine.

The compound has been shown by Wiselogle (1946) to have the following quinine equivalents when tested for suppressive activity :—

P. cathemerium in the canary .	Quinine equivalent		3
P. cathemerium in the duck .	,,	,,	20
P. gallinaceum in the chick .	,,	,,	4
P. lophuræ in the chick . .	,,	,,	6
P. lophuræ in the duck . .	,,	,,	4

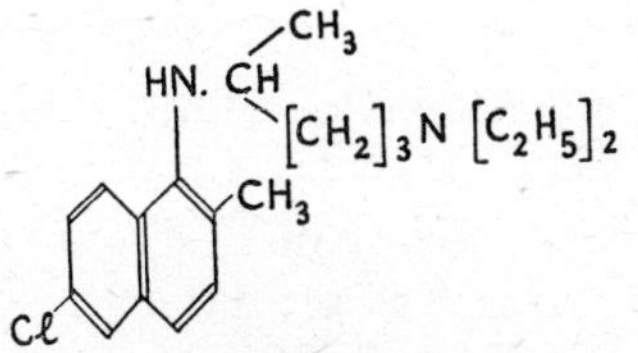

Sontoquine
7-Chloro-4-(4'-diethylamino-1'-methylbutylamino)-
3-methylquinoline.

According to Bovet *et al.* (1948) it is more active than mepacrine against blood-induced *P. gallinaceum* infections. Against *P.*

berghei in mice Schneider *et al.* (1949) found that sontoquine had a chemotherapeutic index of 1 : 150 or 1 : 75. The minimum curative dose subcutaneously in mice against a blood-induced infection is 1 to 2 mgm. per kgm. of body weight. It is active against the asexual erythrocytic forms of *P. falciparum* (McLendon strain), *P. vivax* (McCoy strain) and also against *P. malariæ*. A total dose of 1·8 gm. given as the disulphate monohydrate has been found effective in ending attacks of vivax malaria (Decourt and Schneider, 1947a and b). Gordon *et al.* (1947) gave 3·2 gm. in seven days to eighty-two patients with vivax infection. At the end of twenty-four hours 37 per cent. of patients had no parasitæmia as compared with 53 per cent. of those treated with mepacrine, while fever and symptoms disappeared rapidly. Among the eighty-two patients sixteen showed mild toxic reactions, diarrhœa (six), nausea (five), vomiting (three), and tinnitus (two). Effective suppression has been maintained with doses of 0·1 gm. daily, but even in doses of 0·4 gm. daily SN 6,911 is not a true causal prophylactic against *P. vivax* (St. Elizabeth strain): against blood-induced vivax infection it has a quinine equivalent of four based on total oral dosage when given as the disulphate monohydrate but of only two on the basis of total dosage when given as the salt with 4 · 4′-methylene bis (3-hydroxy-2-naphthoic acid).

In Egypt, Halawani *et al.* (1947b, 1948) found that in ninety-five patients suffering from *P. vivax* infections, forty-six were free from fever and parasites in twenty-four hours, and the remaining forty-nine within forty-eight hours. The dosage employed for adults was 0·5 gm. on the first day, 0·4 gm. on the second day, and 0·3 gm. on the third, fourth, and fifth days. In North Africa, Schneider and Méchali (1948) treated twenty-two patients infected with *P. falciparum* and eleven with *P. vivax*. The dosage was 0·6 gm. on the first day, 0·5 on the second day, and 0·3 gm. on the three following days. In the infections due to *P. falciparum* the duration of fever was 1·57 days, the duration of parasites in the blood stream 2·5 days ; in infections due to *P. vivax* the duration of fever was 1·7 days, the duration of parasites in the blood stream 2·9 days.

Hulshoff (1947), in more than 100 patients, found that doses of

100 mgm. three times daily for five days promptly controlled the clinical symptoms due both to *P. falciparum* and *P. vivax* : The latter infection was not eradicated, although the average time till relapse was sixty-eight days. When sontoquine alone was used 63 per cent. of patients relapsed, when sontoquine and pamaquin were combined only 40 per cent. relapsed. Canet (1948) found sontoquine active in clearing the peripheral blood stream of parasites of *P. vivax* and *P. falciparum* in Northern Indo-China : similar results were obtained by Sohier *et al.* (1948), who noted a reduction in splenomegaly. Ruhe *et al.* (1949b) used the bisulphate monohydrate (0·165 gm. salt = 0·1 gm. base). In patients infected with the St. Elizabeth vivax strain early attacks were treated by 0·8 gm. on the first day, followed by 0·4 gm. per day for five days. Fever fell to normal in two to three days, and parasitæmia was absent in from three to four days. All five volunteers had late relapses in from 269 to 390 days after the original exposure to infection. Late attacks were similarly treated, but in three of four cases relapses took place in thirty-seven to forty-six days. Mean plasma levels varied from 222 to 347 μgm. per litre. Two volunteers suffered from nausea and vomiting on the fourth and fifth days.

The effects of suppressive treatment were studied also by Ruhe *et al.* (1949b). Five volunteers were given 0·8 gm. of base on the fourth day before infection and then 0·4 gm. daily till the sixth day after being bitten, 4·8 gm. in eleven days. Malaria developed in from 277 to 332 days, at the same time as patients protected by mepacrine. Mean plasma concentrations were from 328 to 474 μgm. per litre. Five other volunteers were treated as before but for twenty days after infection. Malaria developed in from 225 to 297 days after exposure. It may therefore be concluded that sontoquine is not a causal prophylactic for vivax malaria. All the patients had fine tremor of the hands, diarrhœa, nausea, anorexia with or without vomiting, epigastric soreness, and eructations. Two had vertigo and four headache, insomnia, and irritability.

Derivatives of Sontoquine

The antimalarial activity of a number of sontoquine derivatives

was studied by Gray and Hill (1949). The chemical relationship
of these compounds, their antimalarial activity against trophozoite-induced infections of *P. gallinaceum*, and their toxicity for
mice is shown in the table in association with the generic formula.

Generic formula.

Compound.	Substitution in quinoline nucleus.					Activity against *P. gallinaceum*. M.E.D. in mgm./kgm.	Toxicity for mice. LD 50 mgm./kgm.
	3	5	6	7	8		
Chloroquine	—	—	—	Cl	—	1·0	250
Sontoquine	CH_3	—	—	Cl	—	5·0	450
Compound I	CH_3	—	—	—	—	10·0	500
,, II	CH_3	—	Cl	—	—	20·0	400
,, III	CH_3	Cl	—	—	—	50·0	800
,, IV	CH_3	—	—	—	Cl	200·0	800
,, V	CH_3	—	—	Cl	CH_3	Inactive	600

All doses are in terms of the hydrochloride.

Compound I was prepared by Andersag *et al.* (1941), compounds
II and IV were prepared by Steck *et al.* (1946), and III and V by
Gray and Hill (1949). Position 7 in the quinoline nucleus, as in
chloroquine, is the optimum one for the chlorine atom, and the
presence of a methyl group in position 3 (sontoquine) reduces
activity, and a second methyl group in position 8 results in
complete inactivity.

Camoquin (Cam-Aqi)

Among the 4-aminoquinolines which have been tested clinically
is 4-(3'-diethylaminomethyl-4'-hydroxyanilino)-7-chloroquinoline
dihydrate dihydrochloride, (4 - (7' - chloro - 4' - quinolyamino) - α -

diethyl-amino-*o*-cresol), SN 10,751, first known as " Cam-Aqi," later as amodiaquin, miaquin or camoquin.

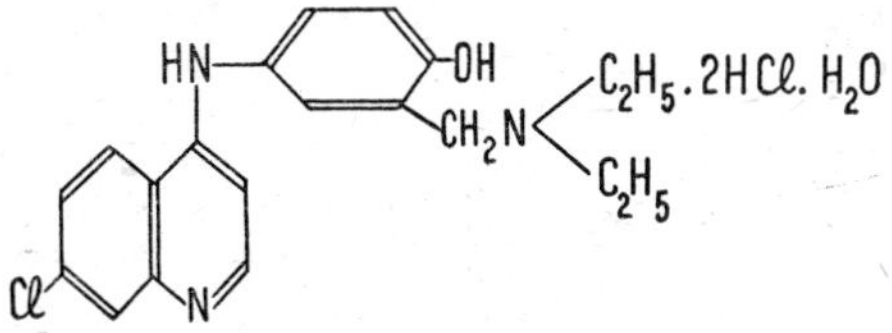

Camoquin.

This compound, which is formed from the interaction of 4, 7-dichloroquinoline and 4-acetamido-α-diethylamino-*o*-cresol, is a yellow crystalline powder, melting at 208° C., and very soluble in water, 1 gm. dissolving in 5 ml. at 25° C. Chronic toxicity tests for seven days, recorded by Wiselogle (1946), showed that in mice the drug was three to four times as toxic as quinine; in eleven-day tests in rats it was five times as toxic as quinine. In unanæsthetised dogs to which the drug was given intravenously total doses of 20 to 30 mgm. per kgm. of body weight were sometimes fatal, convulsions coming on before death. Single oral doses in dogs as small as 75 mgm. per kgm. of body weight were sometimes fatal : if given in capsules larger doses were tolerated. Convulsions and vomiting were caused by a daily oral dose of 50 mgm. per kgm. for three days and 75 mgm. per kgm. daily for three days with death on the sixth day. Bloody diarrhœa was also present associated with petechial hæmorrhages in the gastric mucosa and acute inflammation of the intestine.

Monkeys given a daily oral dose of 50 mgm. per kgm. died in from seventeen to forty-nine days, but one monkey was in good health after sixty-three days, apart from loss of weight and a slight fall in hæmoglobin. Fatty changes were present in the livers of those monkeys that died. Oral doses of 25 mgm. per kgm. of body weight for twenty-five days caused only slight toxic changes in monkeys. SN 10,751 is less toxic in laboratory animals than chloroquine when given in a single dose : similarly, its acute toxicity is about equal to that of mepacrine, but after prolonged administration it is only one-fourth to one-eighth as toxic. In addition to anorexia and vomiting there may be spasticity, clonic convulsions, and death from respiratory failure.

In man, after doses of 0·3 gm. daily, the plasma concentrations in sixteen individuals ranged from 113 to 334 μgm. per litre, with a mean plasma concentration of 189 μgm. per litre.

Mild toxic symptoms occur in about half the persons given 0·3 gm. daily, nausea, vomiting, diarrhœa, tenesmus, headache, palpitation, and fainting, but they tend to disappear rapidly, leaving no after effects. One man has taken 1·0 gm. in a day without developing any symptoms, and a pregnant woman did not abort.

In avian malarias camoquin has no prophylactic activity, but its quinine equivalents in the control of an acute attack are as follows :—

Cathemerium malaria :	canary	. . .	1·0–6·0
	duck	. . .	30
Gallinaceum malaria :	chick	. . .	8·0–30
Lophuræ malaria :	chick	. . .	30
	duck	. . .	15

In Egypt, Halawani et al. (1947a, 1948) treated forty-two patients, three infected with P. falciparum and thirty-nine with P. vivax.

Various dose schedules were used :—

(1) An initial dose of 0·1 gm., followed by 0·05 gm. every twelve hours for seven doses, a total of 0·45 gm.

(2) An initial dose of 0·1 gm. followed by 0·1 gm. every twelve hours for three doses, a total of 0·40 gm.

(3) An initial dose of 0·15 gm. followed by 0·15 gm. after twelve hours and then two doses every twelve hours of 0·1 gm., a total of 0·50 gm.

(4) An initial dose of 0·2 gm. followed by 0·2 gm. after twelve hours, a total of 0·40 gm.

There was little to choose between these schedules : parasites disappeared from the peripheral blood in from twenty-four to forty-eight hours. Among thirty patients followed for from three to five months no relapses occurred. There was no effect on gametocytes of P. falciparum and a very doubtful effect on those of *P. vivax*. Ejercito and Duque (1948) in the Philippines had excellent results with a single dose of 10 mgm. per kgm.

Very similar results were obtained by Simeons and Chhatre (1947) in India, where fifty patients were treated, thirty-nine having infections due to *P. vivax* and eleven due to *P. falciparum*. A single dose of 10 mgm. per kgm. weight was given. The temperature fell to normal in an average of twenty-seven hours for the falciparum cases and twenty-eight hours for the vivax infections : in no instance did it persist for more than forty-eight hours ; asexual parasites disappeared from the blood in forty hours for *P. falciparum* and forty-six hours for *P. vivax* infections. Gametocytes were unaffected. No relapses took place in any patients given 10 mgm. per kgm. of body weight within an observational period of three months, but relapses occurred in two of sixteen patients given 7·5 mgm. per kgm. of body weight and in nine out of eighteen when a dose of 5·0 mgm. per kgm. was given. Doses of 10 to 15 mgm. per kgm. of body weight produced no serious toxic reactions. Chaudhuri (1948), in India, found that camoquin was equally effective in malaria due to all the three parasites. Chaudhuri and Chakravarty (1948) treated twenty-three vivax, twenty-three falciparum, and three malariæ cases. Two regimes were given, 0·1 gm. twice daily for three days and a single dose of 0·5 gm. With the first regime the average duration of fever was twenty-two hours, with the second thirty hours. One falciparum and eight vivax cases relapsed in eight months. Patel and Mehta (1948) similarly found a single dose of 0·25 gm. better than 0·05 gm. twice daily for two days : five falciparum, twenty-two vivax, and five mixed infections were treated, but of twenty patients five relapsed within four months, five vivax and one falciparum. In South America, Mein and Rosado (1948) found that camoquin rapidly removed both *P. vivax* and *P. falciparum* from the blood stream. Coggeshall (1949) treated 100 patients with relapsing vivax infection from the South Pacific area : 1·0 gm. of camoquin in twenty-four hours brought an acute attack to an end in twenty-four hours and chronic cases could be kept parasite-free by 0·5 gm. weekly. Payne *et al.* (1949) showed that camoquin hydrochloride could be given intramuscularly if desired, only very slight induration being caused at the site of injection. In eleven patients infected with the trophozoites of *P. vivax* 0·123 gm. of the base ended parasitæmia in from twenty-four to 192 hours. Three patients relapsed in from fifteen to forty days : among sixteen patients similarly infected with *P. malariæ* the same dose of the base ended parasitæmia in from twenty-four to 132 hours : .four patients relapsed. There is some evidence, which obviously requires confirmation, that a single dose of 10 mgm. per kgm. of body weight may be effective as a suppressive for as long as two months, but camoquin has no action as a true causal prophylactic. Small infants under two years would seem to require 0·1 gm., children of from five to fourteen years 0·3 gm., and adults 0·4 to 0·8 gm., according to the body weight. Camoquin is less toxic even than chloroquine (Hoekenga, 1950).

7-Chloro-4-(3'-diethylamino-2'-hydroxypropylamino)-quinoline diphosphate (SN 8,137)

SN 8,137 has no prophylactic action, according to Wiselogle (1946), against *P. cathemerium* in the canary, *P. gallinaceum* in the chick, and *P. lophuræ* in the turkey. It is active against the asexual erythrocytic forms of *P. vivax* (McCoy strain) and *P. falciparum* (McLendon strain). Gordon *et al.* (1947) gave 2·0 gm. in three days to sixty-three patients : parasites had disappeared from the blood in 48 per cent., as compared with fifty-three per cent. treated with mepacrine. Minor toxic reactions occurred in twenty-one patients, diarrhœa (five), dizziness (four), tinnitus (two), blurring of vision (two), pruritus (two), and urticaria and rashes (two). SN 8,137 had no prophylactic action when given in a dose of 0·4 gm. daily for three days after infection, but it suppressed *P. vivax* infection in a daily dose of 0·25 gm. once weekly. Wiselogle (1946) found that in vivax infections due to *P. vivax* its quinine equivalent, based on total dosage, was between four and five.

SN 8,137 appears incapable of preventing relapses of *P. vivax* infections. Packer (1947) gave twelve patients from 0·125 to o·5 gm. weekly for four weeks. The four patients receiving the highest dosage all had malaria in from 120 to 270 days.

2-*p*-Chlorophenylguanidino-4-β-diethylaminoethylamino-6-methylpyrimidine (3349) and N$_1$-*p*-chlorophenyl-N$_5$-methyl-N$_5$-*iso*propylbiguanide (4430)

In view of their activity in controlling and eradicating bird malarias, compounds 3349 and 4430 were tested in man.

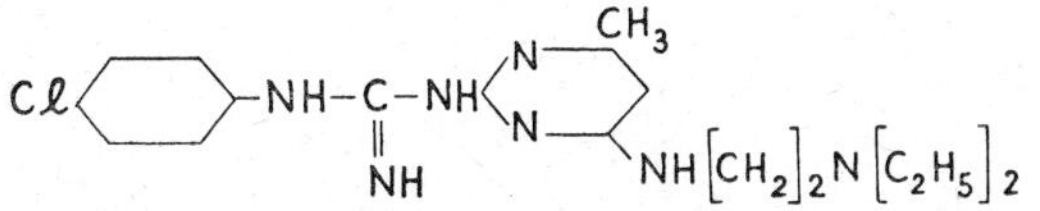

3349

3349 has a high activity against *P. gallinaceum* in chicks but no activity against *P. lophuræ* in ducks : 4430 acts as a causal prophylactic against *P. gallinaceum* but has no action on the asexual blood forms of *P. cathemerium*, although it acts on the blood forms of *P. lophuræ* in chicks.

The antimalarial activity of 3349 in man was tested by Adams and Sanderson (1945a, b, c, d) against infections due to *P. vivax* and *P. falciparum*.

Therapeutic malaria caused by the intravenous injection of *P. vivax* was rapidly controlled by the oral administration of 200 mgm. three times a day and in one case 100 mgm. three times a day ; the temperature in six cases fell to normal in from twenty-four to seventy-two hours, while parasites disappeared from the peripheral blood stream in from forty-eight to ninety-six hours. Two hundred and fifty-nine attacks of vivax malaria were treated. A dosage of 0·1 gm. thrice daily for seven days was often ineffective in controlling attacks, but doses of 0·2 gm. thrice daily were effective. The relapse rate after effective treatment of attacks of benign tertian malaria was over 70 per cent. and bore little or no relation either to the dosage employed or the type of attack, whether primary or one of a series of relapses. The action on *P. vivax* infections of 3349 was very similar to that of mepacrine (Adams and Sanderson, 1945d) ; Adams and Sanderson (1945a, c) also investigated the action of the drug on *P. falciparum*. Here again doses of at least 200 mgm. thrice daily were necessary to control attacks, and even with doses of 500 mgm. twice a day for seven days one of two patients relapsed within three weeks. Only when a single dose of 2·0 gm. was given to two patients in twenty-four hours did both patients fail to react. No action was noted on the gametocytes of either *P. vivax* or *P. falciparum*. The toxic effects of 3349 were mild colic, diarrhœa and frontal headache. One or other, or all three, of these symptoms were encountered in some degree in roughly half of those on a dosage of 0·2 gm. thrice daily, but in no instance were they sufficiently severe to cause interference with the continuance of treatment. With dosages beyond 0·2 gm. toxic symptoms were more severe, and very severe diarrhœa was encountered in a patient who took 1 gm. of the drug. As patients became habituated to the drug the toxic effects were diminished. Das Gupta *et al.* (1945) treated sixty patients with *P. vivax* infections in India : twenty-five patients showed a return of parasitæmia within eight weeks. Among fifty-one patients with *P. falciparum* there were no relapses of the specific parasite for which they had been treated, but eight had attacks of vivax infection. Nausea and vomiting were common and were not eliminated even with daily doses of 400 mgm. Among the 106 patients treated five deaths occurred. In four of these fatal cases serious complications were present before therapy was begun, but in all the fatal cases the drug is believed to have contributed to the final results. Evidence of bronchopneumonia was common. In West Africa, Findlay (1945) found 3349 inferior to mepacrine in the treatment of falciparum infections. In fifty-four European patients the following dosage was given : first and second days 1·0 gm., third and fourth days 800 mgm., fifth, sixth and seventh days 400 mgm. In comparison with mepacrine and quinine the results were as follows :—

Drug.	Average time for disappearance of parasites from the blood in hours.	Average time for cessation of fever in hours.	Average time for disappearance of clinical symptoms in hours.
3349	65·0	69·8	74·8
Mepacrine (0·8 gm. first day)	48·0	66·0	67·8
Quinine (30 gr. daily) . .	25·5	63·3	64·2

Nausea and vomiting was common and five patients had to abandon treatment for this cause, while another had continuous diarrhœa. Five of the forty-nine patients who completed the course relapsed in from four to twenty days, while in three others the drug failed to remove parasites from the blood in seven days. Similar poor results were recorded by the Army Malaria Research Unit (1944).

In view of the close similarity in the chemical structure of 4430, N_1-*p*-chlorophenyl-N_5-methyl-N_5-*iso*propylbiguanide, to proguanil, its effects in human malaria are of considerable interest. A total of forty-four cases of vivax infection were treated by Adams, Townshend and King (1945) with varying dose from 60 mgm. a day for seven days to 1·5 or 3·0 gm. in one day. In every case there was a rapid cure of the clinical attack with a return of the temperature to normal within seventy-two hours and disappearance of the parasites from the blood in ninety-six hours from the commencement of treatment. Gametocytes were observed in the peripheral blood up to six days after the start of treatment. Of the forty-four cases treated no less than twenty-eight relapsed within ten weeks of treatment whatever the dosage employed. Nine cases of naturally acquired *P. falciparum* infections were treated with varying doses of 4430, varying from 300 mgm. for six days to 1·5 gm. daily for seven days. Here again the clinical attack was promptly arrested, fever and asexual forms of the parasite disappearing in under seventy-two hours from the beginning of treatment. Gametocytes persisted in the peripheral blood for a considerable time, in one case for as long as thirty days. One-third of the cases treated were known to relapse. With dosages of under 1·0 gm. daily no toxic effects were noted. With dosages of 1·0 gm. daily and over, nausea and sometimes vomiting occurred in some cases about two hours after each dose. In two patients with *P. vivax* infections receiving in one instance 500 mgm. twice daily and in the other 1·0 gm. thrice in twenty-four hours, each with a low urinary output, severe loin pains, vomiting and profuse sweating occurred with, in the case on the smaller dosage, the passage of scanty urine containing much albumin and some scanty red cells, and in that on the larger dosage oliguria and considerable hæmaturia. In both cases an immediate increase in fluid intake with the establishment of diuresis relieved the symptoms and the urine completely cleared in twenty-four hours. When a liberal fluid intake was subsequently administered no further trouble was encountered when 4430 was given.

The action of 4430 in controlling vivax infections was further studied by Johnstone (1946a) in ninety-seven patients, ninety of whom had been infected in India and Burma and six in the Mediterranean zone. Although the symptoms of the acute attack were promptly controlled, thirty-seven, or 28·9 per cent., of the patients relapsed, the average interval till the first relapse being 1·9 months.

Fairley (1946b) carried out experiments in Australia to determine whether 4430 could act as a causal prophylactic against New Guinea strains of *P. vivax*. From the day previous to exposure to the bites of *Anopheles punctulatus* var. *punctulatus* infected with *P. vivax*, six volunteers received 200 mgm. of 4430 by mouth daily : one control received no drug therapy and the other was given 100 mgm. of mepacrine in the same way, following previous medication with 200 mgm. of 4430 twice daily for four days. Administration of each drug was continued for a further twenty-three days. Nine days later, as shown by subinoculations of their blood, the six receiving 4430 were not harbouring parasites in their blood. During treatment with 4430 and mepacrine no malarial symptoms were seen, but sixteen to fifty-nine days after treatment with 4430 ceased malaria developed in all six patients, while the patient receiving mepacrine developed malaria in twenty-seven days. Thus the exoerythrocytic forms were not eradicated and the drug acts only as a partial causal prophylactic. The eight patients with overt malaria were then given 400 mgm. of 4430 daily for fourteen days. Their bloods became free from parasites in from six to ten days after treatment started ; symptoms abated on an average in five days. Three months later none of the patients had relapsed. No toxic symptoms were observed.

Proguanil

Proguanil (paludrine, chlorguanide, chloriguane (R.P. 3359), palusil, bigumal) was selected for examination in human malaria because of its activity in avian malarias, especially that due to

P. gallinaceum (Curd *et al.*, 1945). Although further investigations are still required on the effects of proguanil in human malaria, enough observations have been made to indicate the possibilities of proguanil as a therapeutic agent.

Proguanil in a dose of 0·6 mgm. per kgm. of body weight protects against blood-induced infections with *P. cynomolgi* (Genther *et al.*, 1948). It is not a causal prophylactic against sporozoite-induced infections (Schmidt *et al.*, 1948). According to Goodwin (1949) the quinine equivalent of proguanil against a blood-induced infection with *P. berghei* in mice is 4·6, whereas against *P. gallinaceum* it is twelve.

The effect on *P. falciparum*, *P. vivax* and *P. malariæ* differs in certain respects.

P. falciparum Infections. *Clinical Cure.* Preliminary observations were made by Maegraith *et al.* (1945) on the effects of treating twenty-two infections due to *P. falciparum* contracted in West and East Africa ; sixteen patients were considered to be suffering from primary attacks. Small doses were at first used as it was thought the drug might be somewhat toxic. Oral doses of 50 mgm. twice daily for fourteen days controlled the clinical attacks effectively and were apparently as satisfactory as doses of 600 mgm. twelve-hourly. Apart from vomiting, no toxic effects were noted. Similar results were recorded by Maegraith *et al.* (1946a). What were possibly radical cures followed 200 to 400 mgm. daily for fourteen days, while clinical cures resulted from 20 mgm. daily for fourteen days or 500 mgm. daily for four days. Thirty patients, the majority of whom had primary infections contracted in West African ports, were followed up for six to seven months in three cases, for eight to twenty-four months in ten cases, and for two to four years for the remainder. No relapses were recorded. Unfortunately there is no record of the length of time of infection before treatment was instituted, a point of importance since after a person has left an endemic malarial area falciparum infections tend to die out spontaneously in from six to eighteen months.

Clinical cure has resulted from single doses of 100 mgm. when dealing with S.-W. Pacific strains (Fairley *et al.*, 1946b), though 100 mgm. thrice daily for fourteen days was more to be relied upon. In most cases asexual parasites were rapidly cleared from

CLINICAL RESPONSE TO ORAL PROGUANIL IN ACUTE FALCIPARUM
MALARIA

Strain.	Daily dose in mgm.	Number of cases.	Therapeutic response.		Authority.
			Mean. Last day of fever.	Mean. Last day of trophozoites.	
West and East Africa .	100 × 14	10	2·2	2·0	Maegraith *et al.*
	1,000 × 14	10	2·2	2·8	(1945)
S.W. Pacific	300 × 10	105	2	1	Fairley *et al.* (1946b)
Belgian Congo	300	253	3	4	Van Riel (1948)
North Africa	300	20	1·77	2·4	Schneider and Méchali (1948)
India . .	300 × 1	93	—	4	Jafar (1947)
West Africa .	300 × 14	5	3·16	3·2	Covell *et al.* (1949a)
	600 × 7	5	2·33	3·0	Covell *et al.* (1949a)
Eritrea	300 × 10	—	2·5	2·9	Ferro-Luzzi (1948)
Panama .	500 × 3	8	3·0	3·0	Rognoni and Puyol (1947)

RESULTS OF PROGUANIL THERAPY IN 105 CASES OF ACUTE
FALCIPARUM INFECTIONS (S.-W. PACIFIC STRAINS).
(Fairley *et al.*, 1946b)

Type of infection.	Number of cases.	Therapeutic response.			
		Secondary attacks.	Last day of tropho-zoites.	Last day of tempera-ture.	Last day of symptoms.
Natural . . .	41	0	1	2	7
Experimental (sporozoite-induced) .	47	1	1	3	7
Experimental (trophozoite-induced)	17	0	1	2	5

the peripheral blood, but the clinical response was described as
" not rapid."

Although the early results have in general been confirmed, it
has been found that in Africa, south of the Sahara, and in Southern
Arabia, proguanil acts less rapidly than elsewhere on falciparum
infections. Van Riel (1948), for instance, in the Belgian Congo,

found that trophozoites continued in the blood stream on the average for four days while fever continued for three days. In the Sudan, Abbott (1949) and others found parasitæmia still persisting after five days though 300 mgm. had been given daily. It is now generally agreed that 100 mgm. daily is too small a dose to control the majority of clinical attacks, but the results with 300 mgm. daily are as good as with 600 or 1,000 mgm. daily. This was certainly the experience of Schneider and Méchali (1948) in North Africa. In Eritrea, Ferro-Luzzi (1948) reported that trophozoites persisted for an average of 2·9 days ; in one case they continued for fifteen days, and 43 per cent. of 112 falciparum cases relapsed in thirty days. In Egypt, Halawani *et al.* (1948) gave 0·3 gm. daily for ten days to six cases. Asexual parasites disappeared, but one patient relapsed after two and a half months. In the Aden Protectorate and Yemen, treatment with 300 to 900 mgm. daily was not as effective in reducing temperature and splenomegaly as quinine. Arab patients relapsed even within five days of the end of a course of 3 gm. (Kay, 1949). In Italy, Raffaele (1948) failed to control infection with daily doses of 400 mgm.

In the Gold Coast, Findlay (1945) found that in five cases daily doses of 300 mgm. for seven days produced a rather slower response than mepacrine as judged by fall of fever and disappearance of parasitæmia. Walls (1948) prefers to give quinine first followed by proguanil to ensure a rapid fall in temperature. Covell *et al.* (1949a, b) also find that proguanil combined with quinine or mepacrine acts more readily on the temperature and parasitæmia caused by a strain of *P. falciparum* from Lagos. The effects with proguanil itself were slow (table, p. 317). Shearer (1949), on the Jos Plateau, in Nigeria, has noted persistence of ring forms in the blood even after 800 mgm. daily for three days. Clinical symptoms also are slow in disappearing.

Some strains of Indian falciparum malaria also appear to react rather slowly to proguanil. On some tea estates, and in Baluchistan, a single dose of 100 mgm. failed to control an attack. Afridi (1947), found that of eighty-one cases from various parts of India seventy-one, or 88 per cent., showed a return to a normal temperature within three days : of 619 cases given 300 mgm. in a single dose 563, or 91 per cent., had a normal temperature within three days, while of 340 cases given more prolonged courses only 293, or 86 per cent., were clinically cured in three days. Jafar (1947), in an area near Calcutta, gave 300 mgm. in a single dose to 119 patients; twenty-three relapsed within twenty-eight days. It must be remembered that in this instance all the patients were Indians, many of whom probably had a considerable degree of immunity to *P. falciparum*. Similar results have been obtained in Malaya with semi-immune populations.

In America also the quinine-resistant Costa strain of *P. falciparum* is rather resistant to proguanil (Shannon, 1949). Total doses of proguanil ranging from 338 to 750 mgm. were given to nine patients, the six-day mean plasma proguanil levels varying from 55 to 106 μgm. per litre. Class III effects (absence of parasitæmia for fourteen days) were seen in two patients having mean plasma drug levels of 78 to 95 μgm. per litre, the remainder of the patients having Class II effects, the parasite-free intervals ranging from two to fourteen days. There was no apparent correlation between effects on the Costa strain of falciparum malaria and drug levels in the range of 55 to 106 μgm. per litre (Earle *et al.*, 1948a). Whereas single-dose regimes may well be of value for those with some degree of immunity, it seems in the light of present evidence that for non-immunes a dose of 300 mgm. should be given daily for ten days.

In Roumania, Ciuca *et al.* (1948b) treated three cases: with daily doses of 200 mgm. the disappearance of asexual parasites did not occur for four days but the temperature was normal in two days.

For children the dosage should be as follows :—

Children under 1 year	.	.	.	25 mgm. for ten days
,, 1–2 years	.	.	.	50 ,, ,, ,,
,, 3–6 ,,	.	.	.	100 ,, ,, ,,
,, 7–9 ,,	.	.	.	150 ,, ,, ,,
,, 10–12 ,,	.	.	.	200 ,, ,, ,,
,, 13–16 ,,	.	.	.	250 ,, ,, ,,

Insufficient evidence is available to determine the relation of proguanil to the genesis of blackwater fever in persons partially immune to *P. falciparum.* Although proguanil has usually been given by mouth, it may, as the acetate or preferably the lactate, be given intravenously. Chaudhuri and Chakravarti (1949) treated eight Indian patients with *P. falciparum* with total doses of 50 to 400 mgm. Three patients, one of whom died, had cerebral malaria and three others had excessive vomiting. Fever was controlled in from twenty-four to seventy-two hours and parasites disappeared in about the same time. Relapses were frequent. It is still uncertain whether intravenous proguanil has any great advantage over intravenous quinine, since most of the patients treated in India had almost certainly some degree of immunity.

CLINICAL CURE OF INDIAN STRAINS OF MALARIA ON DIFFERENT DOSE SCHEDULES OF PROGUANIL

(Clinical cure=subsidence of fever within three days) (Afridi, 1947)

Parasite.	Dosage.								
	0·1 gm. single dose.			0·3 gm. single dose.			All other dosages.		
	Total number of cases.	Number cured.	Per cent.	Total number of cases.	Number cured.	Per cent.	Total number of cases.	Number cured.	Per cent.
Plasmodium falciparum	81	71	88	619	563	91	340	293	86
Plasmodium vivax .	31	23	74	161	133	83	154	123	80
Plasmodium malariæ .	0	0	—	41	37	90	6	3	—
Mixed infections. .	4	3	—	11	10	—	16	8	—
All infections . .	116	97	84	832	743	89	516	427	83

For intravenous injection the drug is dissolved in 7·5 to 10 ml. of distilled water and blood pressure readings before and immediately after injection show no important change (Field, 1947). Mullick and Gupta (1947) gave 300 mgm. as a 2 per cent. solution in normal saline to fifty cases of vivax infection in adult Indians ; no toxic results were recorded and only five patients required a second injection. Maegraith *et al.* (1946b) claim clinical cure of tropho-zoite-induced vivax infections with single intravenous doses of 5 to 20 mgm.

Intramuscular injection in animals causes focal necrosis of muscle, followed by necrosis and inflammation, and leaving an area of fibrosis as a sequela, the results for comparable doses being similar to those with mepacrine. In man, intramuscular injections of from 10 to 100 mgm. did not cause any reaction beyond that which might be expected with any benign injection. As the solubility of proguanil acetate is not great the intramuscular dose of 5 ml. for 100 mgm. is inconveniently large (Innes, 1947).

Radical Cure. Earlier observations made in Liverpool by Maegraith et al. (1945) did not suffice to provide a radical cure rate. Later observations by Maegraith and Andrews (1949) suggested that a radical cure could be attained. The investigations made by Fairley and his colleagues at Cairns also favoured the view that proguanil produces radical cures in patients infected with New Guinea strains of *P. falciparum*. Radical cure was effected in forty-one out of forty-one natural and in forty-six out of forty-seven experimentally-induced sporozoite infections treated with a ten-day course of 100 mgm. thrice daily, and forty-six out of forty-seven experimentally-induced sporozoite infections given 100 mgm. thrice daily for ten days were considered to have been radically cured. Although numerous observations on the clinical cure of malaria have been made in India and Malaya, there is little evidence regarding the radical cure rate. Chaudhuri (1948) drew attention to the existence in India of strains of *P. falciparum* which give rise to infections not radically cured by a dosage of 300 mgm. of proguanil for ten days. He also cited the case of a patient who experienced a second overt attack nine days after the completion of treatment and a third attack eleven days later. The patient was eventually cured by chloroquine. Ferro-Luzzi (1948) found that in Eritrea, after a course of 300 mgm. for ten days, 43 per cent. of patients relapsed. In one case where the infection had been treated with two courses of proguanil the drug exerted no schizonticidal effects at all. Working on neuro-syphilitics, all previously infected with a strain of *P. falciparum* from Lagos, Covell et al. (1949a, c) found that proguanil was a conspicuous failure in bringing about radical cure. Of ten patients given 300 mgm. once or twice daily for fourteen days nine relapsed. It was only when proguanil was reinforced with mepacrine or quinine that there was failure to relapse. The results of treatment obtained by Covell et al. are shown in the table on p. 317. Kay (1949) failed to bring about a radical cure in Aden and the Yemen.

TREATMENT OF A LAGOS STRAIN OF *P. falciparum* WITH PROGUANIL
(Covell *et al.*, 1949a, c)

Group.	Number of patients.	Treatment.	Average duration of fever after treatment.	Average duration of asexual para-sitæmia.	Subsequent history.
1	5	Proguanil 300 mgm. once daily for fourteen days.	76 hours	3·2 days	All relapsed within three weeks and were given 600 mgm. daily for ten days. A second relapse occurred in one case.
	5	Proguanil 300 mgm. twice daily for fourteen days.	68 hours	3·0 days	Four of five cases relapsed within three weeks and were given 600 mgm. daily for ten days. Two cases had a second relapse.
3	5	Proguanil 300 mgm. twice daily for ten days; quinine hydrochloride 10 gr. t.i.d. on the first day of treatment.	78 hours	2·0 days	No relapse in three months.
4	5	Proguanil as in Group 3 but mepacrine 300 mgm. t.i.d. on the first day of treatment.	50 hours	2·5 days	No relapse in three months.
5	5	Quinine hydrochloride 10 gr. twice daily for ten days.	55 hours	2·5 days	No relapse in three months.

These results suggest that to produce a radical cure of West African strains of *P. falciparum* it is necessary to combine proguanil with mepacrine, since the use of quinine is contraindicated in view of its tendency to induce blackwater fever (Findlay and Stevenson, 1944).

Action on Gametocytes. Proguanil has little direct action on the gametocytes of *P. falciparum* which do not disappear as a result of proguanil medication. In fact, in Africans in the Belgian Congo, van Riel (1948) noted that there may be showers of gametocytes, and these may remain in the blood stream for as long as twenty-three days (Ciuca *et al.*, 1948b) or fifty-five days (Chaudhuri, 1948). Ferro-Luzzi (1948) noted them for more than twenty days in Eritrea. Nevertheless there is evidence that proguanil does affect the gametocytes, more especially, in all probability, the female macrogametocytes.

Shute and Maryon (1948) fed *Anopheles maculipennis* var. *atroparvus* daily on a patient given 0·8 gm. of proguanil in divided doses three hours apart two days after gametocytes had appeared in the peripheral blood stream. The mosquitoes were then killed and dissected. In mosquitoes which fed before the sixth day after the dose of proguanil had been given the oöcysts remained very small, and those which fed later contained tiny oöcysts as well as apparently normal ones. Sporozoites were first noted in a mosquito fed eight days before on proguanil. While male gametocytes exflagellate normally in the blood clot in the mosquito and fertilise some of the female gametocytes, it seems that large numbers of female gametocytes must be destroyed or sterilised before fertilisation or before they can penetrate the gut wall. Others penetrate the gut wall but die a few days later. Somewhat similar results had previously been obtained by Black (1947), who showed that proguanil did not inhibit the production of gameto-cytes of *P. falciparum* nor did it influence the numbers or morpho-logy of those already formed. If sporozoites were taken up by the mosquito, a stage of encystment followed but development then ceased. Complete sterilisation of mosquitoes occurred if they were fed one hour after their host had taken 100 mgm. by mouth. No irreversible change occurs in gametocytes, for if they persist in the peripheral blood stream till all the proguanil is excreted they will then develop normally. Full and unimpaired activity was shown twelve, but not ten, days after patients had completed a course of 300 mgm. daily for ten days.

Suppression and **Causal Prophylaxis.** Considerable interest was aroused by the discovery of Fairley and his colleagues (1946b) that proguanil was a powerful suppressive of S.-W. Pacific strains of *P. falciparum* : unfortunately the discovery came too late to be of help in the campaigns in the Pacific theatre of war. When given during the prepatent period the drug was found to sterilise parasites before they reached the red cells ; in other words, primary exo-erythrocytes were destroyed. Proguanil in a daily dose of 100 or 300 mgm. was given for varying periods before, during, and after the normal incubation period. Later, experiments were made by giving single doses at different times during the incubation to ascertain the phase at which the parasite is most sensitive to the drug. In single doses of 100 mgm. or less, proguanil when given between seventy-two and 131 hours after the infecting dose sterilised twenty-five out of twenty-six infections. If given only on the day of exposure a relatively large dose of 1·0 gm. was necessary, but smaller doses such as 10 to 100 mgm. were active during the period from forty-eight to 120 hours after exposure. In a further group of experiments proguanil was given continuously at doses of 100 mgm. or less a day to volunteers who were repeatedly bitten by mosquitoes infected with *Plasmodium falciparum*. The results are summarised in the table :—

EFFECTS OF 100 MGM. PROGUANIL (OR LESS) ON VOLUNTEERS REPEATEDLY BITTEN BY MOSQUITOES INFECTED WITH S.-W. PACIFIC STRAINS OF *P. falciparum* (Fairley *et al.*, 1946b)

Cases.	Dose in mgm. daily.	Days given.	Infective bites.	Biting period in days.
6	100	−1 to 23	20	1
5	100	−1 to 42	41	15
1	100	1 to 42	42	15
1	100	−1 to 53	6	26
1	50	−1 to 42	42	15
1	50	−1 to 53	6	26
1	25	−1 to 42	42	15
1	25	−1 to 53	6	26

Results : (*a*) during administration : no clinical or parasitological evidence of malaria or suppressed malaria. (*b*) After administration : no overt malaria or demonstrable parasites in forty to 119 days' observation.

The true prophylactic efficiency of proguanil was further emphasised in an experiment planned to simulate field conditions. Eight volunteers received in all a total of 130 infective bites from mosquitoes infected with *P. falciparum* and 120 from vivax-infected mosquitoes in sixteen biting sessions over sixty-two days. They were exposed during this period to heavy physical stress, including long marches in hilly country in the tropical climate of Queensland—thirty miles in one day, eighty-nine miles in three days and seventy-two miles in thirty-six hours, with a climb on the longest marches from sea level to 2,500 ft. The soldiers were exposed to extreme cold, one hour at − 10° C. with minimal clothing in a refrigerator. From the day before the first infective bites till twenty-eight days after the last, a total of ninety-two days, they were given 100 mgm. of proguanil daily. The results of this experiment may be summarised as follows :—

(*a*) During proguanil administration :

(i) No volunteer developed overt malaria or signs of suppressed malaria ;

(ii) Parasites were never found in thick blood films while the drug was being taken ;

(iii) No reactions to physical stresses were observed which were not also seen in the normal soldier.

(*b*) After ceasing proguanil administration :

(i) No volunteer showed any evidence of falciparum malaria after ceasing proguanil administration, and no parasites were found in thick blood films.

(ii) All the eight volunteers developed vivax infections in from twenty-four to thirty-three days after the last dose.

The implications of this work are that doses of 100 mgm. given daily for the first week of the incubation period of falciparum malaria completely eliminate infection as the parasites are destroyed in the stage of primary exo-erythrocytic infection. Doses of 100 mgm. given twice daily over a period of two months, when infecting bites are frequently repeated, also give complete protection even under conditions of great physical stress.

Single doses of 100 mgm. timed to coincide with the primary wave of proguanil-sensitive exo-erythrocytic forms, between seventy-two and 130 hours after infecting bites, also sterilise the infection completely. Doses of 100 mgm. daily for fourteen days, beginning immediately after the parasites have reached the blood cells, also eliminate infection.

It thus seems that for S.-W. Pacific strains of *P. faciparum* true causal prophylaxis may be obtained by a dose of 100 mgm. per day. Attempts to confirm these findings in other parts of the world have not been entirely successful. It very soon became apparent that in Africa, south of the Sahara, a single dose of 100 mgm. once a week failed entirely to suppress attacks of fever. Walls (1948), writing from Sierra Leone, finds that attacks of fever occur even with doses of 100 mgm. daily. The prevailing malarial parasite in Sierra Leone is *P. falciparum*. Similar reports have come from other areas in West Africa, where many Europeans have given up proguanil in favour of mepacrine or quinine.

In a controlled experiment in the Belgian Congo, van Riel (1948) failed to find that proguanil is a true causal prophylactic against local strains of *P. falciparum*. Twenty African workmen, who lived in a non-endemic area and whose blood had been persistently negative for malarial parasites, were taken to a hyperendemic area. Ten were left as controls and received no antimalarial drugs ; ten were given 300 mgm. proguanil weekly for the four weeks during which they resided in the hyperendemic region. Of the untreated controls all suffered from falciparum infections in from twenty to twenty-seven days after arriving in the malarious area. Of the treated persons none suffered from a malarial attack while in the hyperendemic area and while still on proguanil. On returning to the malaria-free region and ceasing to take proguanil nine developed malaria. In five the infecting parasite was *P. falciparum*, in two *P. vivax* and in two *P. malariæ*. The latent period between stopping proguanil and developing malaria varied from sixteen to fifty-two days with *P. falciparum*, sixteen to thirty-two days with *P. vivax*, and twenty-five to seventy-six days with *P. malariæ*. It should be noted that administration of proguanil was discontinued approximately forty hours after the last possible exposure to infection, a period which probably leaves little if any margin of safety and can scarcely be regarded as sufficient to ensure adequate protection. Covell and his collaborators (1949a, b) also carried out investigations on causal prophylaxis by proguanil. Twenty-seven patients were arranged in groups, as shown in the table (p. 322). The patients, with the exception of two under quinine prophylaxis, were injected once weekly over a period of six weeks ; each subject was bitten by five to ten heavily infected mosquitoes or received by intravenous injection a suspension of the salivary glands of one infected mosquito. Drug administration was started three days before the first infection in each group and was continued till six days after the last infection. No member of any of the proguanil groups showed parasites in the peripheral blood either during the period of drug administration or subsequently. Ten weeks after the cessation of the drug administration eighteen of twenty individuals who had been on proguanil prophylaxis were inoculated intravenously with sporozoites of the same strain of *P. falciparum*. All developed overt attacks of malaria within a period of seven to ten days, thus showing their susceptibility to the Lagos strain. Two members of the laboratory staff were inoculated intravenously with a suspension of the salivary glands of a heavily infected *Anopheles gambiæ* : they had both taken 100 mgm. of proguanil until and including the day before infection, after which the drug was discontinued ; neither developed malaria.

THE PROPHYLACTIC EFFECT OF PROGUANIL AGAINST *P. falciparum*
(Covell *et al.*, 1949a)

Group.	Number in each group.	Drug.	Dosage.	Results.
I	5	Proguanil	100 mgm. daily.	No infection.
II	5	,,	50 mgm. daily.	,, ,,
III	5	,,	100 mgm. twice weekly.	,, ,,
IV	5	,,	300 mgm. once weekly.	,, ,,
V	1	Quinine hydrochloride	5 gr. (320 mgm.) daily.	Malaria five and seven days after ending suppressive.
	1		10 gr. (650 mgm.) daily	
VI (controls)	5	No drug.		Malaria.

There is thus evidence that proguanil is a true causal prophylactic against a West African strain of *P. falciparum*.

Ciuca *et al.* (1948a) also carried out experiments on causal prophylaxis by means of proguanil, using a strain of *P. falciparum* maintained in the laboratory for some years. Five patients repeatedly inoculated with sporozoites over a period of four weeks were given 300 mgm. every week during the period of the inoculations and for a further two weeks after the final inoculation. None of the five patients developed a febrile attack, observation being carried on for at least twenty-three days after the final inoculation.

When the dose was reduced no causal prophylaxis was apparent. Thus five patients given 100 mgm. once weekly during the period of infection and during the two weeks following the final inoculation all developed infection in from six to eighteen days after the final dose of proguanil. In another experiment four patients were given 100 mgm. on the day of inoculation and for the ensuing six days. Two subjects developed infection thirty-four and thirty-five days after inoculation. Two others failed to develop infection, but in one case the period of observation was only twenty-three days. A dose of 100 mgm. on the day of inoculation and on the three succeeding days protected only two of five patients, three developing infection twenty-nine, thirty-five, and forty-five days after infection.

It is thus obvious that to be effective proguanil must be continued for some days after inoculation.

Robertson (1948), working with partially immune children in Zanzibar, found that the administration of 100 mgm. twice weekly for three months had some beneficial effects on malaria, although the dose was too small to be completely effective. The parasite rate which averaged 50 per cent. before treatment fell to nil in about 150 children given proguanil for three months : in control children the parasitæmia fell to 26·8 per cent. Splenic enlargement fell from 60 to 18 per cent. over the treatment period, but in the untreated children remained at 56 per cent. The hæmoglobin percentages were unchanged in both groups. Shearer (1949), among Europeans and non-immune African children in Nigeria, found that 100 mgm. daily was by no means always effective in preventing clinical attacks and parasitæmia.

P. *vivax* Infections. Proguanil is an active schizonticide in vivax malaria.

The earliest observations on control of acute infections were made by Adams *et al.* (1945), who began with small doses of 10 mgm. twice daily and gradually worked up to 20 mgm. twice daily and thereafter by 25- or 50-mgm. increments to 700 mgm. twelve-hourly. In 147 treated with doses of proguanil the temperature had fallen to normal on the third day and the blood was free from asexual parasites on the fourth day. The patients were infected in India, Burma, and the Mediterranean. Clinical cures were thus readily obtained without any serious toxic effects. Johnstone (1946b) obtained similar results in patients infected in the same areas. In 108 patients given 50 mgm. daily for ten days the average duration of fever after commencing treatment was 1·49 days, while with 500 mgm. daily for the same period the average duration was 1·47 days.

Fairley *et al.* (1946b) recorded the results of treating seventy-six vivax infections contracted in New Guinea or experimentally induced with New Guinea strains. The clinical response and the parasite clearance rate from the blood are shown in the table :—

RESPONSE OF NEW GUINEA STRAINS OF *P. vivax* TO PROGUANIL
(Fairley *et al.*, 1946b)

Type of infection.	Daily dosage in mgm. × days.	Number of cases.	Last day.	
			Trophozoites.	Fever.
Expt. sporozoites	1,000 × 14	43	5	4
Nat. ,,	1,000 × 14	17	4	2
Expt. ,,	300 × 14	4	6	3
Trophozoites .	300 × 10	4	5	2
Sporozoites .	100 × 1	8	7	5

S.-W. Pacific strains have also been investigated in America. Jones *et al.* (1948b), using the Chesson strain, found that proguanil in daily doses of 970 mgm. of the base (equivalent to 1·11 gm. of the monohydrochloride) eventually controlled fever and parasitæmia in ten patients artificially infected with sporozoites, but all subjects had one further paroxysm of fever and one had two paroxysms after the first day of treatment. Earle *et al.* (1948a) gave a total dose of 150 mgm. and found that parasites disappeared from the peripheral blood for fourteen days (a Class III effect), while even 25 mgm. produced the same effect in two of four patients. Proguanil was slightly more effective against the McCoy vivax strain, which is known to be more susceptible than the Chesson strain to the suppressive action of quinine, mepacrine, and chloroquine. Total doses of 50 mgm. produced a Class III effect regularly, and even a total dose of 12·5 mgm. produced the same effect in three of ten patients.

In naturally occurring vivax infections in North Africa, Schneider and Méchali (1948) reported that doses of 300 mgm. a day for five days gave an average duration of parasitæmia of 3·88 days, and of fever of 2·77 days ; twenty patients were studied. In Eritrea, Ferro-Luzzi (1948) found that the average duration of fever was from two to three days, the average duration of trophozoites in the blood was two days. In one patient parasites persisted for eleven days. In Egypt, Halawani *et al.* (1948) gave 300 mgm. daily for ten days to 114 patients. Trophozoites disappeared from the peripheral blood-stream in twenty-four hours. One of ninety-eight patients followed for six months relapsed. In India a number of investigations have been carried out by Chaudhuri and Rai Chaudhuri (1947), and by Afridi (1947), who summarises a long series of reports from India and Assam (Parekh and Boghani, 1947a and b ; De and Datta, 1947a and b ; Srivastava, 1947 ; Lomax, 1947 ; Ghosh, 1947 ; Jafar, 1947 ; Viswanathan, 1947 ; Das Gupta *et al.*, 1947 ; Kutumbiah and Ananthachari, 1947 ; Pisharoty, 1947, and Hamilton, 1947). Of thirty-one cases of *P. vivax* given a single dose of 100 mgm. twenty-three, or 74 per cent., showed a subsidence of fever in three days ; of 161 cases given 300 mgm. as a single dose 133, or 83 per cent., showed a similar response, and of 154 cases given longer courses 123, or 80 per cent., showed the same rapid fall in temperature. All these patients probably had some acquired immunity to vivax infections. Jafar (1947), working in an area near Calcutta, found that though in seventy vivax infections a single dose of 300 mgm. controlled the acute infection yet ten relapsed within twenty-eight days and, in addition, four other patients had fever due to heterologous infections. Woodruff (1947), with fifteen Europeans infected in India and Burma, found that a single dose of 100 mgm. would control the infections but the clinical response was slow. Favourable results on the control of fever and parasitæmia come from Elba where Manfredi (1948) treated sixty-one cases : from Panama, where Rognoni and Puyol (1947) studied five vivax infections, and from Rio de Janeiro where Mein and Rosado (1948) treated seven cases.

Proguanil, according to Mackerras and Ercole (1947), does not inhibit the formation of *P. vivax* trophozoites and its action is limited to the dividing nucleus which is rapidly destroyed, the chromatin breaking up and swelling so as to form irregular diffuse masses. The action on gametocytes is similar to that on *P.*

falciparum gametocytes; proguanil neither influences the morphology of those already formed nor prevents fertilisation in the gut of
the mosquito.   Gametocytes taken up by mosquitoes may reach
the gut wall and encyst, but owing to the persistent effects of the
drugs oöcysts eventually die provided that the human host has
taken 150 mgm. of proguanil within twenty-four hours of the
mosquito's feeding.   In the blood of patients with Eritrean strains
gametocytes may persist for more than twenty days (Ferro-Luzzi,
1948).

Much time and thought has been devoted to discovering a
therapeutic course which would abolish relapses by eradicating
the secondary exo-erythrocytic forms or would at any rate reduce
materially the relapse rate.   The question is more fully discussed
on p. 469 ; it may, however, be said that with proguanil alone no
great reduction in the relapse rate has been noted.   Andrews
et al. (1947) found that there was little difference with 100 and
1,000 mgm. daily for fourteen days, while of seventy-nine patients
given an initial dose of proguanil and thereafter 100 mgm. once
weekly for six months eleven relapsed within six months of
cessation of therapy and four in a slightly longer period.   One
patient described by Maegraith *et al.* (1947) relapsed when on a
weekly dose of 100 mgm. and continued to show parasites in the
blood stream after taking 100 mgm. by mouth, although absorption and blood concentration curves were normal.   A dose of
200 mgm. a week for six months controlled this infection.

In India, according to Afridi (1947), a single dose of 300 mgm.
was followed by a 25 per cent. readmission rate and relapses have
occurred three weeks after the cessation of a suppressive *régime* of
100 mgm. once a week for three months.

In Roumania, Ciuca *et al.* (1948b, 1950) treated patients infected with blood containing a Madagascar strain of *P. vivax* maintained in the laboratory since 1941.   Various dose schedules were
used : eight patients had a single dose of 100 mgm. ; twenty-four
had 200 mgm. daily for seven days, and eight had 300 mgm. daily
for seven days.   Of the eight patients given a single dose of
100 mgm. fever had disappeared in seven within twenty-four
hours ; the remaining patient took three days to become afebrile :
parasites disappeared from the peripheral blood in three to five

days. There is some evidence to suggest that the clinical response
is more rapid after some days of fever, as shown in the table :—

PATIENTS TREATED WITH 200 MGM. PROGUANIL DAILY FOR
SEVEN DAYS (Ciuca *et al.*, 1948b)

Number of patients.	Day of fever on which treatment was started.	Average number of days of treatment before	
		Cessation of fever.	Absence of parasitæmia.
4	4–5	2·5	4·25
11	10–11	1·5	3·5
9	11–17	1·22	3·22

In spontaneous infections due to Balkan strains of *P. vivax*,
given daily doses of 300 mgm. for seven to ten days, parasitæmia
disappeared in all in from two to five days.

Periods of observation were not long enough to determine
whether radical cures had been brought about.

There is general agreement that proguanil does not destroy the
form of *P. vivax* responsible for relapses however long the dose is
continued (Fairley *et al.*, 1946a, b ; Maegraith *et al.*, 1946b, 1947 ;
Johnstone, 1946b, 1947 ; Jones *et al.*, 1948a, b ; Coatney and Cooper,
1948). Coatney and Cooper (1948) in one patient continued the
administration of proguanil for one year ; on stopping the drug
the patient promptly relapsed. Ferro-Luzzi (1948) noted 23 per
cent. of relapses among patients in Eritrea after 300 mgm. for ten
days.

Suppression. Experiments were carried out by Fairley and his
colleagues (1946b) at Cairns, in Queensland, on vivax infections
on the same lines as those used with falciparum infection. True
causal prophylaxis was not attained. Twenty-four volunteers
infected with *P. vivax* received from 100 to 1,000 mgm. of proguanil
daily for differing periods before or soon after infection. Subinoculations made on the ninth day were negative, whereas in
controls they are usually positive on the ninth day. Malarial
attacks, however, developed in nineteen of these twenty-four
volunteers within from eighteen to eighty days after ceasing admini-

stration of proguanil.   When 300 mgm. was given daily for twenty-three days after the infecting bites five out of six volunteers were protected for an observation period of ninety-three to 141 days after exposure to infection.   Unfortunately the later history of these five volunteers is not recorded.

Davey (1946a, b) refers to an unpublished experiment carried out by Adams *et al.* in Liverpool.   The somewhat large prophylactic dose of 400 mgm. was given to four patients daily for seventeen days after bites by mosquitoes infected with *P. vivax* :   three of the patients developed malaria nine months later.

Woodruff (1947) found that 100 mgm. once a week for six months did not suppress attacks, for of twenty patients on this dosage one had a proven attack and two had clinical attacks while actually on the drug, and subsequently when proguanil had been stopped at least one other relapse occurred.

The available data on proguanil in vivax malaria may be summarised as follows :—

(1) The drug is not a true causal prophylactic for vivax infections.   Fairley *et al.* (1946b), with New Guinea strains, suggest that the development of primary exo-erythrocytic forms must be inhibited because of the non-appearance of asexual forms in the red cells while the drug is being taken—a phenomenon which may be described as " partial causal prophylaxis."   In some cases, however, blood forms and a clinical attack have occurred during the time that proguanil is actually being taken, so that the action of proguanil as a causal prophylactic is restricted.

(2) A clinical attack of malaria can sometimes, but not invariably, be brought to an end with doses of 300 mgm. per day and frequently with very much smaller doses, but the infection is not eradicated and the primary attack may be delayed for as long as nine months.

(3) The minimal dose for efficient suppression of all strains of vivax malaria is not yet known.   It is obvious that doses of 100 mgm. once or even twice a week are of value only for a few localised strains.   A dose of 100 mgm. daily is probably the most effective dosage, but it seems doubtful whether even this dosage is more effective than 100 mgm. daily of mepacrine.

The old difficulty of radical cure of vivax malaria thus still remains. The exo-erythrocytic forms which are the cause of relapses in vivax malaria are apparently resistant to proguanil as they are resistant to every other known drug except pamaquin in large and almost toxic doses.

Sporozoites. Proguanil has no direct action on sporozoites and a large dose of proguanil concentrated at the brief period when sporozoites are in the circulation is less active in controlling infection than 100 mgm. given some days later. Sporozoites of *P. gallinaceum* exposed *in vitro* to a solution of 5 mgm. per litre of proguanil at 39° C. are still able to infect chicks one hour later (Davey, 1946b). The indirect action of proguanil on sporozoites is due to its inhibitory action on the development of the oöcyst in the mosquito.

The main value of proguanil in the clinical suppression of acute attacks lies in its low toxicity, especially for pregnant women and children. Often patients with severe symptoms experience a sense of positive well-being within one or two hours of taking the drug. Unpleasant gastro-intestinal effects can be reduced by taking the drug on a full stomach with a glass of water.

***P. malariæ* Infections.** The action of proguanil on *P. malariæ* has received comparatively little intensive study, but all the evidence shows that it acts schizonticidally but less strongly than in the case of *P. falciparum* and *P. vivax*.

Afridi (1947), however, in India, found that thirty-seven of forty-one cases showed subsidence of fever within three days when a single dose of 300 mgm. was administered ; with other more prolonged treatments three of six patients exhibited a similar response. Some cases of *P. malariæ* infection from Assam and Baluchistan failed to react to proguanil and had to be given other treatment. Jafar (1947), after a single dose of 300 mgm., reported that eleven out of twenty-one cases showed disappearance of asexual parasites from the blood in three days and in from three to six days a further five became free from parasites. Ciuca *et al.* (1948b), using a strain of *P. malariæ* originally of African origin, found that it was comparatively resistant to proguanil. In four of twelve cases fever did not abate till after four or five days' treatment despite 600 mgm. daily. Treatment should be continued for ten days. Schneider and Méchali (1949) treated thirteen patients infected by *P. malariæ* in West Africa with daily doses of from 0·3 to 1 gm. Results were as effective with 0·3 as with 1 gm., but proguanil was slower than chloroquine in controlling fever and parasitæmia. The duration of fever after treatment was from one to four days, average three days, and the duration of asexual parasitæmia from 6·5 to 10 days. There was no action on gametocytes.

The trophozoites of *P. malariæ* can grow to full size in tissue culture and are less susceptible than those of *P. vivax* : the action of proguanil seems to be limited to the early stages of schizogony (Mackerras and Ercole, 1947). Schizogony may occur up to the twentieth hour after beginning therapy, and with low dosages the resulting merozoites grow to full size.

Proguanil thus does not appear to have any advantage over other drugs in the treatment of infections due to *P. malariæ*.

In practical application, therefore, proguanil can act as a true causal prophylactic against certain strains of *P. falciparum*. Beyond this it does nothing that cannot be done equally with chloroquine or mepacrine, and in addition it cannot produce a radical cure of falciparum infections. There are, however, strong indications that its mode of action is different and that it may act with some strains against the non-circulating stages immediately preceding the erythrocytic cycle. The only loop-hole in the proof of this statement is the possibility that a highly effective metabolic product of proguanil persists into the period of erythrocytic schizogony, a possibility suggested by Fairley *et al.* (1947). Against this is the fact recorded by Fairley *et al.* (1946b) that positive subinoculation has been secured on the third day of the therapy of acute attacks despite doses of 1·0 gm. of proguanil daily. The actual blood levels of proguanil do not answer the question why there is persistence of effect. Despite the rather rapid decline in the proguanil blood-level, the effect persists for a longer period and is associated, at any rate in avian malaria (Hawking, 1947), with an active metabolic product formed in the animal host.

Much further work will obviously have to be undertaken before the true place of proguanil in antimalarial therapy can be assessed.

In the case of *P. vivax* proguanil is not a true causal prophylactic : it controls clinical symptoms but does not prevent relapses. As a suppressive it appears to have a similar action to mepacrine or chloroquine, but to be effective it must be taken in a daily dose of at least 100 mgm. for adults.

In the case of *P. falciparum*, it acts as a true causal prophylactic. In controlling symptoms and parasitæmia its action is slow and in some cases ineffective.

As a suppressive it appears to act satisfactorily with some strains. There is, however, a wide belt stretching from Nigeria, the Belgian Congo, through the Anglo-Egyptian Sudan to Arabia and possibly India, in which some local strains of *P. falciparum* are not well controlled even by 100 mgm. daily (Abbott, 1949 ; Davey and Smith, 1949 ; Jellife, 1949 ; Kay, 1949). Intercurrent bacterial or helminthic infections from which a high percentage of Africans suffer may decrease the efficacy of proguanil suppression.

In treatment there are few toxic symptoms, and in some cases a feeling of well-being. On the other hand, there have been complaints from those who have taken 100 mgm. daily for some months that lassitude, anorexia, and looseness of stools are common. The possibility that proguanil can produce resistant strains requires further study.

Pamaquin

Pamaquin, synthesised in 1926, was the first of the synthetic drugs to be produced in the laboratory with the object of attacking human malaria. Like so many other drugs, it has suffered from a plethora of names and has been known as plasmoquine, plasmochin, leprochin, præquine, quipényl, and pamaquine. Its action in human malarias was first investigated by Sioli (1926) and Mühlens (1926), who found that it acted on the asexual intraerythrocytic forms of *Plasmodium malariæ* and to a lesser extent on those of *P. vivax*. On the asexual forms of *P. falciparum*, however, it had little effect and it was soon realised that the great schizonticidal activity which it possessed in cathemerium malaria in canaries did not hold good in the human malarias. In addition the numerous toxic reactions appeared to be a limiting factor in its use. Nevertheless it was found that it is an active gametocyticidal agent, more especially in infections due to *P. falciparum*. Against the sexual forms of *P. vivax* it is much less active (Ciuca *et al.*, 1942). Its value in destroying the gametocytes of *P.falciparum* was well brought out by Dick and Bowles (1947). In Somali soldiers who received no treatment gametocytes of *P. falciparum* were present in the blood for more than nine days, and in an untreated group of Somali villagers for more than twelve days. When however pamaquin was given in doses of 0·01 gm. three times a day for five days the mean survival time of gametocytes in the blood was two days in the Somali village group and three days in the Somali askari group.

As a direct gametocyticide pamaquin is still the most active of the synthetic antimalarials. Evidence was also forthcoming that pamaquin could act as a true causal prophylactic against both vivax and falciparum malarias. Doses of 80 mgm. of the base were found by James (1931) and James *et al.* (1931) to be required on the day before infection with sporozoites, on the actual day of infection, and for the six succeeding days. Thus pamaquin was shown to act either on the sporozoites or on the early exo-erythrocytic forms. It should be noted that whereas pamaquin naphthoate contains only 45 per cent. of the active base the hydrochloride contains 90 per cent. The dose of the former is therefore twice that of the latter compound.

In addition, Sinton and Bird (1928) and Sinton *et al.* (1930) showed that if combined with quinine and continued over a considerable period of time pamaquin could eradicate vivax infections, presumably by destroying the exo-erythrocytic forms, the combination of quinine and pamaquin being superior to either drug alone. Thus in one series of cases there were 75 per cent. of relapses in an eight weeks period of observation when quinine alone was administered, 25 per cent. of relapses when pamaquin alone was given, and essentially no relapses at all when the two drugs were given in combination.

Further evidence of the value of quinine and pamaquin in preventing vivax relapses by destruction of the exo-erythrocytic forms is discussed on p. 476.

Soon after pamaquin became available for general use it was realised that the doses which had been recommended prophylactically and curatively verged on the toxic. Rice (1932) and

Brown (1933), for instance, showed that though daily doses of
0·03 or 0·06 gm. would undoubtedly act as a true causal prophylactic against *P. falciparum*, yet toxic reactions were frequent,
and even in the daily dose of 0·02 gm. employed by Henderson
(1934) in the Sudan, though malarial morbidity was reduced by
half, toxic reactions were common.

In the earlier experiments in India, when pamaquin was given
in combination with quinine, it had been usual to continue treatment for fourteen to twenty-one days, the usual period for which,
twenty years ago, quinine was administered. When it was shown
that the therapeutic effects of mapacrine were not enhanced by
continuing treatment for more than seven days the idea gradually
spread that pamaquin too could safely be given for this short
treatment. Thus the Malaria Commission of the League of Nations
recommended that for treatment quinine and pamaquin should
not be given for more than seven days with a daily dose of pamaquin not exceeding 27 mgm. For prophylaxis very small doses of
pamaquin were proposed, not exceeding 10 mgm. per diem, or
alternatively 20 mgm. once or at the most twice a week. In such
a dosage pamaquin has little or no action in controlling an acute
vivax infection although it may still act as a gametocyticide. In
prophylaxis also it was shown by Field (1939) that, at any rate in
Malaya, a dose of 20 mgm. twice a week throughout the year had
no appreciable effect on the incidence of malaria.

When in 1940 war broke out in hyperendemic malarial areas the
curative value of large doses of pamaquin had been forgotten
and the toxic effects alone were remembered ; its prophylactic
administration was regarded as impractical.

More recent investigations have tended to confirm the earlier
views of the value of pamaquin in the treatment of malaria at
any rate in Caucasians.

Feldman *et al.* (1946), for instance, have confirmed that pamaquin naphthoate in doses of 160 to 180 mgm. a day is a true causal
prophylactic against mosquito-induced *P. vivax* (McCoy strain)
and *P. falciparum* infections, although even with slightly higher
doses than were used by James some individuals still showed an
infection. Similarly Jones *et al.* (1948a), using the Chesson strain,
found that only two of five subjects were protected by a daily

dose of 90 mgm. given on the day before infection, the actual day, and for six days thereafter. Berliner *et al.* (1948a) found that daily doses of 30 mgm. or more resulted in temporary suppression of parasites and fever in volunteers infected with blood containing *P. vivax* (McCoy strain), while daily doses of 4 to 20 mgm. for four days caused partial or temporary suppression of parasitæmia in ten of eleven volunteers : the effects obtained were not as clearly related to plasma drug concentration as to the daily dose of the drug. In four patients who were given pamaquin for eight days a radical cure was produced in one subject who received a daily dose of 90 mgm.

With blood-induced falciparum infections due to the McClendon and Costa strains doses of 30 or 60 mgm. daily for six days caused interruption of the fever and diminution in parasitæmia, the blood being completely free from parasites in only two of thirteen subjects. The action of pamaquin in controlling a clinical attack was less marked with the McClendon than with the Costa strain. Thus there are strain differences with *P. falciparum* as well as differences between *P. vivax* and *P. falciparum* in their reaction to pamaquin.

Pamaquin alone probably has a curative action in vivax infections induced by sporozoites if continued for fourteen days (Berliner *et al.*, 1948a), but this action in producing a radical cure becomes definite when pamaquin is combined with quinine (p. 476). The importance of giving quinine concurrently with pamaquin has been re-emphasised by Ruhe *et al.* (1949a).

An attempt at the suppression of malaria by pamaquin alone was begun by Decourt *et al.* (1936) in the region of Cap Bon, in Tunisia : it was continued by Dupoux *et al.* (1939), and after an interval reintroduced in 1946 at Gabès by Schneider *et al.* (1948). Three tablets of 0·01 gm. of pamaquin were given weekly for the first month of the malaria season from May 5th, and after that every ten days till the end of November.

The splenic index in children for the whole region at the beginning of the malaria season was 35·27 per cent. and at the end of the period 17·27 per cent. ; in adults the index fell from 10·27 to 6·5 per cent. The parasite rate for children fell from 14·21 to 0·61 per cent. and for adults 6·87 to 1·25 per cent. Among a population of 32,880 there were only twenty-seven cases of malaria, nine children and eighteen adults, but in two neighbouring areas which were uncontrolled there was an autumnal epidemic of malaria. No cases of toxæmia were seen.

Although pamaquin was first introduced as a result of its action in inhibiting the schizogony of *P. cathemerium* in the canary, further investigations have shown that avian malarias exhibit considerable variation in their reaction to pamaquin.

Thus Dearborn and Marshall (1947) give the quinine equivalent of pamaquin in ducks against *P. circumflexum* as 32, *P. lophuræ*, *P. cathemerium*, and *P. relictum* as 64. In *P. cathemerium* infections in ducks 1·4 mgm. per kgm. a day will bring about a 50 per cent. reduction in parasite counts, but to cure 50 per cent. of ducks 23 mgm. per kgm. per day is required (Walker *et al.*, 1946). Earlier observations on the effects of pamaquin on bird malaria are given by Curd (1943).

In infections due to *Hæmoproteus orizivoræ* (Mazza, 1928 ; Collier and Krause, 1929 ; Kikuth, 1932) and to *H. columbæ* (Godoy and Lacorte, 1928 ; Coatney, 1935 ; Rivero and Ramirez, 1940) the gametocytes are readily attacked but schizonts are unaffected (Kikuth, 1935 ; Kikuth and Schönhöfer, 1935). There is evidence of action on the asexual forms of *P. relictum, P. cathemerium, P. circumflexum, P. elongatum, P. rouxi, P. vaughani, P. gallinaceum, P. hexamerium* and *P. paddæ*, but only with *P. cathemerium* (Russell, 1931a and b), *P. elongatum* (Manwell, 1930a and b, 1934), *P. rouxi* (Manwell, 1932, 1934) and *P. vaughani* (Manwell and Haring, 1938) are there claims to have obtained complete sterilisation.

In *P. knowlesi* infections in rhesus monkeys pamaquin shows an effect on the asexual blood forms which is probably greater than that of quinine or mepacrine, but the infection is not eradicated (Nauck, 1934 ; Fulton and Yorke, 1941).

There is evidence, however, that either alone or in combination with quinine, pamaquin will produce a radical cure of established infections in the monkey due to *P. cynomolgi* (Schmidt *et al.*, 1948).

Against blood infections with *P. berghei* in mice pamaquin has a chemotherapeutic index of 1 : 4. It is active in a dose of 3·25 mgm. per kgm. given subcutaneously, and the LD 50 for mice

is 13 mgm. per kgm. (Schneider *et al.*, 1949).   Goodwin (1949)
found the quinine equivalent against blood-induced infection with
P. berghei to be two, whereas against *P. gallinaceum* in chicks
the quinine equivalent of pamaquin is eighteen.

A curious synergistic effect of pamaquin and other 8-amino-
quinolines with naphthoquinones has been observed by Walker
(1947) in *P. cathemerium* infections in the duck.   The amount of
pamaquin necessary to eradicate infection was the same as the
maximum tolerated dose and the same was found to be true of
other 8-aminoquinolines and of a naphthoquinone such as
SN 12,230.   If pamaquin or one of the other 8-aminoquinolines
and the naphthoquinone were added to the diet of ducks, one-eighth
of the maximum tolerated dose of the aminoquinoline and one-
eighth of the maximum tolerated dose of the naphthoquinone were
sufficient to produce a complete cure : this is equivalent to a four-
fold potentiation.   An eight-fold potentiation has also been
observed, as well as potentiation between pamaquin and two other
naphthoquinones, SN 13,936 and SN 5,949 (2-hydroxy-3-(2-
methyl-octyl)-1, 4-naphthoquinone).

Rhodoquine

Rhodoquine, (Fourneau 710), 6-methoxy-8-diethylamino-*n*-
propylamino-quinoline, was originally prepared by Fourneau *et al.*
(1931 and 1933).   In Java, sparrows infected with *Hæmoproteus
paddæ* it is said to have a chemotherapeutic index of 1 : 100.   The
term rhodoquine was originally applied to all the oxyquinolines
prepared by Fourneau, but it is now restricted to 710.   Rhodoquine
is a yellow powder freely soluble in water.   The Russian product,
plasmocide, is said to be identical with Fourneau 710 and not with
pamaquin.   Bovet and Demanche (1933) found that the action of
rhodoquine on blood-induced infections of *P. relictum* in canaries
was similar to that of mepacrine, but in its action on gametocytes
it is very similar to that of pamaquin.

Rhodoquine has been employed chiefly by French workers.
Monier (1931) claimed good results in vivax infections, but Sautet
(1932), in Corsica, found it of little value except in combination

with quinine and acetarsol, when it was active in vivax, falciparum, and malariæ malaria. Sergent *et al.* (1932) obtained good results in Algeria, but nausea and vomiting were not uncommon.

According to Sicault and Decourt (1934), daily doses of 0·018 to 0·048 gm. (0·3 to 0·8 mgm. per kgm. of body weight) caused rapid disappearance of all parasites except the schizonts of *P. falciparum.* Relapses were prevented only in doses that were toxic. Berny and Nicolas (1936) gave 0·02 gm. of rhodoquine together with 0·3 gm. of mepacrine once a week as a prophylactic : no signs of intolerance were noted, but the value of such a combination is very doubtful.

The Russian compound, plasmocide, was employed by Tanejev (1935), who treated 695 patients and observed toxic reactions, epigastric pain, vomiting, and diarrhœa in 7 per cent. With prophylactic doses at fairly long intervals no toxicity has been observed, but cerebellar ataxia, polyneuritis, and optic atrophy have on occasions been recorded from the therapeutic use of plasmocide.

Tetrahydropamaquin and Related Compounds

Antimalarial action is still retained if the quinoline nucleus of pamaquin or pentaquine is reduced with the formation of 8- (δ - diethylamino - α - methylbutylamino) - 6 - methoxy - 1 : 2 : 3 : 4 -

Compound.	Antimalarial activity against		Toxicity for mice LD 50 mgm./kgm.
	P. gallin- aceum.	*P. relictum.*	
	Minimum effective dose (as base) (mgm./kgm.).		
Tetrahydropamaquin hydrochloride .	2·0	2·5	90
,, naphthoate . .	2·5	2·5	200
Pamaquin hydrochloride . . .	0·5	0·5	16
,, naphthoate . . .	0·625	0·5	50
Tetrahydropentaquine diphosphate .	0·5	4·0	300
Pentaquine monophosphate . . .	0·25	0·5	150
8 - γ - Aminopropylamino - 6 - methoxy - 1 : 2 : 3 : 4 - tetrahydroquinoline hydro- chloride	0·5	4·0	200
8 - γ - Aminopropylamino - 6 - methoxy- quinoline hydrochloride . . .	0·25	2·0	200

tetrahydroquinoline), termed tetrahydropamaquin; 8-(*ω-iso*-propylaminoamylamino)-6-methoxy-1 : 2 : 3 : 4-tetrahydroquinoline, termed tetrahydropentaquine; 8-*γ*-aminopropylamino-6-methoxy-1 : 2 : 3 : 4-tetrahydroquinoline, the tetrahydro-derivative of R 36, 8-*γ*-aminopropylamino-6-methoxyquinoline hydrochloride. Tetrahydropamaquin was first prepared by Barber and Wragg (1946).

The action of these compounds against trophozoite-induced avian infections has been studied by Gray and Hill (1949).

The reduction products were all less active than the parent compounds, but in the case of tetrahydropamaquin and tetrahydropentaquine the toxicity was reduced. Tetrahydropamaquin isethionate has the same activity as pamaquin against *P. falciparum* gametocytes but little or no activity against the trophozoites of *P. vivax*. In man also it is less toxic than pamaquin. Tetrahydropamaquin naphthoate was tested clinically in North Africa and was well tolerated, but its gametocyticidal activity is less than that of pamaquin.

Pentaquine

Of the 8-aminoquinolines which have been investigated in an attempt to find a satisfactory substitute for pamaquin most attention has been directed to pentaquine, SN 13,276, 8-(5′-*iso*-propylaminoamylamino)-6-methoxyquinoline

CH₃O

NH-[CH₂]₅- NH-CH[CH₃]₂

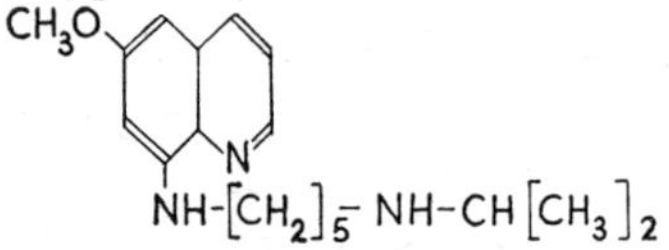

Pentaquine.

In infections in the monkey due to *P. cynomolgi* there is evidence that pentaquine will bring about a radical cure either by itself or in combination with quinine (Schmidt *et al.*, 1948).

In avian malarias, according to Wiselogle (1946), pentaquine has a quinine equivalent of 120 against blood-induced infections of *P. gallinaceum* in the chick and of 150 against *P. lophuræ* in the duck. In tests for prophylactic activity against *P. gallinaceum* it was inactive. For *P. cathemerium* in the duck the curative dose is equal to the maximum tolerated dose. Pentaquine acts synergistically, however, with certain naphthoquinones (Walker, 1947). In man, pentaquine is a true causal prophylactic against the Chesson strain of vivax malaria when given in daily doses of 120 mgm. for at least six days after infection, but this dose produces toxic symptoms in at least half of those subjected to this regime. Jones *et al.* (1948a) found that nine of ten persons infected with sporozoites of the Chesson strain were protected by doses of 120 or 180 mgm. over an observation period of nine to eleven months. The mean plasma concentrations during drug treatment were from 40 to 90 mgm. per litre. As even doses of 60 mgm. daily are liable to cause symptoms, pentaquine is undoubtedly too toxic for use as an ordinary suppressive for long periods (Loeb *et al.*, 1946a). In daily doses of 60 mgm. of the base, equivalent to 80 mgm. of the diphosphate, together with 2 gm. of quinine, in divided doses every four hours for fourteen days, an acute attack is rapidly ended and few relapses occur (*cf.* p. 482). Pentaquine has some curative activity against vivax malaria when administered without quinine. This is discussed on p. 472. Its action against *P. falciparum* requires study.

Pentaquine was tested by Monk (1948) on twenty-five patients suffering from *P. vivax* contracted in India, Burma and the Far East. Rapid clinical cure was produced by 20 mgm. given eight-hourly for ten days, the average duration of pyrexia in the twenty-five patients being 1·2 days, whereas when the same dose of pentaquine was accompanied by 10 gr. of quinine the average duration was 0·73 days.

Other 8-Aminoquinolines

Jones *et al.* (1948a) investigated the therapeutic activity of two other 6-methoxy-8-aminoquinolines, SN 1,452 and SN 11,191. The antimalarial activity of these compounds in comparison with pamaquin is shown in the table at the top of p. 340.

CHEMICAL STRUCTURE, TOXICITY IN THE MONKEY, AND ANTI-
MALARIAL ACTIVITY IN BIRDS OF PAMAQUIN AND OTHER
6-METHOXY-8-AMINOQUINOLINES (Jones *et al.*, 1948a)

Compound.	Aliphatic side-chain in 8-position.	Comparative toxicity in rhesus monkeys.	Quinine coefficient.	
			Gallinaceum in chicks.	Lophuræ in ducks.
Pamaquin .	4-diethylamino-1-methylbutylamino	1	10–40	80
Pentaquine .	5-*iso*propylaminoamylamino .	0·25	100	150
SN 1,452 .	3-aminopropylamino . . .	0·125	40	3
SN 11,191 .	6-diethylaminohexylamino . .	0·5	30	100

The prophylactic action on sporozoite-induced vivax malaria
(Chesson strain) of SN 1,452 and SN 11,191 is shown in the table,
the drugs being given on the day before infection, the day of
infection and three and six days after infection.

PROPHYLACTIC EFFECT OF SN 1,452 AND SN 11,191
(Jones *et al.*, 1948a)

Drug.	Daily dose of base (mgm.).	Number of subjects.	Number protectd.	Period of observation in months.	Parasitic prepatent period in unprotected patients (days).	Mean plasma concentrations (μgm./litre).
SN 1,452	240	3	2	20	21	—
SN 11,191	90	3	2	20	16	⎰120 ⎱110 100

*iso*Pentaquine

*iso*Pentaquine (SN 13,274) is 8-(4'-*iso*propylamino-1'-methyl-
butylamino)-6-methoxyquinoline. It has been studied by Alving
(1948) as the oxalate, which salt contains from 74 to 79 per cent.
of the base. With the Chesson strain of vivax malaria *iso*pentaquine, like pentaquine, will act as a true causal prophylactic if
given for eight days, beginning the day before sporozoite infection.
The dosages required are in the toxic range and its prophylactic
action is thus only of theoretical interest. On blood-induced vivax

malaria the maximum tolerated dose, 240 mgm. of the base daily, given for four days, does not invariably interrupt the erythrocytic cycle in standardised trophozoite-induced infections. *iso*Pentaquine, however, when given intermittently for a few days, will eliminate the gametocytes of *P. falciparum*. The chief value of

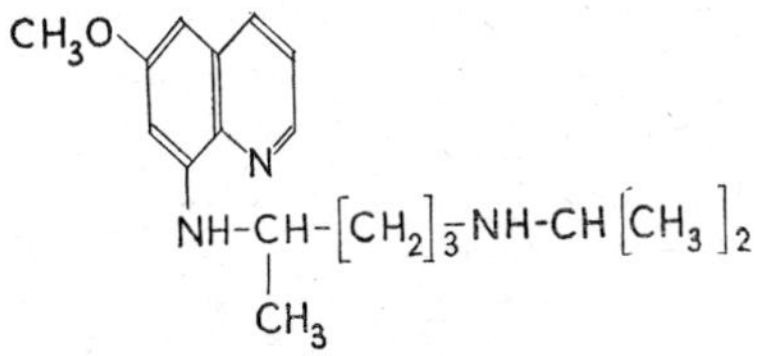

isoPentaquine.

*iso*pentaquine appears to be in its prevention of relapses in vivax infections when given as a dose of 60 mgm. of base daily in association with 2 gm. of quinine sulphate daily for fourteen days during early clinical attacks. There is little to choose between pentaquine and *iso*pentaquine on the basis of their toxicity in doses of 30, 45, and 60 mgm. daily, the last representing the maximum practical therapeutic dose. Acute hæmolytic anæmia has not been observed with *iso*pentaquine, although it appears to be as toxic as pentaquine, but *iso*pentaquine has the advantage over both pamaquin and pentaquine in that the margin between the effective therapeutic dose and the maximum tolerated dose is greater. The maximum tolerated dose in adult white subjects is 240 mgm. per day, or slightly more, and the symptoms at this dosage are equivalent to those observed with 60 mgm. of pamaquin daily. The most marked symptom is methæmalbuminæmia, which can, however, be abolished by the concurrent oral administration of 0·5 gm. of methylene blue daily in divided doses. It is recommended that for an acute primary attack *iso*pentaquine should be given in a daily dose of 60 mgm. of the base in divided doses with 2·0 gm. of quinine sulphate daily for fourteen days : for relapses, 20 to 30 mgm. of the base should be given daily for the same period together with 2·0 gm. of quinine sulphate daily.

Mepacrine

Before the war of 1939–45 very little was known of the activity in malaria of mepacrine, which at various times has been known as atebrin, atabrine, erion or quinacrine (U.S.P.). It has now been clearly demonstrated that mepacrine is not a true causal prophylactic in that it has little action on the schizonts or exo-erythrocytic forms of any malarial parasite, and only in the case of *P. rouxi, P. vaughani,* and *Hæmoproteus orizivoræ,* among the plasmodia attacking birds, is mepacrine capable of rapidly eradicating the infection and producing complete sterilisation (Manwell, 1933 ; Manwell and Haring, 1938 ; Kikuth, 1932, 1935 ; Kikuth and Schönhöfer, 1935). In bird malaria the action is chiefly on the asexual intra-erythrocytic phase. Thus the quinine equivalent of mepacrine hydrochloride, referred to *P. lophuræ* infection in ducks, is *P. circumflexum* 2, *P. lophuræ* 4, *P. cathemerium* 6, *P. relictum* 3 (Dearborn and Marshall, 1947). With *P. knowlesi* mepacrine has given contradictory results. Chopra and Das Gupta (1933, 1934), Christophers and Fulton (1938), Coggeshall and Maier (1941) and Das Gupta and Chopra (1938) all failed to eradicate infection from monkeys, but Malamos (1934) and Nauck (1934 and 1937) found that in occasional animals the parasites were entirely destroyed. *P. cynomolgi* is not radically cured (Schmidt *et al.*, 1948). In doses of 10 mgm. per kgm. of body weight mepacrine will protect against trophozoite-induced infections of *P. cynomolgi* (Genther *et al.*, 1948). Mepacrine has an action on *P. berghei* in mice, the minimum active dose given subcutaneously being 2 to 4 mgm. per kgm. and the toxic dose 230 mgm. per kgm. Thus the chemotherapeutic index is from 1 : 115 to 1 : 57·5 (Schneider *et al.*, 1949). The quinine equivalent against blood-induced infections with *P. berghei* in mice is 7·8 whereas against *P. gallinaceum* in chicks it is 2·0 (Goodwin, 1949). The action of mepacrine on a saurian parasite, *P. floridense,* is solely on young schizonts and merozoites, gametocytes being secondarily affected (Thompson, 1946b).

There is now general agreement that in human malarias mepacrine does not act on the sporozoites or on the exo-erythrocytic forms but solely on the asexual intra-erythrocytic forms. Crucial experiments on human volunteers are recorded by Fairley (1945a). Therapeutic effects in an acute attack are obtained after seven days, and there is no object in administering curative treatment for longer periods. *Plasmodium vivax* infections cannot be eradicated by means of mepacrine. This was clearly shown in the case of New Guinea strains by Fairley (1945a). *P. falciparum*, on the other hand, was sometimes eradicated by continued small doses (Kitchen and Putman, 1942 ; Fairley, 1945b). In West Africa also, *P. falciparum* infections could be entirely eradicated by suitable therapy, as was shown by the reduction in the incidence of blackwater fever (Findlay and Stevenson, 1944 ; Findlay, 1949).

In the treatment of human malarial infections with mepacrine the importance of a large loading dose to obtain a prompt response was first demonstrated by Bryant (1942) in the Anglo-Egyptian Sudan with infections due to *P. falciparum*. On the first day of treatment 0·9 gm. was given, followed by 0·6 gm. on the second day. The superiority of a heavy initial dose of mepacrine, such as 0·8 gm. during the first twenty-four hours, 0·4 gm. on the second and third days, and 0·3 gm. for a further three days, a total of 2·5 gm. in six days, over the more usual 0·3 gm. daily was clearly demonstrated in West Africa (Findlay *et al.*, 1944a and b). Similar results were obtained in carefully controlled experiments by Shannon *et al.* (1944) and Shannon and Earle (1945), in which dosage was correlated with plasma concentrations of mepacrine and with therapeutic effects. It was concluded that the minimum concentration of mepacrine in the plasma necessary for the alleviation of symptoms is 30 μgm. per litre. Ellerbrook *et al.* (1945) found that with a standard course of 2·8 gm. in seven days, plasma concentrations from the second to the eighth day varied from 41 to 52 μgm. per litre ; when 3·2 gm. was given in seven days, the range was 36 to 63 μgm. per litre. Some doubt has since been thrown on the attempted correlation of plasma concentrations and therapeutic response, for Marshall and Dearborn (1946) showed that with *P. lophuræ* infections in the duck parasite response is dependent on the oral dose rather than on the plasma concentration. Similarly, Tonkin and Hawking (1947), in treating trophozoite-induced infections of *P. gallinaceum* in the chick found that the therapeutic response is proportional to the oral dose rather than to the plasma concentration. An eightfold increase in the oral dose causes only a twofold increase in the plasma concentration of mepacrine. The occasional occurrence of parasitæmia in man without symptoms has also been shown by Bang *et al.* (1946a, b) to have no relation to the mepacrine level, since the plasma mepacrine level varied from 10 to 40 μgm. per litre.

In forty patients infected with *P. falciparum* in West Africa and given 2·5 gm. in six days, beginning with 0·8 gm. for the first day, the average duration of fever was 54·9 hours, of symptoms 63·3 hours, and of parasitæmia 43·2 hours (Findlay *et al.*, 1944b) : in the South Pacific area, in patients with *P. vivax* given 2·8 gm. in seven days, beginning with 1·0 gm. on the first day, 64 per cent. had normal temperatures on the second day after treatment and 94 per cent. by the fifth day ; parasites disappeared from the peripheral blood stream in 90 per cent. of cases in thirty-two to forty-eight hours after the initiation of treatment (Ellerbrook *et al.*, 1945). The importance of a large initial dose has been emphasised also by Soviet workers, such as Rotenborg (1945), who perhaps somewhat unnecessarily insist on the administration of 0·3 gm. per os and 0·3 gm. intramuscularly. Baldi and Del Giudice (1948) found 1·5 gm. a day for three days followed by 0·3 gm. for four days superior to 0·3 gm. daily for seven days.

In judging the value of a drug such as mepacrine it is essential to take into consideration the underlying rhythm of the strain of parasite. Some strains of *P. vivax* after an easily suppressed primary attack show a long-latent period followed by a series of late attacks six to eleven months after exposure. Such long-term latency was noted by James, Sinton, and Shute (1937) with Roumanian and Madagascar strains, by Boyd and Kitchen (1945) with the McCoy strain, by Höring (1947) with a Greek strain, and by Cooper *et al.* (1949) with the St. Elizabeth strain. On the other hand, a number of other strains show a much shorter period of latency to relapse. Fairley *et al.* (1945a), with New Guinea strains, reported fourteen to fifty-eight days (mean 29·9 days), Pullman *et al.* (1948) and Coatney *et al.* (1949a) with the Chesson strain forty-four to eighty-eight days. Similar short periods to relapse were noted by Duncan (1945), London *et al.* (1946), Most and Hayman (1946), Bianco *et al.* (1947), with two to four weeks, forty-one days, fifty-three days, and thirty to sixty days as the periods to relapse.

Mepacrine, it seems, does not modify the underlying infection but it modifies the rhythm by increasing the period of latency as a result of the elimination of erythrocytic parasites from the initial wave of invasion. Mepacrine is enabled to do this because of the high concentrations remaining in the body long after administration has ceased. Later attacks are often not controlled with the same ease as the primary attack by mepacrine (Höring, 1947), but Cooper *et al.* (1949), working with the St. Elizabeth strain, showed that if after the first late attack 0·1 gm. of mepacrine were taken daily there were in five volunteers so treated no further attacks. The actual late attacks were treated by 5·2 gm. in twelve days, 0·8 gm. being given on the first day, and 0·4 gm. for the following eleven days.

Just as in man it is advisable to concentrate the drug at the beginning of treatment, so also in the chick infected with *P. gallinaceum*. Tonkin and Hawking (1947) demonstrated that it was advisable to concentrate the drug into the first two days of therapy : with sulphadiazine, on the other hand, the maximum effect is obtained with treatment continued for four days.

If little was known before 1939 of the true capabilities of mepacrine in controlling an acute malarial attack, even less was known of its powers as a suppressive. Earlier experiments of James (1932, 1936) on strains of *P. vivax*, and by Soesilo *et al.* (1933) on *P. falciparum*, had suggested that large doses of mepacrine might destroy sporozoites. Ciuca and his colleagues (1937), however, were able to show that the sporozoites of *P. falciparum* in the salivary glands of Anopheles are able to withstand a concentration of 1 in 2,500 mepacrine for thirty minutes, since they were afterwards able to cause infection in susceptible human subjects. Fairley (1945a), by subinoculation experiments, however, was able to show that mepacrine given at the time of inoculation was not a true causal prophylactic for either *P. vivax* or *P. falciparum*. Confirmatory evidence for the St. Elizabeth strain of *P. vivax* was brought forward by Cooper *et al.* (1949).

Even as a suppressive there was uncertainty before the war as to the effective dose and what was a toxic dose. With indigenous populations living in areas with a definite malarial season there was some evidence that bi-weekly doses of 0·2 gm. of mepacrine given during the malaria transmission season, and for a few weeks afterwards, reduces the number of malarial attacks (Bispham, 1936, and League of Nations, 1937). After the cessation of malaria prophylaxis there was always, however, an excess of cases among those given the drug as compared with attacks among those who had had no prophylactic. This sudden increase in the attack rate must have been due either to delayed primary attacks, the infection having been contracted before prophylaxis began, or to suppression of infection contracted during the period of drug prophylaxis (Field *et al.*, 1937 ; Field and Niven, 1939). Some observers, such as Lambrell (1940) in India, gave 0·2 gm. once a week ; Niven (1938), in Malaya, and Sicault and Messerlin (1937), in Morocco, gave 0·3 gm. once weekly. In Russia, Oganov *et al.* (1937) gave 0·4 gm. every ten days. Field *et al.* (1937) preferred 0·2 gm. on two consecutive days every week. In Malaya 0·3 gm. once a week was more effective than 0·3 gm. a day for five days every five weeks (Field, 1939). Mosna and Canalis (1937), in Sardinia, found that 0·2 gm. twice weekly or 0·05 gm. daily, were both insufficient to prevent all attacks for among 244 persons given the first regimen there were forty-three cases (13·9 per cent.), among 235 given the second regimen fifty-five cases (23.4 per cent.), and among 229 given no prophylactic 161 cases (70·3 per cent.). In Italy, 0·3 gm. twice a week was of some slight value (Canistraci, 1940). Winchester (1937), in the Southern States of America, gave 0·05 gm. daily during the whole of the malaria season. Among 426 persons who took this dose there were no attacks but 202 controls without suppressive had forty-nine attacks.

All these results deal with mepacrine suppression in populations which had either some degree of acquired immunity or a natural resistance against malarial infection. Such factors, as Trager (1947) has pointed out in comparing the effects of mepacrine suppression in European and negro soldiers, are of considerable importance.

With Europeans resident in a hyperendemic area, Junge (1939) showed that it was possible to avoid malarial attacks provided 0·1 gm. of mepacrine was taken daily. Twenty Europeans in Liberia were maintained in health for three and a half years by taking 0·1 gm. and latterly 0·05 gm. daily ; a single dose of 0·3 gm. taken on one day a week was insufficient. Earlier reports from various war zones showed that insufficient doses were being given.

Thus Barber (1943) found that 0·05 gm. daily on week-days and 0·1 gm. on Sundays, a total of 0·4 gm. weekly, was insufficient to prevent acute attacks. Rose (1941) gave 0·06 gm. daily to German soldiers in the Balkan campaign ; these results were uncertain. Findlay and Stevenson (1944) found that under field conditions in West Africa a dose of 0·1 gm. of mepacrine taken on Wednesdays and Saturdays was quite insufficient to protect ; 0·4 gm. weekly, two tablets being taken on Wednesdays and Saturdays, gave some protection for the number of malarial attacks per 1,000 strength among mepacrine takers was 412·4, and among those taking 5 gm. of quinine daily 651·7 per 1,000 strength. When 0·6 gm. was taken weekly the rate of malarial attacks per 1,000 strength fell to 378·8.

For the most part a daily dose of 0·1 gm. was sufficient to suppress malarial infection in the majority of military personnel (Findlay and Stevenson (1944) in West Africa ; Fairley (1945a, b) in New Guinea ; Bang *et al.* (1946a and b) in the South Pacific ; Goldsmith (1946) in Assam).

In a small percentage of instances, however, mepacrine fails to protect against malarial attacks. The reasons for these failures are :—

(1) Failure to take mepacrine regularly.

(2) Arrival in a hyperendemic area with consequent infection before the plasma concentration of mepacrine is sufficiently high.

(3) Failure to absorb mepacrine from the alimentary tract or very rapid destruction in the body.

(4) The strain of parasite.

(5) Inhibition of therapeutic action by competition with essential metabolites.

Studies in New Guinea, West Africa, and Italy (Brown and Rennie, 1946a) show that the most common cause of failure of mepacrine suppression was failure to take the drug regularly, thereby allowing the concentration of the drug in the body to fall to dangerously low levels. Infection could also be established if 0·1 gm. of mepacrine had been taken for an insufficient period before arrival in a hyperendemic zone. A daily dose of 0·1 gm. should almost certainly be taken for twenty-one days before arrival in a hyperendemic zone such as West Africa ; the time can, however, be shortened if 0·3 gm. is taken daily for seven days, or 0·2 gm. daily for fourteen days. The results obtained by the Armored Medical Research Laboratory and Commission on Tropical Diseases (1946) suggest that with a weekly dose of 0·6 gm. (0·1 gm. for six days a week) a period of from three to six weeks is required before the plasma concentration reaches a steady level or " plateau." Becker *et al.* (1946) found fourteen days necessary for stabilisation when 0·1 gm. was taken daily. There is evidence that from personal idiosyncrasy there occur considerable variations in the plasma blood levels of different persons subjected to the same dose-regime ; this variation is distributed logarithmically. There is one small group which shows abnormally high plasma concentrations, and another group, about 7 per cent., which shows abnormally low levels (Armored Medical Research Laboratory, 1946 ; Becker *et al.*, 1946 ; Smith *et al.*, 1946 ; Bang *et al.*, 1946a). These variations in plasma concentrations may be due to defective absorption from the intestine or to the fact, as suggested by Brown and Rennie (1946b), that some persons metabolise mepacrine more rapidly than others.

Some strains of malaria parasite are undoubtedly more resistant to mepacrine than others. As a general rule *P. vivax* is more readily suppressed than *P. falciparum* by 0·1 gm. of mepacrine daily, but whereas on returning from the tropics and ceasing mepacrine suppression it is rare to see attacks of falciparum malaria, vivax attacks are by no means uncommon. Occasional individuals were seen in West Africa in whom *P. falciparum* continued to occur in their blood despite plasma concentrations of more than 30 μgm. per litre. Fairley *et al.* (1946a) found that although faulty discipline was the main cause of failure with mepacrine suppression in New Guinea, in one localised area, Aitaipe-Wewak, there was a local relatively resistant strain of *P. falciparum* for which a double dosage was not too much. This strain was responsible for one-third of the overt attacks of falciparum malaria. This mepacrine-resistant strain was inoculated into volunteers by Fairley *et al.* (1946a), who showed that even 0·2 gm. mepacrine daily was not always effective in suppression, though proguanil in doses of 0·025 to 0·1 gm. daily was a complete causal prophylactic. The strain may have been naturally resistant to mepacrine or may have become resistant in Japanese who were using mepacrine for two years on Wewak (Mackerras, 1946). No evidence of mepacrine-resistant *P. vivax* was obtained in the New Guinea area.

There is a possibility that substances taken in the food or produced in the diet may interfere with the chemotherapeutic action of mepacrine. Thus Seeler (1945) has found that pyridoxine, in a dose of 500 mgm. per kgm. of body weight per os, or 200 mgm. subcutaneously, inhibits the minimal effective dose of mepacrine or quinine against *P. lophuræ* or *P. cathemerium* infection in ducks. Acute toxicity in mice is not affected.

There is no evidence that mepacrine has any direct action on gametocytes. Bang and Hairston (1947) showed that in a body of troops in the South Pacific the gametocyte rate in man and the infection rate in mosquitoes varied in direct relation, but the action of mepacrine in preventing infection is probably an indirect one exercised on the forms which give rise to the gametocytes.

Attention has already been drawn to the fact that when mepacrine was substituted for quinine both in suppression and treatment of malarial attacks, blackwater fever was abolished, among European troops in West Africa. Although mepacrine musonate, or more correctly mepacrine dimethanesulphonate was originally prepared for parenteral administration for which, owing to its extreme solubility in water, it appeared suitable, its toxicity during the Ceylon malaria epidemic of 1934–35 (Briercliffe, 1935) has detracted against its use. It was also generally believed that mepacrine hydrochloride is toxic if given intravenously. Dove (1942) recommended that mepacrine hydrochloride should be given intravenously to patients who were so far gone that absorption after intramuscular injection would be slow. Shannon *et al.* (1944) observed a convulsive seizure in one of five patients given 0·5 gm. of mepacrine hydrochloride intravenously; very similar seizures have, however, been observed in patients with malaria who have never received mepacrine (McGinn and Carmody, 1944). Provided mepacrine hydrochloride is given intravenously in very dilute solution, its toxicity is low. Thus Machella *et al.* (1947) safely gave amounts up to 1 gm. intravenously in falciparum infections, the dose being dissolved in 1 litre of physiological saline and between three and four hours being taken over the injection.

The injection of mepacrine hydrochloride intramuscularly causes considerable necrosis (Hawking, 1943) : this method of administration should therefore be avoided.

2-Chloro-7-methoxy-5-(8-diethylaminobutyl) aminoacridine was tested on *P. knowlesi* infections in doses of 10 to 25 mgm. daily for five days by Siddons and Bose (1944) : it rapidly overcame parasitæmia but in mice it was rather more toxic than mepacrine. No radical cure was obtained.

Suppressive doses of mepacrine may on occasion delay the primary attack due to *P. vivax* for as long as eighteen to twenty-seven months (Bianco *et al.*, 1947 ; Jordan, 1948).

References

ABBOTT, P. H., 1949, Proguanil in the Sudan. *Brit. med. J.*, *i*, 413.

ADAMS, A. R. D., MAEGRAITH, B. G., KING, J. D., TOWNSHEND, R. H., DAVEY, T. H., and HAVARD, R. E., 1945, Studies on synthetic antimalarial drugs. XIII. Results of a preliminary investigation of the therapeutic action of 4888 (paludrine) on acute attacks of benign tertian malaria. *Ann. trop. Med. Parasit.*, **39**, 225.

ADAMS, A. R. D., and SANDERSON, G., 1945a, Studies on synthetic anti-malarial drugs. III. A preliminary investigation of the therapeutic action of 3349 on acute attacks of benign tertian malaria. *Ann. trop. Med. Parasit.*, **39**, 165.

ADAMS, A. R. D., and SANDERSON, G., 1945b, Studies on synthetic anti-malarial drugs. IV. A preliminary investigation of the therapeutic action of 3349 on acute attacks of malignant tertian malaria. *Ann. trop. Med. Parasit.*, **39**, 169.

ADAMS, A. R. D., and SANDERSON, G., 1945c, Studies on synthetic anti-malarial drugs. V. Further investigations of the therapeutic action of 3349 on benign tertian and on malignant tertian malaria infections. *Ann. trop. Med. Parasit.*, **39**, 173.

ADAMS, A. R. D., and SANDERSON, G., 1945d, Studies on synthetic anti-malarial drugs. VI. A comparison of the therapeutic actions of 3349 and of mepacrine hydrochloride on acute attacks of benign tertian malaria. *Ann. trop. Med. Parasit.*, **39**, 180.

ADAMS, A. R. D., TOWNSHEND, R. H., and KING, J. D., 1945, Studies on synthetic antimalarials. XI. An investigation of the therapeutic action of 4430 on benign and malignant tertian malaria. *Ann. trop. Med. Parasit.*, **39**, 217.

AFRIDI, M. K., 1947, A critical review of therapeutic trials on paludrine carried out in India during 1946. *Indian J. Malariol.*, **1**, 347.

ALLEN, W., and THOMSON, T. R. H., 1848, "A narrative of the expedition sent by Her Majesty's Government to the River Niger in 1841, under the command of Captain H. D. Trotter, R.N." 2 Vols. London. R. Bentley.

ANTIMALARIAL DRUGS 351

ALVING, A. S., 1948, Pentaquine (SN 13,276) and *iso*pentaquine (SN 13,274), therapeutic agents effective in reducing relapse rate in vivax malaria. *Proc. 4th Int. Congr. trop. Med. Malariol. Wash.*, Vol. 1, p. 734.

AMANTEA, F., 1922, Il potere curativo della cinconina nella malaria. *Policlinico, sez. prat.*, **29**, 1231.

ANDERSAG, H., BREITNER, S., and JUNG, H., 1941, United States Patent No. 2,233,970.

ANDREWS, W. H. H., GALL, D., and MAEGRAITH, B. G., 1947, Studies on synthetic antimalarial drugs effect of therapeutic courses of paludrine on relapse-rate of vivax malaria. *Ann. trop. Med. Parasit.*, **41**, 375.

APARICO GARRIDO, J., and BENITEZ CALVO, L., 1949, La cloroquina en el tratamiento del paludismo. Acción del medicamento sobre la sintomatologia y la parasitemia. *Med. Colon. Madrid*, **13**, 66.

ARMITAGE, C. H., and MONTANARO, A. F., 1901, "The Ashanti campaign of 1900." London. Sands & Co.

ARMORED MEDICAL RESEARCH LABORATORY AND COMMISSION ON TROPICAL DISEASES, 1946, Plasma quinacrine dosage as a function of dosage and environment. A joint report of the Armored Medical Research Laboratory, Fort, Knox, Ky. and the Commission on Tropical Diseases, Army Epidemiological Board, Preventive Medicine Service, Office of the Surgeon-General, United States Army

ARMY MALARIA RESEARCH UNIT, 1944, Report on 3349. Rept. to Malaria Committee, Medical Research Council. M.L.E. 17.

ASCOLI, V., 1926, Alcuni alcaloidi della china nella cura della malaria. *Policlinico, sez. prat.*, **33**, 370.

BAIKIE, W. B., 1856, "Narrative of an exploring voyage up the Rivers Kwóra and Bínue (commonly known as the Niger and the Tsádda) in 1854." London. J. Murray.

BAKER, G., 1785, Observations on the late intermittent fevers to which is added a short history of the Peruvian Bark, in : "Med. Tracts ; read at the College of Physicians between the years 1767 and 1785. Collected and republished by his son," p. 657 (1818). London. W. Bulmer.

BALDI, A., and DEL GIUDICE, V., 1948, Sui vantaggi delle dosi iniziali alte nella terapia con acridinici (Studio comparativo). *Riv. Malariol.*, **27**, 111.

BALLY, V., 1826, Efficacy of sulphate of cinchonine in intermittent fever. *Lancet*, **9**, 521.

BANG, F. B., and HAIRSTON, N. G., 1947, Studies on atabrine (quinacrine) suppression of malaria. III. The epidemiological significance of atabrine suppression. *Amer. J. trop. Med.*, **27**, 31.

BANG, F. B., HAIRSTON, N. G., MAIER, J., and TRAGER, W., 1946a, Studies on atabrine (quinacrine) suppression of malaria. I. A consideration of the individual failures of suppression. *Amer. J. trop. Med.*, **26**, 649.

BANG, F. B., HAIRSTON, N. G., MAIER, J., and TRAGER, W., 1946b, Studies on atabrine suppression of malaria. II. An evaluation of atabrine suppression in the field. *Amer. J. trop. Med.*, **26**, 753.

BAQUÉ, B., CÉARD, L., KEKESTER, M., and MELNOTTE, P., 1925, Essais de traitement due paludisme par la cinchonine. *Arch. Inst. Pasteur Algér.* **3**, 352.

BARBER, H. J., and WRAGG, W. R., 1946, Contributions to the chemistry of synthetic antimalarials. II. *J. chem. Soc.*, 610.

BARBER, J. F., 1943, A preliminary report on malaria in a combat zone. *Nav. med. Bull. Wash.*, **41**, 977.

BEAVER, P., 1805, "African memoranda relative to an attempt to establish a British settlement on the island of Bulama on the western coast of Africa in the year 1792." London. C. & R. Baldwin.

BECKER, E. R., BURKS, C. S., and KALEITA, E., 1946, Plasma atabrine concentrations attained by subjects taking 0·1 gm. of the drug daily. *J. nat. Mal. Soc.*, **5**, 165.

BECKMAN, H., and SMITH, J., 1944, The apparent advantage of frequently administered quinine in avian malaria infections. *J. Lab. clin. Med.,* 29, 43.

BENNISON, B. E., and COATNEY, G. R., 1948, The sex of the host as a factor in *Plasmodium gallinaceum* infections in young chicks. *Science,* 207, 147.

BERBERIAN, D. A., 1948, Discussion on malaria treatment. *Proc. 4th Int. Congr. trop. Med. Malariol. Wash.,* Vol. I., p. 766.

BERCOVITZ, Z. T., 1945, Malaria complicated by pneumonia : treatment with sulfadiazine and atabrine. *Ann. intern. Med.,* 23, 79.

BERLINER, R. W., EARLE, D. P., Jr., TAGGART, J. V., WELCH, W. J., ZUBROD, C. G., KNOWLTON, P., ATCHLEY, J. A., and SHANNON, J. A., 1948a, Studies on the chemotherapy of the human malarias. VII. The antimalarial activity of pamaquine. *J. clin. Invest.,* 27, Suppl. p. 108.

BERLINER, R. W., EARLE, D. P., Jr., TAGGART, J. V., ZUBROD, C. G., WELCH, W. J., CONAN, N. J., BAUMAN, E., SCUDDER, S. T., and SHANNON, J. A., 1948b, Studies on the chemotherapy of the human malarias. VI. The physiological disposition, antimalarial activity and toxicity of several derivatives of 4-aminoquinoline. *J. clin. Invest.,* 27, Suppl. p. 98.

BERLINER, R. W., TAGGART, J. V., ZUBROD, C. G., WELCH, W. J., EARLE, D. P., Jr., and SHANNON, J. A., 1946, Cinchona alkaloids : I. Appraisal of suppressive antimalarial activity. *Fed. Proc.,* 5, 165.

BERNY, P., and NICOLAS, L., 1936, Note sur la campagne antipaludique effectuée en 1936 à la Crique Anguille (Guyane française) avec la médication mixte (quinacrine-rhodoquine). *Bull. Soc. Path. exot.,* 29, 870.

BIANCO, A. A., SAUNDERS, G. M., LEVINE, A. S., and COHN, R., 1947, Long-term observation of *Plasmodium vivax* malaria in the returned service-man. Part II. Relapses. *Nav. med. Bull. Wash.,* 47, 550.

BINI, G., 1921, La cinconina puó sostituire la chinina. *Policlinico, sez. prat.,* 28, 919.

BISPHAM, W. N., 1936, A report on the use of atabrine in the prophylaxis of malaria. *Amer. J. trop Med.,* 16, 547.

BLACK, R. H., 1947, The effect of antimalarial drugs on *Plasmodium falciparum* (New Guinea strains) developing *in vitro. Trans. R. Soc. trop. Med.,* 40, 163.

BOLDT, T. H., and GOODWINE, C. H., 1949, A second year's field trial with chloroquine suppression of high endemic malaria in a Panamania village. *J. nat. Mal. Soc.,* 8, 238.

BOVET, D., DECOURT, P., SCHNEIDER, J., and MONTEZIN, G., 1948, Activité dans le paludisme aviaire de quelques dérives synthetiques recemment introduits en thérapeutique. *Bull. Soc. Path. exot.,* 41, 268.

BOVET, D., and DEMANCHE, L., 1933, Nouveaux produits actifs dans le paludisme aviaire : une quinoléine de synthèse agissant sur les schizontes et sur les gametes (F. 852). *Ann. Inst. Pasteur,* 51, 528.

BOYD, M. F., and KITCHEN, S. F., 1945, On the employment of quinacrine hydrochloride in the prevention of malaria infections. *Amer. J. trop. Med.,* 25, 307.

BOYLE, J., 1831, " A practical medico-historical account of the western coast of Africa . . . with the causes, symptoms and treatment of the fevers of western Africa." London. S. Highley.

BRAMACHARI, U. N., 1922, Dangers of rapid intravenous injection of concentrated solutions of quinine bihydrochlor. *J. trop. Med. Hyg.,* 25, 209.

BRATTON, A. C., Jr., 1945, Continuous intravenous chemotherapy of *Plasmodium lophuræ* infection in ducks. *J. Pharmacol.,* 85, 103.

BRIERCLIFFE, R., 1935, The Ceylon malaria epidemic, 1934–35. Report by the Director of Medical and Sanitary Services. Sessional papers XXII. Suppl. Colombo. Ceylon Government Press.

BROUGHTON, J., 1871, Chemical and physiological experiments on living cinchona. *Phil. Trans.,* 161, 1.

BROWN, J. Y., 1933, The care, inspection and transportation of live anopheles for use in the malaria therapy of general paralysis. *W. Afr. med. J.*, 1, 78.

BROWN, M., and RENNIE, J. L., 1946a, Suppression of benign tertian malaria with mepacrine : an investigation of 247 cases of apparent failure. *Ann. trop. Med. Parasit.*, 40, 190.

BROWN, M., and RENNIE, J. L., 1946b, Mepacrine metabolism in recurring benign tertian malaria. *Ann. trop. Med. Parasit.*, 40, 337.

BROWNE, SIR THOMAS, 1652, " Pseudodoxia epidemica " in " The works of Sir Thomas Browne," edit. C. Sayle (1912), vol. 2, p. 282. Edinburgh. J. Grant.

BROWNE, SIR THOMAS, 1946, " Letters of Sir T. Browne," edit. Geoffrey Keynes. London. Faber & Faber.

BRUCE-CHWATT, L. J., and BRUCE-CHWATT, J. M., 1950, Antimalarial drugs in West Africa. *Brit. med. J.*, ii, 7.

BRYANT, J., 1942, Heavy atebrin dosage in the treatment of malaria. *E. Afr. med. J.*, 18, 295.

BRYSON, A., 1847, " Report on the climate and principal diseases of the African station ; compiled from documents in the office of the Director-General of the Medical Department, and from other sources, in compliance with the directions of the Right Honorable the Lords Commissioners of the Admiralty, under the immediate direction of Sir William Burnett, M.D., K.C.H., F.R.S." London. W. Clowes & Sons.

CANET, J., 1948, Premiers essais de traitement curatif du paludisme aigu en Cochinchine par un nouveau médicament synthétique : la nivaquine C ou 3038 R P. *Bull. Soc. Path. exot.*, 41, 527.

CANISTRACI, S. C., 1940, Cura e profilassi della malaria con i preparati sintetici. *Riv. Malariol.*, 19, 118.

CHAUDHURI, R. N., 1948, Treatment of malaria. *Indian med. Gaz.*, 83, 225.

CHAUDHURI, R. N., and CHAKRAVARTI, H., 1949, Intravenous " paludrine " (proguanil). *Brit. med. J.*, i, 91.

CHAUDHURI, R. N., and CHAKRAVARTY, N. K., 1948, Clinical trials of Cam-aqi in malaria. *Indian J. Malariol.*, 2, 115.

CHAUDHURI, R. N., and RAI CHAUDHURI, M. N., 1947, Clinical trials of palu-drine. *Indian med. Gaz.*, 82, 247.

CHAUDHURI, R. N., RAI CHAUDHURI, M. N., and CHAKRAVARTY, N. K., 1948, Chloroquine (SN 7,618) in malaria. *Indian J. Malariol.*, 2, 1.

CHEVALIER, A., 1946, Du nouveau sur les plantes à quinquina. *Rev. internat. Bot. appl. Agric. trop. Fr.*, 26, 577.

CHIFFLET (CHIFLETIO), Jean Jacques, 1653, " Pulvis febrifugus Orbis Americani . . . ventilatus." [Louvain.]

CHOMEL, A. F., 1821, Observations sur l'emploi des sulfates de quinine et de cinchonine dans les fièvres intermittentes. *Nouv. J. Méd.*, 10, 257 ; 12, 214.

CHOPRA, R. N., and DAS GUPTA, B. M., 1933, Studies on the action of atebrin in plasmodium infection of monkeys. *Indian med. Gaz.*, 68, 493.

CHOPRA, R. N., and DAS GUPTA, B. M., 1934, Studies on the action of quinine in monkey malaria. *Indian med. Gaz.*, 69, 195.

CHOPRA, R. N., GANGULI, S. K., and ROY, A. C., 1935, On the relationship between the quinine concentration in the circulating blood and parasite count in monkey malaria. *Indian med. Gaz.*, 70, 62.

CHOPRA, R. N., SEN, B., and ROY, A. C., 1937, Individual variations in the effectiveness of synthetic antimalarial drugs (a preliminary note). *Indian med. Gaz.*, 72, 131.

CHRISTOPHERS, S. R., and FULTON, J. D., 1938, Observations on the course of *Plasmodium knowlesi* infection in monkeys (*Macacus rhesus*) with notes on its treatment by (1) atebrin and (2) 1 : 11 normal undecane diamidine together with a note on the action of the latter on bird malaria. *Ann. trop. Med. Parasit.*, 32, 257.

CIUCA, M., BALLIF, L., CHELARESCU, M., and CRISTESCU, A., 1942, Contribution experimentale à la thérapeutique contre le gamétocyte à l'aide de la plasmoquine. Recherches expérimentales sur la dévitalisation des gamétocytes de *P. vivax*. *Arch. roumaines Path. Microbiol.*, 12, 411.

CIUCA, M., BALLIF, L., CHELARESCU, M., ISANOS, M., and GLASER, L., 1937, On drug prophylaxis in therapeutic malaria. *Trans. R. Soc. trop. Med. Hyg.*, 31, 241.

CIUCA, M., BALLIF, L., CHELARESCU, M., TIMISESCO, A., VASILIU-MUNTEANU, F., and VRABIE TROFIM, M., 1948a, Trials of causal prophylaxis of malaria with paludrine. *Bull. World Hlth. Organ.*, 1, 297.

CIUCA, M. BALLIF, L., CHELARESCU, M., TIMISESCO, A., VASILIU-MUNTEANU, F., and VRABIE TROFIM, M., 1950, Paludrine treatment of experimental malaria infection ; effective minimum doses. *Trans. R. Soc. trop. Med. Hyg.*, 43, 435.

CIUCA, M., IRIMESCO, G., MANOLIU, E., ALEXA, —, and CONSTANTINESCO, P., 1925, Essais comparatifs sur l'action thérapeutique de la quinine, de la cinchonine et du quietum dans la malaria. *Bull. Soc. Path. exot.*, 18, 770.

CIUCA, M., SOFLETTE, A., CONSTANTINESCO, P., and TERITEANU, N., 1948b, Preliminary note on the therapy of malaria with paludrine in experimental infection by inoculation of infected blood. *Bull. World Hlth. Organ*, 1, 301.

COATNEY, G. R., 1935, The effect of atebrin and plasmochin on the hæmoproteus infection of the pigeon. *Amer. J. Hyg.*, 21, 249.

COATNEY, G. R., and COOPER, W. C., 1948, The chemotherapy of malaria in relation to our knowledge of exoerythrocytic forms. *J. Parasit.*, 34, 275.

COATNEY, G. R., COOPER, W. C., RUHE, D. S., JOSEPHSON, E. S., YOUNG, M. D., and BURGESS, R. W., 1948, Studies in human malaria. VII. The protective and therapeutic action of quinine sulphate against St. Elizabeth strain vivax malaria. *Amer. J. Hyg.*, 47, 120.

COATNEY, G. R., COOPER, W. C., RUHE, D. S., and YOUNG, M. D., 1949a, Studies in human malaria. XVII. Trials of quinacrine, colchicine (SN 12,080) and quinine against Chesson strain vivax malaria. *Amer. J. Hyg.*, 49, 194.

COATNEY, G. R., RUHE, D. S., COOPER, W. C., JOSEPHSON, E. S., and YOUNG, M. D., 1949b, Studies in human malaria. X. The protective and therapeutic action of chloroquine (SN 7,618) against St. Elizabeth strain of vivax malaria. *Amer. J. Hyg.*, 49, 49.

COGGESHALL, L. T., 1949, quoted by PAYNE *et al.*, 1949, *Amer. J. trop Med.*, 29, 353.

COGGESHALL, L. T., and MAIER, J., 1941, Determination of the activity of various drugs against the malaria parasite. *J. infect. Dis.*, 69, 108.

COLLIER, W. A., and KRAUSE, M., 1929, Zur Chemotherapie der Halteridieninfektion des Reisfinken. *Z. Hyg. InfektKr.*, 110, 522.

COOPER, W. C., RUHE, D. S., COATNEY, G. R., JOSEPHSON, E. S., and YOUNG, M. D., 1949, Studies in human malaria. VIII. The protective and therapeutic action of quinacrine against St. Elizabeth strain vivax malaria. *Amer. J. Hyg.*, 49, 25.

CORDES, W., 1924, Ueber den therapeutischen Wert des Cinchonins bei malaria tropica. *Arch. Schiffs-u. Trop. Hyg.*, 28, 120.

COVELL, G., NICOL, W. D., SHUTE, P. G., and MARYON, M., 1949a, Paludrine (proguanil) in prophylaxis and treatment of malarial infections caused by a West African strain of *P. falciparum*. *Brit. med. J.*, i, 88.

COVELL, G., NICOL, W. D., SHUTE, P. G., and MARYON, M., 1949b, Studies on a West African strain of *Plasmodium falciparum*. The efficacy of paludrine (proguanil) as a prophylactic. *Trans. R. Soc. trop. Med. Hyg.*, 42, 341.

COVELL, G., NICOL, W. D., SHUTE, P. G., and MARYON, M., 1949c, Studies on a West African strain of *Plasmodium falciparum* ; the efficacy of paludrine as a therapeutic agent. *Trans. R. Soc. trop. Med. Hyg.*, 42, 465.

CRAIG, C. F., 1909, " The malarial fevers, hæmoglobinuric fever and the blood protozoa of man." London. J. & A. Churchill.

CULWELL, W. S., COOPER, W. C., WHITE, W. C., LINTS, H. A., and COATNEY, G. R., 1948, Studies in human malaria. XX. The intramuscular administration of chloroquine. *J. nat. Mal. Soc.*, 7, 311.

CURD, F. H. S., 1943, The activity of drugs in the malaria of man, monkeys and birds. *Ann. trop. Med. Parasit.*, 37, 115.

CURD, F. H. S., DAVEY, D. G., and ROSE, F. L., 1945, Studies on synthetic antimalarial drugs. X. Some biguanidine derivatives as new types of antimalarial substances with both therapeutic and causal prophylactic activity. *Ann. trop. Med. Parasit.*, 39, 208.

DAS GUPTA, B. C., BALANKHE, G. T., KOWSHIK, G. N., and HEDGE, M. V., 1947, Paludrine treatment in malaria. Quoted by AFRIDI, M. K., 1947. *Indian J. Malariol.*, i, 347.

DAS GUPTA, B. M., and CHOPRA, R. N., 1938, Studies on the action of synthetic drugs on simian malaria ; sulphonamide derivatives. *Indian med. Gaz.*, 73, 665.

DAS GUPTA, B. M., LOWE, J., and CHAKRAVARTI, H., 1945, M 3349 (Paludrine) in the treatment of human malaria. *Indian med. Gaz.*, 80, 241.

DAVEY, D. G., 1946a, Use of avian malaria for discovery of drugs effective in treatment and prevention of human malaria ; drugs for clinical treatment and clinical prophylaxis. *Ann. trop. med. Parasit.*, 40, 52.

DAVEY, D. G., 1946b, Use of avian malaria for discovery of drugs in treatment and prevention of malaria, drugs for causal prophylaxis and radical cure and chemotherapy of exoerythrocytic forms. *Ann. trop. Med. Parasit.*, 40, 453.

DAVEY, F., and SMITH, M., 1949, Malaria prophylaxis with proguanil. *Brit. med. J.*, i, 956.

DAWSON, W. T., and GARBADE, F. A., 1930, Idiosyncrasy to quinine, cinchonidine and ethylhydrocupreine and other lævorotatory alkaloids of the cinchona series. *J. Amer. med. Ass.*, 94, 704.

DE, M. N., and DATTA, P. N., 1947a, A clinical study of paludrine. *Indian med. Gaz.*, 82, 257.

DE, M. N., and DATTA, P. N., 1947b, Final report on the study of 58 cases of malaria treated with paludrine. *Indian. J. Malariol.*, 1, 373.

DEARBORN, E. H., 1948, A comparison of one dose per day with six doses per day of quinine in the suppression of lophuræ malaria in the duck. *J. Pharmacol.*, 94, 178.

DEARBORN, E. H., and MARSHALL, E. K., Jr., 1947, The susceptibility of different species of avian malarial parasites to drugs. *Amer. J. Hyg.*, 45, 25.

DECOURT, P., MARINI, C., and HENRY, C., 1936, Expériences sur la prophylaxie collective du paludisme réalisées à Menzel-Temime (Cap Bon Tunisien) en 1935. *Bull. Soc. Path. exot.*, 29, 480.

DECOURT, P., and SCHNEIDER, J., 1947a, Traitement curatif du paludisme par divers sels du 3-méthyl-4 (diethylaminopentyl) amino-7-chloroquinoléine (nivaquine). *Bull. Soc. Path. exot.*, 40, 14.

DECOURT, P., and SCHNEIDER, J., 1947b, Tolérance de l'homme pour le chlorhydrate de 3-methyl 7 chloro 4 (diéthylaminopentyl) aminoquinoléine (nivaquine). *Bull. Soc. Path. exot.*, 40, 179.

DELAHOUSSE, J., 1947, Essai d'étude de l'activité thérapeutique de la nivaquine (3038 R.P.) sur le paludisme à *Plasmodium falciparum*. *Bull. Méd. Afrique Occidentale Française*, 4, 203.

DICK, G. W. A., and BOWLES, R. V., 1947, The value of plasmoquine as a gametocide in sub-tertian malaria. *Trans. R. Soc. trop. Med. Hyg.*, 40, 447.

356   *CHEMOTHERAPEUTIC TREATMENT*

DON, C. S. D., and MEYER, P. F., 1944, An unusual case of cerebral malaria. *Brit. med. J.*, *i*, 149.

DOUCET, G., 1948, Note préliminaire sur l'emploi du SN 7,618 en milieu malarien hyperendemique. *Ann. Soc. belge Méd. trop.*, **27**, 341.

DOVE, W. S., 1942, The treatment of malaria. *Amer. J. trop. Med.*, **22**, 227.

DREISBACH, R. H., 1949, Antagonists for fatal and non-fatal doses of quinine intravenously in depressed circulatory states and in hyperthermia. *J. Pharmacol.*, **95**, 347.

DREISBACH, R. H., and HANZLIK, P. J., 1945, Antagonists for the circulatory depression of quinine injected intravenously and the implied cholinergic action, and nature and importance of the vasodilation in the depression. *J. Pharmacol.*, **83**, 167.

DUNCAN, G. G., 1945, Quinacrine hydrochloride as a malaria-suppressive for combat troops. *War Med.*, **8**, 305.

DUPOUX, R., BARTHAS, R., ANTOINE, A., and GARALI, T., 1939, Nouveaux résultats des expériences de prophylaxie collective antipaludique en Tunisie. *Bull. Acad. Med. Paris*, **121**, 591.

DURAND, J. B. L., 1806, " A voyage to Senegal, or historical, philosophical and political memoirs relating to the discoveries, establishments and commerce of Europeans in the Atlantic Ocean from Cape Blanco to the River of Sierra Leone ; to which is added an account of a journey from Isle de St. Louis to Galam." London. R. Phillips.

DUTROULAU, A. F., 1868, "Traité des maladies des Européens dans les pays. chauds (régions tropicals)." 2me Edit. Paris. J. B. Bailliere.

EAMES, W. J., 1861, Fever on the Niger. *Lancet*, *ii*, 604.

EARLE, D. P., Jr., BERLINER, R. W., TAGGART, J. V., ZUBROD, C. G., WELCH, W. J., BIGELOW, F. S., KENNEDY, T. J., Jr., and SHANNON, J. A., 1948a, Studies on the chemotherapy of the human malarias. X. The suppressive antimalarial effect of paludrine. *J. clin. Invest.*, **27**, Suppl., p. 130.

EARLE, D. P., Jr., WELCH, W. J., and SHANNON, J. A., 1948b, Studies on the chemotherapy of the human malarias. IV. The metabolism of cinchonine in relation to its antimalarial activity. *J. clin. Invest.*, **27**, Suppl., p. 87.

EJERCITO, A., and DUQUE, M., 1948, Preliminary report on Cam-Aqi dihydrochloride (miaquin camoquin) in the treatment of human malaria. *J. Philipp. med. Ass.*, **24**, 33.

EJERCITO, A., and SANTOS, G. O., 1937, The Philippine totaquina in the treatment of human malaria : preliminary report. *Mon. Bull. Bur. Hlth., Philippines*, **17**, 219.

ELLERBROOK, L. D., LIPPINCOTT, S. W., CATENO, C. F., GORDON, H. H., and MARBLE, A., 1945, Plasma quinacrine concentration in treatment of *Plasmodium vivax* malaria acquired in the South Pacific. *Arch. intern. Med.*, **76**, 352.

ELMENDORF, J. E., Jr., 1948, Second and supplementary report on field experiments to demonstrate effectiveness of various methods of malaria control. *Amer. J. trop. Med.*, **28**, 425.

ENRIQUEZ-NAVARRO, A. F., and ROGNONI, M., 1948, Uso del aralen (Cloroquina Winthrop) en el tratamiento de la malaria aguda en niños. *Arch. Hospital Santo Tomás*, **3**, 35.

FAIRLEY, N. H., 1945a, Chemotherapeutic suppression and prophylaxis in malaria : an experimental investigation undertaken by medical research teams in Australia. *Trans. R. Soc. trop. Med. Hyg.*, **38**, 311.

FAIRLEY, N. H., 1945b, Medicine in jungle warfare. *Proc. R. Soc. Med.*, **38**, 195.

FAIRLEY, N. H., 1946a, Malaria in the South-West Pacific, with special reference to its chemotherapeutic control. *Med. J. Aust.*, *ii*, 145.

FAIRLEY, N. H., 1946b, The value of M 4430 as a suppressive drug in volunteers exposed to experimental mosquito-transmitted malaria (*P. vivax*—New Guinea strains). Australian Army Medical Research Unit, Cairns, Queensland. R.F.A.(46).5.

FAIRLEY, N. H., BLACKBURN, C. R. B., ANDREW, R. R., MACKERRAS, M. J., ROBERTS, F. H. S., ALLMAN, S. L. W., GREGORY, T. S., BACKHOUSE, T. C., TONGE, J. I., BLACK, R. H., LEMERLE, T. H., ERCOLE, Q. N., POPE, K. G., DUNN, S. R., SWAN, M. S. A., AKHURST, T. A. F., and ROBERTS, E. M., 1947, Sidelights on malaria in man obtained by subinoculation experiments. *Trans. R. Soc. trop. Med.*, **40**, 621.

FAIRLEY, N. H., BLACKBURN, C. R. B., MACKERRAS, M. J., GREGORY, T. S., BLACK, R. H., LEMERLE, T. H., ERCOLE, Q. N., POPE, K. G., DUNN, S. R., SWAN, M. S. A., AKHURST, T. A. F., MACDONALD, I. C., and TONGE, J. I., 1946a, Atebrin susceptibility of the Aitaipe-Wewak strains of *P. falciparum* and *P. vivax*—a field and experimental investigation by L.H.Q. Medical Research Unit, Cairns. *Trans. R. Soc. trop. Med. Hyg.*, **40**, 229.

FAIRLEY, N. H., BLACKBURN, C. R. B., MACKERRAS, M. J., GREGORY, T. S., TONGE, J. I., BLACK, R. H., LEMERLE, T. H., ERCOLE, Q. N., POPE, K. G. DUNN, S. R., SWAN, M. S. A., and AKHURST, T. A. F., 1946b, Researches on paludrine (M 4888) in malaria : an experimental investigation under-taken by the L.H.Q. Medical Research Unit (A.I.F.), Cairns, Australia. *Trans. R. Soc. trop. Med. Hyg.*, **40**, 105.

FELDMAN, H. A., PACKER, H., MURPHY, F. D., and WATSON, R. B., 1946, Pamaquine naphthoate as a prophylactic for malarial infections. *Fed. Proc.*, **5**, 244.

FERRO-LUZZI, G., 1948, La " paludrina " nella terapia della malaria in Eritrea. *Bol. Soc. italiana Med. Ig. trop.*, **8**, 19.

FIELD, J. W., 1934, Notes on totaquina. *Malay med. J.*, **9**, 26.

FIELD, J. W., 1939, " Malaria." *Rep. Inst. med. Res. F.M.S.*, 1938, p. 97.

FIELD, J. W., 1947, Paludrine : a general review. Malaria Advisory Board, Malayan Union. Medical No. 3. Kuala Lumpur. Malayan Union Govern-ment Press.

FIELD, J. W., and NIVEN, J. C., 1939, Malarial chemoprophylaxis. Field observations on post-prophylactic epidemicity. *Compt. rend. Dixième Congrès. Far East. Ass. trop. Med., Hanoi*, Nov. 26th–Dec. 2nd, **2**, 959.

FIELD, J. W., NIVEN, J. C., and HODGKIN, E. P., 1937, The prevention of malaria in the field by the use of quinine and atebrin. Experiments in clinical prophylaxis. *Quart. Bull. Hlth Org. L.o.N.*, **6**, 236.

FIGUEROA, I., 1942, Breve estudio sobre las quinas colombianas. *Bol. Inst. Nac. Hig. Samper Martinez. Bogota.* No. 5, p. 9.

FILIPELLA, P., 1923, Contributo allo studio sulla terapia della malaria con la cinconina. *Policlinico, sez. prat.*, **30**, 464.

FINDLAY, G. M., 1945, Investigations in the chemotherapy of malaria in West Africa. Treatment with paludrine (3349). Rept. to Malaria Committee, Medical Research Council.

FINDLAY, G. M., 1949, Blackwater fever in West Africa, 1941–45. I. Black-water fever in European military personnel. *Ann. trop. Med. Parasit.*, **43**, 140.

FINDLAY, G. M., MARKSON, J. L., and HOLDEN, J. R., 1944a, Investigations in the chemotherapy of malaria in West Africa. I. Treatment with quinine and mepacrine. *Ann. trop. Med. Parasit.*, **38**, 139.

FINDLAY, G. M., MARKSON, J. L., and HOLDEN, J. R., 1944b, Investigations in the chemotherapy of malaria in West Africa. III. Further investiga-tions on treatment with quinine and mepacrine. *Ann. trop. Med. Parasit.*, **38**, 201.

FINDLAY, G. M., and STEVENSON, A. C., 1944, Investigation in the chemo-therapy of malaria in West Africa. II. Malaria suppression—quinine and mepacrine. *Ann. trop. Med. Parasit.*, **38**, 168.

FitzHugh, T., Jr., Pepper, D. S., and Hopkins, H. U., 1944, The cerebral form of malaria. *Bull. U.S. Army med. Dept.*, No. 83, p. 39.

Fletcher, W., 1923, "Notes on the treatment of malaria with the alkaloids of cinchona." London. John Bale, Sons & Danielsson Ltd.

Fletcher, W., 1925, Further notes on the treatment of malaria with cinchona febrifuge, quinidine and cinchoninine. *Bull. Inst. med. Res., F.M.S.*, No. 3.

Fletcher, W., 1934, The therapeutic efficacy of totaquina in human malaria. II. Critical analysis of the results achieved. *Quart. Bull. Hlth Org. L.o.N.*, 3, 344.

Fletcher, W., and Travers, E. A. O., 1923, Quinine idiosyncrasy and cinchonine. *Brit. med. J.*, i, 629.

Fourneau, E., Tréfouel, J., Tréfouel, Madame, Bovet, D., and Benoit, G., 1931, Contribution à la chimiothérapie du paludisme. Essais sur les calfats. *Ann. Inst. Pasteur.*, 46, 514.

Fourneau, E., Tréfouel, J., Tréfouel, Madame, Bovet, D., and Benoit, G., 1933, Contribution à la chimiothérapie du paludisme. Essais sur les calfats (deuxième mémoire). *Ann. Inst. Pasteur*, 50, 731.

Fulton, J. D., and Yorke, W., 1941, Studies in chemotherapy. XXIX. The development of plasmoquine-resistance in *Plasmodium knowlesi*. *Ann. trop. Med. Parasit.*, 35, 233.

Genther, C. S., Squires, W., Fradin, R., and Schmidt, L. H., 1948, Malaria chemotherapy. I. The response of trophozoite-induced infections with *Plasmodium cynomolgi* to various antimalarial drugs. *Fed. Proc.*, 7, 221.

Ghosh, B. N., 1947, Preliminary report on the result of treatment of malaria with paludrine. *Indian J. Malariol.*, 1, 369.

Godoy, A., and Lacorte, J. G., 1928, Action d un noyau de l'oxyamino-quinoléine sur les gamètes et les sporozoites de l'*Halteridium* du pigeon. *C.R. Soc. Biol. Paris*, 98, 617.

Goldsmith, K., 1946, A controlled field trial of SN 7,618–5 (chloroquine) for the suppression of malaria. *J. Malaria Inst. India*, 6, 311.

Goodwin, L. G., 1949, Response of *Plasmodium berghei* to antimalarial drugs. *Nature, Lond.*, 164, 1133.

Gordon, H. H., Dieuaide, F. R., Marble, A., Christianson, H. B., and Dahl, L. K., 1947, Treatment of *Plasmodium vivax* malaria of foreign origin : a comparison of various drugs. *Arch. intern. Med.*, 79, 365.

Gray, A., and Hill, J., 1949, Antimalarial studies in the quinoline series. *Ann. trop. Med. Parasit.*, 43, 32.

Gray, W., and Dochard, —, 1825, "Travels in Western Africa, in the years 1818–21, from the River Gambia, through Woolli, Bondoo, Galam, Kasson, Kaarta and Foolidoo, to the River Niger." London. J.Murray.

Green, R. A., 1945, Totaquine in the treatment of malaria. *Bull. U.S. Army med. Dept.*, No. 84, p. 51.

Halawani, A., Baz, I., and Morkos, F., 1947a, A preliminary report on the antimalarial CAM-AQI. *J. R. Egypt med. Ass.*, 30, 99.

Halawani, A., Baz, I., and Morkos, F., 1947b, On the antimalarial activity of nivaquine C. *J. R. Egypt med. Ass.*, 30, 665.

Halawani, A., Baz, I., and Morkos, F., 1948, Field trials with new anti-malarial drugs in Egypt. *Ann. trop. Med. Parasit.*, 42, 304.

Halliday, A., 1821, "Memorial to the Honorable the Court of Directors for the affairs of the East India Company." Calcutta.

Hamilton, K. S. P., 1947, Paludrine prophylactic and treatment investigation. Quoted by Afridi, M. K., 1947. *Indian J. Malariol.*, 1, 347.

Hanzlik, P. J., and Cutting, C. C., 1945, Clinical trials with quinine-epinephrine intravenously. *J. Amer. med. Ass.*, 129, 1241.

Harned, B. K., and Cole, V. V., 1942, A therapeutic incompatibility between sulfapyridine and quinine. *J. Pharmacol.*, 74, 42.

HAWKING, F., 1943, Intramuscular injection of mepacrine (atebrin). Histological effect. *Brit. med. J.*, *ii*, 198.

HAWKING, F., 1947, Activation of paludrine *in vitro*. *Nature, Lond.*, **159**, 409.

HAYMAN, J. R., Jr., MOST, H., LONDON, I. M., KANE, C. A., LAVIETES, P. H., and SCHROEDER, E. F., 1946, Chloroquine (SN 7,618), a new highly effective antimalarial drug for routine use in treatment of acute attacks of vivax malaria. *Trans. Ass. Amer. Phys.*, **59**, 82.

HENDERSON, L. H., 1934, Prophylaxis of malaria in the Sudan with special reference to the use of plasmoquine. *Trans. R. Soc. trop. Med. Hyg.*, **28**, 157.

HESSE, O., 1872, On chinamine, a new cinchona alkaloid. *Chem. News*, **25**, 191.

HICKS, E. P., and CHAND, D., 1935, The relative clinical efficacy of totaquina and quinine. *Rec. Malar. Surv. India*, **5**, 39.

HOEKENGA, M. T., 1950. Camoquin treatment of malaria : a preliminary report. *Amer. J. trop Med.*, **30**, 63.

HÖRING, R. O., 1947, Induced and war malaria. *J. trop. Med. Hyg.*, **50**, 150.

HOWIE, J. W., and MURRAY-LYON, R. M., 1943, Tanret reaction in subtertian malaria. *Lancet*, *ii*, 317.

HULSHOFF, A. A., 1947, Therapie van malaria. *Acta Leiden. Scholæ Med. trop.* (1948), **18**, 142.

HUTCHINSON, T. J., 1855, " Narrative of the Niger, Tshadda and Binue exploration, including a report on the position and prospects of trade up those rivers, with remarks on the malaria and fevers of Western Africa." London. Longman, Brown, Green and Longmans.

INDIA. SECRETARY OF STATE (1866–70), "Correspondence . . . relating to the cultivation of chinchona plants." London. Ordered by the House of Commons to be printed.

INNES, J. R. M., 1947, The effect of intramuscular injection of paludrine and mepacrine in experimental animals. *Ann. trop. Med. Parasit.*, **41**, 46.

JAFAR, M., 1947, Preliminary report on the result of treatment of malaria with paludrine. *Indian J. Malariol.*, **1**, 365.

JAMES, S. P., 1931, Some general results of a study of induced malaria in England. *Trans. R. Soc. trop. Med. Hyg.*, **24**, 477.

JAMES, S. P., 1932, Synthetic antimalarial remedies and quinine. *Trans. R. Soc. trop. Med. Hyg.*, **26**, 105.

JAMES, S. P., 1936, " Consecutive reports on the antimalarial chemotherapeutic tests carried out at the Devon Mental Hospital from 1932–35." Devon Mental Hospital Printing Press. Exminster.

JAMES, S. P., NICOL, W. D., and SHUTE, P. G., 1931, On the prevention of malaria with plasmoquine. *Lancet*, *ii*, 341.

JAMES, S. P., NICOL, W. D., and SHUTE, P. G., 1932, Study of induced malignant tertian malaria. *Proc. R. Soc. Med.*, **25**, 1153.

JAMES, S. P., SINTON, J. A., and SHUTE, P. G., 1937, in : The treatment of malaria : a study of synthetic drugs, as compared with quinine, in the therapeutics and prophylaxis of malaria. Fourth General Rept. Malaria Commission. *Quart. Bull. Hlth Org. L. o. N.*, **6**, 895.

JAMES, W. M., 1913, The Canal Zone treatment of malaria. *Sth. med. J.*, *Nashville*, **6**, 347.

JELLIFE, D. B., 1949, Proguanil prophylaxis and intercurrent infection. *Lancet*, *i*, 1052.

JESUITS, 1743, "Travels of the Jesuits, into various parts of the world : compiled from their letters. Now first attempted in English . . . by Mr. Lockman." London. J. Noon. 2 Vols. [principally translated from " Lettres édifiantes et curieuses," edit. C. Le Gobien].

JOHNSON, JAMES, 1813, " The influence of tropical climates, more especially the climate of India, on European constitution ; the principal effects and diseases thereby induced, their prevention or removal and the means of preserving health in hot climates, rendered obvious to Europeans of every capacity. An essay." London. J. J. Stockdale.

JOHNSTONE, R. D. C., 1946a, Relapsing benign tertian malaria treated with 4430. *Ann. trop. Med. Parasit.*, 40, 330.

JOHNSTONE, R. D. C., 1946b, Relapsing benign tertian malaria treated with paludrine. *Lancet, ii*, 825.

JOHNSTONE, R. D. C., 1947, Paludrine in relapsing benign tertian malaria; further trials. *Lancet, i*, 674.

JONES, R., Jr., CRAIGE, B., Jr., ALVING, A. S., WHORTON, C. M., PULLMAN, T. N., and EICHELBERGER, L., 1948a, A study of the prophylactic effectiveness of several 8-aminoquinolines in sporozoite-induced vivax malaria (Chesson strain). *J. clin. Invest.*, 27, Suppl., p. 6.

JONES, R., Jr., PULLMAN, T. N., WHORTON, C. M., CRAIGE, B., Jr., ALVING, A. S., and EICHELBERGER, L., 1948b, The therapeutic effectiveness of large doses of paludrine in acute attacks of sporozoite-induced vivax malaria (Chesson strain). *J. clin. Invest.*, 27, Suppl., p. 51.

JORDAN, W. S., Jr., 1948, Primary attack of vivax malaria occurring twenty-seven months after infection. *New Engl. J. Med.*, 239, 397.

JUNGE, W., 1939, Zur Dauervertraglichkeit und Dosierung der Atebrin-Prophylaxe. *Arch. Schiffs-u. Tropenhyg.*, 43, 409.

KAHN, N. E., 1945, Cerebral malaria. *J. R. Army med. Corps.*, 84, 263.

KAMAL, A. M., and ABDEL MESSIH, G., 1947, Aralen, a new antimalarial compound, SN 7618. *J. Egypt. publ. Hlth. Ass.*, 22, 31.

KAY, H. E. M., 1949, Resistance to proguanil. *Lancet, i*, 712.

KELSEY, F. E., OLDHAM, F. K., CANTRELL, W., and GEILING, E. M. K., 1946, Antimalarial activity and toxicity of a metabolic derivative of quinine. *Nature, Lond.*, 157, 440.

KIEGEL, B., and SHERWOOD, L. T., Jr., 1949, The resolution of chloroquine SN 7,618. *J. Amer. chem. Soc.*, 71, 1129.

KIERLAND, R. R., and McCREIGHT, W. G., 1948, The termination of therapeutic malaria with chloroquine. *Amer. J. Syph.*, 32, 57.

KIKUTH, W., 1932, Chemotherapeutische Versuche mit neuen synthetischen Malariamitteln in ihrer Bedeutung für die Bekämpfung der Malaria. *Zbl. Bakt. I. Orig.*, 127, 172.

KIKUTH, W., 1935, Die experimentelle Chemotherapie der Malaria. *Dtsch. med. Wschr.*, 61, 573.

KIKUTH, W., 1945, Zur Weiterentwicklung der Malariatherapie : Sontochin ein neues synthetisches Malaria heilmittel. Pharmaceuticals : Research and Manufacture at I.G. Farbenindustrie. Final Rept. No. 116. Append. 4. Brit. Int. Objectives Subcommittee. London. H.M. Stationery Office.

KIKUTH, W., and SCHÖNHÖFER, F., 1935, Das Plasmochin und Atebrin. *Münch. med. Wschr.*, 82, 304.

KITCHEN, S. F., and PUTMAN, P., 1942, Observations on mechanisms in falciparum malaria. *Amer. J. trop. Med.*, 22, 361.

KLIGLER, I. J., SHAPIRO, J. M., and WEITZMAN, I., 1924, Malaria in rural settlements in Palestine. *Trans. R. Soc. trop. Med. Hyg.*, 17, 259.

KNOPPERS, A. T., 1948, Le problème du totaquina. *Rev. Palud.*, 6, 97.

KUTUMBIAH, P., and ANANTHACHARI, M. D., 1947, Report on the treatment of malaria with paludrine. Quoted by AFRIDI, M. K., 1947. *Indian J. Malariol., i*, 347.

LAIRD, M., and OLDFIELD, R. A. K., 1837, " Narrative of an expedition into the interior of Africa, by the River Niger, in the steam-vessels *Quorra* and *Alborkah*, in 1832, 1833 and 1834." 2 Vols. London. R. Bentley.

LAMBRELL, B. A., 1940, Quinine and atebrin in the control of malaria ; with special emphasis on the practical and economic view points. *Indian med. Gaz.*, **75**, 266.

LANDER, R., and LANDER, J., 1832, " Journal of an expedition to explore the course and termination of the Niger ; with a narrative of a voyage down that river to its termination." (Edited by A. B. B., *i.e.*, A. B. Becher.) London. J. Murray.

LEAGUE OF NATIONS, 1933, Third general Report of the Malaria Commission. The therapeutics of malaria : principles of treatment based on the results of controlled experiments. *Quart. Bull. Hlth Org. L.o.N.*, **2**, 181.

LEAGUE OF NATIONS, 1937, Fourth general Report of the Malaria Commission. The treatment of malaria ; study of synthetic drugs, as compared with quinine, in the therapeutics and prophylaxis of malaria. *Quart. Bull. Hlth Org. L.o.N.*, **6**, 895.

LIND, JAMES, 1768, "An essay on diseases incidental to Europeans in hot climates." London. T. Becket and P. A. de Hondt.

LIND, JAMES, 1777, "An essay on the diseases incidental to Europeans in hot climates." 3rd Edition. London. T. Becket.

LINDSAY, D. K., 1943, Guidance notes on pernicious malaria. *Trans. R. Soc. trop. Med. Hyg.*, **37**, 63.

LOBATO PARAENSE, W., 1947, Ação patogênica das formas exo-eritrocritarias do *Plasmodium gallinaceum*. 3. Algumas caracteristicas das hemácias nas infecções tratadas com quina. *Mem. Inst. Osw. Cruz.*, **45**, 345.

LOEB, R. F., CLARK, W. M., COATNEY, G. R., COGGESHALL, L. T., DIEUAIDE, F. R., DOCHEZ, A. R., HAKANSSON, E. G., MARSHALL, E. K., Jr., MARVEL, C. S., McCOY, O. R., SAPERO, J. J., SEBRELL, W. H., SHANNON, J. A., and CARDEN, G. A., Jr., 1946a, Activity of a new antimalarial agent, pentaquine (SN 13,276). Statement approved by a Board for Co-ordination of Malarial Studies. *J. Amer. med. Ass.*, **132**, 321.

LOEB, R. F., CLARK, W. M., COATNEY, G. R., COGGESHALL, L. T., DIEUAIDE, F. R., DOCHEZ, A. R., HAKANSSON, E. G., MARSHALL, E. K., Jr., MARVEL, C. S., McCOY, O. R., SAPERO, J. J., SEBRELL, W. H., SHANNON, J. A., and CARDEN, G. A., Jr., 1946b, Activity of new antimalarial agent, chloroquine (SN 7,618) : statement approved by Board for Co-ordination of Malarial Studies. *J. Amer. med. Ass.*, **130**, 1069.

LOMAX, P. H., 1947, Paludrine treatment enquiry in Assam. *Indian J. Malariol.*, **1**, 389.

LONDON, I. M., KANE, C. A., SCHROEDER, E. F., and MOST, H., 1946, Delayed primary attack of vivax malaria. *New Engl. J. Med.*, **235**, 406.

LUCENA, D. T., 1948, Tratamento da malária pelo aralen. *Rev. brasil. Med.*, **5**, 269.

MACBRIDE, D., 1777, " A methodical introduction to the theory and practice of the art of Medicine," 2nd edit., 2 vols. Dublin. W. Watson.

McCARRISON, R., and CORNWALL, J. W., 1919, Pharmaco-dynamics of quinine. *Indian J. med. Res.*, **6**, 248.

MACGILCHRIST, A. C., 1915, The relative therapeutic value in malaria of the cinchona alkaloids—quinine, cinchonine, quinidine, cinchonidine and quinoidine and the two derivatives—hydro-quinine and ethyl-hydro-cupreine. *Indian J. med. Res.*, **3**, 1.

McGINN, S., and CARMODY, J. T. B., 1944, Cerebral symptoms in malaria. *Nav. med. Bull. Wash.*, **43**, 1157.

MACHELLA, T. E., KIMMELMAN, L. J., and LEWIS, R. A., 1947, The intravenous administration of atabrine in falciparum malaria. *Bull. U.S. Army med. Dept.*, **7**, 1009.

MACKERRAS, I. M., 1946, Malaria in the South-West Pacific. *Med. J. Aust.*, **ii**, 249.

MACKERRAS, M. J., and ERCOLE, Q. N., 1947, Observations on the action of paludrine on malarial parasites. *Trans. R. Soc. trop. Med. Hyg.*, **41**, 365.

McWILLIAM, J. O., 1843, " Medical history of the Niger expedition during the years 1841–42, comprising an account of the fever which led to its abrupt termination." London. J. Churchill.

MAEGRAITH, B. G., ADAMS, A. R. D., KING, J. D., TOWNSHEND, R. H., DAVEY, T. H., and HAVARD, R. E., 1945, Studies on synthetic antimalarial drugs. XIV. Results of a preliminary investigation of the therapeutic action of 4888 (paludrine) on acute attacks of malignant tertian malaria. *Ann. trop. Med. Parasit.*, **39**, 232.

MAEGRAITH, B. G., ADAMS, A. R. D., KING, J. D., TOTTEY, M. M., RIGBY, D. J., and SLADDEN, R. A., 1946a, Paludrine in the treatment of malaria. *Brit. med. J.*, i, 903.

MAEGRAITH, B. G., ADAMS, A. R. D., KING, J. D., RIGBY, D. J., SLADDEN, R. A., and TOTTEY, M. M., 1946b, Treatment of B.T. and M.T. malaria with paludrine. *Trans. R. Soc. trop. Med. Hyg.*, **40**, 1.

MAEGRAITH, B. G., ADAMS, A. R. D., ANDREWS, W. H., and TOTTEY, M., 1947, Relapse of benign tertian malaria during a course of 100 mgm. paludrine weekly. *Trans. R. Soc. trop. Med. Hyg.*, **40**, 366.

MAEGRAITH, B. G., and ANDREWS, W. H. H., 1949, Proguanil and falciparum malaria. *Brit. med. J.*, i, 545.

MALAMOS, B., 1934, Die Rolle des Retikulo-Endothetialen Systems, insbesondere der Milz bei Affenmalaria. *Arch. Schiffs.-u. Tropenhyg.*, **38**, 326.

MANFREDI, M., 1948, Prove di trattamento con paludrina (Farma 01015) nella malaria da vivax. *Acta med. ital.*, **3**, 205.

MANWELL, R. D., 1930a, Further studies on the effect of quinine and plasmo chin on the avian malarias. *Amer. J. trop. Med.*, **10**, 379.

MANWELL, R. D., 1930b, The varying effects of quinine and plasmochin on the different avian malarias. *J. Parasit.*, **17**, 110.

MANWELL, R. D., 1932, Quinine and plasmochin therapy in *Plasmodium rouxi* infections, with further notes on the effects of these drugs on the other avian malarias. *Amer. J. trop. Med.*, **12**, 123.

MANWELL, R. D., 1933, Effect of atebrine on avian malarias. *Proc. Soc. exp. Biol., N.Y.*, **31**, 198.

MANWELL, R. D., 1934, Quinine and plasmochin therapy in infections with *Plasmodium circumflexum*. *Amer. J. trop. Med.*, **14**, 45.

MANWELL, R. D., and HARING, A. T., 1938, Plasmochin and atebrin therapy in *Plasmodium vaughani* infections. *Riv. Parassitol.*, **2**, 207.

MARANON, J., PEREZ, A., and RUSSELL, P. F., 1935, Philippine totaquina. *Philipp. J. Sci.*, **56**, 229.

MARSHALL, E. K., Jr., 1949, The significance of drug concentration in the blood as applied to chemotherapy, in " Evaluation of Chemotherapeutic Agents," edited by C. M. MACLEOD. Symposia of the section on Microbiology No. 2, p. 3. New York Acad. Med., New York. Columbia University Press.

MARSHALL, E. K., Jr., and DEARBORN, E. H., 1946, The relation of the plasma concentration of quinacrine to its antimalarial activity. *J. Pharmacol.*, **88**, 142.

MARSHALL, P. B., 1945, Loss of antimalarial properties in quinine degradation products. *Nature, Lond.*, **156**, 505.

MARSHALL, P. B., and ROGERS, E. W., 1948, The determination of quinine degradation product in blood and its absorption in the chick. *Biochem. J.*, **43**, 414.

MATTHEWS, J., 1788, " A voyage to the River Sierra Leone on the coast of Africa : containing an account of the trade and productions of the country and of the civil and religious customs and manners of the people, in a series of letters to a friend in England during his residence in that country in the years 1785, 1786 and 1787." London. B. White and Son, and J. Sewell.

ANTIMALARIAL DRUGS 363

MAZZA, S., 1928, Acción de la plasmoquine sobre los gametocitos de infecciones
espontáneas por hemoproteus. *Prensa méd. Argent.*, 15, 55.
MEDICAL RESEARCH COUNCIL, 1925, Clinical comparisons of quinine and
quinidine. *Spec. Rept. Ser. med. Res. Coun. Lond.*, No. 96.
MEIN, R. M., and ROSADO, P. N. S., 1948, Experiência com novos medica-
mentos contra a malária da Amazonia. *Rev. Serv. especial Saudé publ.
Rio de Janeiro*, 1, 1059.
MONIER, H. M., 1931, Essais thérapeutiques du 710 Fourneau dans quelques
cas de paludisme. *Bull. Soc. Path. exot.*, 24, 97.
MONK, J. F., 1948, Results of an investigation of the therapeutic action of
pentaquin on acute attacks of benign tertian malaria. *Trans. R. Soc.
trop. Med. Hyg.*, 41, 663.
MORALES, A. L., 1949, Paludismo y nivaquina-B (cloroquina). Estudio
clínico, parasitológico y epidemiológico. *Rev. San. Hig. Pub.*, 23, 705.
MOSNA, E., and CANALIS, A., 1937, Profilassi e terapia della malaria coi
prodotti sintetici. (Esperienze coordinate dal Comitato d'Igiene della
S.d.N.). *Riv. Malariol.*, 16, Sez. 1, Suppl. No. 3.
MOST, H., and HAYMAN, J. M., 1946, Relative efficiency of quinacrine
(atabrine) and quinine in treatment of acute attacks of vivax malaria.
Amer. J. med. Sci., 211, 320.
MOST, H., LONDON, I. M., KANE, C. A., LAVIETES, P. H., SCHROEDER, E. F.,
and HAYMAN, J. M., Jr., 1946, Chloroquine for treatment of acute attacks
of vivax malaria. *J. Amer. med. Ass.*, 131, 963.
MÜHLENS, P., 1926, Die Behandlung der natürlichen menschlichen Malaria-
infektionen mit Plasmochin. *Arch. Schiffs-u. Tropenhyg.*, 30, Beiheft
No. 3, 25.
MULLICK, K. B., and GUPTA, J. C., 1947, Intravenous paludrine in malaria.
Indian med. Gaz., 82, 666.
MURGATROYD, F., FINDLAY, G. M., and MacCALLUM, F. O., 1939, Long-latent
infection with *Plasmodium ovale* becoming manifest after yellow-fever
vaccination. *Lancet, i*, 1262.
NAUCK, E. G., 1934, Chemotherapeutische Versuche bei Affenmalaria (*Pl.
knowlesi*). *Arch. Schiffs-u. Tropenhyg.*, 38, 313.
NAUCK, E. G., 1937, Die Bedeutung der experimentellen Affenmalaria für die
Malariaforschung, in: "Festschrift Bernhard Nocht zum 80 Geburtstag,"
p. 394. Hamburg. J. J. Augustin.
NIVEN, J. E., 1938, "Malaria." *Rept. Inst. med. Res. F.M.S.*, 1937, p. 99.
OGANOV, L. I., YEFIMOV, I. A., and MILOVIOROVA, E. I., 1937, [Acriquine as
an antimalarial prophylactic]. *Med. Parasitol. Moscow*, 6, 209.
PACHECHO, O., URCUYO, G. F., GONZÁLEZ, A., JIMÉNEZ, A., BUTTS, D. C. A.,
and HERNAN PAÉZ, L., 1946, Informe preliminar de un ensayo con
neuvo antimalárico SN 7618. *Rev. Med. Costa Rica*, 13, 118.
PACKER, H., 1947, Experimental field-type suppression with SN 7,618 (chloro-
quine), SN 8,137 and SN 12,837 (paludrine). *J. nat. Mal. Soc.*, 6, 147.
PAMPANA, E. J., 1934, The therapeutic efficacy of totaquina in human malaria.
I. Clinical tests carried out under the auspices of the Malaria Commission.
Quart. Bull. Hlth Org. L.o.N., 3, 328.
PAREKH, J. G., and BOGHANI, B. P., 1947a, Clinical trials of paludrine in
malaria. *Indian med. Gaz.*, 82, 253.
PAREKH, J. G., and BOGHANI, B. P., 1947b, Report on the use of paludrine
tablets. *Indian J. Malariol.*, 1, 383.
PARK, MUNGO, 1815–16, "Travels in the interior districts of Africa performed
in the years 1795, 1796, 1797 with an account of a subsequent mission to
that country in 1805." 2 Vols. London. J. Murray.
PARROT, L., CATANEI, A., and AMBIALET, R., with CLASTRIER, J., 1937,
Comparative experiments in mass prophylaxis of malaria by means of
quinine and of synthetic drugs (quinacrine and praequine). *Quart. Bull.
Hlth Org. L.o.N.*, 6, 683.

PÂRVULESCU, G., CONSTANTINESCO, N., and BOERIU, V., 1934, Efficacité comparée du totaquina dans le paludisme humaine (infection naturelle). *Arch. roum. Path. exp. Microbiol.*, **7**, 523.

PATEL, J. C., and MEHTA, J. M., 1948, Clinical trials of Cam-Aqi in malaria. *Indian J. med. Sci.*, **2**, 675.

PAYNE, E. H., SHARP, E. A., and NICKEL, K. C., 1949, Parenteral use of camoquin hydrochloride as an antimalarial. *Amer. J. trop. Med.*, **29**, 353.

PEPPER, W., 1853, On the use of berberine and cinchonia in the treatment of intermittent fever. *Amer. J. med. Sci.*, N.S., **25**, 13.

PERRINE, H., 1826, Fever treated with large doses of sulphate of quinine in Adams County, near Natchez, Mississippi. *Philad. med. phys. J.*, **13**, 36.

PREMUDA, L., 1947, Sull' attuazione di una cura antimalarica per via endovenosa con il solfato di chinina nell'anno 1831. *Minerva med.*, **38**, 260.

PISHAROTY, —, 1947, Report on the treatment of malaria with paludrine hydrochloride. Quoted by AFRIDI, M. K., 1947, *Indian J. Malariol.*, **1**, 347.

PULLMAN, T. N., CRAIGE, B., Jr., ALVING, A. S., WHORTON, C. M., JONES, R., Jr., and EICHELBERGER, L., 1948, Comparison of chloroquine, quinacrine (atabrine) and quinine in the treatment of acute attacks of sporozoite-induced vivax malaria (Chesson strain); preliminary report. *J. clin. Invest.*, **27**, Suppl., p. 46.

RAFFAELE, G., 1948, Discussion on malaria treatment. *Proc. 4th int. Congr. trop. Med. Mal. Wash.*, Vol. I., p. 767.

RAYMOND, W. D., 1946, Totaquina and its rivals. *E. Afr. med. J.*, **23**, 301.

REIMANN, H. A., 1947, Infectious diseases : thirteenth annual review of significant publications. *Arch. intern. Med.*, **80**, 514.

RICE, J. B., 1932, Experiments on plasmoquine as a prophylactic among West African negroes exposed to bites of *A. costalis* infected with subtertian malaria. *Ann. trop. Med. Parasit.*, **26**, 555.

RICHARDSON, A. P., HEWITT, R. I., SEAGER, L. D., BROOKE, M. M., MARTIN F., and MADDUX, H., 1946, Chemotherapy of *Plasmodium knowlesi* infections in *Macaca mulatta* monkeys. *J. Pharmacol.*, **87**, 203.

RIVERO, Maria de los Dolores, and RAMIREZ, E., 1940, La infección por el *Hœmoproteus columbœ* en la investigación de la actividad antimalarica. *Rev. Inst. Salubridad y Enfernedad. Trop.*, **1**, 245.

ROBERTSON, J. D., 1948, Paludrine treatment of school children. *Zanzibar, Med. San. Rep. for year ended 31st December*, 1947. *Appendix* II, p. 24.

ROGNONI, M., and PUYOL, L. M., 1947, Informe de los primeros 15 casos tratados con paludrina en el Hospital Santo Tomás. *Arch. Hospital Santo Tomas*, **2**, 391.

ROSE, —, 1941, Malaria prophylaxic mit Atebrin, ihre Dosierung und Angeblichen Komplikationen. *Dtsch. med. Wschr.*, **67**, 1306.

ROTENBURG, S. S., 1945, [Treatment of malaria with acriquine by administration of a single massive dose on the first day (0·3 gm. per os and 0·3 gm. intramuscularly)]. *Med. Parasitol. Moscow*, **14**, 62.

ROW, R., DALAL, N. P., and GOLLERKERI, G. V., 1933, On the effects of quinine, atebrin, and plasmoquin on experimentally induced malaria in the macacus monkey and on some of the pathological changes observed. *Indian J. med. Res.*, **21**, 295.

RUHE, D. S., COOPER, W. C., COATNEY, G. R., and JOSEPHSON, E. S., 1949a, Studies in human malaria. XIII. The therapeutic action of pamaquine (plasmochin) against St. Elizabeth strain vivax malaria. *Amer. J. Hyg.*, **49**, 367.

RUHE, D. S., COOPER, W. C., COATNEY, G. R., JOSEPHSON, E. S., and YOUNG, M. D., 1949b, Studies in human malaria. IX. The protective and therapeutic action of SN 6,911 (Sontochin) against St. Elizabeth strain vivax malaria. *Amer. J. Hyg.*, **49**, 41.

RUSSELL, A. J. H., 1937, Quinine supplies in India. *Rec. Malar. Sur. India,* **7**, 233.

RUSSELL, P. F., 1931a, Avian malaria studies. I. Prophylactic plasmochin in inoculated avian malaria. *Philipp. J. Sci.,* **46**, 305.

RUSSELL, P. F., 1931b, Avian malaria studies. II. Prophylactic plasmochin *versus* prophylactic quinine in inoculated avian malaria. *Philipp. J. Sci.,* **46**, 347.

SANDERS, J. P., 1935, Treatment of malaria with a short course of quinidine. *Amer. J. trop. Med.,* **15**, 651.

SANDERS, J. P., and DAWSON, W. T., 1932, Efficacy of quinidine in malaria. *J. Amer. med. Ass.,* **99**, 1773.

SAUTET, J., 1932, Traitement du paludisme par le 710 et le 574 associés ou non à la quinine ou au quinostovarsol. *Bull. Soc. Path. exot.,* **25**, 1074.

SCHMIDT, L. H., FRADIN, R., SQUIRES, W., and GENTHER, C. S., 1948, Malaria chemotherapy. II. The response of sporozoite-induced infections with *Plasmodium cynomolgi* to various antimalarial drugs. *Fed. Proc.,* **7**, 253.

SCHNEIDER, J., DECOURT, P., and MONTÉZIN, G., 1949, Sur l'utilisation d'un nouveau plasmodium (*Pl. berghei*) pour l'étude et la recherche de médicaments antipaludiques. *Bull. Soc. Path. exot.,* **42**, 449.

SCHNEIDER, J., DIGNAT, M., VORON, —, and SFAR, M., 1948, Prophylaxic collective du paludisme par la prémaline dans la région de Gabès (Mai–Novembre, 1946). *Bull. Soc. Path. exot.,* **41**, 194.

SCHNEIDER, J., and MÉCHALI, D., 1948, Traitement curatif du paludisme. Étude de l'activité comparée de quatre nouveaux dérivés synthétiques. *Bull. Soc. Path. exot.,* **41**, 274.

SCHNEIDER, J., and MÉCHALI, D., 1949, Traitement curatif du paludisme à *Pl. malariæ* par le chloriguane (chlorhydrate N_1-*p*-chlorophenyl-N_5-*iso*propyl diguanide). *Bull. Soc. Path. exot.,* **42**, 156.

SEELER, A. O., 1945, The inhibitory effect of pyridoxine on the activity of quinine and atabrine against avian malaria. *J. nat. Mal. Soc.,* **4**, 13.

SERGENT, ET., SERGENT, ED., and CATANEI, A., 1925, Etude expérimentale du paludisme des oiseaux (*Plasmodium relictum*). Suite des essais de traitement préventif ou curatif par des produits autres que la quinine : cinchonine (xxx note) action de la cinchonine sur les plasmodium pendant la période aiguë. *Arch. Instit. Pasteur Algér.,* **3**, 122.

SERGENT, ET., SERGENT, ED., TRENSZ, F., and VOGT, D., 1932, Essais de traitement du paludisme à *Plasmodium præcox* par le 710 Fourneau, seul ou associé à la quinine, chez des paludéens d'Algérie. *Arch. Inst. Pasteur Algér.,* **10**, 1.

SHANNON, J. A., 1943, Relationship between chemical structure and physiological disposition of series of substances allied to sulfanilamide. *Ann. N.Y. Acad. Sci.,* **44**, 455.

SHANNON, J. A., 1946, Rationale underlying the clinical evaluation of antimalarial drugs. In : " A Survey of Antimalarial Drugs 1941–45," edited by F. Y. Wiselogle. Vol. 1, Chap. 4, p. 177. Ann Arbor. Michigan. J. W. Edwards.

SHANNON, J. A., 1949, Evaluation of antimalarial drugs, in " Evaluation of Chemotherapeutic Agents," edited by C. M. Macleod. Symposia of the Section on Microbiology, No. 2. New York Acad. Med., New York. Columbia University Press.

SHANNON, J. A., and EARLE, D. P., Jr., 1945, Recent advances in the treatment of malaria. *Bull. N.Y. Acad. Med.,* **21**, 467.

SHANNON, J. A., EARLE, D. P., Jr., BRODIE, B. B., TAGGART, J. V., and BERLINER, R. W., 1944, The pharmacological basis of the rational use of atabrine in the treatment of malaria. *J. Pharmacol.,* **81**, 307.

SHEARER, G., 1949, Second thoughts on proguanil. *Brit. med. J.,* **i**, 774.

366   CHEMOTHERAPEUTIC TREATMENT

SHUTE, P. G., 1946, Latency and long-term relapses in benign tertian malaria. *Trans. R. Soc. trop. Med. Hyg.*, **40**, 189.

SHUTE, P. G., and MARYON, M., 1948, The gametocytocidal action of paludrine upon infections due to *Plasmodium falciparum*. *Parasitology*, **38**, 264.

SICAULT, G., and DECOURT, P., 1934, Observations sur 25 paludéens traités par la rhodoquine (710 F). *Bull. Soc. Path. exot.*, **27**, 146.

SICAULT, G., and MESSERLIN, A., 1937, Vues nouvelles sur les prophylaxies medicamenteuses du paludisme. *Riv. Malariol.*, **16**, Sez. 1, 480.

SIDDONS, L. B., and BOSE, A. N., 1944, The action of 2-chloro-7-methoxy-5 (δ-diethyl-amino-butyl) aminoacridine on simian malaria. *Indian med. Gaz.*, **79**, 101.

SILVESTRI, S., 1921, La cinconina nella cura della malaria. *Policlinico, sez. med.*, **28**, 529.

SIMEONS, A. T. W., and CHHATRE, K. D., 1947, Preliminary report on a new synthetic antimalarial. *Indian med. Gaz.*, **82**, 255.

SIMPSON, W. M., and SAGEBIEL, J. L., 1943, Cerebral malaria. A report of twelve cases encountered at a U.S. naval base hospital. *Nav. med. Bull. Wash.*, **6**, 1596.

SINTON, J. A., and BIRD, W., 1928, Studies in malaria with special reference to treatment. IX. Plasmoquine in the treatment of malaria. *Indian J. med. Res.*, **16**, 159.

SINTON, J. A., SMITH, S., and POTTINGER, D., 1930, Studies in malaria, with special reference to treatment. Part XII. Further researches into the treatment of chronic benign tertian malaria with plasmoquine and quinine. *Indian J. med. Res.*, **17**, 793.

SIOLI, F., 1926, Prüfung des Plasmochins bei der Impfmalaria der Paralytiker. *Arch. Schiffs-u. Tropenhyg.*, **30**, Beiheft No. 3, 19.

SLATINEANU, A., CIUCA, M., BALTEANU, I., ALEXA, E., ALEXA, I., FRANCKE, M., and RUGINA, I., 1934, Efficacité thérapeutique des alcaloïdes totaux de l'écorce de quinquina dans le paludisme humain (infection naturelle). *Bull. Soc. Path. exot.*, **27**, 723.

SMITH, H. F., DY, F. J., and CABRERA, D. J., 1949, Studies on the efficiency of chloroquine and chloroguanide as antimalarials. II. As curative agents against Philippine strains of plasmodia. *Acta med. Philipp.*, **6**, 137.

SMITH, H. F., DY, F. J., and DEOGRACIAS, J. C., 1948, Studies on the efficiency of chloroquine and chlorguanide as antimalarials. I. As suppressants. *Acta med. Philipp.*, **5**, 1.

SMITH, P. K., GALLUP, B. N., and CAIN, L. J., 1946, Blood plasma atabrine levels obtained with suppressive and therapeutic doses of atabrine dihydrochloride. *J. Pharmacol.*, **87**, 360.

SOESILO, R., GILBERT, A. P. W., and BAGINDO, Z. G. S., 1933, Een en ander over malaria prophylaxe en Atebrin (eerste mededeeling). *Geneesk. Tijdschr. Ned-Ind.*, **73**, 153.

SOHIER, R., GREGOIRE, J., and RANC, A., 1948, Traitement du paludisme à *Pl. vivax* par le dichlorhydrate de méthyl 3 (diethylamino-pentyl amino 4-chloro-7-quinoléine) (3030 R.P. ou nivaquine C) et le sulfate neutre de diéthyl amino-pentyl) amino-4-chloro-7-quinoléine (3377 R.P. ou nivaquine B). *Bull. Soc. Path. exot.*, **41**, 482.

SRIVASTAVA, R. S., 1947, Final report on the field trials of " Paludrine " in selected hyperendemic malarious areas of Naini Tal Tarai in the United Provinces (September 11th to December 31st, 1946). *Indian J. Malariol.*, **1**, 361.

STECK, E. A., HALLOCK, L. L., and HOLLAND, A. J., 1946, Quinolines, I., II. *J. Amer. chem. Ass.*, **68**, 129, 132.

STRAHAN, J. H., 1948, Quinine by continuous intravenous drip in the treatment of acute falciparum malaria. *Trans. R. Soc. trop. Med. Hyg.*, **41**, 669.

STURM, ROLAND, 1659, Febrifugi Peruviani vindicarum . . . Sectio prima, p. 8. Delphis. P. Oosterhout.

SURGEON-GENERAL, U.S. ARMY OFFICE OF, 1943, The drug treatment of malaria, suppressive and clinical. *J. Amer. med. Ass.*, **123**, 205.

SURREY, A. R., and HAMMER, H. F., 1946, Some 7-substituted 4-amino-quinoline derivatives. *J. Amer. chem. Soc.*, **68**, 113.

SYDENHAM, THOMAS, 1677, " The works. . . . Translated from the Latin edition of Dr. Greenhill with a life of the author by R. G. Latham (1848–50)." 2 Vols. London. Sydenham Society

TAGGART, J. V., BERLINER, R. W., ZUBROD, C. G., WELCH, W. J., EARLE, D. P., Jr., and SHANNON, J. A., 1946, Cinchona alkaloids. 3. Physiological disposition in man. *Fed. Proc.*, **5**, 206.

TAGGART, J. V., EARLE, D. P., Jr., BERLINER, R. W., ZUBROD, C. G., WELCH, W. J., WISE, N. B., SCHROEDER, E. F., LONDON, I. M., and SHANNON, J. A., 1948, Studies on the chemotherapy of the human malarias. III. The physiological disposition and antimalarial activity of the cinchona alkaloids. *J. clin. Invest.*, **27**, Suppl., 80.

TALBOR (TALBOT), ROBERT, 1672, " Pyretologia : a rational account of the cause and cure of agues." London. R. Robinson.

TALBOR (TALBOT), ROBERT, 1682, " The English Remedy : or Talbor's wonderful secret, for cureing of agues and feavers." London. J. Wallis.

TANEJEV, E., 1935, Efficacité des dérivés synthétiques antipaludéens fabriques en U.R.S.S. Note dactylographiée. (Quoted in Fourth General Rept. Malaria Commission League of Nations.) *Quart. Bull. Hlth Org. L.o.N.*, 1037, **6**, 017.

THOMAS, J. W., and SYDENSTRICKER, V. P., 1938, Further notes on pernicious malaria. *Sth. med. J., Nashville*, **31**, 300.

THOMPSON, P. E., 1946a, Effects of quinine on saurian malaria parasites. *J. infect. Dis.*, **78**, 160.

THOMPSON, P. E., 1946b, The effects of atabrine on the saurian malarial parasite, *Plasmodium floridense*. *J. infect. Dis.*, **79**, 282.

TONKIN, I. M., and HAWKING, F., 1947, The technique of testing chemotherapeutic action on *Plasmodium gallinaceum*. *Brit. J. Pharmacol.*, **2**, 221.

TORTI, FRANCESCO, 1712, " Therapeutice specialis ad febres quasdam perniciosas, inopinato ac repente lethales, una vero china china, peculiari methodo ministrata, sanabiles. . . ." Mutinæ. B. Soliani.

TRAGER, W., 1947, The rate of asymptomatic malarial infection in white and negro service troops taking suppressive atabrine. *Amer. J. Hyg.*, **46**, 336.

TUCKEY, J. K., 1818, " Narrative of an expedition to explore the River Zaire, usually called the Congo, in South Africa, in 1816, under the direction of Captain J. K. Tuckey, R.N." London. J. Murray.

U.S. ARMY MEDICAL DEPARTMENT, 1947a, Clinical evaluation of chloroquine. *Bull. U.S. Army med. Dept.*, **7**, 835.

U.S. ARMY MEDICAL DEPARTMENT, 1947b, Chloroquine-diphosphate—a newly standardised antimalarial drug. *Bull. U.S. Army med. Dept.*, **7**, 834.

VAN RIEL, —, 1948, Essai de prophylaxie causale et de traitement de la tierce tropicale par la paludrine. *Ann. Soc. belge Méd. trop.*, **28**, 85.

VISWANATHAN, K. S., 1947, A brief summary of the field experiments conducted with paludrine by the malaria organisation of the Madras Public Health Department up to October 31st, 1946. Quoted by AFRIDI, M. K., 1947. *Indian J. Malariol.*, **1**, 347.

VRIJ, J. E. DE, 1874, On quinamine. *Pharm. J.*, **4**, 609.

WALKER, H. A., 1947, Potentiation of the curative action of antimalarial agents, with special reference to 8-aminoquinolines and naphthoquinones. *J. Bact.*, **54**, 669.

WALKER, H. A., STAUBER, L. A., and RICHARDSON, A. P., 1946, Pamaquine naphthoate, quinacrine hydrochloride and quinine bisulfate as curative agents in *Plasmodium cathemerium* infections of the duck. *Fed. Proc.*, 5, 210.

WALLS, E. S., 1948, Paludrine. *Brit. med. J.*, *ii*, 275.

WARTHIN, T. A., LEVINE, S. A., and EVANS, R. R., 1948, Malaria observations on treatment with chloroquine (SN 7,618) and combined quinine and plasmochin. *New Engl. J. Med.*, 238, 467.

WELCH, W. J., TAGGART, J. V., BERLINER, R. W., ZUBROD, C. G., EARLE, D. P., Jr., and SHANNON, J. A., 1946, Cinchona alkaloids : 6. Suppressive antimalarial activity of cinchonine carbostyril. *Fed. Proc.*, 5, 216.

WILLIS, THOMAS, 1659, " Diatribæ duæ medico-philosophicæ, quarum prior agit de fermentatione sive de motu intestino particularum in quovis corpore, altera de febribus sive de motu earundum in sanguine animalium ; his accessit dissertatio espistolica de urinis." Londoni. T. Roycroft.

WINCHESTER, M. E., 1937, Individual chemoprophylaxis of malaria. Report of and second year's investigation. *Sth. med. J.*, *Nashville*, 30, 1172.

WINCKEL, C. W. F., 1947, Quinine injections in malaria. *J. trop. Med. Hyg.*, 50, 201.

WINCKEL, C. W. F., 1949, The efficacy of quinacrine and quinine in the treatment of *Plasmodium malariæ* infections. *Document. neerland. indon. Med. trop.*, 1, 93.

WISELOGLE, F. Y., edited by, 1946, "A survey of antimalarial drugs, 1941–45." 2 vols. Ann Arbor. Michigan. J. W. Edwards.

WOODRUFF, A. W., 1947, The suppressive and schizonticidal value of paludrine (100 mg.) in vivax malaria. *Trans. R. Soc. trop. Med. Hyg.*, 41, 263.

WRIGHT, T. E., 1915, Thirty cases of malaria, estivo-autumnal, treated with quinine intravenously. *Sth. med. J.*, *Nashville*, 8, 196.

YEAGER, O. W., REIDER, R. F., and McDANIEL, G. E., 1946, Evaluation of totaquine in treatment of malaria in endemic malarious areas. *J. Amer. pharm. Ass.*, 35, 337.

YORKE, W., and MACFIE, J. W. S., 1924, Observations on malaria made during treatment of general paralysis. *Trans. R. Soc. trop. Med. Hyg.*, 18, 13.

YOUNG, M. D., and EYLES, D. E., 1948, The efficacy of chloroquine, quinacrine, quinine and totaquine in the treatment of *Plasmodium malariæ* infections (Quartan malaria). *Amer. J. trop. Med.*, 28, 23.

ZUBROD, C. G., BERLINER, R. W., TAGGART, J. V., WELCH, W. J., EARLE, D. P., Jr., and SHANNON, J. A., 1946, Cinchona alkaloids. 2. Comparative suppressive antimalarial activity. *Fed. Proc.*, 5, 216.

CHAPTER VIII

THE CHEMOTHERAPEUTIC TREATMENT OF PLASMODIAL INFECTIONS (*Continued*)

METALLIC COMPOUNDS

FROM time to time there have been reports that metallic compounds have some influence on malarial infections. The first observations were made by Fowler (1786), Fauvres (1804), and Fodéré (1810) with arsenic. M'Lean (1797) was the first to state that arsenic was of value only in intermittents, and during the Peninsular War army surgeons employed arsenic in preference to cinchona bark, which produced little effect on the prevailing fevers.

Mercury in the form of mercuric chloride, mercurochrome, and mercurophen has been used but without any definite therapeutic results, and the same is true of M3, a compound said to be composed of manganese iodomercurate with an extract of spleen (Torres Munõz, 1939 ; Chopra *et al.*, 1940).

Antimony preparations were at one period thought to have some value. Emetics were for long believed to aid in the cure of malaria. Dr. John Hall, Shakespeare's son-in-law, cured that " excellent poet Drayton " of an ague by emetic infusions and " one ounce of syrup of violets," but this emetic was Oxymel scyllæ (Hall, 1657). The Antidotarium Gandavense of 1663, however, contains a prescription for fever known as pulvis indicus sive catholicus, containing scammony, antimony, and crystallised tartrate. Rogers (1917) believed that tartar emetic acted on gametocytes, but the gametocytes of *P. falciparum* tend to disappear spontaneously in those who have acquired some degree of immunity, and it is doubtful whether antimony salts have any action in human malaria (Stephens *et al.*, 1917), although in *P. lophuræ* infections in ducks they are active in doses which are toxic.

Bismuth was first tested by Schwartz (1939) : the most effective compound is sodium bismuth thioglycollate, $Bi(SCH_2COONa)_3$, thiobismol, with a metallic content of 38 per cent. When given intramuscularly by Cole *et al.* (1940) to ninety-two patients with vivax infections, therapeutically induced, there were only four in whom a single injection did not have some effect on the course of treatment ; usually in prolonged fever a single injection caused a forty-eight hours' respite after which paroxysms returned on alternate days ; a single injection converts a quotidian (double tertian) fever into a simple tertian and repeated injections will frequently arrest the fever for a considerable period. Brunsting and Love (1940) and Young *et al.* (1945) obtained similar results. Spector *et al.* (1945) failed to obtain satisfactory results in acute and chronic vivax infections, but Kaplan and Read (1948) both attach value to thiobismol for regulating therapeutically induced malaria due to *P. malariæ* or *P. vivax*.

The action of thiobismol is apparently limited to an inhibition of half-grown forms of *P. vivax*. Kaplan *et al.* (1946) have shown that the effect of injections of 0·1 and 0·2 gm. into patients given *P. malariæ* therapeutically is very similar to that seen with *P. vivax* infections. In patients with true quartan periodicity a temporary interruption of symptoms occurred in 42 per cent. ; in patients with double and quotidian quartan malaria 87·5 per cent of the patients exhibited a temporary interruption and/or a reduction in the frequency of the paroxysms. As in the case of *P. vivax*, the parasites which are inhibited are only those which are half developed ; very young and mature parasites are not affected. In patients with a very heavy density of parasites, such as more than 10,000 per c.mm., thiobismol reduces the number of parasites very considerably. Thus thiobismol may be of value in enabling patients with neurosyphilis to tolerate more easily complete courses of quartan malaria administered for therapeutic purposes.

In *P. gallinaceum* infections in chicks sodium bismuth iodate has been found to clear parasites from the blood stream by inhibiting the development of the young merozoites ; it does not affect the exo-erythrocytic forms (Guerra *et al.*, 1944).

Paludex, or as it is now called Cuprochin, is described as a " copper mercury oxyquinoline sulphonate of soda " ; claims were originally made for it in the treatment of vivax, falciparum, and malariæ infections in the Belgian Congo by van Nitsen (1936 and 1937), and van Nitsen and Serra (1936). Van Riel (1938) was unable to confirm these results so far as *P. falciparum* is concerned, and Rodhain and Hendrix (1937) failed to show any activity against *Halteridium oryzivoræ, P. cathemerium, P. gonderi* or *P. knowlesi*. More recently cuprochin has contained quinine, to which it doubtless owes some therapeutic action.

Arsenical Compounds ; Arsphenamine and Neoarsphenamine. Shortly after the introduction of arsphenamine for syphilis an attempt was made to determine whether it had any value in malaria (Werner, 1910, 1912a ; Tuschinsky, 1912). Kopanaris (1911) was unable to demonstrate any effect on *P. præcox* (= *P. relictum*) infections in canaries ; atoxyl also was valueless. Lourie (1934) obtained negative results with arsphenamine on *P. cathemerium*. Later neoarsphenamine was employed in human infections (Werner, 1912b ; Iversen and Tuschinsky, 1912 ; Summa, 1913 ; Baetge, 1913). Since then neoarsphenamine has in areas such as the Balkans enjoyed a high reputation in the control of chronic malarial infections ; others have failed to obtain any striking results in natural malarial infections (Stephens *et al.*, 1918, 1919 ; Pratt-Johnson *et al.*, 1921 ; Whittingham, 1925). In the Netherlands, neoarsphenamine has been used with some success for terminating attacks of vivax infection therapeutically induced, for though it cannot compare with quinine in ending a paroxysm, it does retard the development of the parasites. According to Winckel (1941), Madagascar strains of *P. vivax* are more susceptible than those from the Netherlands. In blood-induced infections with Dutch strains of *P. vivax* a single intravenous injection of 0·15 gm. of neoarsphenamine given immediately after an attack of fever is sufficient to convert a quotidian into a simple tertian fever : if the injection is given on an afebrile day the attack of fever will be aborted for some days and a series of injections of 0·3, 0·45, and 0·6 gm. will usually terminate the fever. With the Madagascar strain doses of 0·075 and 0·1 gm. are enough to bring about the same results. Field *et al.* (1948) failed to obtain any evidence that neoarsphenamine influenced the relapse rate of vivax malaria. Infections due to *P. malariæ* are unaffected by neoarsphenamine, and so are those caused by *P. falciparum*. One of the worst infections with algid symptoms due to *P. falciparum* seen in West Africa during the war years was in a patient who was receiving a course of neoarsphenamine combined with bismuth for syphilis. Giemsa *et al.* (1926) found neoarsphenamine without action on *P. relictum* in canaries.

Oxophenarsine (mapharsen, mapharside). The value of oxophen-arsine in malaria is doubtful. Goldman (1938) claimed that it was of value in both induced and naturally acquired malaria. His work was confirmed by Cleveland and Turvey (1939) in a series of cases with therapeutic malaria. Good results were also reported by Dao (1944), Lowe (1944) and Stewart (1945). Oxophenarsine added to quinine appeared to shorten convalescence. Niven (1940), in Malaya, gave two intravenous injections of 0·04 and 0·06 respectively at an interval of five to seven days. In vivax malaria the effect on the parasites appeared to be more rapid than that of quinine by mouth. The rate of reproduction of the asexual stages was apparently altered by elimination of the half-grown stages. Gibbs (1940) obtained only indifferent results in the Southern United States, while Kay (1945) found oxophenarsine quite useless in relapsing vivax malaria. Spector *et al.* (1945) had similar results in patients with frequent relapses.

There is general agreement that oxophenarsine has no action on *P. malariæ* or *P. falciparum*, while its action on *P. vivax* would seem to differ according to the strain and to the method of inducing the infection. Its main value is in the control of therapeutically induced vivax infections. Bratton (1945) found that in *P. lophuræ* infections in the duck oxophenarsine was effective in a dose of 32 mgm. per kgm. of body weight when given intravenously, but it was also toxic in this dose. Against *P. knowlesi* in monkeys neither oxophenarsine nor neoarsphenamine was of value in therapeutic doses (Das Gupta and Siddons, 1944).

Carbarsone was ineffective in relapsing vivax malarias (Spector *et al.*, 1945).

Melarsen oxide has been used by Payne *et al.* (1946) in Brazil, 25 mgm. being given intravenously daily for seven days. Among forty patients given the full course, the symptoms subsided on or about the fourth to fifth day of treatment ; tenderness in the upper abdomen decreased and enlarged spleens became smaller. The delayed response renders melarsen oxide unsuitable for the treatment of the acute stages of malaria.

Acetarsol (stovarsol, acetylarsen), the sodium salt of 3-acetyl-amino-4-hydroxyphenylarsinic acid, although originally investigated by Ehrlich and Hata (1911), was not tested against malarial infections till 1924, when Valenti and Tomaselli showed that acetarsol by mouth cleared the blood in infections due to *P. malariæ* and *P. vivax*, although the patient with a quartan infection rapidly relapsed. Marchoux and Cohen (1925) also tested the results of injecting 1 gm. of acetarsol in 10 ml. of saline intravenously. The results were remarkable in infections due to *P. vivax* as parasites disappeared from the peripheral blood within twenty-four hours of the injection. Marchoux (1925) showed that acetarsol acted on the larger pigmented trophozoites in the blood stream, the smaller forms being more resistant. Acetarsol did not produce a fragmentation of the parasite but caused condensation of the chromatin and, later, loss of staining power of the chromatin. In the end the nucleus disappears, leaving the red cells intact but full of Schüffner's dots. These results were confirmed by Sinton (1927), who believed that acetarsol either prevented the normal increase in size of the young trophozoites or destroyed them when they had reached a certain stage of development.

Acetarsol does not prevent relapses of vivax infections, and, like other arsenicals, it is valueless in infections due to *P. falciparum* (Guérin *et al.*, 1927 ; Freiman, 1927 ; van Nitsen, 1927). Acetarsol does not reduce splenomegaly as readily as quinine. Hegner *et al.* (1928) were unable to detect any action on *P. cathemerium* infections in canaries : Sergent *et al.* (1925) obtained similar negative results with *P. relictum*.

A combination of quinine and acetarsol has been tested, but the relapse rate in vivax infections, according to Sinton, Bird, and Eate (1928), is no better than in those treated with cinchona alkaloids. Quinine troposan, the quinine salt of 5-acetylamino-2-hydroxyphenylarsinic acid, and quinine dimethylarsinate have been tested by Sinton, Bird, and Orr (1928), Puyal (1928), Navarro-Martin (1928), and Alvarez-Cienfuegos (1928). The results do not seem to be any better than those obtained with quinine.

It may be noted that levels of radioactivity as high as 1·1 micro-curie per ml. of blood, induced by injection of radioiron, are without effect on the course of blood-induced *P. cathemerium* infections in the canary (Thompson *et al.*, 1949).

References

ALVAREZ-CIENFUEGOS, J. M., 1928, Ensayo terapéutico del paludismo (1). *Med. Paises calidos*, 1, 547.

BAETGE, P., 1913, Behandlung der Malaria tertiana mit Neosalvarsan. *Münch. med. Wschr.*, 60ii, 2776.

BRATTON, A. C., Jr., 1945, Continuous intravenous chemotherapy of *Plasmodium lophuræ* infection in ducks. *J. Pharmacol.*, 85, 103.

BRUNSTING, L. A., and LOVE, W. R., 1940, The tempering effect of sodium bismuth thioglycollate (thio-bismol) on therapeutic malaria. *Proc. Mayo Clin.*, 15, 285.

CHOPRA, R. N., ROY, D. N., HAYTER, R. T. M., and SEN, B., 1940, M3, a new drug in the treatment of malaria. *Indian med. Gaz.*, 75, 19.

CLEVELAND, D. E. H., and TURVEY, S. E. C., 1939, Use of mapharsen for terminating malaria artificially produced by inoculation. *Arch. Derm. Syph., Chicago*, 39, 1043.

COLE, H. N., DEOREO, G. A., DRIVER, J. R., JOHNSON, H. H., and SCHWARTZ, W. F., 1940, Use of bismuth injections to manage course of therapeutic malaria. *J. Amer. med. Ass.*, 115, 422.

DAO, L. L., 1944, Resultados clinicos obtenidos con el marfarside en el tratamiento del paludismo. *Rev. Policlín. Caracás*, 13, 339.

DAS GUPTA, B. M., and SIDDONS, L. B., 1944, Organic arsenicals in the treatment of simian malaria. *Indian med. Gaz.*, 79, 99.

EHRLICH, P., and HATA, S., 1911, "Die experimentelle Chemotherapie der Spirillosen. (Syphilis, Rückfallfieber, Hühnerspirillose, Främbösie.)" Berlin. J. Springer.

FAUVRES, R., 1904, "Recherches cliniques sur les effets de l'arsenic dans le traitement des fièvres intermittentes." Paris.

FIELD, J. W., JOHNSTON, R. S., and SMITH, H., 1948, Failure of neoarsphenamine in relapsing vivax malaria. *Trans. R. Soc. trop. Med.*, 41, 677.

FODÉRÉ, F. E., 1810, "Recherches experimentales faites a l'hôpital civil et militaire de Martiques, sur la nature des fièvres à periodes et sur la valeur des différens remèdes substitués au quinquina ; spécialement sur les propriétés médicales de l'arséniate de soude souivies d'une notice sur l'extrait de pavots des jardins, pour remplacer l'opium oriental." Marseille. J. Mossy.

FOWLER, T., 1786, "Medical reports on the effects of arsenic in the cure of agues, remitting fevers and periodic headaches." London. J. Johnson.

FREIMAN, M., 1927, Stovarsol in treatment of malaria. *J. trop Med. Hyg.*, 30, 127.

GIBBS, O. S., 1940, Some pharmacological problems of malaria. *Mississippi Dr.*, 18, 331.

GIEMSA, G., WEISE, W., and TROPP, C., 1926, Chemotherapeutische Studien mit Vogelmalaria (*Plasmodium præcox*). *Arch. Schiffs-u. Tropenhyg.*, 30, 334.

GOLDMAN, D., 1938, The use of mapharsen in the treatment of malaria. *Amer. J. Med. Sci.*, 196, 602.

Guérin, F., Borel, E., and Advier, M., 1927, Stovarsol et paludisme. *Bull. Soc. Path. exot.*, **20**, 331.

Guerra, F., Beltran, E., De La Garza, F., and Larenasm, R., 1944, La accion del yodobismutito de sodio sobre el paludismo aviario. *Rev. Inst. Salubr. Enferm. trop.*, **5**, 59.

Hall, John, 1657, "Select observations on English bodies ; or cures, both empericall and historicall, performed upon very eminent persons in desperate diseases. First written in Latine by Mr. John Hall living at Stratford-upon-Avon in Warwickshire, where he was very famous, as also in the counties adjacent, as appeares by these observations drawn out of severall hundreds of his, as choysest. Now put into English for common benefit by James Cooke." London. J. Sherley.

Hegner, R., Shaw, E. H., Jr., and Manwell, R. D., 1928, Methods and results of experiments on the effects of drugs on bird malaria. *Amer. J. Hyg.*, **8**, 564.

Iversen, J., and Tuschinsky, M., 1912, Neosalvarsan bei Malaria tertiana. *Münch. med. Wschr.*, 59ii, 1606.

Kaplan, L. I., and Read, H. S., 1948, Technical aspects of therapeutic malaria. *Amer. J. Med.*, **4**, 846.

Kaplan, L. I., Read, H. S., and Becker, F. T., 1946, The action of thiobismol on therapeutic quartan malaria. *J. Lab. clin. Med.*, **31**, 735.

Kay, C. F., 1945, Failure of mapharsen as an adjuvant to atabrine in the treatment of relapsing tertian malaria. *J. Amer. med. Ass.*, **127**, 984.

Kopanaris, P., 1911, Die Wirkung von Chinin, Salvarsan und Atoxyl auf die *Proteosoma—(Plasmodium praecox)*—Infektion des Kanarienvogels. *Arch. Schiffs-u. Tropenhyg.*, **15**, 586.

Lourie, E. M., 1934, Studies on chemotherapy in bird malaria. II. Observations bearing on the mode of action of quinine. *Ann. trop. Med. Parasit.*, **28**, 255.

Lowe, J., 1944, Novarsenobillon and mapharside in the treatment of the attack of malaria. *Indian med. Gaz.*, **79**, 97.

Marchoux, E., 1925, Action exclusive de l'arsenic (stovarsol) sur le paludisme à *Plasmodium vivax*. *Ann. Inst. Pasteur*, **39**, 197.

Marchoux, E., and Cohen, —, 1925, Le stovarsol est contre le paludisme au moins aussi actif que la quinine. *C. R. Soc. Biol. Paris*, **92**, 132.

M'Lean, Hector, 1797, "An enquiry into the nature and causes of the great mortality among the troops at St. Domingo ; with practical remarks on the fever of that island ; and directions for the conduct of Europeans on their first arrival in warm climates." London. T. Cadell Jun. and W. Davies.

Navarro-Martin, A., 1928, Ensayo de toxicidad. *Med. Paises calidos*, **1**, 547.

Niven, J. C., 1940, Mapharside in the treatment of malaria. *Bull. Inst. Med. Res. F.M.S.*, No. 6.

Payne, E. H., Balthazar, E., and Bezerra, D. A., 1946, Preliminary observations on use of melarsen oxide in malaria. *Sth. med. J., Nashville*, **39**, 970.

Pratt-Johnson, J., Gilchrist, K., and Hay-Michel, —, 1921, On the action of certain special preparations on malarial parasites and their employment in the treatment of malaria. *Brit. med. J.*, i, 80.

Puyal, J., 1928, El dimetilarsinato de quinina en el paludismo agudo y crónico. *Med. Paises cálidos*, **1**, 546.

Rodhain, J., and Hendrix, H., 1937, Essais de traitement du paludisme des oiseaux et des singes au moyen du "paludex." *Bull. Inst. col. belge*, **8**, 137.

Rogers, L., 1917, Disappearance of malignant tertian crescents from the blood following the intravenous injection of tartar emetic. *Brit. med. J.*, i, 6.

SCHWARTZ, W. F., 1939, The effect of thiobismol on therapeutic malaria. *J. Pharmacol.*, **65**, 175.

SERGENT, ET., SERGENT, ED., and CATANEI, A., 1925, Étude experimentale du paludisme des oiseaux (*Plasmodium relictum*) : suite des essais de traitement par des produits autre que la quinine : le stovarsol. *Arch. Inst. Pasteur, Algér.*, **3**, 124.

SINTON, J. A., 1927, Studies in malaria with special reference to treatment. Part VII. The intravenous injection of sodium stovarsol in the treatment of benign tertian malaria. *Indian J. med. Res.*, **15**, 287.

SINTON, J. A., BIRD, W., and EATE, S. N., 1928, Studies in malaria with special reference to treatment. Part VIII. The oral administration of quinine stovarsol in the treatment of chronic benign tertian malaria. *Indian J. med. Res.*, **15**, 595.

SINTON, J. A., BIRD, W., and ORR, W. B. F., 1928, Studies in malaria with special reference to treatment. Part X. Quinine-tropozan in the treatment of chronic benign tertian malaria. *Indian J. med. Res.*, **16**, 333.

SPECTOR, S., HAVILAND, J. W., and COGGESHALL, L. T., 1945, The ineffectiveness of intensive mapharsen, bismuth and carbarsone as curative drugs in chronic malaria. *Amer. J. trop Med.*, **25**, 463.

STEPHENS, J. W. W., YORKE, W., BLACKLOCK, B., MACFIE, J. W. S., and COOPER, C. F., 1917, Studies in the treatment of malaria. [I. Intravenous injections of tartar emetic.] *Ann. trop. Med. Parasit.*, **11**, 91.

STEPHENS, J. W. W., YORKE, W., BLACKLOCK, B., MACFIE, J. W. S., COOPER, C. F., and CARTER, H. F., 1918, Studies in the treatment of malaria. XVI. Intravenous injections of novarsenobillon in simple tertian malaria. *Ann. trop. Med. Parasit.*, **12**, 211.

STEPHENS, J. W. W., YORKE, W., BLACKLOCK, B., MACFIE, J. W. S., COOPER, C. F., and CARTER, H. F., 1919, Studies in the treatment of malaria. XXV. Arsenic in malignant tertian malaria. *Ann. trop. Med. Parasit.*, **13**, 75.

STEWART, W. H., 1945, Treatment of malaria with arsenicals. *Nav. med. Bull. Wash.*, **44**, 991.

SUMMA, —, 1913, Zwei Malaria-tertiana-Rückfälle unmittelbar nach energischer Salvarsanbehandlung. *Arch. Schiffs-u. Tropenhyg.*, **17**, 836.

THOMPSON, P. E., MCGINTY, D. A., WILSON, M. L., and BAYLES, A., 1949, Further studies on radioiron in avian malaria. *J. Parasit.*, **35**, 215.

TORRES MUÑOZ, A., 1939, El yodomercurato de manganeso en el paludismo. *Rev. Med. trop. Parasit.*, **5**, 31.

TUSCHINSKY, M., 1912, Ueber die Behandlung der Malaria mit Salvarsan. *Dtsch. med. Wschr.*, **38**, 548.

VALENTI, F., and TOMASELLI, A., 1924, Lo stovarsolo nella cura della malaria. II. Nota. *Policlinico, sez. prat.*, **32**, 1629.

VAN NITSEN, R., 1927, L'action du stovarsolate de quinine sur les infections à *Plasmodium falciparum*. *Bull. Soc. Path. exot.*, **20**, 727.

VAN NITSEN, R., 1936, Le traitement de la malaria par le paludex nouveau dérivé quinoléinique (étude basée sur 1,000 observations d'indigènes). *Ann. Soc. belge Méd. trop.*, **16**, 387.

VAN NITSEN, R., 1937, Contribution à la chimiothérapie du paludisme. *Brux.-méd.*, **17**, 587.

VAN NITSEN, R., and SERRA, D., 1936, Le paludisme chez les Européens traités par le paludex. *Ann. Soc. belge Méd. trop.*, **16**, 409.

VAN RIEL, J., 1938, Essai de traitement de la malaria per le cuprochin. *Ann. Soc. belge Méd. trop.*, **18**, 339.

WERNER, H., 1910, Das Ehrlich-Hata Mittel 606 bei Malaria. *Dtsch. med. Wschr.*, **36**, 1982.

WERNER, H., 1912a, Weitere Beobachtungen über die Wirkung von Salvarsan bei Malaria. *Arch. Schiffs-u. Tropenhyg.*, **16**, Bhft. No. 1, 18.

SULPHONAMIDES 377

SULPHONAMIDES 377

SULPHONAMIDES 377

SULPHONAMIDES 377

SULPHONAMIDES

SULPHONAMIDES 377

Werner, H., 1912b, Ueber Neosalvarsan bei Malaria. *Dtsch. med. Wschr.*, **38**, 2068.
Whittingham, H. E., 1925, The treatment of malaria by novarsenobillon. *Proc. R. Soc. Med.* (War Section), **18**, 23.
Winckel, C. W. F., 1941, Neoarsphenamine to manage course of fever in therapeutic malaria. *J. Amer. med. Ass.*, **116**, 2660.
Young, M. D., McLendon, S. B., and Smarr, R. G., 1943, The selective action of thio-bismol on induced malaria. *J. Amer. med. Ass.*, **122**, 492.

SULPHONAMIDES AND SULPHONES

Since Díaz de León (1937 and 1938) first claimed to have produced a clinical cure in fifteen cases of vivax infection by means of rubiazol (6-carboxy-4-sulphamido-2'-4'-diaminoazobenzene) a very considerable amount of work has been carried out with sulphonamides and sulphones on the malarias of man, monkeys and birds. This research did not produce results of first-class importance, although it showed that the search for true causal prophylactics was by no means hopeless, since sulphanilamide acts as a true causal prophylactic against *P. knowlesi* in rhesus monkeys, while sulphadiazine acts similarly against *P. gallinaceum*. In addition, the fact that the antimalarial action of sulphonamides is inhibited by *p*-aminobenzoic acid has shed fresh light on the metabolic requirements of plasmodia. The mode of action of sulphonamides on malaria parasites is discussed on p. 549. Full references to earlier work on sulphonamides and malaria are given by Curd (1943).

Malaria in Man

Plasmodium falciparum. Ninety-three patients were treated by intramuscular injections of 10 ml. of prontosil soluble every twelve hours; after four injections marked improvement occurred. No relapses are recorded and no reactions were observed (Hill and Goodwin, 1937). Similar results were reported in India by Chopra *et al.* (1939a). Menk and Mohr (1939), however, obtained very poor results on parasitæmia in seven patients with prontosil; this they suggest may have been due to the fact that their patients possessed no immunity.

Sulphanilamide by mouth has been shown to exert some action on schizonts and on the duration of fever (Niven, 1938; Menk and Mohr, 1939, and Díaz de León, 1940); Díaz de León gave sulphanilamide intravenously. Similar results on the asexual erythrocytic forms of *P. falciparum* have been demonstrated with the following compounds :—

Compound.	Reference.
Soluseptazine (Disodium-*p*-(γ-phenyl-propylamino)-benzene sulphonamide-αγ-disulphonate).	Farinaud and Ragiot (1938); Farinaud and Eliche (1939).
Promin (Diamino diphenylsulphone-N, N′didextrose sulphonate).	Coggeshall, Maier and Best (1941).
Sulphapyridine.	Chopra, Hayter and Sen (1939b).
Sulphadiazine	Coggeshall, Maier and Best (1941); Findlay, Maegraith, Markson and Holden (1946); Wiselogle (1946).
Proseptazine (*p*-benzylaminobenzene-sulphonamide).	Farinaud and Eliche (1939); Sinton, Hutton, and Shute (1939).
Rubiazole	Farinaud and Eliche (1939); González Barreras (1939).
Sulphathiazole	Findlay, Maegraith, Markson, and Holden (1946).
Sulphamezathine	Findlay, Maegraith, Markson, and Holden (1946).
Sulphapyrazine	Findlay, Maegraith, Markson, and Holden (1946).
Sulphamerazine	Findlay, Maegraith, Markson, and Holden (1946); Schneider and Caruana (1948).
Succinylsulphathiazole . . .	Findlay, Maegraith, Markson, and Holden (1946).
The cinnamylidine Schiff's base of diaminodiphenyl sulphone with four sulphonic acid groups . . .	Findlay, Maegraith, Markson, and Holden (1946).

The effects of different sulphonamides vary considerably. Coggeshall *et al.* (1941) found that of five patients treated with sulphadiazine, two were unaffected by the drug, fever and parasites still persisting ; in the other three, parasites disappeared from the peripheral blood in one, two, and three days, whereas fever disappeared in one, one, and three days respectively. With West African strains, of eighteen patients given 6 gm. of sulphadiazine in twenty-four hours and thereafter 4 gm. daily for five days (total 26 gm.) two failed to respond, the average duration of parasitæmia was fifty-eight hours and the variation from twelve to 156 hours.

The relative efficiency of certain sulphonamides on West African strains of *P. falciparum* is shown in the table :—

THE EFFECT OF SULPHONAMIDES ON WEST AFRICAN STRAINS OF
Plasmodium falciparum (Findlay *et al.*, 1946)

Drug.	Number of patients.	Dosage in gm. × days.	Average duration of fever in hours.	Average duration of parasites in peripheral blood in hours.
Sulphathiazole . .	18	6 × 1 : 4 × 5 (26)	48	63
Sulphadiazine . .	18	,, ,, ,,	60	58
Sulphamezathine . .	40	,, ,, ,,	55	62
Sulphapyrazine . .	20	,, ,, ,,	101	96
Sulphamerazine .- .	20	,, ,, ,,	86	68
Succinylsulphathiazole .	10	18 × 6 (108)	72	79
The cinnamylidene Schiff's base of diamino-diphenyl sulphone with four sulphonic acid groups (W.F. 301).	10	5 × 3 4 × 2 (26) 1 × 1	89	16
Quinine	.	. . .	63	25
Quinine and mepacrine .		. . .	60	41
Mepacrine 0·9 gm. initial dose		. . .	75	67
Mepacrine 0·6 gm. ,, ,,		. . .	64	63
Mepacrine 0·8 gm. ,, ,,		. . .	66	48

Saini (1947), in Italy, found 4 : 4'-diamidinodiphenyl sulphone inactive in falciparum infections in children, whereas Secreto (1946) concluded that it was of some value. Ardias (1948) believed that it shortened the period of fever and was equal to quinine against all Italian strains.

With North African strains of *P. falciparum* Schneider and Caruana (1948) believed that sulphamerazine (sumédine) was of value as four of six cases were cured and did not relapse ; for adults the daily dose was 3 gm. a day for five days.

There is general agreement that prontosil and sulphanilamide do not directly affect the gametocytes of *P. falciparum* (Chopra and Basu, 1939 ; Díaz de Léon, 1940 ; González Barreras, 1939). Chopra and Basu (1939), for instance, gave five crescent carriers doses up to 20 gm. and fed on them 511 laboratory-bred *Anopheles stephensi* : no interference with the development cycle in the mosquito was noted. Farinaud and Ragiot (1938) noted that when 10 ml. of soluseptazine was given night and morning for ten days the schizonts disappeared in six days, but the gametocytes, so far from decreasing, actually increased considerably in number. The infectivity of these gametocytes for mosquitoes was not tested. Findlay *et al.* (1946) found that of twenty-five patients treated with sulphamezathine nineteen showed very numerous gametocytes in their blood. Feeding experiments with *Anopheles gambiæ* indicated that these drug-treated gametocytes were not capable of completing the sexual cycle in the mosquito.

Sulphonamides as a rule do not act as true causal prophylactics against *P. falciparum*. Wiselogle (1946) found that sulphadiazine has no true causal prophylactic action against falciparum malaria.

Sinton *et al.* (1939) have, however, produced very suggestive results with proseptazine (N^4-benzylsulphanilamide). Eight patients were bitten by from fifteen to twenty heavily infected *Anopheles maculipennis* var. *atroparvus*. In the first experiment three patients were given 7·5 gm. in twenty-four hours before infection and 4·5 gm. in the eight hours after infection : two had no fever or parasitæmia, the third had one parasite in the peripheral blood stream twelve days later. A patient given no drug had a clinical attack on the eleventh day. In the second experiment two patients were given 12 gm. in the twenty-four hours before infection and 15 gm. in the thirty-two hours following infection. One patient remained free from fever and parasitæmia, the other had an attack twenty-two days after the infected feed.

In a third experiment three patients were given 3 gm. three times at an interval of four hours.

One patient was bitten immediately after the last dose; fever occurred fifteen days later ; the second patient was bitten twenty-four hours after the last dose, he remained free from infection; a third patient was bitten forty-eight hours after the last dose, he had an attack of fever after sixteen days. Thus of eight patients bitten by infected mosquitoes five remained free from a clinical attack.

These experiments therefore indicate either that proseptazine attacks the primary exo-erythrocytic forms of *P. falciparum* or that it destroys the earliest schizonts and eventually leads to " suppressive cure " (Coatney *et al.*, 1947a) or " medicocurative prophylaxis."

That suppressive cure may be brought about in falciparum infections is shown by experiments carried out during the war by

Fairley *et al.* (1945) in Australia, and by Coatney *et al.* (1947b) in America, on sporozoite-induced infections under laboratory conditions, and by Findlay (1948) under field conditions in West Africa.

In Australia, Fairley *et al.* (1945), working with New Guinea strains of *P. falciparum,* found that the administration of 1 gm. daily for twenty-three days after exposure to infection of either sulphadiazine, sulphamerazine or sulphamethazine was sufficient to suppress the infection in twenty out of twenty-one volunteers and to eradicate the infection in seventeen out of the twenty-one volunteers. Coatney *et al.* (1947a) independently carried out somewhat similar experiments with the McLendon strain of *P. falciparum* ; this strain was originally isolated in South Carolina. Employing sulphadiazine, it was found that in doses at the limit of tolerance (12 gm. per day) and continued for forty-six hours after exposure, it did not act as a causal prophylactic, although the prepatent and incubation periods were doubled. Four grams of sulphadiazine daily for six days after exposure, or 2 gm. daily for five or ten days, likewise produced only delay in the prepatent period. Four grams of sulphadiazine daily for eleven days after exposure, however, prevented infection in four of five subjects. Four grams of sulphadiazine daily for forty-two days after exposure permanently protected all of ten subjects ; 2 gm. daily for the same period protected eight of nine, and 0·5 gm. daily for forty-two days protected three of five subjects from patent parasitæmia. The minimum blood concentrations of sulphadiazine associated with suppression were approximately 1·0 mgm. per 100 ml. With sulphapyrazine 0·5 gm. daily for forty-two days gave the same results as the same dose of sulphadiazine. Renal complications occurred only with the highest doses and in only two patients was there drug fever, accompanied, in one instance, by a severe skin reaction, in volunteers taking 2 and 4 gm. sulphadiazine.

In 1942, in West Africa, field experiments were carried out with doses of 0·5 gm. daily of either sulphapyrazine, sulphamethazine or sulphamerazine as compared with mepacrine hydrochloride 0·6 or 0·7 gm. weekly. The results are shown in the table. It will be seen that sulphapyrazine gave results which were superior to those with mepacrine, sulphamethazine results about equal to those with mepacrine, and sulphamerazine results inferior to those with mepacrine. In a further experiment carried out during the whole of 1944, involving a single military unit in West Africa, 129 persons took 0·1 gm. daily of mepacrine and 102 persons took 0·5 gm. sulphapyrazine daily. Among the mepacrine takers there were twenty attacks of fever with parasites in the blood and fourteen with fever but no parasites in the blood ; among the sulphapyrazine takers there was one attack of fever with parasites and six of fever without parasites in the blood. No toxic results were seen in those who took sulphapyrazine even up to a period of eighteen months (Findlay, 1948). Further investigations into the suppressive cure of malaria by sulphonamides are required. In the treatment of acute falciparum infections the sulphonamides are obviously inferior to many other drugs. Occasionally, however, there are persons who fail to react to quinine or mepacrine and continue to show parasites in the blood. The administration of sulphonamides to such individuals occasionally has a highly beneficial effect (Findlay *et al.*, 1946). Livadas and Sphangos (1944) also concluded that sulphonamides in combination with quinine had a beneficial action.

Plasmodium vivax. Results on the clinical cure of vivax infections with various sulphonamides show that their action is not as marked as with falciparum infections. Chopra, Das Gupta, Sen, and Hayter (1939a) obtained good results with prontosil in India, as did Hill and Goodwin (1937) in seven patients given intramuscular injections. Menk and Mohr (1939) and Read and Pino (1938) failed to demonstrate any satisfactory response to prontosil, prontosil soluble or sulphanilamide. Other compounds which have been employed in acute attacks with somewhat variable success are are shown in the table on page 383.

In addition, in terminating induced attacks of vivax malaria, therapeutically induced, prontosil and proseptazine (Pakenham-Walsh and Rennie, 1938), sulphapyridine (Pakenham-Walsh and Rennie, 1939), and sulphathiazole (Pakenham-Walsh and Rennie, 1940) have all been used with success, as has promin (Coggeshall *et al.*, 1941). Hall (1938) found that sulphanilamide gave extremely poor results, as did Saini (1947) working with 4 : 4′-diamidino-diphenylsulphone. In blood-induced vivax malaria due to the McCoy strain, sulphadiazine had a quinine equivalent of 0·1 (Wiselogle, 1946). Sulphamethazine, sulphamerazine, and sulpha-

Promin (Diamino diphenylsulphone-N, N¹-didextrose sulphonate).		Coggeshall, Maier and Best (1941).
Soluseptazine	.	Farinaud and Elche (1939).
Proseptazine	.	Motzfeldt (1938) ; Farinaud and Ragiot (1938) ; Farinaud and Elche (1939).
Sulphapyridine	.	Chopra, Hayter and Sen (1939b).
Sulphadiazine	.	Coggeshall, Maier and Best (1941) ; Johnson (1943) ; Coxon and Hayes (1945) ; Wiselogle (1946) ; Coatney, Cooper, Young, Burgess and Smarr (1947b).
Sulphathiazole	.	Schwartz, Furst and Flippin (1941).
Sulphanilamide	.	Sorley and Currie (1938) ; Niven (1938).
Sulphamerazine	.	Wiselogle (1946) ; Schneider and Caruana (1948).
Sulphapyrazine	.	Wiselogle (1946).
Sulphamethazine	.	Wiselogle (1946).
1-Sulphanilamido-3 : 5, dibromobenzene and its chloro analogue 6-Sulphanilylmetanilamide	.	Ishii (1948).

pyrazine have quinine equivalents of less than 0·1, based on total oral dosage, against the McCoy strain of vivax malaria (Wiselogle, 1946). Sulphamerazine was useless in controlling North African strains of *P. vivax* (Schneider and Caruana, 1948). Coggeshall, Martin, and Bates (1945) found that sulphadiazine was useless in preventing relapses of vivax malaria after the acute attack had been controlled with quinine or mepacrine. Coatney *et al.* (1947b) showed that sulphadiazine given in total daily doses of 3 gm. for two days before and forty-two days after exposure to infected mosquitoes failed to prevent infection with the St. Elizabeth strain of *P. vivax* in any of ten volunteers. Mean blood concentrations of over 5 mgm. per 100 ml. were, however, suppressive, and in four out of the ten individuals exposed to infection malaria did not appear for from nine to eleven months after exposure. With total daily doses of 2 gm. for a similar period infection occurred in all five volunteers, either shortly after ceasing to take the drug or after a latent period of twelve months. In a total daily dose of 1 gm. sulphadiazine was even less effective, as was sulphapyrazine in doses of 1 or 0·5 gm. daily. Compared with mepacrine and quinine, sulphadiazine and sulphapyrazine are relatively poor suppressives of the St. Elizabeth strain (a temperate-zone strain) of *P. vivax*. Similarly, Fairley *et al.* (1945) showed that sulpha-diazine, sulphamerazine, and sulphamezathine given in doses of 1·0 gm. daily for twenty-three days after exposure failed to protect against infection by New Guinea strains. Twenty-one out of twenty-four volunteers developed overt malaria during the period of drug administration and the remaining three volun-teers had attacks shortly after drug administration had ceased.

Sulphonamides have no action on the gametocytes of *P. vivax*. Vivax malaria, as a rule, is thus more resistant to sulphonamides than falciparum malaria.

Plasmodium malariæ. Relatively few investigations have been carried out on strains of quartan malaria with sulphonamides. Van der Wielen (1937) found that prontosil rapidly terminated acute attacks of quartan malaria, but Faget *et al.* (1938) were unable to confirm these results.

The following sulphonamides have been found to have a slight action in reducing fever and overcoming the parasitæmia due to *P. malariæ* :—

Prontosil rubrum . . .	Chopra, Das Gupta, Sen and Hayter (1939a).
Soluseptazine . . .	Farinaud and Ragiot (1938).
Sulphanilamide . . .	Gardner and Dexter (1938).
Sulphapyridine . . .	Chopra, Hayter and Sen (1939b).
Sulphadiazine . . .	Coggeshall, Maier and Best (1941) ; Coxon and Hayes (1945) ; Wiselogle (1946).
Sulphamerazine 6-Sulphanilyl-metanilamide .	Wiselogle (1946).

4 : 4′-Diamidinodiphenylsulphone was inactive in quartan infec-tions in Italy (Secreto, 1946).

There is no evidence that any of the sulphonamides is capable of eradicating infections due to *P. malariæ* either by destroying the hypothetical exo-erythrocytic forms or by suppressive cure. The gametocytes of *P. malariæ* are unaffected by sulphonamides.

It is to be noted that when sulphadiazine and mepacrine are administered together the tissue levels of mepacrine are slightly lower than they would have been with the same doses of mepacrine alone. When sulphathiazole and mepacrine are given together the mepacrine levels are considerably lower than with mepacrine

alone. Mepacrine had no effect on the blood levels of either free
or total sulphathiazole or sulphadiazine.

The dangers of sulphonamides in malaria are the same as those
in other acute infections similarly treated. Renal involvement is
undoubtedly the greatest hazard.

Malaria in Monkeys

The three simian parasites on which information of the
effects of sulphonamides is available are *Plasmodium knowlesi*,
P. cynomolgi, and *P. inui*. No experiments appear to have been
carried out with *P. kochi*, in which an exo-erythrocytic stage has
been found by Garnham (1947). The majority of the observations
relate to *P. knowlesi* in rhesus monkeys, a parasite which Chopra
and Das Gupta (1938) first showed was susceptible to soluseptazine,
two injections of 2 ml. at twenty-four hours' interval removing the
parasitæmia. *P. knowlesi* is of particular interest because, as
Coggeshall (1938a) originally showed, not only is the incubation
period prolonged and the parasite/time level reduced by sulphanilamide, but with suitable dosage, usually 1 gm. daily by mouth
for one to three days, it is possible to obtain complete sterilisation
as shown by the non-infectivity of the blood to other monkeys
and the possibility of reinfection (Coggeshall, 1938a and b, 1940,
1941 ; Coggeshall and Maier, 1941). The doses employed by
Rodhain (1938), although they influenced the parasite levels, were
insufficient to cause complete sterilisation of the infection.
Elimination of parasites due to *P. knowlesi* from the blood stream
was, however, obtained by Coggeshall *et al.* (1941) with prontosil
rubrum, rodilone, and promin, while Coggeshall and Maier (1941)
found that sulphathiazole, sulphapyridine, and sulphadiazine had
an effect on the asexual blood forms. With the sodium salt of
sulphanilyl sulphanilic acid the incubation period was prolonged
and the parasite level in the blood reduced, but there was no
eradication of the infection (Coggeshall, 1938a). Chopra and Das
Gupta (1939) and Jaswant Singh and Harwant Singh (1939) also
found that infections due to *P. knowlesi* were eradicated by
sulphapyridine.

The action of sulphadiazine depends on the actual dose administered. Richardson *et al.* (1946), using a standard injecting dose

of 50 million parasites per kgm. given intravenously in rhesus monkeys, found that daily doses up to 0·06 mgm. of sulphadiazine per kgm. produced no consistent effect, but doses of 0·12 mgm. per kgm. caused an effect comparable to that of 22·2 mgm. per kgm. of quinine base. On the basis of oral dosage, sulphadiazine is thus 175 times as effective as quinine. The concentration of sulphadiazine required to control infection is below 0·5 mgm. per cent.

When 30 mgm. per kgm. of body weight of *para*-aminobenzoic acid is given to rhesus monkeys the minimal effective dose of sulphadiazine was found to be between 6 and 37·5 mgm. per kgm. of body weight per day ; at least 100 times as much sulphadiazine is thus required in the presence of this dose of *para*-aminobenzoic acid to produce an antimalarial effect as in the absence of it.

Soluseptazine was found by Chopra and Basu (1938) to reduce the parasite level in the blood stream when given in two doses of 2 ml. at an interval of twenty-four hours, but the infection was not eradicated : prontosil soluble produced similar results (Das Gupta and Chopra, 1938 ; Coggeshall *et al.*, 1941), as did sulphathiazole in the hands of Dikshit and Ganapathi (1940).

Plasmodium cynomolgi is less susceptible to sulphonamide compounds than *P. knowlesi*. Sulphanilamide lowers the parasite level but does not lead to complete eradication : on the other hand, promin appears to bring about complete sterilisation (Coggeshall *et al.*, 1941). Sulphathiazole acts like sulphanilamide and reduces the parasite level but does not eliminate the infection (Coggeshall and Maier, 1941).

Plasmodium inui is still more resistant, for although there is a reduction in the parasites in the blood (Coggeshall, 1941) there is no evidence that the infection is destroyed (Coggeshall, 1940 ; Coggeshall *et al.*, 1941). Sulphathiazole has an exactly similar action (Coggeshall and Maier, 1941 ; Coggeshall *et al.*, 1941), while even promin, which eradicates *P. cynomolgi*, does not affect *P. inui*. If a monkey is given a mixed infection of *P. knowlesi* and *P. inui* the former infection is eliminated by 1 gm. of sulphanilamide, the latter remains as a chronic infection.

Further work is required to determine the effect of sulphonamides on monkey malarias transmitted by mosquitoes.

Coggeshall and Maier (1941) point out that there is no correlation between the action of sulphonamides on these simian malaria parasites and their *in vitro* oxygen consumption.

Avian Malarias

Qualitative experiments with a number of the earlier sulphonamides were carried out on experimental bird malaria by many observers; the majority of the sulphonamides tested were found to influence the parasite level in the peripheral blood stream (Curd, 1943).

With more accurate methods of assessing antimalarial activity it has been possible to show that the same sulphonamide acts differently in different avian malarias. Thus Manwell *et al.* (1941) found that in the canary sulphapyridine was without action against *P. relictum* and *P. nucleophilum* but active against *P. circumflexum*. Similarly Dearborn and Marshall (1947) found that the quinine equivalents of sulphadiazine against blood infections in ducks are as follows :—

P. circumflexum	1·0
P. lophuræ	3·0
P. cathemerium	0·15
P. relictum	0·075

Wiselogle (1946) gives the following quinine equivalents against the blood forms of various avian malarias :—

	Sulpha-pyrazine.	Sulpha-merazine.	Sulpha-methazine.	N'-2-Quin-oxyalylsul-phanilamide.	6-Sulphani-lylmetanil-amide.
P. cathemerium in the canary	0·008	—	<0·008	0·04 very slight	0·002
„ „ „ duck	—	<0·15	—	2	0·06
P. gallinaceum in the chick .	3	0·1–0·4	0·4	8	0·06–0·15
P. lophuræ in the chick .	—	—	—		0·6
„ „ „ duck .	0·02–4	1·0	active	2	0·6

Not only does the same species of plasmodium react differently in different host species, in some cases a difference may be noted in different host strains.

Cantrell *et al.* (1949), for instance, have noted a difference in the behaviour of *P. gallinaceum* to sulphadiazine in two strains of chicken.

Although sulphonamides are capable of reducing parasitæmia their action is often slower than that of quinine. Brackett *et al.* (1945), for instance, found sulphanilamides slower in acting against *P. gallinaceum* than quinine, and similarly in *P. lophuræ* infections in ducks sulphadiazine is slower than quinine (Marshall *et al.*, 1946). This slower action is correlated with the fact that inhibition of *P. lophuræ* in ducks does not begin to be noticeable before the parasites have been exposed to sulphadiazine for seventy-two hours. *P. gallinaceum* begins to be inhibited after from twenty-four to thirty-six hours' exposure to sulphadiazine.

ACTIVITY OF SULPHONAMIDE DERIVATIVES IN CHICKENS AND CANARIES ON ERYTHROCYTIC FORMS OF MALARIAL PARASITES
(P. B. Marshall, 1945)

Derivative.	Action on *Plasmodium gallinaceum* in chicks. (Approx. sulphadiazine equivalents.)	Action on *Plasmodium cathemerium* in canaries.
Sulphanilamide	0·5	trace
Sulphapyridine	trace	inactive
Sulphadiazine	1·0	,,
Sulphamezathine	1·0	,,
Sulphathiazole	0·5	,,
5-Sulphanilamido-quinoline . .	trace	slight activity
8-Sulphanilamido-quinoline . .	,,	inactive
8-Sulphanilamido-6-methoxy-quinoline	,,	trace
2-Sulphanilamido-benzamide . .	0·1	inactive
3-Sulphanilamido-benzamide . .	0·2	,,
4-Sulphanilamido-benzamide . .	0·2	,,
N^1-(6'-quinoxalyl) sulphanilamide .	0·2	,,

The fact that sulphonamides are so much more active against the blood forms of *P. gallinaceum* in the chick than against other avian malarial species in canaries is probably due to the different blood concentrations of sulphonamides in the two species of birds. In chickens, as Marshall (1945) has pointed out, antimalarial activity varies with the blood concentration attained. Sulphadiazine and sulphamezathine in doses of 50 mgm. per kgm. of body weight are the most effective against *P. gallinaceum* : they also give rise to the highest blood concentrations which can be maintained at fairly high levels for about sixteen hours. Sulphanilamide and sulphathiazole have about half the antimalarial activity of sulphadiazine and the blood concentrations of these two drugs are correspondingly lower. The sulphanilamido-benzamides (Henry and Gorvin, 1944) and N^1-(6'-quinoxalyl)-sulphanilamide show about one-fifth the activity of sulphadiazine. The blood concentrations are low and, except in the case of 2-sulphanilamido-benzamide, fall to zero within sixteen hours. The three sulphanilamido-quinoline compounds have low blood concentration curves and only a trace of antimalarial activity. Sulphapyridine has only slight antimalarial activity, and though initially it produces high blood concentrations, these fall to low levels within seven hours.

The red blood cell concentrations in chicks are as a rule the same or slightly higher than the whole blood levels. Exceptions are sulphadiazine and sulphathiazole with which the concentrations in red cells are lower, with sulphathiazole so low in fact as to appear hardly in agreement with the observed antimalarial activity.

On the whole in chicks there is a considerable degree of agreement between the blood concentration curves and the order of antimalarial activity.

In canaries the red blood cell concentrations for sulphamezathine and the sulphanilamido-benzenes are much higher than the corresponding curves in chickens but the blood concentration curves fall away more rapidly. These drugs are quite inactive against *P. cathemerium* in doses equivalent to those given to chickens, but by maintaining canaries on frequently repeated doses of sulphadiazine so that the whole blood concentrations are between 50 to 100 mgm. per 100 ml., infection can be suppressed as long as treatment continues. Thus very much higher concentrations of sulphadiazine are necessary to inhibit *P. cathemerium* in canaries than *P. gallinaceum* in chicks. If sufficiently high blood concentrations could be given to canaries many other sulphonamides would undoubtedly inhibit *P. cathemerium* were they not too toxic. The very slight activity exhibited by the sulphanilamido-quinolines (Choudhury *et al.*, 1937 ; Bobranski, 1939 ; Winterbottom, 1940) in a dose of 250 to 500 mgm. per kgm. of body weight may be due to the action of the quinoline part of the molecule.

Causal Prophylaxis. The first demonstration that a sulphon-amide could act on the exo-erythrocytic forms was given by Coatney and Cooper (1944), who showed that in the domestic fowl sulpha-diazine destroyed the primary exo-erythrocytes of *P. gallinaceum* resulting from a sporozoite-induced infection following the bites of infected *Aëdes ægypti*. When sulphadiazine was given in a dose of 1·0 mgm. per kgm. of body weight twice daily for eight days or at a dosage of 0·5 mgm. per kgm. of body weight for four days beginning just prior to infection, none of the treated birds deve-loped malaria. When sulphaguanidine was given according to the same dosage two of twenty birds receiving the higher dose and five of twelve receiving the lower dose became infected. Similar findings were reported by Coggeshall *et al.* (1944) and Americano Freire and Paraense (1944). Infections were perma-nently prevented even when the last dose of the drug was given less than thirty-six hours after exposure. Coggeshall *et al.* (1944), using a technique involving repeated brain biopsies, produced direct evidence that it was the exo-erythrocytic forms which are destroyed by sulphadiazine whereas they are largely uninfluenced by quinine or mepacrine. Zuckerman (1946), by exposing exo-ery-throcytic forms of *P. gallinaceum* to solutions of sulphadiazine *in vitro* and then implanting them on the chorio-allantoic mem-brane of chick embryos was able to show that there was a marked suppressive action, as judged by the subsequent development of infection in the embryos.

Sulphapyrazine and, according to Coatney and Cooper (1948), at least thirty-four other sulphonamide derivatives, listed in the table on p. 393, are capable of acting on the exo-erythrocytic forms of avian malaria.

Once the infection has become established in the chick sulpha-diazine does not eradicate the infection, thus demonstrating that secondary exo-erythrocytes differ from primary forms in their reactions to chemotherapeutic drugs.

Sulphadiazine also acts to a much slighter degree as a causal prophylactic against *P. cathemerium* in the canary and *P. lophuræ* in the turkey : it has little if any action against *P. lophuræ* in the chick or *P. cathemerium* in the duck.

ACTIVITY AGAINST INFECTIONS IN CHICKS WITH SPOROZOITES OF
Plasmodium gallinaceum : TREATMENT BEGUN ON THE DAY
OF INFECTION (Davey, 1946)

Compound.	Treatment.				Results.
Sulphadiazine . .	25	mgm. b.i.d.	× 4		Radical cure.
	12·5	,,	,,	× 4	Some radical cures.
	6·25	,,	,,	× 4	Marked delay in infection ; no cures.
	1·0	,,	,,	× 4	Marked delay in infection in some chicks.
	0·5	,,	,,	× 4	No effect on mortality rate.
Sulphamezathine . .	25	,,	,,	× 4	Cure in most chicks.
	12·5	,,	,,	× 4	Marked delay in infection ; no cures.
	4·0	,,	,,	× 4	Marked delay in infection ; no cures.
	2·0	,,	,,	× 4	Delay in death in some chicks ; no cures.
Sulphamerazine . .	25	,,	,,	× 4	Marked delay in infection ; no cures.
Sulphanilamide . .	25	,,	,,	× 4	Marked delay in infection ; some cures.
Sulphathiazole . .	25	,,	,,	× 4	Marked delay in infection ; no cures.
Sulphapyridine . .	25	,,	,,	× 4	Marked delay in infection ; no cures.
Mepacrine hydrochloride .	8	,,	,,as long as possible.		No effect on mortality rate.
Proguanil hydrochloride .	3	,,	,,	× 5	Radical cure.
	2	,,	,,	× 5	Some radical cures.
	1	,,	,,	× 5	Marked delay in infection.
	0·25	,,	,,	× 6	Death delayed some days.
	0·1	,,	,,	× 6	Death delayed some days in some chicks.

The comparative effect of a number of sulphonamides on sporozoite-induced infections of *P. gallinaceum* has been studied by Davey (1946), treatment being begun on the day of infection. The results in comparison with those obtained with mepacrine and proguanil are shown in the table.

Wiselogle (1946) found that against *P. cathemerium* in the canary sulphamethazine, sulphamerazine, and N^1-2-quinoxalylsulphanil amide were inactive as causal prophylactics : sulphadiazine and sulphapyrazine had some action but with 6-sulphanilylmetanilamide such action was very slight. Against *P. lophuræ* in the turkey, sulphadiazine, sulphapyrazine, and N^1-2-quinoxalylsulphanilamide were active.

The close correlation between persistence in the blood stream and prophylactic action against *P. gallinaceum* was emphasised by Cantrell *et al.* (1949). The mean concentrations required to protect 50 per cent. of chickens were as follows :—

Sulphapyrazine . . . . 2·6 mgm. per ml.
Sulphadiazine . . . . 3·1 ,, ,, ,,
Sulphamethazine . . . . 4·7 ,, ,, ,,
Sulphamerazine . . . . 7·0 ,, ,, ,,

In addition to these compounds nineteen of sixty-one other sulphonamides tested were found to protect chickens against infection. Derivatives of sulphapyridine are particularly active. Of sulphadiazine derivatives those in which the alkyl substituents are connected to the pyrimidine ring through an ether linkage are poor in activity, but similar derivatives of N'-4-pyrimidyl sulphanilamide are active. All derivatives of sulphathiazole were active. Derivatives of 1-sulphanilyl-2-thiopseudourea were less active than similar concentrations of sulphadiazine.

Another compound which is said to act as a true causal prophylactic against *P. gallinaceum* is aluminium *para*-aminobenzene sulphonate, " sulfalumin," which has been used by León (1944) to treat certain cases of human malaria, apparently with good results. When given by mouth in doses of 500 mgm. per kgm. of body weight twice a day to chicks infected by sporozoites of *P. gallinaceum* sulfalumin is said to act as a causal prophylactic if the administration is continued from the first to the sixth day after infection. When treatment is delayed till after parasites have appeared in the blood the parasite level is decreased but the infection is not eradicated (León *et al.*, 1945).

Sulphonamides have no direct gametocyticidal action nor do they directly affect sporozoites. Davey (1946) exposed sporozoites of *P. gallinaceum* to a concentration of sulphadiazine of 5 mgm. per litre and found that they were still capable of inducing infection.

Bergeim *et al.* (1947) prepared a series of aminosulphanilamides which have some action in avian malaria, and English *et al.* (1946a) have found halogenated sulphanilamidoheterocycles active.

The mode of action of sulphonamide drugs on malaria parasites and the inhibition of such action by *p*-aminobenzoic acid is discussed on p. 549.

Synergistic Action. Investigations by Greenberg *et al.* (1948) have shown that proguanil and sulphadiazine potentiate each other's action against sporozoite-induced infections of *P. gallinaceum* in the chick. The results of various dosages of proguanil and sulphadiazine when combined and given prophylactically are shown in the table. The effective dose of proguanil can be reduced to one-quarter when combined with $\frac{1}{32}$ to $\frac{1}{64}$ the effective dose of sulphadiazine. Although the concurrent administration of the two drugs leads to higher plasma levels for sulphadiazine, the potentiation cannot be accounted for by the concentrations of the drugs in blood. The toxicity of the two drugs in combination is additive.

THE EFFECT OF PROGUANIL AND SULPHADIAZINE, ALONE AND IN COMBINATION, ON SPOROZOITE-INDUCED *Plasmodium gallinaceum* INFECTIONS IN CHICKS. (Greenberg, Boyd, and Josephson, 1948)

Dose of proguanil in mgm./gm. b.i.d.	Doses of sulphadiazine in mgm./gm. b.i.d.									
	None.	0·00195	0·0039	0·0078	0·0156	0·03125	0·0625	0·125	0·05	0·5
None . .	0/30	—	—	—	0/10	0/10	1/10	6/29	6/30	2/10
0·0009375 .	—	—	—	—	0/10	—	—	—	—
0·001875 . .	—	—	—	—	0/9	—	—	—
0·00375 . .	—	—	—	—	0/10	—	—	—	—
0·0075 . .	—	—	—	—	0/10	—	—	—	—
0·015 . .	0/20	2/20	2/10	7/10	19/24	15/16	5/5	6/6	—	—
0·03 . .	6/29	—	—	—	—	—	—	—	—
0·06 . .	5/9	—	—	—	—	—	—	—	—

[Number of birds showing no parasitæmia for thirty-five days after inoculation/number of birds treated.]

SULPHONAMIDES FOR WHICH THERE IS DIRECT OR INDIRECT EVIDENCE OF ACTIVITY AGAINST EXO-ERYTHROCYTIC FORMS OF MALARIAL PARASITES (Coatney and Cooper, 1948)

Chemical name.	Other designation.
N[1]-2-thiazolylsulphanilamide	Sulphathiazole
N[1]-2-pyridylsulphanilamide	Sulphapyridine
N[1]-2-pyrimidylsulphanilamide	Sulphadiazine
N[1]-(4-methyl-2-pyrimidyl)sulphanilamide . . .	Sulphamerazine
p-aminobenzenesulphonamide	Sulphanilamide
Sulphanilyl guanidine	Sulphaguanidine
N[1]-2-pyrazinylsulphanilamide	Sulphapyrazine
N[1]-(4, 6-dimethyl-2-pyrimidyl)sulphanilamide . .	{ Sulphamethazine / Sulphamezathine
N[4]-benzylsulphanilamide	Proseptazine
N[1]-3-pyridylsulphanilamide.	
N[1]-(6-chloro-2-pyrazinyl)sulphanilamide.	
N[1]-2-quinoxylylsulphanilamide	Sulphaquinoxaline
N[1]-(5-chloro-2-pyrazinyl)sulphanilamide.	
N[1]-(5-bromo-4, 6-dimethyl-2-pyrimidyl)sulphanilamide.	
N[1]-(5-bromo-4-methyl-2-thiazolyl)sulphanilamide.	

Chemical name.	Other designation.
N^1-(3-methyl-2-pyrazinyl)sulphanilamide.	
p-(2-pyrimidylsulphamyl)acetanilide.	
N^1-(5-methyl-1, 3, 4-thiadiazol-2)sulphanilamide.	
N^1-(4, 5, 6-trimethyl-2-pyrimidyl)sulphanilamide.	
N^1-(6-bromo-3-pyridyl)sulphanilamide.	
N^1-(5-bromo-4-methyl-2-pyrimidyl)sulphanilamide.	
N^1-(4-amino-2-pyrimidyl)sulphanilamide.	
N^1-(5-bromo-2-pyrimidyl)sulphanilamide.	
N^1-(5-chloro-2-pyrimidyl)sulphanilamide.	
N^1-(5-chloro-4-methyl-2-thiazolyl)sulphanilamide.	
N^1-(4-amino-5-bromo-2-pyrimidyl)sulphanilamide.	
4-amino-N-2-pyrimidyl-o-toluenesulphonamide.	
N^1-(5-bromo-2-thiazolyl)sulphanilamide.	
N^1-(5-chloro-2-thiazolyl)sulphanilamide.	
3'-sulphamylsulphanilanilide.	
N^1-(5-chloro-2-pyridyl)sulphanilamide.	
N^1-methyl-N'-2-pyrimidylsulphanilamide.	
N^1-2-benzoxazolylsulphanilamide.	
N^1-(5-iodo-2-pyrimidyl)sulphanilamide.	
6-sulphanilylmetanilamide.	
N^1-2-pyrimidylmetanilamide.	
N^1-2-pyrazinylmetanilamide.	
N^1-(5-chloro-2-pyrimidyl)metanilamide . . .	Metachloridine.
5 - amino - N - (5 - bromo - 2 - pyrimidyl) - o - toluene-sulphonamide.	
N^1-(5-bromo-2-pyridyl)metanilamide.	
m-(5-chloro-2-pyrimidylsulphamyl)acetanilide.	
N^1-3-pyridylmetanilamide.	
N^1-(5-bromo-2-pyrimidyl)metanilamide.	
N^1-(5-chloro-2-pyrazinyl)metanilamide.	
N^1(5-iodo-2-pyrimidyl)metanilamide.	
2-[(dimetanilyl)amino]-5-chloropyrimidine.	
3'-(5-chloro-2-pyrimidylsulphamyl)benzanilide.	
N^1-2-benzoxazolylmetanilamide.	
N^1-(5-bromo-4-methyl-2-pyrimidyl)metanilamide.	
m-[(5-chloro-2-pyrimidyl)sulphamyl]phenylurea.	
2 - [(bis - N^3 N^3-dimethylmetanilyl)amino] - 5 - chloro-pyrimidine.	
N^1-(5-chloro-2-pyrimidyl)-m-nitrobenzene-sulphonamide.	

METANILAMIDES

Derivatives of metanilic acid were first investigated for anti-malarial action by English *et al.* (1946a and b), who discovered that 2-sulphanilamido-5-chloropyrimidine was active. Further investigations resulted in the production of N^1-(5-chloro-2-pyrimidyl) metanilamide, [2-metanilamido-5-chloropyrimidine]. This compound, now known as metachloridine (SN 11,437), is at least sixteen times as active, weight for weight, against *P. gallinaceum* in chickens as sulphadiazine. The bromo- and iodo-analogues are also active.

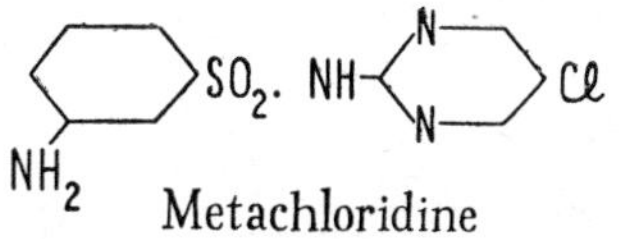

Metachloridine

N¹-(5-chloro-2-pyrimidyl) metanilamide

As in the case of sulphadiazine, this derivative of metanilic acid acts as a true causal prophylactic against *P. gallinaceum* in the chick (Brackett and Waletzky, 1946a and b), *P. cathemerium* in canaries (Gingrich *et al.*, 1946 ; Gingrich, 1948) and *P. lophuræ* in the turkey. With five days of treatment of the canary, doses of 0·5 to 1 gm. per kgm. of body weight are required to eradicate infection, but with ten days of treatment the same effects on *P. cathemerium* are observed with as little as 1 mgm. per kgm. of body weight. Metachloridine is incapable of eradicating an established blood infection by these parasites even when given in the maximum tolerated dose which is 2,000 times the minimum effective dose. The quinine equivalents for suppressive activity against the erythrocytic forms of bird malaria are as follows :—

Cathemerium infection in canaries .		.	33
,,	,,	,, ducks .	60
Gallinaceum	,,	,, chicks .	15
Lophuræ	,,	,, ,, .	15
,,	,,	,, ducks .	30

Against sporozoite-induced infections of *P. cathemerium* metachloridine when given in daily doses of 20 mgm. for ten days affords complete protection and even if the same dose is given for only four days the prepatent period is increased by four days (Hughes and Brackett, 1946).

Single oral doses of 1, 2 or 3 gm. produce maximum blood concentrations in four hours.

The greater part of a dose of metachloridine administered by mouth is found in the urine, showing that absorption is essentially complete. Renal excretion is accelerated by the administration of sodium bicarbonate. Concentrations of the drug in whole blood average only 70 per cent. of the concentrations in the plasma, indicating that there is probably little or no fixation by the cellular elements of the blood. Traces of the drug can still be found in the plasma four to seven days after a single dose of from 1 to 2 gm. Removal from the plasma is quickened by the simultaneous administration of sodium bicarbonate, the concurrent administration tripling the amount of metachloridine required to maintain a given plasma concentration. No acetylation occurs in man as with other sulphonamides.

In mice fed with metachloridine it was found to be about one and a half times as toxic as sulphadiazine on the basis of drug intake and less toxic than sulphadiazine on the basis of blood level. In the rat a diet containing 1 per cent. of the drug was fatal in seven to eleven days. The toxic symptoms were hypoprothrombinæmia with subcutaneous and intestinal hæmorrhages and severe anæmia. The hypoprothrombinæmia can be prevented by the addition of vitamin K, but after ten to fourteen days, even with vitamin K, the skin of the tail, feet, and around the mouth became œdematous and ulcerated : in addition, conjunctivitis developed and opacity of the lens and cornea. These changes in the skin and eyes could not be cured by the addition of biotin, folic acid, liver extract, rice-polishings, wheat-germ concentrate or yeast autolysate. Concretions in the kidneys or bladder were not uncommon, while the thyroid gland was enlarged and hyperactive. Dogs showed gastric ulcers, ulcers on the lips and gums, conjunctivitis and clouding of the cornea when given 0·3 to 0·6 gm. per kgm. body weight. Monkeys on daily doses of 0·15 to 0·5 gm. per kgm. body weight showed few toxic changes except an increase in the clotting time of the blood.

Experiments on patients who were already infected with the Chesson strain of vivax malaria or were given metachloridine before infection showed that a single weekly dose of 0·125 gm. or less failed to suppress clinical attacks, but a weekly dose of 0·25 gm. or more completely suppressed clinical evidence of infection.

With *P. falciparum* infections a weekly dose of 1 gm. failed to suppress infection, and a weekly dose of 2 gm. showed only slight suppressive activity. Curative experiments with the McCoy, Chesson, and St. Elizabeth strains of vivax showed that with the former only four of twenty-seven failed to relapse in from fourteen to 148 days ; with the latter only two of ten failed to relapse in from twenty-two to fifty-eight days. Doses varied from 22 to 40 gm. in six days to 14 to 58 gm. in fourteen days. Cooper *et al.* (1949) failed to cure patients infected with the St. Elizabeth strain of vivax by a twelve-day course of metachloridine alone or in combination with quinine : 2·0 gm. of metachloridine and 2·0 gm. of quinine were given daily : recurrence occurred in five cases in from thirty-one to forty-six days.

Against *P. falciparum* metachloridine shows very little activity (Wiselogle, 1946). However, Kenney and Brackett (1947) found that in British Guiana doses of 1 to 2 gm. weekly in two, three or five doses partially suppressed parasitæmia due to *P. falciparum*. The same doses completely suppressed infection due to *P. malariæ*, the results being better than those against *P. vivax*.

Schneider and Méchali (1948) treated ten patients infected with *P. vivax* and sixteen with *P. falciparum*. With doses of 1 to 2 gm. daily the symptoms were relieved very slowly and it was only with doses of 4 to 6 gm. that more rapid results were obtained. In the vivax infections the duration of fever was 3·4 and the duration of parasitæmia 4·4 days ; in the falciparum infections 2·8 and 3·6 days. Pullman *et al.* (1948) found metachloridine slower than quinine in overcoming parasitæmia due to the Chesson strain of *P. vivax* ; five to twelve as against three to six days. With a total dose of 1·0 gm. or more for a four-day period, giving a mean plasma concentration of 2·2 mgm. per 100 ml. or more, cure was obtained. A partial effect with temporary diminution of either parasitæmia or fever or both was obtained with total doses as small as 0·02 gm.

Metachloridine thus does not prevent relapses in vivax malaria, and it has no action against *P. falciparum*, including the Costa strain.

As a prophylactic its only action, according to Pullman *et al.* (1948), is to prolong the prepatent period by a time which was approximately equal to the duration of drug administration. Thus in untreated controls the prepatent period for the Chesson strain was ten to sixteen days ; in four patients treated for six days after inoculation parasitæmia appeared in twenty, twenty, twenty-four, and thirty-two days ; in those treated for twenty days parasitæmia occurred in thirty-four, thirty-four, thirty-six, and thirty-seven days.

Metachloridine is inferior to the aminoquinolines as well as to proguanil.

Toxic reactions in man were seen when daily doses of 4 to 5 gm. were given together with sodium bicarbonate (Wiselogle, 1946). Epistaxis and urethral bleeding were associated with a prolonged bleeding time. Although bleeding stopped within twenty-four hours of giving vitamin K the prolonged bleeding time persisted for several days after the drug was discontinued. Other toxic reactions were hæmaturia, nausea and vomiting, and transient leucopenia. Two patients, who had previously received metachloridine, developed purpuric rashes on the second and third day of a second course of the drug, probably due to capillary fragility (Cooper *et al.*, 1949). Schneider and Méchali (1948) noted sleepiness, anorexia, cyanosis, and digestive upsets in those given more than 4 gm. daily. Pullman *et al.* (1948) observed only four mild toxic reactions among seventy-three patients. There were no changes in whole blood counts, electrocardiogram, blood non-protein nitrogen, and phenolsulphonphthalein excretion tests.

English *et al.* (1946b) have suggested that metachloridine has a double antimalarial action due to the presence of 5-chloropyrimidine and metanilamide in the molecule. Its activity is not inhibited by *p*-aminobenzoic acid.

Certain other metanilamides have been investigated and, in all, seventeen of them are prophylactic against *P. gallinaceum* in the chick (Coatney and Cooper, 1948) ; 6-sulphanilylmetanilamide (SN 132) only delays patent infection in *P. gallinaceum* (Coatney and Sebrell, 1946 ; Maier, 1946), though Coggeshall and Porter (1946) obtained complete prophylaxis. Against *P. cathemerium* in the canary, Gingrich (1946) described only slight delay, and Coggeshall and Porter (1946) produced no evidence of prophylactic activity against *P. lophuræ* in the turkey. N^1-2-pyrimidylmetanilamide (SN 11,435) was found by Gingrich (1946) to produce an appreciable delay in the appearance of blood infections by

P. cathemerium in the canary. Coggeshall and Porter (1946) demonstrated complete prophylaxis against *P. lophuræ* in the turkey. N^1-(5-chloro-2-pyrimidyl)metanilamide (SN 11,437) showed a greater range of activity, giving complete prophylaxis against *P. cathemerium* in the canary (Gingrich, 1946 ; Gingrich *et al.*, 1946), *P. lophuræ* in the turkey (Coggeshall and Porter, 1946) and *P. gallinaceum* in the chick (Coatney and Sebrell, 1946).

References

AMERICANO FREIRE, S., and PARAENSE, W. L., 1944, The prophylactic and curative action of sulfadiazine (2-sulfanilamide-pyrimidine), sulfapyridine (2-sulfanilamide-pyridine) and sulfanilamide (*p*-aminobenzo-sulfonamide) on erythro and exoerythrocytic cycles of " *Plasmodium gallinaceum* " (therapeutic and parasitological aspects). *Rev. Bras. Biol.*, **4**, 27.

ARDIAS, A., 1948, La solfonoterapia della malaria. *Arch. i a . Sci. Med. colon.*, **29**, 115.

BERGEIM, F. H., LOSEE, K., and LOTT, W. A., 1947, Aminosulfanilamides, *J. Amer. chem. Soc.*, **69**, 583.

BOBRANSKI, B., 1939, Synthetische Versuche in der Reihe der chemotherapeutisch Wirksamen Derivate von Sulfanilsäuramid. *Arch. Pharm. Berl.*, **277**, 75.

BRACKETT, S., and WALETZKY, E., 1946a, The inability of drugs with both causal prophylactic and suppressive action to cure established infections with avian malaria. *J. Parasit.*, **32**, Sect. 2 (Suppl.), 8.

BRACKETT, S., and WALETZKY, E., 1946b, The antimalarial activity of metachloridine (2-metanilamido-5-chloropyrimidine) and other metanilamide derivatives in test infections with *Plasmodium gallinaceum*. *J. Parasit.*, **32**, 325.

BRACKETT, S., WALETZKY, E., and BAKER, M., 1945, The rate of action of sulfadiazine and quinine on the malarial parasite *Plasmodium gallinaceum*. *J. Pharmacol.*, **84**, 254.

CANTRELL, W., KELSEY, F. E., and GEILING, E. M. K., 1949, Sulfonamide blood levels in prophylactic trials against *Plasmodium gallinaceum*. *J. infect. Dis.*, **84**, 32.

CHOPRA, R. N., and BASU, B. C., 1938, Studies on the effect of antimalarial drugs upon the infectivity of patients to mosquitoes. *J. mal. Inst. India*, **1**, 351.

CHOPRA, R. N., and BASU, B. C., 1939, Studies on the effect of antimalarial drugs upon the infectivity of patients to mosquitoes. III. " Prontosil." *J. mal. Inst. India*, **2**, 153.

CHOPRA, R. N., and DAS GUPTA, B. M., 1938, A note on the therapeutic efficiency of soluseptazine in simian malaria (*P. knowlesi*). *Indian med. Gaz.*, **73**, 395.

CHOPRA, R. N., and DAS GUPTA, B. M., 1939, M. & B. 693 (2-sulphanilyl-amino-pyridine) in ape malaria. *Indian med. Gaz.*, **74**, 201.

CHOPRA, R. N., DAS GUPTA, B. M., SEN, B., and HAYTER, R. T. M., 1939a, Prontosil in Indian strains of malaria. *Indian med. Gaz.*, **74**, 321.

CHOPRA, R. N., HAYTER, R. T. M., and SEN, B., 1939b, M. & B. 693 in Indian strains of malaria. *Indian med. Gaz.*, **74**, 658.

CHOUDHURY, A. K., DAS GUPTA, P., and BASU, U., 1937, Sulfonamides. *J. Indian chem. Soc.*, **14**, 733.

COATNEY, G. R., and COOPER, W. C., 1944, The prophylactic effect of sulfa-diazine and sulfaguanidine against mosquito-borne *Plasmodium gallinaceum* infection in the domestic fowl (preliminary report). *Publ. Hlth Rep., Wash.*, 59, 1455.

COATNEY, G. R., and COOPER, W. C., 1948, Symposium on exoerythrocytic forms of malarial parasites. III. The chemotherapy of malaria in relation to our knowledge of exoerythrocytic forms. *J. Parasit.*, 34, 275.

COATNEY, G. R., COOPER, W. C., YOUNG, M. D., and McLENDON, S. B.,1947a, Studies in human malaria. I. The protective action of sulfadiazine and sulfapyrazine against sporozoite-induced falciparum malaria. *Amer. J. Hyg.*, 46, 84.

COATNEY, G. R., COOPER, W. C., YOUNG, M. D., BURGESS, R. W., and SMARR, R. G., 1947b, Studies in human malaria. II. The suppressive action of sulfadiazine and sulfapyrazine against sporozoite-induced vivax malaria (St. Elizabeth strain). *Amer. J. Hyg.*, 46, 105.

COATNEY, G. R., and SEBRELL, W. H., 1946, in : "A survey of antimalarial drugs, 1941–45," edited by Wiselogle, F. Y. 2 Vols. Ann Arbor, Michigan. J. W. Edwards.

COGGESHALL, L. T., 1938a, Prophylactic and therapeutic effect of sulphonamide compounds in experimental malaria. *Proc. Soc. exp. Biol., N.Y.*, 38, 768.

COGGESHALL, L. T., 1938b, The cure of *Plasmodium knowlesi* malaria in rhesus monkeys with sulphanilamide and their susceptibility to reinfection. *Amer. J. trop. Med.*, 18, 715.

COGGESHALL, L. T., 1940, The selective action of sulfanilamide on the parasites of experimental malaria in monkeys *in vivo* and *in vitro*. *J. exp. Med.*, 71, 13.

COGGESHALL, L. T., 1941, Infection of *Anopheles quadrimaculatus* with *Plasmodium cynomolgi*, a monkey malaria parasite, and with *Plasmodium lophurœ*, an avian malaria parasite. *Amer. J. trop. Med.*, 21, 525.

COGGESHALL, L. T., and MAIER, J., 1941, Determination of the activity of various drugs against the malaria parasite. *J. infect. Dis.*, 69, 108.

COGGESHALL, L. T., MAIER, J., and BEST, C. A., 1941, The effectiveness of two new types of chemotherapeutic agents in malaria, sodium p, p'-diamino-diphenylsulfone N, N'-didextrosesulfonate (promin) and 2-sulfanilamido pyrimidine (sulfadiazine). *J. Amer. med. Ass.*, 117, 1077.

COGGESHALL, L. T., MARTIN, W. B., and BATES, R. D., Jr., 1945, Sulfadiazine in treatment of relapsing malarial infections due to *Plasmodium vivax*. *J. Amer. med. Ass.*, 128, 7.

COGGESHALL, L. T., and PORTER, R. J., 1946, in : "A survey of antimalarial drugs, 1941–45," edited by Wiselogle, F. Y. 2 Vols. Ann Arbor, Michigan. J. W. Edwards.

COGGESHALL, L. T., PORTER, R. J., and LAIRD, R. L., 1944, Prophylactic and curative effects of certain sulfonamide compounds on exoerythrocytic stages in *Plasmodium gallinaceum* malaria. *Proc. Soc. exp. Biol., N.Y.*, 57, 286.

COOPER, W. C., RUHE, D. S., COATNEY, G. R., and JOSEPHSON, E. S., 1949, Studies in human malaria. XIII. The therapeutic action of metachlori-dine (SN 11,437) against St. Elizabeth strain vivax malaria. *Amer. J. Hyg.*, 49, 355.

COXON, R. V., and HAYES, W., 1945, Investigation into efficacy of sulpha-diazine in treatment of malaria. *Trans. R. Soc. trop. Med. Hyg.*, 39, 196.

CURD, F. H. S., 1943, The activity of drugs in the malaria of man, monkeys and birds. *Ann. trop. Med. Parasit.*, 37, 115.

DAS GUPTA, B. M., and CHOPRA, R. N., 1938, Studies on the action of synthetic drugs on simian malaria : sulphonamide derivatives. *Indian Med. Gaz.*, 73, 665.

DAVEY, D. G., 1946, The use of avian malaria for the discovery of drugs effective in the treatment and prevention of human malaria. II. Drugs for causal prophylaxis and radical cure or the chemotherapy of exo-erythrocytic forms. *Ann. trop. Med. Parasit.*, **40**, 453.

DEARBORN, E. H., and MARSHALL, E. K., Jr., 1947, The susceptibility of different species of avian malarial parasites to drugs. *Amer. J. Hyg.*, **45**, 25.

DÍAZ DE LEÓN, A., 1937, Primeros casos de paludismo tratados por un derivodo de la sulfanilamida. *Bol. Ofic. sanit. pan-amer.*, **16**, 1039. [English trans. *Publ. Hlth Rep., Wash.*, 1937, **52**, 1460.]

DÍAZ DE LEÓN, A., 1938, Las sulfanilamidas en el tratamiento del paludismo. *Medicina Méx.*, **18** 89.

DÍAZ DE LEÓN, A., 1940, El paludismo y su tratamiento intravenoso por las sulfanilamidas. *Medicina, Méx.*, **20**, 551.

DIKSHIT, B. B., and GANAPATHI, K., 1940, Sulphathiazole in monkey malaria. *J. Mal. Inst. India*, **3**, 525.

ENGLISH, J. P., CLARK, J. H., CLAPP, J. W., SEEGER, D., and EBEL, R. H., 1946a, Studies in chemotherapy. XIII. Antimalarials. Halogenated sulfanilamidoheterocycles. *J. Amer. chem. Soc.*, **68**, 453.

ENGLISH, J. P., CLARK, J. H., SHEPHERD, R. G., MARSON, H. W., KRAPCHO, J., and ROBLIN, R. O., Jr., 1946b, Studies in chemotherapy. XIV. Antimalarials. Synthesis of substituted metanilamides and related compounds. *J. Amer. chem. Soc.*, **68**, 1039.

FAGET, G. H., PALMER, M. R., and SHERWOOD, R. O., 1938, Unsuccessful treatment of malaria with sulfonamide compounds. *Publ. Hlth Rep., Wash.*, **53**, 1364.

FAIRLEY, N. H., ANDREW, R. R., BLACKBURN, C. R. B., MACKERRAS, M. J., ROBERTS, F. H. S., ALLMAN, S. L. W., BACKHOUSE, T. C., GREGORY, T. S., POPE, K. C., DUNN, S. R., WOOD, I. J., PEDLAR, J., FORSYTH, L., TONGE, J. I., FERRIS. A. A., FREEMAN, M. J., OFFICER, R., ROBERTS, E. M., WHEELER, R., and BRENTON, B., 1945, Chemotherapeutic suppression and prophylaxis in malaria. *Trans. R. Soc. trop. Med. Hyg.*, **38**, 311.

FARINAUD, E., and ELICHE, J., 1939, Nouvelles observations sur le traitement du paludisme par les dérivés de la sulfamide. *Bull. Soc. Path. exot.*, **32**, 674.

FARINAUD, E., and RAGIOT, C., 1938, Recherches sur l'emploi des dérivés de la sulfamide dans le traitement du paludisme. *Bull. Soc. Path. exot.*, **31**, 907.

FINDLAY, G. M., 1948, Investigations in the chemotherapy of malaria in West Africa. VI. " Suppressive cure " of malaria. *Ann. trop. Med. Parasit.*, **43**, 1.

FINDLAY, G. M., MAEGRAITH, B. G., MARKSON, J. L., and HOLDEN, J. R., 1946, Investigations in the chemotherapy of malaria in West Africa. V. Sulphonamide compounds. *Ann. trop. Med. Parasit.*, **40**, 358.

GARDNER, W. A., and DEXTER, L., 1938, A case of quartan malaria following transfusion and treated with sulfanilamide. *J. Amer. med. Ass.*, **111**, 2473.

GARNHAM, P. C. C., 1947, Exoerythrocytic schizogony in *Plasmodium kochi* Laveran. A preliminary note. *Trans. R. Soc. trop. Med. Hyg.*, **40**, 719.

GINGRICH, W., 1946, in : "A survey of antimalarial drugs," 1941–45, edited by Wiselogle, F. Y. 2 Vols. Ann Arbor, Michigan. J. W. Edwards.

GINGRICH, W., 1948, The prophylactic and suppressive antimalarial effect of metachloridine with *Plasmodium cathemerium* in the canary. *J. Parasit.*, **34**, Sect. 2 (Suppl.), 36.

GINGRICH, W., SCHOCH, E. W., and TAYLOR, C. A., 1946, Therapeutic, prophylactic and curative tests in avian malaria (*Plasmodium cathemerium*) with metachloridine. *J. Parasit.*, **32**, Sect. 2 (Suppl.), 9.

GONZÁLEZ BARRERAS, P., 1939, Colorantes azoiceos y paludismo. *Bol. Ofic. Sanit. pan-amer.*, **18**, 753.

GREENBERG, J., BOYD, B. L., and JOSEPHSON, E. S., 1948, Synergistic effect of chlorguanide and sulfadiazine against *Plasmodium gallinaceum* in the chick. *J. Pharmacol.*, **94**, 60.

HALL, W. E. B., 1938, The sulphanilamides in tertian malaria. *J. Pharmacol.*, **63**, 353.

HENRY, T. A., and GORVIN, J. H., 1944, British Patent No. 562349.

HILL, R. A., and GOODWIN, H. M., Jr., 1937, " Prontosil " in treatment of malaria : report of 100 cases. *Sth. med. J.*, *Nashville*, **30**, 1170.

HUGHES, C. O., and BRACKETT, S., 1946, The prevention of sporozoite-induced infections of *Plasmodium cathemerium* in the canary by metachloridine. *J. Parasit.*, **32**, 340.

ISHII, N., 1948, Researches on the chemotherapy of protozoal infections. *Jap. med. J.*, **1**, 30.

JASWANT SINGH and HARWANT SINGH, 1939, Treatment of simian malaria with M. and B. 693. *J. mal. Inst. India*, **2**, 181.

JOHNSON, C. E., Jr., 1943, Status of sulfonamide therapy in malaria. *Amer. J. med. Sci.*, **206**, 327.

KENNEY, M., and BRACKETT, S., 1947, The effectiveness of metachloridine in suppressing natural infections with *Plasmodium malariæ* and *P. falciparum* in British Guiana. *Amer. J. trop. Med.*, **27**, 493.

LEÓN, A. P., 1944, *para*-Amino-bencene-sulfonato de aluminio. Sulfalumin. Un nuevo compuesto anti-infeccioso. *Rev. Inst. Salubrid. Enferm. trop.*, **5**, 255.

LEÓN, A. P., BELTRAN, E., and LARENAS, M. R., 1945, Accion del sulfalumin sobre los parasitos del paludismo experimental de los pullos, *P. gallinaceum*. *Rev. Inst. Salubrid. Enferm. trop.*, **6**, 137.

LIVADAS, G., and SPHANGOS, J., 1944, [Combination of sulphonamides and small doses of quinine in malaria treatment]. *Akad. Iatr.*, p. 1 (June).

MAIER, J., 1946, in : " A survey of antimalarial drugs, 1941-45," edited by Wiselogle, F. Y., 2 Vols. Ann Arbor, Michigan. J. W. Edwards.

MANWELL, R. D., COUNTS, E., and COULSTON, F., 1941, Effect of sulfanilamide and sulfapyridine on the avian malarias. *Proc. Soc. exp. Biol.*, *N.Y.*, **46**, 523.

MARSHALL, E. K., Jr., LITCHFIELD, J. T., Jr., and WHITE, H. J., 1946, The antimalarial action in ducks of certain sulfanilamide derivatives. *J. Pharmacol.*, **86**, 273.

MARSHALL, P. B., 1945, The absorption of sulphonamides in the chick and the canary, and its relationship to antimalarial activity. *J. Pharmacol.*, **84**, 1.

MENK, W., and MOHR, W., 1939, Zur Frage der Wirksamkeit des Prontosils bei akuter Malaria. *Arch. Schiffs-u. Tropenhyg.*, **43**, 117.

MOTZFELDT, K., 1938, Sulfanilamid ved malaria. *Norsk. Mag. Lægevidensk.*, **99**, 872.

NIVEN, J. C., 1938, Sulphanilamide in the treatment of malaria. *Trans. R. Soc. trop. Med. Hyg.*, **32**, 413.

PAKENHAM-WALSH, R., and RENNIE, A. T., 1938, Sulphonamides in malaria. *Lancet*, **ii**, 79.

PAKENHAM-WALSH, R., and RENNIE, A. T., 1939, M. and B. 693 in malaria. *Lancet*, **i**, 1382.

PAKENHAM-WALSH, R., and RENNIE, A. T., 1940, Sulphathiazole in malaria. *Lancet*, **ii**, 485.

PULLMAN, T. N., ALVING, A. S., JONES, R., Jr., WHORTON, C. M., CRAIGE, B., Jr., and EICHELBERGER, L., 1948, A study of the prophylactic, curative and suppressive activity of SN 11,437 (metachloridine) in standardised infections of vivax malaria. *Amer. J. trop Med.*, **28**, 413.

READ, H., and PINO, J. O., 1938, Versuche mit den Sulfonamid-Präparaten bei der Malaria behandlung. *Arch. Schiffs-u. Tropenhyg.*, **42**, 132.

RICHARDSON, A. P., HEWITT, R. I., SEAGER, L. D., BROOKE, M. M., MARTIN, F., and MADDUX, H., 1946, Chemotherapy of *Plasmodium knowlesi* infections in *Macaca mulatta* monkeys. *J. Pharmacol.*, 87, 203.

RODHAIN, J., 1938, *para*Aminophenylsulfamide et plasmodium des singes. *Ann. Soc. belge. Med. trop.*, 18, 255.

SAINI, M., 1947, Sulla cura della malaria infantile con sulfoni. *Minerva Med., Torino*, 1, 52.

SCHNEIDER, J., and CARUANA, M., 1948, Essais de traitement curatif du paludisme par la sulfaméthyldiazine (sumédine). *Bull. Soc. Path. exot.*, 41, 478.

SCHNEIDER, J., and MÉCHALI, D., 1948, Traitement curatif du paludisme. Étude de l'activité comparée de quatre nouveaux dérivés synthétiques. *Bull. Soc. Path. exot.*, 41, 274.

SCHWARTZ, L., FURST, W., and FLIPPIN, H. F., 1941, Sulfathiazole as an antimalarial. *Amer. J. Hyg.*, 34C, 160.

SECRETO, E., 1946, Il diaminodifenilsulfone nelle malaria. *Arch. Sci. med.*, 81, 139.

SINTON, J. A., HUTTON, E. L., and SHUTE, P. G., 1939, Some successful trials of proseptasine as a true causal prophylactic against infection with *Plasmodium falciparum. Ann. trop. Med Parasit.*, 33, 37.

SORLEY, E. R., and CURRIE, J. G., 1938, Notes on the experimental use of prontosil album in the treatment of malaria. *J. R. nav. med. Serv.*, 24, 322.

VAN DER WIELEN, Y., 1937, Prontosil en malaria quartana. *Ned. Tijdschr. Geneesk.*, 81, 2905.

WINTERBOTTOM, R., 1940, Sulfanilyl derivatives of pyridine and quinoline amines. *J. Amer. chem. Soc.*, 62, 160.

WISELOGLE, F. Y., edited by, 1946, " A survey of antimalarial drugs, 1941–45." 2 Vols. Ann Arbor, Michigan. J. W. Edwards.

ZUCKERMAN, A., 1946, Infections with *Plasmodium gallinaceum* in chick embryos induced by exoerythrocytic and blood stages. *J. infect. Dis.*, 79, 1.

SULPHABIGUANIDINES

Sulphabiguanidines of types A and B, having different aryl substituents at N^1 of the biguanide residue were prepared by Bami *et al.* (1947, 1948a). These compounds show a very feeble tendency to chelation, possibly because of the electronegative nature of the substituents. Nevertheless these compounds exhibit antimalarial activity, thus showing that chelation is not essential for antimalarial action. Bami *et al.* (1948b) have prepared compounds of metachloridine and 2-metanilamido-5-chloropyrimidine.

Type A.

$$\text{X--NH--}\underset{\underset{NH}{\|}}{C}\text{--NH--}\underset{\underset{NH}{\|}}{C}\text{--NH}\bigcirc\text{SO}_2\text{ NH}\underset{\underset{N}{\|}}{C}\overset{N\text{--C.CH}_3}{\underset{=CH}{\underset{\|}{C}}}\text{CH.HC}\ell$$

Type B.

X = substituted aryls (phenyl; *p*-chlorophenyl; 2-4-dichloro-phenyl; *p*-bromophenyl; *p*-iodophenyl; *p*-methylphenyl; 3, 4-dimethylphenyl; *p*-methoxyphenyl; *p*-nitrophenyl).

References

BAMI, H. L., IYER, B. H., and GUHA, P. C., 1947, Antimalarials. V. Some sulfabiguanide derivatives. *J. Ind. Inst. Sci.*, 29A, 15.

BAMI, H. L., IYER, B. H., and GUHA, P. C., 1948a, Studies on antimalarials : sulphabiguanidine derivatives. *Current Sci.*, 17, 90.

BAMI, H. L., IYER, B. H., and GUHA, P. C., 1948b, Metachloridine-substituted aryl biguanides as possible antimalarial compounds. *Nature, Lond.*, 162, 146.

ANTIBIOTICS

The majority of antibiotics are completely inactive against malarial parasites. Tyrothricin, however, has been found by Taliaferro *et al.* (1944) to be effective curatively against *P. galli-naceum* in chickens both with sporozoite- and blood-induced infections. The antibiotic is best given intravenously in a 9·5 per cent. alcoholic solution to chickens. It produces a predominantly parasiticidal effect, especially on extracellular merozoites produced at segmentation and to a lesser extent growth and reproduction-inhibiting effects when given daily in doses of 0·2 mgm. per 100 gm. of body weight. The incubation period of blood-induced infections is lengthened if daily treatment is given from the beginning of infection and in addition the peak of the acute infection and fatal relapses in both sporozoite- and blood-induced infections are modified. Tyrothricin is not effective when given intravenously in distilled water, when given intraperitoneally in 9·5 per cent. alcohol or in distilled water, or when given in capsules by mouth. It does not act prophylactically and thus probably does not act either on the sporozoites or exo-erythrocytic forms. When given in twelve daily doses intravenously in a 9·5 per cent. alcoholic solution, tyrothricin has a quinine equivalent of approxi-mately four when quinine is given in a similar manner in distilled water. The effective amount, however, is near the toxic level, for about half the chickens die when given multiple doses of 0·3 mgm. of tyrothricin. Such doses more effectively suppress blood-induced than sporozoite-induced infections.

Relatively large doses of penicillin fail to alter in any way the course of therapeutically induced vivax infections in man (Lyons, 1943; Hindle *et al.*, 1945). Both crude and pure sodium penicillins were without action on *P. lophuræ* infections in ducks (Bratton, 1945). Large doses of streptomycin fail to suppress the blood-induced infections due to *P. cathemerium*, *P. lophuræ*, and *P. gallinaceum*, but they have some inhibitory action on the course of sporozoite-induced infections caused by the last parasite (Seeler *et al.*, 1946).

Tonkin (1946) found that in tissue cultures of the exo-erythrocytic forms of *P. gallinaceum* streptothricin and streptomycin inhibited growth in concentrations of 2·5 mgm. per 100 ml. (= 10 units per ml.) and 250 mgm. per 100 ml. (= 500 units per ml.) respectively. Chloramphenicol has no action on *P. lophuræ* in ducks (Smith *et al.*, 1948).

McLean *et al.* (1949) find that chloramphenicol has a quinine equivalent of <0·05 against *P. lophuræ* in ducks and 0·1 in chicks. The daily dose was 200 and 537 mgm. per kgm. per day for five days. The most striking results, however, have been obtained with aureomycin. Against blood-induced infections of *P. gallinaceum* in chicks, aureomycin has a quinine equivalent of 0·25 : in tests for causal prophylaxis aureomycin is able to prevent infection and in tests against late exo-erythrocytic forms aureomycin prevents death. Its action is thus similar to certain 8-aminoquinolines, proguanil, and sulphadiazine (Coatney *et al.*, 1949).

Against vivax malaria (Chesson strain) aureomycin was ineffective (Cooper *et al.*, 1949), but Levaditi and Vaisman (1950) found it effective against *P. berghei*.

An extract of a lichen, *Parmelia parietina*, was at one time thought to have a curative action in malaria (Sander, 1815 ; Monkewitz, 1817 ; Styx, 1817). Some attempts at chemical analysis, in the circumstances inconclusive, were carried out by Mannhardt (1818).

Carlson *et al.* (1946) found that watery extracts of buttercup, sagebrush, dwarf waterleaf, mountain pasque, and juniper when mixed and kept at room temperature for six hours with the blood of chickens containing *P. gallinaceum* inactivated the plasmodia, as shown by the results of subsequent intravenous injection of chickens.   Sagebrush and dwarf waterleaf extracts had some action on the exo-erythrocytic phase of the parasites as well as diminishing the established blood infection.

Tetanus Toxoid

The possible use of tetanus toxoid was suggested by the chance observation that infection due to *Clostridium welchii* caused the disappearance of *P. vivax* in forty-eight hours from the blood stream.   Garcia (1948) therefore tested the effects of two injections of tetanus toxoid on the relapse rate of patients infected with *P. vivax* or *P. falciparum*.   Each patient during an acute exacerbation was given mepacrine or chloroquine as a routine, and in addition two injections of 2 ml. of tetanus toxoid at an interval of twenty-one days.   Controls were given mepacrine or chloroquine without tetanus toxoid.   Of sixty-one patients with *P. falciparum* given malaria treatment and tetanus toxoid none relapsed ; of twenty-five not given tetanus toxoid twenty-one relapsed, the average interval to relapse in two series being 105 and 120 days respectively.   Of 193 patients with *P. vivax* infection fifteen relapsed after tetanus toxoid, the average interval to relapse being 315 days : of forty patients with *P. vivax* given only the course of mepacrine or chloroquine thirty-six relapsed in from 105 to 120 days.   If these claims are true it would thus appear that tetanus toxoid with mepacrine or chloroquine can cure every case of falciparum infection and from 90 to 94 per cent. of vivax infections.   It is suggested that the anti-relapse effect of tetanus toxoid injected subcutaneously is such as to stimulate the reticulo-endothelial system that it becomes capable of attacking the exoerythrocytic stages of the parasites.   Tetanus toxoid alone, without the action of antimalarial drugs, is unable to prevent relapses.   Boyd and Coelho (1949) have similarly shown that a patient suffering from infection due to *Clostridium welchii* reacted feebly to a therapeutically induced infection due to *P. falciparum*. Presumably the soluble exotoxin adversely affects the plasmodium.

PANTOTHENIC ACID

References

BOYD, M. F., and COELHO, R. D., 1949, A note on the apparent antagonism of a bacterial intoxication to a plasmodial infection. *Amer. J. Trop. Med.*, **29**, 199.

BRATTON, A. C., Jr., 1945, Continuous intravenous chemotherapy of *Plasmodium lophuræ* in ducks. *J. Pharmacol.*, **85**, 103.

CARLSON, H. J., BISSELL, H. D., and MUELLER, M. G., 1946, Antimalarial and antibacterial substances separated from higher plants. *J. Bact.*, **52**, 155.

COATNEY, G. R., GREENBERG, J., COOPER, W. C., and TREMBLEY, H. L., 1949, The antimalarial activity of aureomycin against *Plasmodium gallinaceum* in the chick. *J. Parasitol.*, **35** (No. 6, Sect. 2), 25.

COOPER, W. C., COATNEY, G. R., and IMBODEN, C. A., Jr., 1949, Aureomycin in experimental Chesson strain vivax malaria. *Proc. Soc. exp. Biol.*, *N.Y.*, **72**, 587.

GARCIA, E. Y., 1948, The inhibition of malarial relapses by toxoid of *Clostridium tetani*. *Ann. New York Acad. Sci.*, **50**, 171.

HINDLE, J. A., ROSE, A. S., TREVETT, L. D., and PROUT, C., 1945, The effect of penicillin on inoculation malaria. A negative report. *New Engl. J. Med.*, **232**, 133.

LEVADITI, C., and VAISMAN, A., 1950, Activité anti-paludique (*Plasmodium berghei*) de l'aureomycin. *C. R. Acad. Sci. Paris*, **230**, 1908.

LYONS, C., 1943, Penicillin therapy of surgical infections in the U.S. Army. *J. Amer. med. Ass.*, **123**, 1007.

McLEAN, I. W., Jr., SCHWAB, J. L., HILLEGAS, A. B., and SCHLINGMAN, A. S., 1949, Susceptibility of micro-organisms to chloramphenicol (chloromycetin). *J. clin. Invest.*, **28**, 953.

MANNHARDT, J., 1818, "*Lobariæ Parietinæ* seu *Lichenis parietini* L. analysis chemica denuo instituta." Kiliæ. C. F. Mohr.

MONKEWITZ, J. H., 1817, "Chemisch medizinische Untersuchung über die Wandflechte (*Lichen parietinus*) und über die gebräuchlichsten Chinarinden. Eine akademische streitschrift." Dorpat. J. C. Schünmann.

SANDER, G. C. H., 1815, "Die Wandflechte, ein Arzneimittel welches die peruvianische Rinde nicht nur entbehrlich macht, sondern sie auch an gleichartigen Heilkräften übetrifft." Sundershausen. B. F. Voigt.

SEELER, A. O., MALANGA, C., and PIERSON, J., 1946, Effect of streptomycin on avian malaria. *Proc. Soc. exp. Biol.*, *N.Y.*, **59**, 291.

SMITH, R. M., JOSLYN, D. A., GRUHZIT, O. M., McLEAN, I. W., Jr., PENNER, M. A., and EHRLICH, J., 1948, Chloromycetin : biological studies. *J. Bact.*, **55**, 425.

STYX, M. E., 1817, "Ueber die Heilkräfte der Wandflechte als neuentdeckter, inländischer Substitut der Chinarinde." Dorpat.

TALIAFERRO, L. G., COULSTON, F., and SILVERMAN, M., 1944, The antimalarial activity of tyrothricin against *Plasmodium gallinaceum*. *J. infect. Dis.*, **75**, 179.

TONKIN, I. M., 1946, The testing of drugs against exoerythrocytic forms of *P. gallinaceum* in tissue culture. *Brit. J. Pharmacol.*, **1**, 163.

Pantothenic Acid Derivatives

Although pantothenic acid derivatives have not yet found a place in the treatment of human malarial infections, the study of this group of compounds illustrates the principle of biological competition in relation to malarial parasites.

The addition of calcium pantothenate to an appropriate medium containing red cells parasitised by *Plasmodium lophuræ* was found by Trager (1943) to lengthen the time of survival of the parasites.

As a consequence of the work of Snell (1941), Kuhn *et al.* (1941) and McIlwain (1942), it was known that pantoyltaurine and pantoyltauramide could inhibit the growth of those bacteria which require pantothenic acid as an essential metabolite.

These two substances, pantoyltaurine and pantoyltauramide, and several closely related derivatives were inactive when given by mouth to chicks with blood-induced infections due to *P. gallinaceum* or ducks infected with *P. lophuræ*. However, if pantoyltauramide-4-chlorobenzene is given intravenously to chicks in large doses of 2 gm. or more per kgm. per day, it has a marked suppressive effect on the growth of *P. gallinaceum*, being at least four times as active as quinine (Brackett *et al.*, 1946). The effect of pantothenic acid analogues on blood-induced infections of *P. gallinaceum* is seen in the table on p. 409. Phenylpantothenone, N-(2-benzoylethyl)-α,γ-dihydroxy-β,β-dimethyl butyramide,which Woolley (1944) found to be a competitive antagonist of pantothenic acid is lacking in antimalarial activity in ducks infected with *P. lophuræ* but capable of suppressing the parasitæmia in chicks infected with *P. gallinaceum* or *P. lophuræ*, the quinine equivalents being 1·0 and 2·0 (Woolley and Collyer, 1945). The inability of phenylpantothenone to influence infection by *P. lophuræ* in ducks while suppressing blood-induced infections of *P. gallinaceum* in chicks is due to some peculiarity not of the parasite but of the host, for according to Trager (1943) the pantothenic acid content of duck and hen red cells is not significantly different. Curiously enough pantothenic acid inhibitors do not suppress the development of sporozoite-induced infections of *P. gallinaceum* (Woolley and Collyer, 1945).

The antimalarial activity of phenylpantothenone is thus due to an interference with the metabolism of pantothenic acid, for it can be overcome by giving chicks infected with *P. gallinaceum* relatively enormous amounts of calcium pantothenate. Pantoyl-taurylamide can also be inhibited by calcium pantothenate. Thus the antimalarial effect of 400 mgm. per kgm. against *P. gallinaceum*

Plasmodium gallinaceum of SEVEN DAYS' DURATION. (Brackett et al., 1946)

No.	Compound.* R	Intake mgm./kgm./day	Activity.†	Quinine equivalent
1	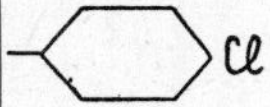 (benzene ring) Cl	3·7, 1·4, 0·9	<0·5, 0·5, 2·0	16
2	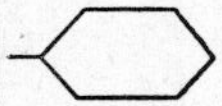 (benzene ring)	4·3, 1·7, 1·0	<0·5, 4·0, 4·0	12
3	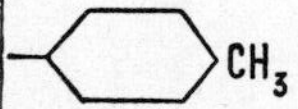 (benzene ring) CH₃	45·0, 5·0	<0·1, 0·25	4
4	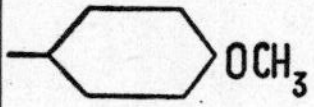 (benzene ring) OCH₃	42, 5·5	<0·1, 1·0	2
5	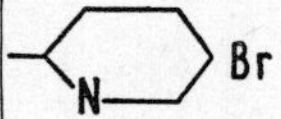 (pyridine ring) Br	70, 30, 10	<0·5, 4·0, 40	1
6	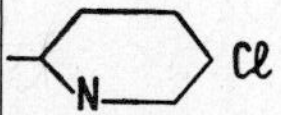 (pyridine ring) Cl	80, 16	<0·5, 8·0	1
7	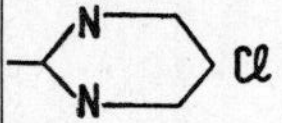 (pyridine ring) Cl	70, 17	<0·5, 1·5	1
8	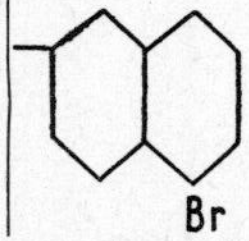 (naphthalene ring) Br	80, 18	<0·5, 20	0·5

No.	Compound.* R	R'	Intake mgm./kgm./day	Activity.†	Quinine equivalent
9	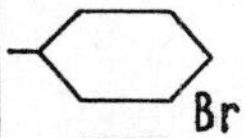 (benzene ring)		80, 17	1, 100	0·25
10	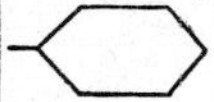 (benzene ring) Br		75, 15	<0·5, 40	1
11	(quinoline ring)	C₂H₅			
12	(quinoline ring)		135, 70, 33	<0·5, 2·0, 43·0	0·5
13	(benzene ring) SO₂NH₂		680, 140	1·0, 14·0	0·25
14	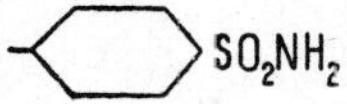 (pyrimidine ring) Br		175, 20	<0·1, 10·0	0·5 (as DL mixture)
15	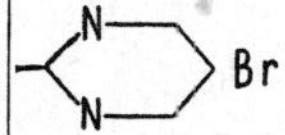 (pyrimidine ring)		1,150	<1	active
	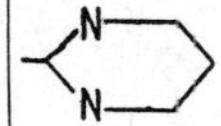		2,800	2	active

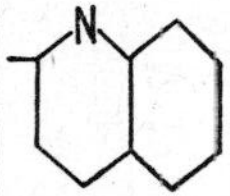

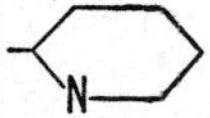

* $CH_2OH-\overset{CH_3}{\underset{CH_3}{C}}-CHOH-CONH(CH_2)_2SO_2N\underset{R'}{\overset{R}{<}}$

† Expressed as $\dfrac{\text{parasitæmia of test birds.}}{\text{parasitæmia of control birds.}}$

is completely nullified by 100, 50 or 25 mgm. per kgm. calcium pantothenate (Cantrell, 1949). As in the case of the antibacterial action of pantothenic acid antagonists, any modification of the pantoyl moiety of such substances leads to complete loss of anti-malarial activity. Phenylpantothenone prepared from D-pantoyl-lactone has no antimalarial activity. On the other hand, a variety of changes can be made in the nature of that moiety of the panto-thenic acid antagonist which corresponds with β-alanine without a marked loss of activity, provided an acyl group (CO, SO, SO_2, S) occupies the same position relative to the molecule as a whole that the carbonyl group of β-alanine occupies in pantothenic acid (Wiselogle, 1946).

The toxicity of SN 13,592, N-2-(phenyl-mercapto-)-ethyl-α, γ-dihydroxy-β, β-dimethyl butyramide, an analogue of phenyl pantothenone, is low. The lethal dose per os for rats is more than 10 gm. per kgm. (Singher *et al.*, 1948) : intravenous injection of 397 mgm. per kgm. in dogs caused no ill effects, but continued oral doses caused some anæmia ; in mice daily doses of more than 270 mgm. per kgm. caused death.

Since the action of pantothenic acid as an essential metabolite for the tubercle bacillus is inhibited by salicylic acid and p-amino-salicylic acid, Deschiens and Pick (1949) tested the effect of p-aminosalicylic acid on *P. gallinaceum* in the chick. The appear-ance of erythrocytic forms in the blood was greatly delayed and the degree of infection was very low.

In this connection it is not without interest that in 1764 the Rev. Edmund Stone, a clergyman of Chipping Norton, Oxfordshire, reported that he had treated some fifty persons suffering from ague with an infusion of either the bark of the common willow or of willow bark and cinchona bark combined. When willow bark and cinchona bark were mixed a synergistic action was observable and one-fifth the usual dose of cinchona bark was then required to control the fever.

References

BRACKETT, S., WALETZKY, E., and BAKER, M., 1946, The relation between pantothenic acid and *Plasmodium gallinaceum* infections in the chicken and the antimalarial activity of analogues of pantothenic acid. *J. Parasit.*, **32**, 453.

CANTRELL, W., 1949, Antagonism of calcium pantothenate for the antimalarial effect of pantoyltaurylamide. *J. Parasit.*, **35**, 219.

DESCHIENS, R., and PICK, F., 1949, Action de certains antagonistes de l'acide pantothénique sur le paludisme aviaire à *Plasmodium gallinaceum.* *C. R. Soc. Biol. Paris*, **144**, 662.

KUHN, R., WIELAND, T., and MÖLLER, E. F., 1941, Synthese des (a-γ-Dioxy-β, β-dimethyl-butyryl)-taurins eines spezifischen Hemmstoffes für Milchsäure bakterien. *Ber. dtsch. chem. Ges.*, **74ii**, 1605.

MCILWAIN, H., 1942, Bacterial inhibition by metabolite analogues. 3. Pantoyl-taurine. The antibacterial index of inhibitors. *Brit. J. exp. Path.*, **23**, 95.

SINGHER, O. H., MILLMAN, N., and BOSWORTH, M. R., 1948, Toxicity and pharmacology of SN 13,592 : an analogue of phenyl pantothenone. *Proc. Soc. exp. Biol.*, *N.Y.*, **67**, 388.

SNELL, E. E., 1941, Growth inhibition by N-(a, γ-dihydroxy-β, β-dimethyl-butyryl) taurine and its reversal by pantothenic acid. *J. biol. Chem.*, **141**, 121.

STONE, E., 1764, An account of the success of the bark of the willow in the cure of agues. *Gen. Mag. Arts Science, Lond.*, **10**, 588.

TRAGER, W., 1943, Further studies on the survival and development *in vitro* of a malarial parasite. *J. exp. Med.*, **77**, 411.

WISELOGLE, F. Y. (editor), 1946, "A survey of antimalarial drugs, 1941–45." 2 Vols. Ann Arbor, Michigan. J. W. Edwards.

WOOLLEY, D. W., 1944, Some new aspects of the relationship of chemical structure to biological activity. *Science*, **100**, 579.

WOOLLEY, D. W., and COLLYER, M. L., 1945, Phenyl pantothenone an antago-nist of pantothenic acid. *J. biol. Chem.*, **159**, 263.

Undecane-1 : 11-diamidine

Although aromatic amidines have found a place in the treatment of trypanosomiasis and leishmaniasis, very little has been done to explore their possibilities in malaria. Glyn-Hughes, Lourie, and Yorke (1938), however, found that undecane-1 : 11-diamidine was capable of controlling the fever and parasitæmia in blood-induced benign tertian and quartan malaria. Relapses nevertheless occurred after a comparatively short latent period. Christophers and Fulton (1938) also found that in knowlesi infections in rhesus monkeys, the blood parasite level/time curve was lowered but no sterilisation occurred. *P. relictum* infection in the canary showed no prolongation of the incubation or prepatent period (Christophers and Fulton, 1938 ; Bishop, 1942). The ethyl ester of *p*-guanyl-benzoic acid (SN 7,266) was shown by Ruhe *et al.* (1949) to have no action on the St. Elizabeth strain of vivax malaria.

s-Triazines

Two *s*-triazines, 2,4-diamino-6-heptyl-*s*-triazine and 2,4-diamino-6-hexyl-*s*-triazine, compounds with three nitrogen atoms arranged symmetrically in the basic ring, have been reported as having a true causal prophylactic action against *P. gallinaceum* (Brackett and Waletsky, 1946). Further investigations on these compounds have been made by Curd, Landquist, and Rose (1947) and by Cuthbertson and Moffatt (1948).

Cuthbertson and Moffatt (1948) studied derivatives of 1 : 3 : 5-triazine with the general formula

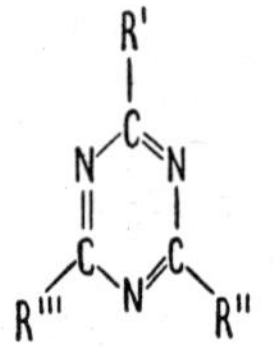

Three types of derivatives were prepared : (a) 6-methoxy-8-quinolylamino-, (b) δ-diethylamino-α-methylbutylamino-, and (c) p-chloranilino-. None of these was active against *Trypanosoma equiperdum*, and of those with some activity against *P. gallinaceum* the only one of interest was when R' = p-chloranilino, R'' = isopropylamino and R''' = H.

Dicoumarin

A curious effect of dicoumarin (3 : 3'-methylene-*bis*-4-hydroxycoumarin) on *P. lophuræ* infections in ducks is recorded by Rigdon and McCain (1948). When doses of from 25 to 100 mgm. were given on five to seven occasions to white Pekin ducks infected with *P. lophuræ* the degree of parasitæmia was reduced, the onset of parasitæmia was delayed but deaths occurred at an earlier stage than in treated birds. The mechanism by which these results were obtained is uncertain : in ducks uninfected with malaria but treated with dicoumarin, anæmia, acidosis, and hæmorrhage into subcutaneous tissues were found.

References

BISHOP, A., 1942, Chemotherapy and avian malaria. *Parasitology*, **34**, 1.
BRACKETT, S., and WALETZKY, E., 1946, The inability of drugs with both causal prophylactic and suppressive action to cure established infections with avian malaria. *J. Parasit.*, **32** (Sect. 2), 8.
CHRISTOPHERS, S. R., and FULTON, J. D., 1938, Observations on the course of *Plasmodium knowlesi* infection in monkeys (*Macacus rhesus*), with notes on its treatment by (1) atebrin and (2) 1 : 11 normal undecane diamidine, together with a note on the action of the latter on bird malaria. *Ann. trop. Med. Parasit.*, **32, 257.**

CURD, F. H. S., LANDQUIST, J. K., and ROSE, F. L., 1947, Synthetic anti-malarials. Part XII. Some 1 : 3 : 5-triazine derivatives. *J. chem. Soc.*, 154.

CUTHBERTSON, W. W., and MOFFATT, J. S., 1948, Contributions to the chemistry of synthetic antimalarials. VI. Some derivatives of 1 : 3 : 5-triazine. *J. chem. Soc.*, 561.

GLYN-HUGHES, F., LOURIE, E. M., and YORKE, W., 1938, Studies in chemotherapy. XVII. Action of undecane diamidine in malaria. *Ann. trop. Med. Parasit.*, **32**, 103.

RIGDON, R. H., and McCAIN, B. E., 1948, Effect of 3, 3'-methylene bis (4 hydroxy-coumarin) " dicumarol " on *P. lophuræ* infection in ducks. *J. nat. Mal. Soc.*, **7**, 38.

RUHE, D. S., COOPER, W. C., COATNEY, G. R., and JOSEPHSON, E. S., 1949, Studies in human malaria. XIV. The ineffectiveness of colchicine (SN 12,080), SN 7,266 and SN 8,557 as curative agents against St. Elizabeth strain vivax malaria. *Amer. J. Hyg.*, **49**, 361.

INDIGENOUS DRUGS

In almost all tropical and in many non-tropical countries there are plants which are reputed to have a curative action in malaria. Even in Great Britain, feverfew, *Chrysanthemum Parthenium* Pers., for long enjoyed this reputation. Many of these plants have merely a diaphoretic action and fail to attack malarial plasmodia directly.

Ch'ang Shan

For many centuries in China, and certainly since the time of the Han dynasties (206 B.C.–A.D. 221), the roots known in the Chung King area as Ch'ang Shan and the leaves as Shun Chi have enjoyed a reputation in the cure of malaria. There is now general agreement that the indigenous pharmaceuticals are derived from *Dichroa febrifuga*, a shrub of the family *Saxifragaceæ*, indigenous in Yunnan and Szechuan Provinces. Early observers, such as Stuart (1911), had identified Ch'ang Shan with *Orixa japonica*, a plant which probably has no antimalarial action.

Dichroa febrifuga, both root and leaves, have now been examined chemically and alkaloids have been isolated by three groups of workers :—

(1) Koepfli *et al.* (1947, 1949) isolated febrifugine and *iso*-febrifugine. Febrifugine is dimorphic and the bases are readily interconvertible.

(2) Chou *et al.* (1947, 1948) reported three isomeric alkaloids called α-, β-, and γ-dichroines.

(3) Kuehl *et al.* (1948) isolated two isomeric alkaloids to which they did not assign names.

(4) Jang *et al.* (1946, 1948) obtained five alkaloids and two neutral principles.

Unfortunately these alkaloids have not been accurately compared. It seems probable, however, that the *iso*febrifugine modification of febrifugine is the same as α-dichroine and that β- and γ-dichroine correspond to the two crystalline forms of febrifugine. It is to be noted that Kuehl *et al.* (1948) and Chou *et al.* (1948) originally assigned the same composition, $C_{16}H_{19}N_3O_3$, to the alkaloids they had obtained : later the Chinese workers produced an amended formula differing by two atoms of hydrogen. Jang *et al.* (1948), in addition to the three dichroine alkaloids, obtained dichroidine and quinazoline (4-keto-dihydroxyquinazoline). Workers who have reported an absence of alkaloids in Ch'ang Shan have probably been led astray because of the fact that the alkaloidal content of the root material is small, 0·05 to 0·1 per cent., and Meyer's reagent is relatively insensitive to febrifugine and *iso*febrifugine. Material from India contains much less alkaloid than material from China. The melting points of the two crystalline forms of febrifugine are 139–140° C. and 154–156° C. The melting point for γ-dichroine is given as 160° C.

The LD 50 of febrifugine by the oral route for mice is 2·5 to 3·0 mgm. per kgm. Toxic doses two to four hours after administration give rise to urinary incontinency, sweating, respiratory symptoms, and a corrosive effect on the gastric mucosa. In monkeys a daily dose of 0·3 mgm. per kgm. of body weight caused no untoward symptoms ; 0·75 mgm. per kgm. daily caused death on the ninth day with hyperæmia of the gastric mucosa. Febrifugine does not affect the formed elements of the peripheral blood or bone marrow nor does it cause cyanosis or methæmalbuminæmia. γ-Dichroine is roughly three and a half times as toxic to mice by mouth as intravenously ; the LD 50 by the intravenous route is 10·0 ± 0·5 mgm. per kgm. of body weight. Parenchymatous degeneration of the kidneys and hydrophilic degeneration of the liver may occur. Dogs given 4 mgm. per kgm. intravenously showed a fall in blood pressure ; in anæsthetised dogs duodenal peristalsis is stimulated.

Antimalarial Activity. Jang and Chou (1943) reported that a crude extract of the roots was effective clinically in human malaria. Later Wang *et al.* (1945) found that crude extracts of the root and leaves of the shrub were effective in chicks infected with *P. gallinaceum*, leaves being some five times more active than the root. An alkaloidal fraction of the root showed antimalarial activity, but further purification involved a considerable loss of activity (Wang *et al.*, 1945). Tonkin and Work (1945) also reported considerable activity against a trophozoite-induced infection of *P. gallinaceum* in chicks on the part of an extract of the roots : the growth of the exo-erythrocytic forms was not prevented. Spencer *et al.* (1947) similarly showed that extracts of roots, leaves, and stems had antimalarial activity against trophozoite-induced infections and to a lesser extent against sporozoite-induced infections of *P. gallinaceum*.

With the possible exception of α-dichroine, β-dichroine, γ-dichroine and quinazoline all three show antimalarial activity in blood-induced infections of *P. gallinaceum*, the activity decreasing in the order given. Kuehl *et al.* (1948) found that in monkeys γ-dichroine in a dose of 1·6 mgm. per kgm. of body weight cleared the blood stream of *P. cynomolgi*. Against *P. lophuræ* in ducks the median suppressive dose, SD 50, is 0·064 mgm. per kgm. of body weight, and against *P. relictum* in canaries 0·146 mgm. per kgm. ; the corresponding figures for quinine are 9·49 mgm. per kgm. and 20·0 mgm. per kgm. Koefli *et al.* (1949) reported that *iso*febrifugine, when given intravenously three times a day to ducks infected with *P. lophuræ*, had a quinine equivalent of one, but febrifugine has a quinine equivalent of 100 against *P. lophuræ* in ducks and of sixty-four against *P. gallinaceum* in chicks ; when tested against trophozoite-induced infections of *P. cynomolgi* in monkeys febrifugine is at least 100 times as active as quinine.

Tsu (1947) prepared an aqueous extract of *Dichroa febrifuga* and on treating this with alcohol obtained an alcohol-soluble fraction. On evaporating this to dryness and again dissolving it in water a therapeutically active suspension was obtained. Eighty-one patients were thus treated with a 6 per cent. solution of Ch'ang Shan. Five doses of 5 ml., corresponding to 25 gm. of dried root, were given daily for from ten to fifteen days in vivax infections and for twenty days in falciparum infections. If more than 5 ml. were given at a time there were symptoms of abdominal discomfort or vomiting. Oral administration is preferred to intramuscular injection. Of sixty-seven patients with vivax infections symptoms are said to have subsided in from three to seven days ; six relapsed but in twenty-five the size of the spleen remained unaffected. In fourteen patients with falciparum infection signs and symptoms disappeared more slowly and three patients were quite unaffected.

Other Plant Extracts

According to Jang *et al.* (1948) another Chinese herb known as Tou Ch'ang Shan also exhibits activity against *P. gallinaceum* in chickens. It has been provisionally identified as *Hydrangea umbellata* Rheder., and if that is the case it belongs to the same family, *Saxifragaceæ*, as *Dichroa febrifuga*. Its active fraction certainly contains alkaloids, though further investigations are required to determine whether or not alkaloids are the active antimalarials.

In Southern Yunnan, since the early part of this century, the root and bark of an indigenous tree has been used in the treatment of malaria. The tree concerned is probably *Fraxinus malacophylla* Hemsley which is known as Pai-chi'ang-kan or Ken-ken-yao. An alkaloid sinine has been isolated from the bark and is claimed by Liu *et al.* (1941) to have some action in human malaria. Altogether thirty-four patients were treated with 9·9 gm. of the dried powder daily. Within eight days both *P. falciparum* and *P. vivax* had disappeared from the blood stream. Chronic infections were less amenable than more acute cases. Reduction in size of the spleen required prolonged treatment.

The therapeutic dose is not far removed from the toxic dose, and, in children especially, twice the therapeutic dose will cause nausea, vomiting, and tinnitus. Tonkin and Work (1945) were unable to determine that *Fraxinus malacophylla* had any action whatsoever against *P. gallinaceum* infections in chicks. Certain Indian plants have been examined for antimalarial action, notably *Alstonia scholaris* F. Br. and *Cæsalpina bonducella* Flemming. The bark of the former, known in Hindi as chhatim, was found by Mukerji *et al.* (1942) to have no activity against malaria in man or monkey ; mixed with quinine it has been used in cases of human malaria by Roy and Chatterjee (1944), but the activity is solely that of quinine. The seeds of *Cæsalpina bonducella* were shown by Mukerji *et al.* (1943) to be without action on *P. gallinaceum* infections in hens. It is doubtful whether *C. sepiaria*, used in China, is any more active (Chu, 1945). *Fraxinus malacophylla*, *Alstonia scholaris* and *Cæsalpina bonducella* all have an antipyretic action and this is probably the cause of their alleged antimalarial action (Mukerji, 1946).

Burasaine has been tested by Davidson (1945) in East Africa. Burasaine is the total alcoholic extract of the roots of a tree *Burasia madagascarensis* Thouras, which is native to Madagascar. The extract is said to contain alkaloids with the methyl *ortho*quinine-*iso*quinoline ring very similar to that found in hydrastine and berberine. The usual dose was 4·8 gm. in twenty-four hours, but this when taken by mouth caused nausea and vomiting. Although its action is said to be slower than that of quinine, it removed parasites from the blood of seventeen out of eighteen Africans suffering from *P. falciparum* infections. The majority of the Africans are said to have been non-immune, but great caution must be exercised in drawing conclusions from the behaviour of *P. falciparum* in Africans. Rest in bed and a purge, without any specific drug treatment, are often enough to banish parasites from the blood stream.

Encostema littorale Blume has been recommended by Rai (1946), and *Momordica charantia* L. in South America (Vélez-Salas, 1944), but insufficient evidence is available to form any opinion on their antiplasmodial action. *Centaurea* sp. has been claimed to have some action in malaria ; it has long been used as a febrifuge in folk medicine (Danzel, 1948).

Extensive series of tests, however, have been carried out by Carlson *et al.* (1946) and Spencer *et al.* (1947), who have examined extracts from nearly 600 plants. Activity was tested against trophozoite- and sporozoite-induced infections due to *P. gallina-ceum* in chickens and against *P. cathemerium* and *P. lophuræ* in ducklings. The bark of *Cornus florida* yielded a water-insoluble product active against *P. cathemerium ;* it had had little effect against *P. lophuræ* in the duck or *P. gallinaceum* in the chick.

Many of the *Simaroubaceæ* showed activity, especially *Castela tortuosa*, *Simaba cedron*, and *Simarouba amara*. Suppressive activity, however, was not infrequently associated with toxicity. Many bulbs of *Amaryllidaceæ* showed some activity associated with alkaloidal fractions.

Colchicine was reported by Ruhe *et al.* (1949) to be valueless in the treatment of vivax malaria (St. Elizabeth strain). During the eighteenth century many remedies of vegetable origin were proposed in place of the Peruvian bark. Some of these substances, such as a spoonful of the juice of the house leek, *Allium sativum*, are now known to contain antibacterial substances. Other vegetable substances found by Lind (1768) to be in common use were a teaspoonful of pepper in a quarter of a pint of gin ; the same quantity of the juice of a plantain ; a spoonful of spirit of turpentine ; juice of rue, *Ruta graveoleus;* half a pint of the juice of groundsel, *Senecio vulgaris ;* a decoction of cinquefoil, *Potentilla reptans*, or spearmint, *Mentha spicata;* a decoction of horse-radish, *Cochlearia armoracia;* the inner bark of the ash or elm and half a drachm of the root of blackthorn, *Prunus spinosa.* It is possible that some of these remedies had a slight anti-plasmodial action.

References

CARLSON, H. J., BISSELL, H. D., and MUELLER, M. G., 1946, Antimalarial and antibacterial substances separated from higher plants. *J. Bact.*, **52**, 155.

CHOU, T. Q., FU, F. Y., and KAO, Y. S., 1948, Antimalarial constituents of Chinese drug Ch'ang Shan, *Dichroa febrifuga* Lour. *J. Amer. chem. Soc.*, **70**, 1765.

CHOU, T. Q., JANG, C. S., FU, F. Y., KAO, Y. S., and HUANG, K. C., 1947, Dichronine, the antimalarial principle of Ch'ang Shan, *Dichroa febrifuga* Lour. *Chin. med. J.*, **65**, 189.

CHU, W. C., 1945, New specific for malaria. *Cæsalpina sepiaria* Roxb. Preliminary report. *Chin. med. J.*, **63A**, 223.

DANZEL, L., 1948, La centaurelle, un bon antimalarique. *Rev. Palud.*, **6**, 133.

DAVIDSON, S., 1945, Experimental investigation of burasaine in the treatment of malaria. *E. Afr. med. J.*, **22**, 80.

JANG, C. S., and CHOU, T. C., 1943. *Nat. med. J. China*, **29**, 137. [Title in Chinese : quoted by Jang, C. S. *et al.*, *Nature*, *Lond.* (1948), **161**, 400.]

JANG, C. S., FU, F. Y., HUANG, K. C., and WANG, C. Y., 1948, Pharmacology of Ch'ang Shan (*Dichroa febrifuga*), a Chinese antimalarial herb. *Nature*, *Lond.*, **161**, 400.

JANG, C. S., FU, F. Y., WANG, C. Y., HUANG, K. C., LU, G., and CHOU, T. C., 1946, Ch'ang Shan, a Chinese antimalarial drug. *Science*, **103**, 59.

KOEPFLI, J. B., MEAD, J. F., and BROCKMAN, J. A., Jr., 1947, An alkaloid with high antimalarial activity from *Dichroa febrifuga*. *J. Amer. chem. Soc.*, **69**, 1837.

PHENANTHRENE AMINO ALCOHOLS 419

KOEPFLI, J. B., MEAD, J. F., and BROCKMAN, J. A., Jr., 1949, Alkaloids of *Dichroa febrifuga*. I. Isolation and degradative studies. *J. Amer. chem. Soc.*, **71**, 1048.
KUEHL, F. A., Jr., SPENCER, C. F., and FOLKERS, K., 1948, Alkaloids of *Dichroa febrifuga*. *J. Amer. chem. Soc.*, **70**, 2091.
LIND, JAMES, 1768, "An essay on diseases incidental to Europeans in hot climates." London. T. Becket and P. A. de Hondt.
LIU, SHAO-KWANG, CHANG, YAO-TEH, TZE-KWANG, CH'UAN and TAN, SHIH-CHIEH, 1941, The new antimalarial drug sinine : a preliminary report. *Chin. med. J.*, **59**, 575.
MUKERJI, B., 1946, Antimalarial drugs in the indigenous materia medica of China and India. *Nature, Lond.*, **158**, 170.
MUKERJI, B., GHOSH, B. K., and SIDDONS, L. B., 1942, Search for an anti-malarial drug in the indigenous materia medica : *Alstonia scholaris* F. Br. *Indian med. Gaz.*, **77**, 723.
MUKERJI, B., GHOSH, B. K., and SIDDONS, L. B., 1943, The search for an antimalarial drug in the indigenous materia medica : *Cæsalpinia bonducella* Flemming. *Indian med. Gaz.*, **78**, 285.
RAI, B. B., 1946, *Encostema littorale* Blume in malaria. *Indian med. Gaz.*, **81**, 506.
ROY, B. C., and CHATTERJEE, K. D., 1944, Malaria. A preliminary report on the studies on the action of ABN-61 (a preparation of dita-bark and quinine) on cases of human malaria. *J. Indian med. Ass.*, **13**, 193.
RUHE, D. S., COOPER, W. C., COATNEY, G. R., and JOSEPHSON, E. S., 1949, Studies in human malaria. XIV. The ineffectiveness of colchicine (SN 12,080), SN 7,266 and SN 8,557 as curative agents against St. Elizabeth strain vivax malaria. *Amer. J. Hyg.*, **49**, 361.
SPENCER, C. F., KONIUSZY, F. R., ROGERS, E. F., SHAVEL, J., Jr., EASTON, N. R., KACZKA, E. A., KUEHL, F. A., Jr., PHILLIPS, R. F., WALTI, A., FOLKERS, K., MALANGA, C., and SEELER, A. O., 1947, Survey of plants for antimalarial activity. *Lloydia*, **10**, 145.
STUART, G. A., 1911, "Chinese materia medica." Shanghai. American Presbyterian Mission Press.
TONKIN, I. M., and WORK, T. S., 1945, A new antimalarial drug. *Nature, Lond.*, **156**, 630.
TSU, C. F., 1947, Ch'ang Shan in the treatment of malaria. *J. trop Med. Hyg.*, **50**, 75.
VÉLEZ-SALAS, F., 1944, Un nuevo agente antipaludico ; se trata de la *Momordica charantia* L., conocida en Venezuela con el nombre de cundeamor. *Rev. farm. B. Aires*, **86**, 512.
WANG, C. Y., FU, F. Y., and JANG, C. S., 1945, *Nat. med. J. China*, **21**, 159. [Title in Chinese : quoted by Jang C. S. *et al.*, *Nature, Lond.* (1948), **161**, 400.]

PHENANTHRENE AMINO ALCOHOLS

Early in 1942 it was found that a number of amino alcohols derived from phenanthrene and naphthalene were active against *Plasmodium gallinaceum* in the fowl. The group was systematically explored for antimalarial activities, and of the many hundred compounds with this general structure six were tried in blood-induced human malarias and two in sporozoite-induced human malarias. One of these compounds is 9-(2'-diamylamino-1'-hydroxy-

14—2

ethyl)-1, 2, 3, 4-tetrahydrophenanthrene hydrochloride (SN 1,796). This compound was synthesised by May and Mosettig (1946). In gallinaceum malaria in the chick the maximum amount tolerated by mouth over a four-day period was 0·5 mgm. per gm. twice daily, the same dosage as quinine but three times that of mepacrine. Its effective minimal dose was 0·0625 mgm. per gm. twice a day, or four times that of quinine, so that its quinine equivalent is 0·25 (0·3 in terms of base). It was not a causal prophylactic against gallinaceum infections, nor did it destroy exo-erythrocytic forms. Its suppressive activity is of the same order as quinine against the erythrocytic forms of cathemerium malaria in the canary and duck, and lophuræ malaria in the chick and duck.

Toxicity. White rats tolerated 100 mgm. per kgm. of body weight once daily for thirty-five days though they did not gain in weight normally. At autopsy they showed no abnormalities.

Intravenous injections in anæsthetised dogs of 5 to 20 mgm. per kgm. caused lowering of blood pressure, vomiting, and diarrhœa; oral doses up to 150 mgm. per kgm. were well tolerated over a seven-day period. The drug is somewhat poorly absorbed from the intestine but absorption is enhanced by concurrent ingestion of fat. In rhesus monkeys oral doses up to 300 mgm. per kgm. (270 mgm. per kgm. of base) daily for six days cause transient pilomotor stimulation but no permanent ill effects. In man, doses up to 1 gm. daily have been taken by mouth. In most of the volunteers a lowering of the threshold of pilomotor response occurred as evidenced by erection of body hair, goose flesh, and transient sensations of chilliness. Slight malaise was found occasionally, and one volunteer complained of difficulty in urinating.

Cooper and Coatney (1947) have studied the effects of the hydrochloride, which contains 91·2 per cent. of base, on patients infected with *P. vivax* (Elizabeth strain), *P. falciparum* (McLendon strain), and the United States Public Health Service strain of *P. malariæ*.

Fifty-one cases infected with *P. vivax* were studied : two were blood-induced and the remainder were caused by infected mosquito bites. The dosage was 0·25 gm. once daily in seven cases, 0·5 gm. once daily in eight cases, 0·9 or 0·96 gm. daily in thirty-three cases and 1·5 gm. daily in three cases. Doses of 0·5 gm. daily, or more, interrupted clinical attacks and reduced parasitæmia to a sub-clinical level in all patients except one. Relapses almost invariably took place.

Similar results were obtained in thirteen patients with mosquito-induced *P. falciparum* infections. Relapses occurred shortly after the termination of therapy in the majority of patients. In two patients with blood-induced infections due to *P. malariæ* there was clearance of parasitæmia and abolition of fever. No relapses occurred over a period of four years.

Toxic reactions were not uncommon and consisted of (1) lowering of the pilomotor threshold, (2) bradycardia, (3) disturbed bladder control, (4) microscopic hæmaturia. The reactions decreased in frequency in the order named. Bradycardia with a pulse rate below fifty and sometimes as low as thirty-five per minute was not uncommon. It could be relieved to some extent by atropine sulphate. The bladder complaints included dysuria, hesitancy in starting micturition, and difficulty in complete emptying. The scrotum was tightened and the external genitalia numb in one patient. Of sixty-six patients, forty-two had asymptomatic bradycardia without much lowering of blood pressure, eight had bladder difficulties, and seventeen had hæmaturia (Cooper and Coatney, 1947).

An attempt to use SN 1,796 as a causal prophylactic was unsuccessful against the St. Elizabeth strain of *P. vivax*. A dose of 0·3 gm. daily for two days before, seven days during, and twenty-eight days after exposure suppressed parasitæmia and fever, but the toxic effects were unpleasant and all the subjects had delayed primary attacks in from six to ten months after exposure (Coatney *et al.*, 1947).

SN 5,241, α-dinonylaminomethyl-1, 2, 3, 4-tetrahydro-9-phenanthrene methanol was found by Ruhe *et al.* (1949a) to interrupt acute attacks of the St. Elizabeth strain when given in doses of 1·5 gm. for six days. Relapses occurred in from 168 to 262 days later : treatment of late attacks was less effective and clearance of parasitæmia was slow.

The ethyl ester of *p*-guanyl-benzoic acid, and colchicine were shown by Ruhe *et al.* (1949b) to be of no value in treating the St. Elizabeth strain.

References

COATNEY, G. R., COOPER, W. C., YOUNG, M. D., and BURGESS, R. W., 1947, Studies in human malaria. IV. The suppressive action of a phenanthrene amino alcohol, NIH-204 (SN 1,796), against sporozoite-induced vivax malaria (St. Elizabeth strain). *Amer. J. Hyg.*, **46**, 132.

COOPER, W. C., and COATNEY, G. R., 1947, Studies in human malaria. III. The therapeutic effect of a phenanthrene amino alcohol, NIH-204 (SN 1,796) in vivax, falciparum and quartan malaria. *Amer. J. Hyg.*, **46**, 119.

MAY, E. L., and MOSETTIG, E., 1946, Attempts to find new antimalarials. I. Amino alcohols derived from 1, 2, 3, 4-tetrahydrophenanthrene. *J. organ. Chem.*, **11**, 1.

RUHE, D. S., COOPER, W. C., COATNEY, G. R., and JOSEPHSON, E. S., 1949a, Studies in human malaria. XIII. The protective and therapeutic action of SN 5,241 against St. Elizabeth strain vivax malaria. *Amer. J. Hyg.*, **49**, 346.

RUHE, D. S., COOPER, W. C., COATNEY, G. R., and JOSEPHSON, E. S., 1949b, Studies in human malaria. XIV. The ineffectiveness of colchicine (SN 12,080), SN 7,266 and SN 8,557 as curative agents against St. Elizabeth strain vivax malaria. *Amer. J. Hyg.*, **49**, 361.

NON-SPECIFIC TREATMENT WITH SODIUM THIOSULPHATE

Lorant (1946) found that sodium thiosulphate given intravenously had some effect in overcoming an acute attack of vivax malaria. Seventy-nine cases of vivax infection were given from 0·75 to 3·0 gm. of sodium thiosulphate intravenously three times daily for ten days : forty-two cases showed a definite response, the temperature falling to normal within the ensuing six days and the number of parasites in the blood stream decreasing rapidly. The action of sodium thiosulphate in canaries infected with *P. præcox* has been studied by Hirade and Yasui (1948), who found that 0·2 gm. per kgm. of body weight when given one hour before 0·2 ml. of 0·5 per cent. quinine hydrochloride slowed down the development of the parasites so that the infection in treated birds was seventy-two hours behind that in untreated controls. The exact mode of action of sodium thiosulphate is at present unknown.

These observations seem to be a repetition of certain investigations described by Polli (1870), who found that alkaline sulphites and hyposulphites were suppressive and curative in malaria.

References

HIRADE, J., and YASUI, Y., 1948, Thiosulphate as an aid to chemotherapy. *Brit. med. J.*, **i**, 903.

LORANT, S., 1946, The non-specific chemotherapy of malaria. *J. trop. Med. Hyg.*, **49**, 63.

POLLI, G., 1870, " Della Malaria e dei Febbrifugi." Milano.

NAPHTHOQUINONES

A large number of naphthoquinones have been prepared by Fieser, Berliner, and his colleagues (1948a). In 1943 hydrolapachol and two other quinones, originally prepared in 1936 by Hooker, were found to have undoubted antimalarial activities. Some 300 of these compounds have now been prepared and found to possess antimalarial activity against *P. lophuræ* in ducks and possibly, in some instances, against *P. knowlesi* in monkeys.

Naphthoquinones that have been tested in man are either quite inactive or only very slightly active (Wiselogle, 1946 ; Ruhe *et al.*, 1949), but whether this is due to the fact that man metabolises these compounds in a different way from that in birds or whether it denotes a specific action on the part of the naphthoquinones for certain species of plasmodia is unknown (Richardson and Hewitt, 1946 ; Fieser, 1946). Wendel (1946), however, has shown that many of the naphthoquinones depress the oxygen uptake of *Plasmodium lophuræ* and that there is close agreement between *in vivo* antimalarial activity in the duck and *in vitro* depression of respiration and inhibition of carbohydrate metabolism. This agreement holds when the substituent group in position 2 is a normal alkyl radical, an *iso*alkyl radical, a tertiary alkyl radical, a methyl, dimethyl or ethyl substituted alkyl radical, an unsaturated alkyl radical or a *cyclo*alkyl radical. The sera of ducks which have received compounds active *in vivo* and *in vitro* are inhibitory of *P. lophuræ* respiration. The oxygen uptake of parasites treated with naphthoquinones is very sensitive to variations in pH. Over a range of pH which includes physiological values, a unit decrease in pH produces approximately a ten-fold increase in anti-respiratory activity in eight compounds tested. Inhibition of oxygen uptake by plasmodia results principally from interference with carbohydrate oxidation. Whereas normally a suspension of cells containing *P. lophuræ* does not show aerobic glycolysis, lactic acid accumulates in suspensions containing an active naphthoquinone in proportion to the degree of respiratory inhibition. Oxidation of lactate to pyruvate is inhibited by effective naphthoquinones. The respiratory and carbohydrate metabolisms of normal duck red cells are influenced by naphthoquinones in essentially the same manner as those of parasitised cells. However, more than 100 times as high a concentration of certain naphthoquinones is required to inhibit the respiration of normal duck red cells by 50 per cent. as is necessary to affect equally the oxygen uptake of cells containing *P. lophuræ*. It has not been ascertained whether human red cells are affected in the same way by naphthoquinones. It is, however, known that degradation products accumulate in the blood of patients to whom these compounds have been given. Fieser *et al.* (1948b) have established that the rapid and extensive degradation consists in oxidation of the hydrocarbon side-chain with the production of metabolites that are distinctly more hydrophilic than the compounds administered. Several of the metabolites were isolated and found to be secondary alcohols, tertiary alcohols or carboxylic acids. Gastro-intestinal irritation, diarrhœa, nausea, and malaise were produced by certain compounds. The relation of the side-chain to development of symptoms in non-malarial human subjects is shown in the table (p. 428). Fieser *et al.* (1948c) found that the mouse shows the closest parallelism to man in the retention and degradation of the naphthoquinones.

The plasma of patients given naphthoquinones contains a pigment. This pigment has anti-respiratory activity, and by evaluating this anti-respiratory activity Fieser *et al.* (1948c) have evolved a method of evaluating naphthoquinones as possible anti-malarial drugs with respect to plasma levels, extent of metabolic deactivation, and persistence of active material.

Compounds with hydrocarbon side-chains terminating in a ring are rapidly metabolised to products hydroxylated in this ring. The metabolites retain 10 to 60 per cent. of the original activity, and often persist in the blood for long periods. In some instances they may exert a therapeutic effect.

Optimum antimalarial activity apparently requires a certain balance between lipophilic and hydrophilic character. Hydroxylation of the side-chain is attended with a very marked hydrophilic displacement. A compensating shift in the opposite direction can be achieved by an increase in the size of the hydrocarbon side-chain. One compound of this type, M 2350, has a hydroxylated C_{19}-side-chain and shows considerable resistance to metabolic deactivation.

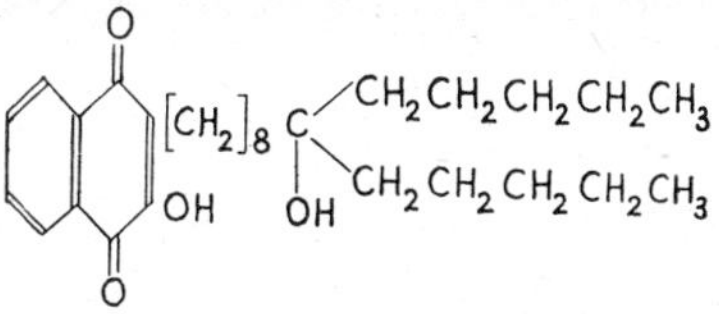

M 2350

However, it is not absorbed efficiently from the gut and has potentialities as a therapeutic agent only if given parenterally.

Naphthoquinones are bound to plasma proteins. Heymann and Fieser (1948) have shown that, as judged by dialysis experiments, the binding power of plasma is in the order: human > monkey > duck. Protein antagonism to drug action as measured by the depression of the inhibitory action of naphthoquinones on the respiration of parasitised red cells decreases in the order: human serum > chicken serum > duck serum. The difference in protein antagonism between chicken and duck plasma possibly accounts for differences in the antimalarial potency of naphthoquinones in these species.

One of the most promising of these compounds is 2-[3'-(decahydro-β-naphthyl)propyl]-3-hydroxy-1, 4-naphthoquinone (SN 8,557): it probably consists of four isomers with *cis* forms predominating. This compound has been used in the treatment of infections due to *P. cathemerium* in the canary. The maximum tolerated dose for canaries appears to be about 150 mgm./kgm. a day; no deaths occurred when this dose was given by mouth for five or ten days, but occasional birds succumbed if it was continued for fifteen days.

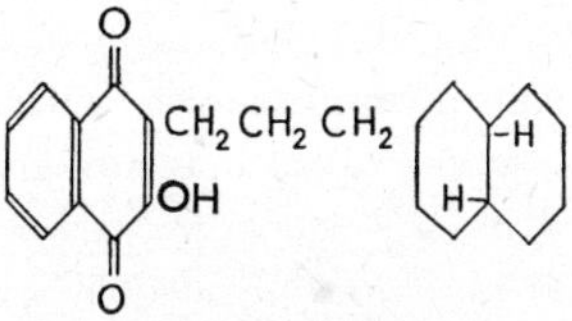

M 297 (SN 8,557)

Gingrich *et al.* (1947) found that in the canary infected with *P. cathemerium* the drug had a quinine equivalent of one in that 0·24 mgm. per day of both SN 8,557 and quinine base produce approximately the same reduction of parasitæmia. Prophylactic tests with 150 to 200 mgm. per kgm. a day caused a few days' delay in the appearance of blood parasites but did not prevent infection. Administration of the drug for fifteen days apparently cured twenty-eight of thirty-six birds, including some with latent sporozoite-induced infections. In latent infections susceptibility to cure is related to the duration of latency as well as to the particular strain of *P. cathemerium*. The duration of immunity to *P. cathemerium* after cure by SN 8,557 is less than five months.

Wiselogle (1946) states that SN 8,557 shows activity against blood-induced vivax (McCoy) malaria. Relapses occurred in from thirty-three to thirty-five days after doses of from 1·0 to 2·4 gm. daily for twelve days. In vivax infections it has a quinine equivalent of less than 0·15, based on total oral dose. The drug showed no prophylactic activity against either falciparum or vivax malaria. There is also evidence of toxicity : two subjects receiving 2·4 gm. per day showed fever, confusion, and diarrhœa, while one subject receiving 1 gm. daily had diarrhœa and abdominal cramps. All subjects receiving the drug exhibited a pink discoloration of the skin which lasted for about one week after administration of the drug had been discontinued. In combination with quinine it did not prevent relapses of the St. Elizabeth vivax strain (Ruhe *et al.*, 1949). It did not act as a suppressive against sporozoite-induced *P. vivax* (McCoy strain) or *P. falciparum* (Costa strain).

Other naphthoquinones referred to by Wiselogle (1946) and Fieser *et al.* (1948 *a, b*) include hydrolapachol (SN 3,529) (Hooker, 1936), hydrolapachol propionate (SN 8,307), 2-(3′-*cyclo*hexylpropyl)-3-hydroxy-1, 4-naphthoquinone (SN 5,090) and 2-hydroxy-3-(2′-methyloctyl)-1, 4-naphthoquinone (SN 5,949). All these compounds exhibit some prophylactic activity against cathemerium malaria in the canary, gallinaceum malaria in the chick, and lophuræ malaria in the turkey. SN 3,529 has a quinine equivalent of 0·15 against blood-induced vivax malaria, based on the total oral dose. It showed, however, no prophylactic activity against the McCoy strain of vivax malaria in a dose of 2·0 gm. daily, and in this amount it was toxic to man, causing nausea, vomiting, anorexia, and weakness as well as the pink discoloration of the skin.

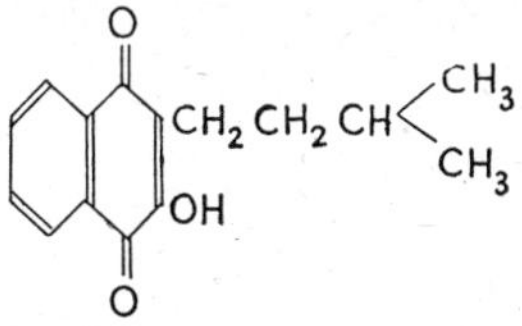

Hydrolapachol (M 1523, SN 2,527)

SN 8,307 also has a slight activity in blood-induced vivax malaria, but a quinine equivalent of less than 0·1 based on total oral dose. In addition to the toxic symptoms noted with SN 3,529, doses of 2 to 3 gm. daily in man caused hæmaturia and albuminuria.

Although SN 5,090 exhibited slight activity in blood-induced falciparum and vivax malarias, in the latter infection it had a quinine equivalent of less than 0·1 based on a total oral dose. It showed no prophylactic action against the McCoy strain of vivax malaria when a daily dose of 2·5 gm. was given for one day beyond the day of infection. In this dosage, however, there were no manifestations of toxicity.

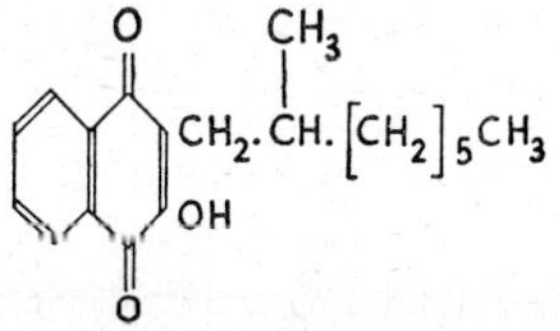

2-(*Hydroxy-3-2'-methyloctyl*)-
1, 4-*naphthoquinone*
(*SN 5,949*).

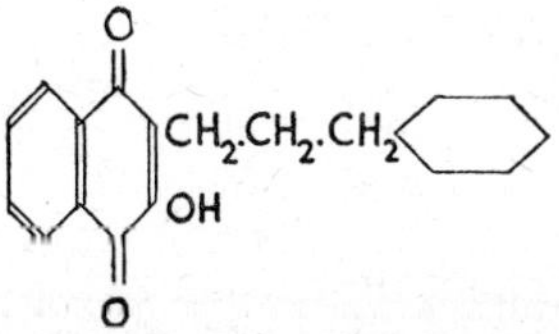

2-(3'-cyclo*Hexylpropyl*)-3-
hydroxy-1, 4-*naphthoquinone*
(*SN 5,090*).

Although SN 5,949 exhibited no activity against blood-induced falciparum or vivax malaria in a daily dose of 2 gm., doses of 1 gm. daily caused no toxic reactions in man.

Clarke and Theiler (1948) found that 2-hydroxy-3-β-decalylpropyl-1, 4-naphthoquinone (M-2279), which may contain either the original isomer or a mixture of the eight possible *cis* isomers, will destroy the sporozoites of *P. gallinaceum* in the chick ; it also acts on the erythrocytic stages and may clear parasites from the blood stream. The action of the same compound on the mosquito cycle has been studied by Whitman (1948).　When given to *Aëdes ægypti* forty-eight hours before an infective feed fewer oöcysts and sporozoites develop and a second dose forty-eight hours after the infective feed still further depresses oöcyst formation.　No oöcysts developed when the drugs were mixed with heparinised infected blood but given four to seven days after an infecting feed; when oöcysts have developed it had no effect on the subsequent development and infectivity of sporozoites.　When taken at the time of rupture of oöcysts, eight or nine days after an infecting feed, the number of sporozoites was reduced.　Once sporozoites had reached the salivary glands of the mosquito they were unaffected by the naphthoquinone.　The synergistic action of certain naphthoquinones and pamaquin or other 8-aminoquinolines, described by Walker (1947), is discussed on p. 336.

ADMINISTRATION OF NAPHTHOQUINONES TO HUMAN SUBJECTS
(Fieser *et al.*, (1948b)

Quinone M-	Side-chain.	Number of cases.	Dose.		Symptoms.	Peak levels of quinone pigment.	
			gm.	days.		Plasma per litre, mgm.	Urine per 24 hours, mgm.
1916	—(CH₂)₃C₆H₁₁—Cy	13	0·5-2·7	1-14	3/13 G.I.	12-20	>100
	Acetate	1	2·3	4	None.	29	372
	Propionate	2	1·8-2·4	1	2/2 M., N.	24	90
	Hydroquinone triacetate	1	1·9	2	None.	18	34
1971	—(CH₂)₄C₆H₁₁—Cy	4	2-2·8	1-3	2/3 N.	5-9	206
1956	—(CH₂)₅C₆H₁₁—Cy	2	2	2	2/2 G.I., N.	10-15	10-48
285	—CH₂CH(CH₃)C₆H₁₃n	2	1·3-2	1-2	2/2 D.	15	174
		2	0·7-1	1-2	1/2 D.	10	207
1523	—(CH₂)₃CH(CH₃)₂	7	1-4	1-4	2/7 G.I.	6-21	204
	Propionate	3	1·3-2·5	1-3	3/3 M.	13	358
	Caprylate	2	2	1	None.	5-7	
1711	—(CH₂)₃CH(CH₃)₂, Acetate	1	4·1	1	None.	7·7	184
1929	—(CH₂)₄CH(CH₃)₂	7	1-4	1-2	3/7 N., D.	6-9	about 100
287	—(CH₂)₅CH(CH₃)₂, Acetate	2	2-3	—	None.	8·7	116
273	—C₁₀H₂₁—n, Acetate	1	2·4	3	None.	19	364
1941	—CH₂CH(CH₃)(CH₂)₃CH(CH₃)₂ Acetate	1	3	2	Slight.	1·2	22
1933	—(CH₂)₂CH(CH₃)(CH₂)₃—CH(CH₃)₂ Acetate	1	2·3	2	1/1 D.	1·5	50
1538	—CH=CHC₆H₁₁—n	1	1	2	None.	4·8	14
289	—(CH₂)₆CH=CH₂	1	2	2	1/1 G.I.	3·2	133
374	—(CH₂)₃—Δ^2-cycloHexenyl	2	2	1-2	None.	6·8	
297	—(CH₂)₃—β-Decalyl-*trans*	8	2-3	1-16	None.	12-14	8-61
	acetate	1	2	1	None.	0	
	Hydroquinone triacetate	1	3·5	1	None.	0	
2279	—(CH₂)₃—β-decalyl-*cis*	5	2-3	1-11	3/5 M.D.	10-14	low
1952	—(CH₂)₃—C₆—H₄CH₃—p	2	2-3	1-2	None.	8-10	28
295	—(CH₂)₃—β-tetralyl	1	1·8	2	1/1 N.	4·6	
266	—cycloHexyl	1	0·6 i.v.	—	None.	—	—

G.I. = Gastro-intestinal irritation.　　D. = diarrhœa.　　N. = nausea.　　M. = malaise.

Mode of Action

It is possible that the hydroxyalkylnaphthoquinones act by inhibiting the respiration of parasitised red blood corpuscles. Wendel (1946) found that at a concentration of the order of 1×10^6 M, M 1916 is able to bring about a 50 per cent. inhibition of the respiration of parasitised red cells from a duck infected with *P. lophuræ*. Determinations of the relative anti-respiratory activities of 158 naphthoquinones show that the *in vitro* test can be used as an alternative to screening *in vivo*. The compounds presumably interfere with carbohydrate metabolism and cause the accumulation of lactic acid in the organisms. The power to inactivate respiratory activity, however, is bound up with rapidity of drug degradation. Both M 285 and M 1916, for instance, are degraded very extensively and rapidly in the human organism. M 285 yields the carboxylic acid (I), formed by the elimination of the terminal carbon atom and oxidation at the next position. The metabolite (I) is devoid of anti-respiratory activity and several synthetic acids are inactive in this test and also in assays against *P. lophuræ*.

M 1916 (SN 5,090)   M 285 (SN 5,949).

M 1916 is degraded to two isomeric secondary alcoholic derivatives, one of which is the *trans*-4'-hydroxy derivative (II). The hydroxyl group in the side-chain causes a shift in pE from 9·45 to 6·40. These more hydrophilic substances are well tolerated by the organism and persist in the blood for several days. The presence of a hydroxyl substituent, however, depresses antimalarial activity.

Many efforts have been directed to discover a side-chain more resistant to metabolic oxidation by examining and characterisation of substances derived from urine extracts. Although the decalylalkyl derivatives M 297 and M 2279 were recognised as substances of the M 1916 type but of higher antimalarial activity only very minute amounts of naphthoquinone pigment were excreted in the urine.

The drug activity can, however, be determined accurately, relative to a standard (M 1916), by finding in the Warburg apparatus the concentration necessary to produce a 50 per cent. inhibition of the respiration of parasitised duck red cells. The course of the metabolic deactivation of a drug given intravenously or orally can be followed by removing samples of blood at intervals and determining the naphthoquinone pigment and the anti-respiratory activity per colorimetric equivalent of pigment. A comparison of the activity of the plasma pigment with that of the drug administered gives an exact measure of the degree of degradation. Thus a study of M 1916 shows that four hours after an intravenous injection the activity of the plasma is reduced by one-tenth, persisting at this level for some twenty hours. The two hydroxylated metabolites isolated were then found to possess anti-respiratory activity one-tenth that of M 1916. Thus the suppressive action of M 1916 observed in the clinical trials is due to the activity of the persisting alcoholic metabolites.

A hydroxyl group in the hydrocarbon side-chain thus provides protection against metabolic attack. Investigations have shown that the reduction in antimalarial activity produced by oxygen substitution can be offset by an increase in the number of carbon atoms in the side-chain. Thus the p-phenoxyphenylpropyl derivative M 2309 with a C_{15} side-chain possesses antimalarial activity and is more resistant to metabolic deactivation than quinones with oxygen-free side-chains. In compounds with very large hydroxylated side-chains such as $-(CH_2)_8C(OH)R_2$ anti-respiratory activity was found to increase with increasing carbon content to a maximum of 2·2 times that of M 1916 in a compound with a C_{19} side-chain, (M 2350)

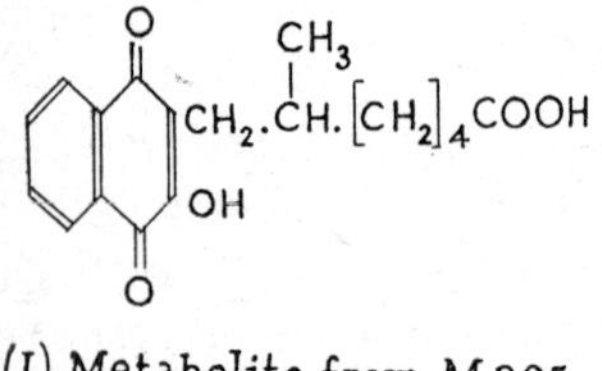

(I) Metabolite from M 285 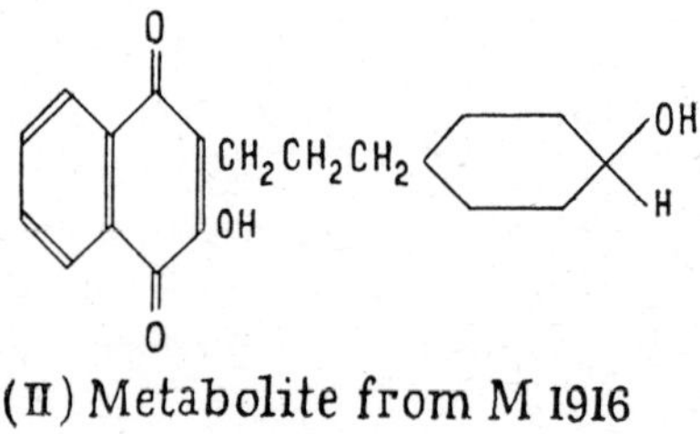   (II) Metabolite from M 1916

When given orally M 2350 shows low antimalarial activity, but intramuscularly it possesses high potency. In man and animals it is considerably more resistant to degradation than quinones with hydrocarbon side-chains, and parenterally administered it gives effective plasma levels of the drug for several hours.

A further factor apparently influences the chemotherapeutic activity of the naphthoquinones. Plasma proteins, particularly albumin, bind the naphthoquinones in the form of dialysis-resistant complexes, and quinones so bound are less active in the inhibition of parasitised red cells than are free quinones. Differences in the susceptibility to antagonism by the plasma proteins of different species probably account for variations in the dosage necessary in different species to produce a given response. A marked alternation in molar anti respiratory activity from homologue to homologue is seen in several species. Alternation also is found in susceptibility to human-protein antagonism ; the homologues of highest potency are the most susceptible to this antagonism. It is suggested that there exists a competition for naphthoquinone between plasma proteins and a respiratory enzyme; the odd or even character of the side-chain seems to promote firmness of binding to both proteins. The site of action of the naphthoquinones is not clear, for no diffusion of naphthoquinone into the red cells has been detected. Since hæmoglobin does not exert an inhibitory action, the effect on respiration may be due to the diffusion of an amount of material too small for detection by the methods at present in vogue. Ball *et al.* (1947) suggest that naphthoquinones inhibit succinic dehydrogenase.

References

BALL, E. G., ANFINSEN, C. B., and COOPER, O,. 1947, The inhibitory action of naphthoquinones on respiratory processes. *J. biol. Chem.*, **168**, 257.

CLARKE, D. H., and THEILER, M., 1948, Studies on parasite-host interplay between *Plasmodium gallinaceum* and the chicken as influenced by hydroxynaphthoquinones. *J. infect. Dis.*, **82**, 138.

FIESER, L. F., 1946, quoted by Wendel, W. B., 1946. *Fed. Proc.*, **5**, 406.

FIESER, L. F., BERLINER, E., BONDHUS, F. J., CHANG, F. C., DAUBEN, W. G., ETTLINGER, M. G., FAWAZ, G., FIELDS, M., FIESER, M., HEIDELBERGER, C., HEYMANN, H., SELIGMAN, A. M., VAUGHAN, W. R., WILSON, A. G., WILSON, E., WU, M-I., LEFFLER, M. T., HAMLIN, K. E., HATHWAY, R. J., MATSON, E. J., MOORE, E. E., MOORE, M. B., RAPALA, R. T., and ZAUGG, H. E., 1948a, Naphthoquinone antimalarials. I. General survey. *J. Amer. chem. Soc.*, **70**, 3151.

FIESER, L. F., CHANG, F. C., DAUBEN, W. G., HEYMANN, H., and SELIGMAN, A. M., 1948b, Naphthoquinone antimalarials. XVIII. Metabolic oxidation products. *J. Pharmacol.*, **94**, 85.

FIESER, L. F., HEYMANN, H., and SELIGMAN, A. M., 1948c, Naphthoquinone antimalarials. XX. Metabolic degradation. *J. Pharmacol.*, **94**, 112.

GINGRICH, W., SCHOCH, E. W., SCHWAB, M., and SHEPHERD, C. C., 1947, Radical cure of avian malaria (*Plasmodium cathemerium*) with SN 8,557, a naphthoquinone derivative. *Amer. J. trop. Med.*, **27**, 147.

HEYMANN, H., and FIESER, L. F., 1948, Naphthoquinone antimalarials. XIX. Anti-respiratory study of protein binding. *J. Pharmacol.*, **94**, 97.

HOOKER, S. C., 1936, The constitution of lapachol and its derivatives. Part IV. Oxidation with potassium permanganate. *J. Amer. chem. Soc.*, **58**, 1163.

RICHARDSON, A. P., HEWITT, R., 1946, quoted by Wendel, W. B., 1946, *Fed. Proc.*, **5**, 406.

RUHE, D. S., COOPER, W. C., COATNEY, G. R., and JOSEPHSON, E. S., 1949, Studies in human malaria. XIV. The ineffectiveness of colchicine (SN 12,080), SN 7,266 and SN 8,557 as curative agents against St. Elizabeth strain vivax malaria. *Amer. J. Hyg.*, **49**, 361.

WALKER, H. A., 1947, Potentiation of the curative action of antimalarial agents with specific reference to 8-aminoquinolines and naphthoquinones. *J. Bact.*, **54**, 669.

WENDEL, W. B., 1946, The influence of naphthoquinones upon the respiratory and carbohydrate metabolism of malarial parasites. *Fed. Proc.*, **5**, 406.

WHITMAN, L., 1948, The effect of artificial blood meals containing the hydroxynaphthoquinone M 2279 on the development cycle of *Plasmodium gallinaceum* in *Aëdes ægypti*. *J. infect. Dis.*, **82**, 251.

WISELOGLE, F. Y., edit. by, 1946, " A survey of antimalarial drugs," 1941–45. 2 Vols. Ann Arbor, Michigan. J. W. Edwards.

ANALOGUES OF METHIONINE AND VITAMINS

Up to the present so little has been known of the metabolism of malaria parasites that no attempt has been made to employ analogues of essential metabolites as antimalarial agents. McKee *et al.* (1947) found that *P. knowlesi* requires the addition of methionine for its *in vitro* growth and multiplication, and *P. knowlesi* infection in rhesus monkeys can be controlled by starving the animal. If DL-methionine is given in the diet the malarial infection recurs. The *in vitro* growth of *P. knowlesi* is markedly inhibited by methoxinine and ethionine and the inhibition is overcome by the addition of additional methionine (McKee and Geiman, 1948). It is of some interest to note that during the severe Bengal famine of 1943–44 people in a condition of extreme emaciation developed severe malaria two to three weeks after having been placed on a high protein diet, although during the stage of acute starvation no febrile reaction was seen. On the other hand, frequent attacks of malaria such as occur in hyperendemic malarial areas may lower the methionine content of the blood and thus help in the production of the cirrhosis of the liver which is so common in tropical Africa. Seeler and Ott (1946) found that with *P. lophuræ* infections in chicks parasitæmia was less in well-nourished chicks than in those fed on a diet containing a deficiency of protein. In experimental animals various dietary deficiencies have been shown to affect the course of malaria. Biotin deficiency apparently increases the severity of lophuræ malaria in chicks (Tragar, 1943a and b, 1947 ; Seeler *et al.*, 1944). Trager (1947) believes that the diminished resistance in biotin deficiency is due to decreased formation of an active antimalarial factor, lipid in nature and associated with the serum proteins. Injection of plasma proteins rich in this factor inhibits multiplication of malarial parasites. Riboflavin deficiency was found to decrease the severity of *P. lophuræ* infections in chicks as judged by parasite counts (Seeler and Ott, 1944) ; the administration of riboflavin during the course of the infection increased the severity of the infection. As chicks receiving an adequate amount of riboflavin but whose total food intake was restricted to one-half that of the control group developed an even heavier infection than did the controls, the reduced parasite count is apparently specifically due to the lack of vitamin rather than to the lowered consumption of other dietary factors. The addition of an excess of riboflavin to a diet already adequately supplied with the vitamin has no effect on the disease. In this connection it is of interest that the chemical structures of riboflavin and mepacrine are very similar and, as Madinaveitia (1946) has shown, mepacrine antagonises the effect of riboflavin on the growth of certain bacteria. Folic acid deficiency also appears to decrease the severity of the parasitæmia due to *P. lophuræ*. Vitamin A deficiency does not influence lophuræ infections in ducks so far as the time of maximal parasitæmia or the degree of parasitæmia is concerned (Rigdon, 1946). In the case of aneurin, the parasitæmia, according to Seeler and Ott (1946), is lower in chicks receiving the minimal dietary requirements for normal growth than in chicks with severe deficiency or excess of aneurin in the diet. Deficiencies in pyridoxine, riboflavin, biotin or folic acid also reduce parasitæmia to some degree (Seeler, 1944 ; Seeler and Ott, 1944, 1945, 1946). It would seem that with a diet containing neither a gross deficiency nor an excess of dietary essentials the hen is best able to cope with a malarial infection. Possibly some unknown factors are of importance for parasitæmia is less in chicks fed on a diet of natural foodstuffs than in those given purified diets complete in all nutrients at present recognised.

The administration of nicotinic acid to patients suffering from cerebral malaria is generally regarded as being of value owing to the vasodilator action of nicotinic acid. Trupp (1946) has suggested, on somewhat slender evidence, however, that massive destruction of available nicotinic acid occurs in malaria during the phase of parasite multiplication. There would thus occur competitive activity between the host and the parasites. Becker *et al.* (1949) have shown that in chicks *P. lophuræ* infections may precipitate dietary deficiency.

References

BECKER, E. R., BRODINE, C. H., and MAROUSEK, A. A., 1949, Eyelid lesions of chicks in acute dietary deficiency resulting from blood-induced *Plasmodium lophuræ* infection. *J. infect. Dis.*, 85, 230.

McKEE, R. W., and GEIMAN, Q. M., 1948, Methionine in the growth of the malarial parasite, *Plasmodium knowlesi*. *Fed. Proc.*, 7, 172.

McKEE, R. W., GEIMAN, Q. M., and COBBEY, T. S., Jr., 1947, Amino acids in the nutrition and metabolism of malaria parasites. *Fed. Proc.*, 6, 276.

MADINAVEITIA, J., 1946, Antagonism of malaria drugs by riboflavin. *Biochem. J.*, 40, 373.

RIGDON, R. H., 1946, Effect of vitamin A deficiency on *Plasmodium lophuræ* infection in ducks. *J. infect. Dis.*, 79, 272.

SEELER, A. O., 1944, Effect of pyridoxine on activity of quinine and atabrine against *Plasmodium lophuræ* infections. *Proc. Soc. exp. Biol., N.Y.*, 57, 113.

SEELER, A. O., 1944, Effect of riboflavin deficiency on the course of *Plasmodium lophuræ* infection in chicks. *J. infect. Dis.*, 75, 175.

SEELER, A. O., and OTT, W. H., 1945, Studies on nutrition and avian malaria : deficiency of " folic acid " and other unidentified factors. *J. infect. Dis.*, 77, 181.

SEELER, A. O., and OTT, W. H., 1946, Effect of deficiencies in vitamins and in proteins on avian malaria. *J. nat. Mal. Soc.*, 5, 123.

SEELER, A. O., OTT, W. H., and GUNDEL, M. E., 1944, Effect of biotin deficiency on course of *Plasmodium lophuræ* in chicks. *Proc. Soc. exp. Biol., N.Y.*, 55, 107.

TRAGER, W., 1943a, The influence of biotin upon susceptibility to malaria. *Science*, 97, 206.

TRAGER, W., 1943b, The influence of biotin upon susceptibility to malaria. *J. exp. Med.*, 77, 557.

TRAGER, W., 1947, The relation to the course of avian malaria of biotin and a fat-soluble material having the biological activities of biotin. *J. exp. Med.*, 85, 663.

TRUPP, M., 1946, Metabolism in cerebral malaria (practical and theoretical considerations). *Dis. nerv. System*, 7, 368.

HORMONES

Although hormones have not been employed in the treatment of malaria, there is some evidence that in birds hormones may influence the degree of parasitæmia.

Trager (1947, 1948) has found that a plasma lipoprotein plays a *rôle* in the resistance of birds to avian malaria parasites. Ducks with actively functioning ovaries inoculated with *P. lophuræ* inhibit the multiplication of the parasites whereas those with inactive ovaries and males showed a high degree of parasitæmia and the lipoprotein content of the plasma of ducks with active ovaries is higher than that of ducks with inactive ovaries. A similar increase in lipids can be produced by the injection of œstrogenic hormones into immature male as well as female chickens (Entenman *et al.*, 1940). The responsible factor is present in the euglobulin fraction of hen plasma (Trager and McGhee, 1950). Urinary œstrogens, it may be noted, increase the bactericidal effects of the blood serum of male rabbits on *Salmonella typhi* (Tsao, 1941). Bennison and Coatney (1948) found that female chicks six to eight days old showed slightly higher densities of *P. gallinaceum*, a poorer response to treatment with quinine, and earlier appearance of exo-erythrocytic forms in the brain than did males. Hauschka (1947), on the other hand, found that when brother and sister mice were inoculated with *Trypanosoma cruzi* the infection in the males attained parasite densities twice as great as those seen in the females.

References

BENNISON, B. E., and COATNEY, G. R., 1948, The sex of the host as a factor in *Plasmodium gallinaceum* infections in young chicks. *Science*, **107**, 147.

ENTENMAN, C., LORENZ, F. W., and CHAIKOFF, I. L., 1940, The endocrine control of lipide metabolism in the bird. III. The effects of crystalline sex hormones on the blood lipides of the bird. *J. biol. Chem.*, **134**, 495.

HAUSCHKA, T. S., 1947, Sex of host as a factor in Chagas' disease. *J. Parasit.*, **33**, 399.

TRAGER, W., 1947, The relation to the course of avian malaria of biotin and a fat-soluble material having the biological activities of biotin. *J. exp. Med.*, **85**, 663.

TRAGER, W., 1948, The resistance of egg-laying ducks to infection by the malaria parasite *Plasmodium lophuræ*. *J. Parasit.*, **34**, 389.

TRAGER, W., and McGHEE, R. B., 1950, Factors in plasma concerned in natural resistance to an avian malaria parasite (*Plasmodium lophuræ*). *J. exp. Med.*, **91**, 365.

TSAO, T. N., 1941, Bacterial property of blood serum of male rabbits treated with urinary estrogens. *Proc. Soc. exp. Biol., N.Y.*, **48**, 38.

ANIMAL TISSUE EXTRACTS

The possibility that animal tissues contain substances which act against the malarial parasite was first suggested by Jacobs (1947), who believed that as part of their defence mechanism animals developed substances which destroyed their own parasitised red cells. Whitman (1948), however, demonstrated the prolonged viability of sporozoites of *P. gallinaceum* in extracts of washed chicken erythrocytes. Trager and McGhee (1949) believed that some factor developed in the tissues with age, for if young chickens were injected with 3 ml. of adult hen plasma they developed less severe infections than untreated young chicks. The same result was obtained by the injection of 3 ml. of 6 per cent. bovine albumin in saline. The most definite results were reported by Haas *et al.* (1948). Saline extracts of lymph nodes, spleen, and liver of white mice were found to inactivate sporozoites and blood forms of *P. gallinaceum* after suitable contact *in vitro*. Against exo-erythrocytic forms only extract of spleen was active. Similar extracts from the white rat, the rice rat *Oryzomys palustris*, the cotton rat *Sigmodon hispidus*, and the cow showed an equal inactivating effect against erythrocytic stages, but extracts from the spleens of fowls and pigs were less potent than extracts from the spleens of rats and cows. Of 367 chicks inoculated with fowl red cells parasitised by *P. gallinaceum* only 26 per cent. developed microscopically detectable parasitæmia during a period of three weeks' observation ; of 213 chicks inoculated with untreated red cells infected with *P. gallinaceum* 87 per cent. developed parasitæmia in the same period.

Bovine spleen extract concentrated by ethyl alcohol precipitation had an effect on sporozoite-induced gallinaceum infection *in vivo*. Of 170 treated chicks 64 per cent. developed parasitæmia in three weeks whereas of 146 control chicks 97 per cent. became patently infected. In treated chicks parasitæmia, when it did develop, was slower in onset than in controls. Bovine spleen extract is toxic to chicks, but extracts of bovine red cells are less toxic and quite as effective in reducing parasitæmia. Thus of 162 chicks treated with bovine red cell extract 79 per cent. developed patent infections, but of ninety-eight controls 93 per

cent. became infected.   Concentrated extracts of bovine plasma
or serum had no action on malaria in chickens.   There is some
evidence to show that the active substance in bovine blood cell
extracts is a protein or a substance closely bound up with proteins.
   Very little has yet been done to determine whether the tissues
of lower animals contain active antimalarial substances.   However,
from the wings of the Philippine butterfly, *Terias hecabe* Linn.,
Garcia (1948) has isolated a yellow pterin after the wings have
been boiled in normal saline.   The extract has hæmostatic properties, but in addition Garcia (1949) has found that it has an
anti-plasmodial action, since it removes the asexual parasites of
P. falciparum, *P. vivax*, and *P. malariæ* from the blood-stream of
human patients.   Precise details of its action are not available,
but it is suggested that hecabepterin combines with *p*-aminobenzoic
acid and later glutamic acid to form pteroyl glutamic acid.   Thus
the parasites are starved of *p*-aminobenzoic acid.   It may be
recalled that up to the beginning of last century a much-esteemed
remedy for malaria was a common spider gently bruised and
wrapped up in a raisin, taken either in the cold fit or on three
successive mornings.   An alternative treatment was 5 grains of
cobwebs mixed with breadcrumbs twice a day (MacBride, 1777).
Cobwebs are still looked upon as a valuable remedy for ague in
Spanish Morocco (Más y Guindal, 1932).   Possibly cobwebs may
contain pterins.

References

GARCIA, E. Y., 1948, The strong anti-hæmorrhagic property of hecabepterin,
    the yellow pigment in the Philippine butterfly *Terias hecabe* Linnæus.
    J. Philipp. med. Ass., **24**, 515.
GARCIA, E. Y., 1949, Extract of the wings of the Philippine butterfly *Terias
    hecabe* Linnæus, a new antibiotic for malaria.   *J. Philipp. med. Ass.*,
    25, 279.
HAAS, V. H., WILCOX, A., and COLEMAN, N., 1948, Modification of *Plasmodium
    gallinaceum* infections by certain tissue extracts.   *J. nat. Mal. Soc.*, **8**, 85.
JACOBS, H. R., 1947, Consideration of anti-erythrocytic factors in resistance
    to malaria.   *Quart. Bull. Nthwest Univ. med. Sch.*, **21**, 52.
MACBRIDE, D., 1777, " A methodical introduction to the theory and practice
    of the art of medicine."   2 vols.   2nd Edit.   Dublin.   W. Watson.
MÁS Y GUINDAL, J., 1932, " Farmacognosia y Terapéutica musulmana-
    herbraica."   Madrid.
TRAGER, W., and MCGHEE, R. B., 1949, Passive transfer of age-resistance to
    an avian malarial parasite.   *Fed. Proc.*, **8**, 373.
WHITMAN, L., 1948, The prolonged viability of sporozoites of *Plasmodium
    gallinaceum* in extracts of washed chicken erythrocytes.   *J. Immunol.*,
    59, 285.

CHAPTER IX

DRUG RESISTANCE AND IMMUNITY

RESISTANCE OF PLASMODIA AGAINST ANTIMALARIAL DRUGS

THE question of the development of resistance by plasmodia to commonly used antimalarial drugs is obviously of considerable importance since the same drugs are so frequently administered therapeutically and prophylactically over long periods.

Quinine. Attempts to produce quinine-resistant strains of plasmodia have not been very satisfactory. Sergent and Sergent (1921a and b) were the first to claim that resistance had been induced in *P. relictum*, but their experimental evidence was meagre. Kritschewski and Rubinstein (1932) brought forward rather more convincing evidence. Kritschewski and Halperin (1933) found that sometimes, but not invariably, resistance persisted after the passage of *P. relictum* through the mosquito *Culex pipiens*. Some degree of resistance against quinine was recorded by Nauck (1934) in *P. knowlesi* in rhesus monkeys. Lourie (1935) failed to induce any appreciable degree of resistance to quinine in *P. cathemerium* in canaries after seventeen months' exposure to the drug. Williamson *et al.* (1947) and Williamson and Lourie (1947) also failed to produce resistance against quinine in *P. gallinaceum* in chicks over an experimental period of $2\frac{1}{2}$ years. Knoppers (1947), by using doses of 10 mgm. per kgm. of body weight for sixteen weeks, followed by 20 mgm. per kgm. of body weight for a further sixteen weeks, claimed to have produced a two-fold resistance to quinine in *P. gallinaceum*. After a single mosquito-passage in *Aëdes ægypti* resistance to quinine was partially lost. The quinine-resistant strain was not resistant to mepacrine, chloroquine or proguanil, but some resistance was present against the 8-aminoquinolines, pamaquin and pentaquine. Later Knoppers (1949) reported that the strain of *P. gallinaceum* resistant to quinine maintained its resistance through an exo-erythrocytic stage carried out in tissue culture. The resistant strain was resistant also to the lævo-rotatory cinchonidine but had a decreased resistance to the dextro-rotatory alkaloids cinchonine and quinidine. An increased sensitivity developed also against the 8-aminoquinolines, pamaquin, pentaquine and *iso*pentaquine.

Pamaquin. Some evidence of resistance to *P. knowlesi* was obtained by Nauck (1934), a finding confirmed by Fulton and Yorke (1941) with a blood-passaged strain of *P. knowlesi*. Bishop and Birkett (1948) also produced a strain of *P. gallinaceum* which after eight months' exposure to the drug had gained sufficient resistance to withstand the minimum effective dose (0·08 mgm.) of pamaquin. Lourie (1935) failed to induce pamaquin-resistance in *P. cathemerium* in canaries after 9½ months, and Fulton (1942) was similarly unsuccessful with *P. gallinaceum* after 15½ months' exposure to pamaquin. It is thus obviously far from easy to produce any degree of resistance to pamaquin. The effect of mosquito transmission on pamaquin resistance has not been studied.

Mepacrine. Difficulty has also been experienced in producing mepacrine-resistant strains of plasmodia. Bishop and Birkett (1947) failed with *P. gallinaceum* over a period of six months, and Williamson *et al.* (1947) and Williamson and Lourie (1947) had no better success after exposing *P. gallinaceum* for 2½ years to mepacrine methane sulphonate. Piekarski (1948), however, claims to have induced a mepacrine-resistant strain of *P. cathemerium* in the canary.

Camoquin. A slight but not very definite increase in resistance to camoquin was produced in *P. lophuræ* by Thompson (1948).

Proguanil. Unlike the older antimalarial drugs, proguanil appears to give rise to resistant strains of *P. gallinaceum* with comparative ease. Bishop and Birkett (1947) and Williamson *et al.* (1947), working independently, succeeded in producing proguanil-resistant strains of *P. gallinaceum*. Bishop and Birkett (1947) produced a forty-fold increase in resistance to proguanil and the resistance was still demonstrable after five transmissions through *Aëdes ægypti*, thus showing that drug resistance could survive when the plasmodia lived in the tissues of the mosquito, an environment quite unlike that in which the drug resistance was originally acquired. Williamson *et al.* (1947) and Williamson and Lourie (1947), after exposure of *P. gallinaceum* to increasing doses of proguanil in the chick, found that the strains were from twenty to forty times more resistant to proguanil. With one strain the appearance of resistance was so sudden as to suggest very strongly the selection of a new mutant. No loss of proguanil resistance occurred after one passage through *Aëdes ægypti*. Knoppers (1948) in three months increased the resistance of *P. gallinaceum* thirty or forty times. Greenberg (1949) found that proguanil resistance persisted after repeated passage in the absence of proguanil. A strain of *P. relictum* made resistant to proguanil was shown by Redmond and Fincher (1949) to produce more exo-erythrocytic forms than a normal strain. Rollo *et al.* (1948) failed to produce resistance of latent infections by prolonged treatment, presumably because exo-erythrocytic forms are not actively multiplying.

There is now evidence that proguanil-resistant strains of *P. falciparum* and *P. vivax* can be obtained (Adams and Seaton, 1949 ; Lourie and Seaton, 1949 ; Seaton and Lourie, 1949). In the case of *P. vivax* resistance was more than eighty times greater than normal and the length of time required to develop resistance was short. Resistance persists through mosquito passage. Seaton and Adams (1949), by passaging a West African strain of *P. falciparum* by injections of blood, succeeded in raising the resistance of the strain so that it was unaffected by 1 gm. of proguanil daily for ten days, the largest dose which could be tolerated by patients. Attempts were made to infect batches of *Anopheles stephensi* by feeding the mosquitoes on patients harbouring *P. falciparum* of the eleventh and twelfth blood-passages. The first two batches of mosquitoes thus fed failed to permit the development of the parasites beyond the oöcyst stage though neither of the patients had ever taken proguanil. A third batch of mosquitoes, however, allowed full development of the parasites and with the sporozoites thus produced fresh volunteers could be infected. The infection then produced was quite resistant to 1 gm. proguanil daily. Proguanil resistance, having once been induced, can therefore obviously be transmitted through the mosquito. It remains to be seen whether such an increase in proguanil resistance

Proguanil Resistance Experimentally Produced in Malarial Infections

Malarial species.	Host.	Months to acquire resistance indicated.	Blood passage at which resistance appeared.	Degree of resistance.	Persistence after mosquito passage.	Authors
P. gallinaceum	Chick.	4½	23rd	+ + +	Yes.	Bishop and Birkett (1947, 1948).
,,	,,	—	—	× 20–40	Yes.	Williamson *et al.* (1947).
,,	,,	3	—	× 30–40	—	Knoppers (1948).
P. lophuræ	Duck.	7	60th	× 4	—	Thompson *et al.* (1948).
P. cynomolgi	Monkey	14	Same animal. 3rd	+ + + × 2,000	— Yes.	Hawking and Perry (1948). Schmidt *et al.* (1949).
P. vivax	Man.	20	27th	× 80	Yes.	Seaton and Lourie (1949).
P. falciparum	,,	10	10th	+ + +	Yes.	Adams and Seaton (1949); Seaton and Adams (1949).

+ + + = Dose resisted by parasite close to limit of tolerance.

will often occur in populations given proguanil as a prophylactic or suppressive. The existence of strains of *P. falciparum* over a wide area of Africa with a naturally high resistance to proguanil has already been mentioned. Covell (1949) emphasises the fact that a strain brought to England from Lagos had never been exposed to proguanil and the writer in Accra in 1945 had a similar experience with naturally resistant strains of *P. falciparum*. That some degree of resistance may be acquired is suggested by the observation of Field and Edeson (1949) and Edeson and Field (1950) in Malaya. In 1947 all of twenty-six cases of acute falciparum infection were cured clinically by a single tablet of 100 mgm. and in all the parasitæmia cleared within four days. In the first half of 1949 one in four of the cases treated from the Tampin district with 250 to 300 mgm. failed to respond, and from May to July, 1949, seven infections resisted proguanil in doses as great or greater than a standard therapeutic course of 300 mgm. daily for seven to ten days. Local strains had been exposed to the drug, regularly or sporadically, for two years. If these results are confirmed from other areas the prophylactic or suppressive use of proguanil may render its therapeutic employment impossible. Hawking and Perry (1948) found in a monkey that after fourteen months' treatment with small doses of proguanil the resistance of *P. cynomolgi* to this drug had been increased one-thousand-fold. Schmidt *et al.* (1949) obtained a two-thousand-fold increase which was transmissible through mosquitoes.

Thompson (1948) found a ten-fold increase in resistance to proguanil on the part of *P. lophuræ*. The resistant strain showed no change in sensitivity to quinine, mepacrine, chloroquine, camoquin, and pamaquin.

Sulphonamides. Williamson *et al.* (1947) failed to render *P. gallinaceum* resistant to sulphadiazine. This resistance was, however, induced by Bishop and Birkett (1948), though the development of resistance was slow and the degree obtained not very great. Later, Bishop and McConnachie (1948) obtained a strain of *P. gallinaceum* in young chicks in which the resistance to sulphadiazine was thirty-two times greater than that of the untreated strain. Whereas the minimum dose of sulphadiazine which affected the normal strain was 0·625 mgm. per 20 gm. of body weight given twice daily on successive days, in the resistant strain growth of the parasites occurred in chicks receiving 20 mgm. twice daily. This strain, with a thirty-two-fold resistance, took approximately twelve months to produce. No loss of resistance was noted after passage through *Aëdes ægypti*.

Cross-resistance. The strain of *P. gallinaceum* rendered resistant to proguanil by Bishop and Birkett (1947) was not resistant to mepacrine or pamaquin but was resistant to the methyl homologue of proguanil, N^1-*p*-chlorophenyl-N^5-methyl-N^5-*iso*propylbiguanide (4430). Williamson *et al.* (1947) found that their proguanil-resistant strain was just as sensitive as before to quinine, mepacrine, sulphadiazine, and to 2-*p*-chlorophenylguanidino-4-β-diethylaminoethylamino-6-methyl-pyrimidine (3349). These workers failed entirely to produce resistance to 3349 in *P. gallinaceum*. The strains of *P. gallinaceum* rendered highly resistant to sulphadiazine by Bishop and McConnachie (1948) were resistant, as might be expected, to sulphathiazole, sulphapyridine and sulphanilamide; they were, however, resistant also to proguanil. In addition, a proguanil-resistant strain was found to be resistant to sulphadiazine. Further investigation showed that resistance to sulphadiazine develops later than resistance to proguanil; this probably explains why Williamson *et al.* (1947) and Williamson and Lourie (1947) failed to determine sulphadiazine resistance in their proguanil-resistant strain. Greenberg (1949) found that a strain of *P. gallinaceum* resistant to proguanil became from four to eight times as sensitive as the parent strain to sulphadiazine. The proguanil-resistant strain was still hypersensitive to sulphadiazine at the fifth passage carried out in the absence of proguanil.

The absence of acquired resistance to 3349 on the part of the proguanil-resistant strain, coupled with the failure to induce resistance to 3349, is of interest since both proguanil and 3349 possess the very similar prototropic possibilities stressed by Curd, Davey and Rose (1945) as associated with antimalarial activity in compounds of this general type. Both proguanil and 4430, N^1-p-chlorophenyl-N^5-methyl-N^5-*iso*propylbiguanide, lack the pyrimidine ring present in 3349. Williamson *et al.* (1947) suggest that the presence or absence of a pyrimidine ring in such compounds as 3349 and proguanil may be a factor in determining the existence of drug resistance.

Sulphadiazine, however, also contains a pyrimidine ring and the resistance between it and proguanil is reciprocal. On the other hand, Williamson and his co-workers (1947) failed to produce resistance to 3349, which has a pyrimidine ring. Thus in these compounds the presence or absence of a pyrimidine ring does not appear to have any relationship to the formation of drug-resistant strains of *P. gallinaceum*.

If human plasmodia can be rendered drug resistant to proguanil as readily as *P. gallinaceum*, then the value of proguanil as a malarial suppressive on a large scale will be greatly reduced. Evidence for the development of resistance to proguanil in human plasmodia is, unfortunately, already accumulating.

The evidence at present available goes to show that it is not easy to produce resistant strains of human plasmodia to quinine, mepacrine or pamaquin. It is curious that whereas trypanosomes pathogenic for man acquire drug resistance with comparative ease against many different chemical compounds, plasmodia fail to produce comparably resistant strains with the same rapidity and ease.

References

ADAMS, A. R. D., and SEATON, D. R., 1949, Resistance to paludrine developed by a strain of *Plasmodium falciparum*. *Trans. R. Soc. trop. Med. Hyg.*, 42, 314.

BISHOP, A., and BIRKETT, B., 1947, Acquired resistance to paludrine in *Plasmodium gallinaceum*. Acquired resistance and persistence after passage through the mosquito. *Nature, Lond.*, 159, 884.

BISHOP, A., and BIRKETT, B., 1948, Drug resistance in *Plasmodium gallinaceum*, and the persistence of paludrine resistance after mosquito transmission. *Parasitology*, **39**, 125.

BISHOP, A., and MCCONNACHIE, E. W., 1948, Resistance to sulphadiazine and paludrine in the malaria parasite of the fowl (*P. gallinaceum*). *Nature, Lond.*, **162**, 541.

COVELL, G., 1949, The Lagos strain of *Plasmodium falciparum* and paludrine. *Trans. R. Soc. trop. Med. Hyg.*, **43**, 350.

CURD, F. H. S., DAVEY, D. G., and ROSE, F. L., 1945, Studies on synthetic antimalarial drugs. X. Some biguanide derivatives as new types of antimalarial substances with both therapeutic and causal prophylactic activity. *Ann. trop. Med. Parasit.*, **39**, 208.

EDESON, J. F. B., and FIELD, J. W., 1950, Proguanil-resistant falciparum malaria in Malaya. *Brit. med. J.*, i, 147.

FIELD, J. W., and EDESON, J. F. B., 1949, Paludrine-resistant falciparum malaria. *Trans. R. Soc. trop. Med. Hyg.*, **43**, 233.

FULTON, J. D., 1942, Attempts to prepare in fowls a strain of *Plasmodium gallinaceum* resistant to plasmoquine. *Ann. trop. Med. Parasit.*, **36**, 75.

FULTON, J. D., and YORKE, W., 1941, Studies in chemotherapy. XXIX. The development of plasmoquine-resistance in *Plasmodium knowlesi*. *Ann. trop. Med. Parasit.*, **35**, 233.

GREENBERG, J., 1949, Hypersensitivity to sulfadiazine of a chlorguanide-resistant strain of *Plasmodium gallinaceum*. *J. nat. Mal. Soc.*, **8**, 30.

HAWKING, F., and PERRY, W. L. M., 1948, Resistance to proguanil (paludrine) in a mammalian malaria parasite. *Lancet*, ii, 850.

KNOPPERS, A. T., 1947, Acquired resistance (two-fold) to quinine in *Plasmodium gallinaceum*. *Nature, Lond.*, **160**, 606.

KNOPPERS, A. T., 1948, Relatieve ongevoeligheid van *Plasmodium gallinaceum* voor kinine door regelmatige toediening daarvan. *Ned. Tijdschr. Geneesk.*, **92**, 3034.

KNOPPERS, A. T., 1949, Two-fold resistance of *Plasmodium falciparum* induced by regular administration of the drug. *Document. nederl. indon. Morb. trop.*, **1**, 55.

KRITSCHEWSKI, I. L., and HALPERIN, E. P., 1933, Ueber die Medikament-festigkeit der Erreger der Vogelmalaria (*Plasmodium præcox*). 11. Der Einfluss des geschlechtlichen Vermehrungszyklus auf die Medikament-festigkeit. *Z. ImmunForsch.*, **76**, 149.

KRITSCHEWSKI, I. L., and RUBINSTEIN, P. L., 1932, Ueber die Medikament-festigkeit der Erreger von Vogelmalaria (*Plasmodium præcox*). 1. Mitteilung. *Z. ImmunForsch.*, **76**, 506.

LOURIE, E. M., 1935, Studies on chemotherapy in bird malaria. IV. Failure to promote drug-resistance in *Plasmodium cathemerium* by prolonged administration of quinine or plasmochin. *Ann. trop. Med. Parasit.*, **29**, 421.

LOURIE, E. M., and SEATON, D. R., 1949, Resistance to paludrine developed by a strain of *Plasmodium vivax*. *Trans. R. Soc. trop. Med. Hyg.*, **42**, 315.

NAUCK, E. G., 1934, Chemotherapeutische Versuche bei Affenmalaria (*Pl. knowlesi*). *Arch. Schiffs-u. Tropenhyg.*, **38**, 313.

PIEKARSKI, G., 1948, Experimentelle Untersuchungen zur Frage der Atebrin-festigkeit der Malariaparasiten. *Z. Hyg. InfektKr.*, **127**, 501.

REDMOND, W. B., and FINCHER, E. L., 1949, Exoerythrocytic forms in relation to paludrine administration in pigeons infected with *Plasmodium relictum*. *J. Parasitol.*, **35** (No. 6, Sect. 2), 25.

ROLLO, I. M., WILLIAMSON, J., and LOURIE, E. M., 1948, Acquired paludrine resistance in *Plasmodium gallinaceum*. II. Failure to produce such resistance by prolonged treatment of latent infections. *Ann. trop. Med. Parasit.*, **42**, 241.

SCHMIDT, L. H., GENTHER, C. S., FRADKIN, R., and SQUIRES, W., 1949, Development of resistance to chlorguanide (paludrine) during treatment of infections with *Plasmodium cynomolgi*. *J. Pharmacol.*, **95**, 382.

SEATON, D. R., ADAMS, A. R. D., 1949, Acquired resistance to proguanil in *Plasmodium falciparum*. *Lancet, ii*, 323.

SEATON, D. R., and LOURIE, E. M., 1949, Acquired resistance to proguanil (paludrine) in *Plasmodium vivax*. *Lancet, i*, 394.

SERGENT, ET., and SERGENT, ED., 1921a, Avantages de la quininisation preventive demontrès et précisés expérimentalement (paludisme des oiseaux). *Ann. Inst. Pasteur*, **35**, 125.

SERGENT, ET., and SERGENT, ED., 1921b, Etude expérimentale du paludisme. Paludisme des oiseaux (*Plasmodium relictum*). *Bull. Soc. Path. exot.*, **14**, 72.

THOMPSON, P. E., 1948, On the ability of *Plasmodium lophuræ* to acquire resistance to chlorguanide, "camoquin" and chloroquine. *J. infect. Dis.*, **83**, 250.

WILLIAMSON, J., BERTRAM, D. S., and LOURIE, E. M., 1947, Effects of paludrine and other antimalarials. *Nature, Lond.*, **159**, 885.

WILLIAMSON, J., and LOURIE, E. M., 1947, Acquired paludrine-resistance to *Plasmodium gallinaceum*. I. Development of resistance to paludrine and failure to develop resistance to certain other antimalarials. *Ann. trop. Med. Parasit.*, **41**, 278.

IMMUNITY AND CHEMOTHERAPY

When a man is infected with malaria he will, if entirely untreated by chemotherapeutic drugs, either die or develop resistance to the parasites. Two forms of acquired resistance occur :—

(1) Tolerance : the host limits the degree of reaction to a given infecting dose.

(2) Specific immunity : the host limits the infection developed or, in other words, inhibits the development of the parasites.

In addition, as Garnham (1949) has emphasised, among those peoples who have lived for generations in a hyperendemic area there is a racial or phylogenetic resistance, and some degree of immunity also is transmitted passively from immune mothers to their offspring. Some degree of innate tolerance may be exhibited by chicks to *P. lophuræ* (Reilly *et al.*, 1949). There is a suggestion that some races, such as the Indonesians, do not obtain such a high degree of immunity as Africans. Whether this is due to a racial difference or to a difference in the strain of parasite is uncertain (Swellengrebel, 1949).

It has long been recognised that those who have been born and bred in one malarial area, and have attained to adult life, rarely suffer from severe symptoms though parasites may be present in their blood stream in considerable numbers. In patients with general paralysis treated by injections of *P. vivax* tolerance usually develops before specific immunity (Yorke and Macfie, 1924; Boyd and Kitchen, 1936; Boyd, 1938, and Blackburn, 1948). James (1931), Boyd and Stratman-Thomas (1933), and Blackburn (1948) all showed that immunity is strain-specific whereas tolerance or innate resistance may be developed to heterologous strains of *P. vivax*. In other words, there is a differentiation from the patient's point of view of " malarial disease and malarial infection " (Sinton, 1945). Some species of animals apparently owe their innate resistance to infection, not to specific immune bodies which have developed as a result of adequate exposure to the particular parasite, but to the presence of antiplasmodial substances in their blood. It has never been possible to infect fowls with *P. cathemerium* because, according to Beckman (1948), the blood of fowls contains a substance which inhibits the formation of exo-erythrocytic forms from the sporo-zoites of *P. cathemerium*. Whether similar substances occur in the blood of man apart from exposure is unknown but improbable. Some exceptional Europeans, however, fail to react to infection with malarial parasites, and it has long been recognised that negroes possess a natural tolerance to *P. vivax*. This has been demonstrated in America where *P. vivax* cannot be used for the treatment of neurosyphilis in negroes even in the non-malarial Northern States : it was shown also during the second world war when West African soldiers failed to exhibit symptoms when exposed to Indian strains of *P. vivax* with which they could never previously have come in contact. Trager and McGhee (1949) suggest that fowls develop a factor in the serum with age since old hens have less severe infections than young chicks when first inoculated with *P. gallinaceum*.

In connection with the question of increased tolerance to infection, it is of interest to note that in 1917 Abrami and Sénevet came to the conclusion that the acute malarial attack was essentially allergic in character, a view to which support has been lent by the later work of Sinton *et al.* (1928), Sapero (1946), Danielopolo (1946), Fourrier (1949) and others. With this theory in view, Thiodet and Fourrier (1948, 1949) have treated patients suffering from relapsing vivax malaria with intradermal injections of the patient's own globulins prepared by bubbling carbon dioxide through the patient's own serum diluted with saline, in order to produce desensitisation. While such injections have no action on the number of parasites in the red cells they are said to lead to a rapid disappearance of the fever, shivering, and headache characteristic of the acute paroxysm : in other words, they lead to increased tolerance.

Theoretically, unless sporozoites are destroyed before they have time to infect the cells of the host some degree of immunity is bound to occur and such immunity should help to modify the subsequent reaction of the host to the action of malarial parasites.

In practice, however, if the disease is terminated shortly after infection, little immunity is demonstrable. In man only a very feeble immunity results from a single infection unless the continued development of the parasites is uninhibited by chemotherapy. Redmond (1941) suggests that the infection must continue untreated for at least one year. Both experimentally (Blackburn, 1948), and under natural conditions, it would seem that repeated infections at comparatively short intervals are necessary for the development of any degree of immunity. In most hyperendemic areas there is little difficulty in ensuring that such repeated reinfections occur, but it must always be remembered that even in a hyperendemic area there may be several strains of malarial parasite which may induce some degree of general tolerance but little specific heterologous immunity.

The investigations on man made by Blackburn (1948) show that the presence of exo-erythrocytic forms in the tissues does not result in either tolerance or immunity. Minor trophozoite waves during a suppressive regimen induce a greater degree of tolerance than the absence of such waves; the greatest tolerance, however, develops as a result of considerable trophozoite experience. The question how long it takes to lose an effective immunity to a particular strain of plasmodium is not easy to answer. In the case of some strains of *P. falciparum* immunity is usually lost in about two years. With vivax infections effective immunity after apparent cure has been demonstrated after as long as two years and three and a half years by James (1933) and Boyd *et al.* (1936) respectively : in Boyd's case subinoculation of blood was negative. It would therefore seem that with *P. vivax* immunity can persist for some time after the disappearance of the parasites as demonstrated by subinoculation but that such immunity eventually dies out. Coggeshall *et al.* (1948) believe that after the cure of vivax malaria the duration of immunity is variable but in general short. After radical cure with pentaquine and quinine, immunity varied from three and a half to twenty-one months.

It is obvious that if experience of trophozoites is the deciding factor in the induction and persistence of immunity the continued application of suppressive drugs may well prevent the development of immunity or increase the rate at which it is lost.

According to Taliaferro *et al.* (1948) and Taliaferro and Taliaferro (1949), the *rôle* of a drug such as quinine in relation to chemotherapy is somewhat complex. Quinine does not increase the phagocytosis of malarial parasites by macrophages ; it does not act as an opsonin nor does it appear to stimulate either inherent tolerance or acquired immunity. In hens in which the spleen has been removed the blood level of quinine, following a standard dose, is considerably higher than in intact birds, but quinine is, curiously enough, less effective against *P. gallinaceum* in splenectomised than in normal hens. It is therefore concluded that during quinine treatment three independent factors operate : (1) innate tolerance ; (2) specific immunity, and (3) the antimalarial action of quinine. In splenectomised birds the acquired immunity is so much reduced that the increased antimalarial activity resulting from an increased quinine blood level is nullified. When monkeys infected with *P. knowlesi* are examined it is found that the malarial process *per se* depresses very considerably the phagocytic activity of the reticulo-endothelial system : when, as a result of the administration of quinine, parasites are removed from the peripheral blood stream the phagocytic activity of the reticulo-endothelial system at once increases (Gupta and Ganguly, 1944). In man, Bang *et al.* (1947) have shown that when once some degree of immunity is acquired smaller doses of a chemotherapeutic drug are required than in non-immunes.

These findings on the relationship between tolerance, specific immunity, and chemotherapeutic administration are obviously of very considerable importance, especially in relation to the treatment of malaria in indigenous populations. Here the aim of treatment must obviously be to develop tolerance as soon as possible so that the clinical reaction is restricted, whereas tropho-zoites must be allowed to appear in the peripheral blood stream in sufficient numbers so that specific immunity to the local strains develops. Specific acquired immunity is not necessary for the efficient action of the drug, but it is necessary to prevent relapse after the cessation of treatment.

If in an indigenous population immunity is allowed to wane but the possibility of reinfection is not entirely eliminated, serious reactions may occur. African students who have spent some years in Europe or America find that after returning to Africa they are liable to severe attacks. Walton (1949) has noted the same phenomenon among Africans resident in Freetown, Sierra Leone, and Findlay (1949) has correlated the high rate of blackwater fever in African troops in West Africa with loss of immunity to local strains of *P. falciparum*.

The action of the reticulo-endothelial system, and especially of the spleen, has long been recognised as playing an important *rôle* in chemotherapy. Krishnan *et al.* (1933) studied the course of infection with a strain described as *P. inui* (probably *P. knowlesi*) in splenectomised and in normal monkeys, *Macaca mulatta*, *M. irus* and *M. radiata*. Removal of the spleen resulted in more severe infections and a poorer response to treatment. Rodhain (1949) obtained similar results with *P. berghei* in splenectomised cotton rats. Klinger (1949), in a splenectomised man, found mepacrine and quinine useless. Kritschewski and Demidowa (1934) found that infections of *P. præcox* (= *P. relictum*) responded to quinine, pamaquin, and arichin (SN 5,341) better in untreated canaries than in birds " blockaded " with trypan blue.

These results were confirmed by Taliaferro and Kelsey (1948) and Taliaferro, Taliaferro, and Kelsey (1948), using *P. gallinaceum*. Splenectomy increases mortality and parasitæmia to about the same extent in chickens treated with quinine and in those un-treated. It therefore seems that the spleen is not directly con-cerned with increasing the suppressive action of quinine but simply adds an additional antimalarial factor. This added factor appears to be an acquired immunity but not an innate tolerance. Quinine might act indirectly by stimulating either innate tolerance or acquired immunity or by an opsonin-like effect on the parasite which renders the parasite more easily phagocytised. As phago-cytosis of macrophages is not increased during quinine therapy the drug cannot act by (1) stimulating acquired immunity, (2) stimulating non-specifically the reticulo-endothelial system and thereby increasing innate immunity, (3) acting as an opsonin on the parasite.

Many earlier observers believed that quinine acted as a stimulus to acquired immunity. Yorke and Macfie (1924) suggested that quinine destroys directly or indirectly a large number of parasites which set free soluble antigens and these antigens in turn stimulate the formation of specific antibodies which then, if high enough in titre, destroy the remaining parasites. Krishnan (1933) similarly postulated that quinine, though it may act directly on the parasite, owes its chief importance to its capacity to increase antibody for-mation by the reticulo-endothelial cells. Lourie (1934a, b) studied the possible relation of quinine chemotherapy to acquired immunity by comparing the effects of the drug and of immunity on the asexual reproduction of bird malaria. The reproductive cycle of the parasite was found to be profoundly disturbed by quinine as evidenced by inhibition of the growth of the parasite, by a decrease in the synchronism of reproduction, and by a reduction in the number of merozoites. Acquired immunity did not have any such effect either at the time of crisis or after heavy super-infections. He therefore concluded that it need not be postulated that quinine stimulates the defence mechanism residing in the macrophages. Lourie's conclusions with respect to acquired immunity must be modified in view of the findings (Boyd and Allen, 1934 ; Boyd, 1939 ; Boyd and Gilkerson, 1942, and Taliaferro and Taliaferro, 1944) that the number of merozoites formed by each segmenting parasite (*a*) gradually decreases during infection with *P. cathemerium*, (*b*) reaches a minimal value at about the time of the crisis in initial infections, and (*c*) is slightly lower during superinfection than during the acute rise of initial infections. These changes are probably due to acquired immunity. Lourie's conclusion may therefore be restated as follows : the changes due to the most intense immune reactions are minor compared to those following treatment with a therapeutic dose of quinine. Nevertheless, acquired immunity is of considerable importance in effecting cures, as stressed by Yorke and Macfie (1924), especially when suppressive drugs are discontinued before the infection is completely eradicated. Many clinicians at one time believed that quinine is more effective when given after a patient has undergone several paroxysms rather than early in the infection : the benefit from waiting to apply the drug may be due to the development of acquired immunity.

It seems that in the development of acquired immunity there is an optimum amount of antigen which can be utilised at any one time. Sinton (1938), for instance, believes that small amounts of antigen given repeatedly over a considerable period are probably more effective than a single large dose of antigen. On the other hand, intense quinine therapy may greatly suppress the acquisition and hence the supplemental value of acquired immunity by reducing the amount of antigen absorbed in a given time. The degree to which quinine therapy affects immunity varies probably as a result of the interplay of a number of factors such as antigenicity, virulence, and number of parasites. Infections due to *P. cathemerium* seldom relapse, but when heavily suppressed by quinine they give rise to a high degree of immunity. In infections such as those due to *P. gallinaceum* in the chick, antigenic stimulation is minimal, as evidenced by frequent relapses and by the small amount of immunity developed in infections suppressed by quinine (Taliaferro, 1948, Taliaferro and Taliaferro, 1948). However, specific activation of the lymphoid-macrophage system by a previous infection with *P. lophuræ*, which gives a slight cross immunity with *P. gallinaceum*, results in a greater degree of malaria suppression with a standard dose of quinine. Thus the addition of acquired immunity increases the suppression during quinine treatment just as its reduction decreases it.

Non-specific activation of the lymphoid-macrophage system by multiple injection of sheep serum did not affect the degree of malarial suppression with a given dose of quinine, nor did it materially alter the quinine blood level (Taliaferro and Kelsey, 1948). It is thus most unlikely that the reticulo-endothelial system plays any direct part in absorbing and redistributing quinine so as to facilitate a better contact between parasite and drug.

15—2

References

ABRAMI, P., and SÉNEVET, G., 1917, Recherches de la pathogènie du paludisme à *Plasmodium falciparum*; rôle de l'immunité; la réaction schizontolytique; mécanisme de rechutes. *Bull. Mém. Soc. méd. Hôp. Paris*, **33**, 519.

BANG, F. B., HAIRSTON, N. G., TRAGER, W., and MAIER, J., 1947, Treatment of acute attacks of vivax and falciparum malaria. Comparison of atabrine and quinine. *Bull. U.S. Army med. Dept.*, **7**, 75.

BECKMAN, H., 1948, Infectivity of sporozoites of *Plasmodium cathemerium* 3 H exposed *in vitro* to hen and canary bloods. *Proc. Soc. exp. Biol.*, *N.Y.*, **67**, 172.

BLACKBURN, C. R. B., 1948, Observations on the development of resistance to vivax malaria. *Trans. R. Soc. trop. Med. Hyg.*, **42**, 117.

BOYD, G. H., 1939, Study of rate of reproduction in avian malaria parasite, *Plasmodium cathemerium*. *Amer. J. Hyg.*, **29C**, 119.

BOYD, G. H., and ALLEN, L. H., 1934, Adult size in relation to reproduction of avian malaria parasite, *Plasmodium cathemerium*. *Amer. J. Hyg.*, **20**, 73.

BOYD, G. H., and GILKERSON, S. W., 1942, Influence of conditions of latency upon merozoite production and gametocyte survival in *Plasmodium cathemerium* infections of canaries. *Amer. J. Hyg.*, **36**, 1.

BOYD, M. F., 1938, The threshold of parasite density in relation to clinical activity in primary infection with *Plasmodium vivax*. *Amer. J. trop. Med.*, **18**, 497.

BOYD, M. F., and KITCHEN, S. F., 1936, On the efficiency of the homologous properties of acquired immunity. *Amer. J. trop. Med.*, **16**, 447.

BOYD, M. F., and STRATMAN-THOMAS, W. K., 1933, Studies on benign tertian malaria. I. On the occurrence of acquired tolerance to *Plasmodium vivax*. *Amer. J. trop Med.*, **17**, 55.

BOYD, M. F., STRATMAN-THOMAS, W. K., and KITCHEN, S. F., 1936, On the duration of acquired homologous immunity to *Plasmodium vivax*. *Amer. J. trop Med.*, **21**, 245.

COGGESHALL, L. T., RICE, F. A., and YOUNT, E. H., Jr., 1948, The cure of recurrent vivax malaria and status of immunity thereafter. *Proc. 4th Int. Congr. trop Med. Mal. Washington*, p. 749.

DANIELOPOLU, D., 1946, " Phylaxie, paraphylaxie (immunité-anaphylaxie) et maladie specifique (maladie du sérum, maladies infectiéuses).'' Paris. Masson et Cie.

FINDLAY, G. M., 1949, Blackwater fever in West Africa, 1941–45. II. In African military personnel. *Ann. trop. Med. Parasit.*, **43**, 213.

FOURRIER, A., 1949, Pathogénie des accès palustres. Aspects théoriques et corollaires thérapeutiques. Thèse. Alger.

GARNHAM, P. C. C., 1949, Malarial immunity in Africans : effects in infancy and early childhood. *Ann. trop. Med. Parasit.*, **43**, 47.

GUPTA, J. C., and GANGULY, S. C., 1944, The effect of quinine and stilbamidine (M. & B. 744) on the reticulo-endothelial system as measured by the Congo-red index. *Indian med. Gaz.*, **79**, 104.

JAMES, S. P., 1933, Antimalarial chemotherapeutic tests at Devon Mental Hospital. *J. trop. Med. Hyg.*, **19**, 289.

KLINGER, W., 1949, Milzextirpation und Malaria. *Z. Tropanmed.*, **1**, 195.

KRISHNAN, K. V., 1933, Observations on the mode of action of quinine in malaria. *Indian J. med. Res.*, **21**, 343.

KRISHNAN, K. V., SMITH, R. O. A., and LAL, C., 1933, Contributions to protozoal immunity : immunity to malaria in monkeys and effect of splenectomy on it. *Indian J. med. Res.*, **21**, 639.

KRITSCHEWSKI, I. L., and DEMIDOWA, L. W., 1934, Ueber eine noch unbekannte Funktion des reticuloendothelialen Systems : ueber die Bedeutung des retikuloendothelialen Systems in der Therapie der Malaria. *Z. Immun-Forsch.*, **84**, 14.

LOURIE, E. M., 1934a, Studies on chemotherapy in bird malaria ; acquired immunity in relation to quinine treatment in *Plasmodium cathemerium* infections. *Ann. trop. Med. Parasit.*, **28**, 151.

LOURIE, E. M., 1934b, Studies on chemotherapy in bird malaria : observations bearing on mode of action of quinine. *Ann. trop. Med. Parasit.*, **28**, 255.

REDMOND, W. B., 1941, Immunity to human malaria ; characteristics of immunity : in " A Symposium on Human Malaria," edited by F. R. MOULTON, p. 231. Amer. Ass. Adv. Sci., Publ. No. 15, Washington.

REILLY, J., CHEN, G., and GEILING, E. M. K., 1949, An evaluation of anti-malarials with *Plasmodium lophuræ* in the chick. *J. inf. Dis.*, **85**, 205.

RODHAIN, J., 1949, Le comportement du cotton rat vis-à-vis du *Plasmodium berghei* (Vincke and Lips). *Ann. Soc. belge Méd. trop.*, **29**, 483.

SAPERO, J. J., 1946, The malaria problem to-day : influence of wartime experience and research. *J. Amer. med. Ass.*, **132**, 623.

SINTON, J. A., 1938, The effects of treatment upon the development and degree of immunity acquired in malarial infections. *Acta Convent. tertii de trop. atque. malar. Morbis.*, **2**, 312.

SINTON, J. A., 1945, quoted by Blackburn, C. R. B., 1948, Observations on the development of resistance to vivax malaria. *Trans. R. Soc. trop. Med. Hyg.*, **42**, 117.

SINTON, J. A., ORR, W. B. F., and AHMAD, B., 1928, Physico-chemical changes in the blood in malaria. *Indian J. med. Res.*, **16**, 341.

SWELLENGREBEL, N. H., 1949, Stages in the development of collective immunity in malaria. *Docum. neder indon. Morb. trop.*, **1**, 165.

TALIAFERRO, W. H., 1948, The rôle of the spleen and the lymphoid-macrophage system in the quinine treatment of gallinaceum malaria. I. Acquired immunity and phagocytosis. *J. infect. Dis.*, **83**, 164.

TALIAFERRO, W. H., and KELSEY, F. E., 1948, The rôle of the spleen and lymphoid-macrophage system in the quinine treatment of gallinaceum malaria. II. Quinine blood levels. *J. infect. Dis.*, **83**, 181.

TALIAFERRO, W. H., and TALIAFERRO, L. G., 1944, Effect of immunity on asexual reproduction of *Plasmodium brasilianum*. *J. infect. Dis.*, **75**, 1.

TALIAFERRO, W. H., and TALIAFERRO, L. G., 1948, Reduction in immunity in chicken malaria following treatment with nitrogen mustard. *J. infect. Dis.*, **82**, 5.

TALIAFERRO, W. H., and TALIAFERRO, L. G., 1949, The rôle of the spleen and lymphoid-macrophage system in the quinine treatment of gallinaceum malaria. III. The action of quinine and of immunity on the parasite. *J. infect. Dis.*, **84**, 187.

TALIAFERRO, W. H., TALIAFERRO, L. G., and KELSEY, F. E., 1948, Rôle of the spleen and phagocytosis in the quinine treatment of malaria. *Fed. Proc.*, **7**, 311.

THIODET, J., and FOURRIER, A., 1948, L'accès palustre, considéré comme un choc, peut-il être traité par des injections intradermiques de CO_2-globulines de paludéen (médication antichoc). *Bull. Mém. Soc. méd. Hôp. Paris*, **64**, 928.

THIODET, J., and FOURRIER, A., 1949, La pathogénie de l'accès palustre. Rapports avec le choc anaphylactique. Corollaires thérapeutiques. *Bull. Mem. Soc. méd. Hôp. Paris*, **65**, 798.

TRAGER, W., and McGHEE, R. B., 1949, Passive transfer of age resistance to an avian malaria parasite. *Fed. Proc.*, **8**, 373.

WALTON, G. A., 1949, On the control of malaria in Freetown, Sierra Leone. II. Control methods and the effects upon the transmission of *Plasmodium falciparum* resulting from the reduced abundance of *Anopheles gambiæ*. *Ann. trop. Med. Parasit.*, **43**, 117.

YORKE, W., and MACFIE, J. W. S., 1924, Observations on malaria made during treatment of general paralysis. *Trans. R. Soc. trop. Med. Hyg.*, **18**, 13.

CHAPTER X

THE TREATMENT OF MALARIA IN MAN

IT is now possible to evaluate the *rôle* of drugs in the chemo-therapeutic control of malaria in man. The drugs available are quinine and totaquina ; 8-aminoquinolines such as pamaquin, pentaquine, and *iso*pentaquine ; mepacrine ; chloroquine ; certain other 4-aminoquinolines such as nivaquine and camoquin ; proguanil, and combinations of these drugs.

Before discussing the drugs to be employed it is necessary to emphasise two points. Firstly, not only are there four different human malarial parasites with differing susceptibilities to chemo-therapeutic drugs, but each species of parasite has various strains which differ considerably in their reactions to drugs. Secondly, the populations which suffer from malaria are divisible into two unequal groups :—

(1) Indigenous inhabitants who are exposed repeatedly to the same strain or strains of parasite and constitute the overwhelming majority of those infected.

(2) Immigrants who arrive in a malarial zone without previous exposure to the local strains and are only temporarily exposed to infection, with the possibility of escaping reinfection.

Although most of the indigenous inhabitants of the tropics are included in Group (1) this group is not homogeneous, for though adults in a malarious region may have some degree of immunity, children in each generation are forced, sometimes at the peril of their lives, to acquire this immunity. In addition, the geographical distribution of any one strain of malaria parasite is frequently small, a matter of considerable significance now that roads have become more common and other means of communica-tion have become far more rapid. During the second World War Belgian troops stationed in Nigeria had a higher malarial rate than Nigerian troops, and Gold Coast troops stationed in Gambia a higher rate than Gambian troops. Many tribes who dwell in mountainous non-malarial areas dislike visiting the plains because of their fear of contracting malaria. Under natural conditions infections with more than one species of parasite may occur ; two or more strains of the same species of *P. vivax* may be present (Boyd and Kitchen, 1948) ; *P. falciparum* tends to suppress *P. vivax*.

The second group is composed largely, though not exclusively, of Europeans who arrive in the tropics as young adults and pass the greater part of their working lives in a malarial area or, in the case of military personnel, only a few months or years. Non-Europeans who live in an uninfected zone of a malarious continent also fall into Group (2), as do those originally immune, especially to falciparum infections, who return to an endemic zone after some years in a non-endemic area.

The object of drug treatment naturally differs in the two groups.

In Group (1) the aim must be to allow the development of immunity without permitting acute attacks to endanger the life of the individual or even to interfere with his normal enjoyment of existence. If the development of immunity is prevented during childhood the non-immune or partially immune individual becomes liable to severe attacks of malaria during adult life ; in fact, he becomes a member of the second group, and where *P. falciparum* is prevalent he then runs the risk of developing blackwater fever. If, on the other hand, acute attacks of malaria are insufficiently treated, in addition to the risks of cerebral malaria from which many die, the small child suffers from chronic ill-health which saps his vitality. If, for example, as is the case with *P. knowlesi*, methionine is essential also for the development of the human species of malarial parasite, recurrent attacks of malaria may increase the drain on methionine, an amino acid which is already deficient in the diet of many indigenous peoples ; thereby the risk of nutritional liver disease and cirrhosis is increased.

In the case of the European in Group (2), the object is (*a*) to prevent the development of acute attacks by the use of a suppressive drug which should, if possible, be a true causal prophylactic capable of inhibiting the growth of the primary exo-erythrocytic forms, (*b*) to control acute attacks as rapidly as possible, (*c*) to eradicate the persisting erythrocytic forms in the case of *P. falciparum* and the exo-erythrocytic forms in the case of *P. vivax*, thus preventing relapses.

Theoretically it should be a help in reducing the malaria rate to destroy the gametocytes in the blood. In practice, however, with the drugs available it is doubtful whether the use of specific gametocyticidal compounds is justified.

In the case of people in Group (2), as Sinton (1939) has pointed out, there should be radical cure of infections and clinical prophylaxis if true causal prophylaxis is impossible.

In assessing the value of antimalarial drugs it is therefore important to keep in mind the object for which the drug is being administered and the type of person to whom it is being administered. In addition, in comparing different drugs, comparisons can be valid only when the same strains of parasite are compared. Failure to take this into account and attempts to apply to all strains what holds good for only one has led, and may again lead, to failure and disappointment.

In comparing antimalarial drugs it is necessary to assess their action in :—

(1) Controlling acute attacks.
(2) Preventing relapses and eradicating infection.
(3) Suppressing infections and acting as true causal prophylactics.
(4) Destroying gametocytes.

INFECTIONS DUE TO *P.* FALCIPARUM

The control of acute attacks due to *P. falciparum* can be carried out by a number of drugs—quinine, mepacrine, chloroquine, camoquin, and proguanil. In view of the serious symptoms which may develop during the course of an attack of falciparum malaria it is of the utmost importance that the attack should be brought under control as rapidly as possible. There is now ample evidence to show that, provided a " loading dose " of mepacrine is first administered, as first recommended in East Africa by Bryant (1942), parasitæmia and fever are controlled as quickly or even more quickly by mepacrine than by quinine. This has been amply demonstrated by comparison of the effects of quinine and mepacrine on West African strains (Findlay *et al.*, 1944a and b), and on New Guinea strains (Bang *et al.*, 1947 ; Maier *et al.*, 1948) in non-immune populations. Mepacrine has the advantage over quinine in that if continued it brings about permanent cure, " curative suppression " (Kitchen and Putman, 1942 ; Fairley, 1945). This is at least one of the reasons why mepacrine used as a routine suppressive does not precipitate blackwater fever, while the substitution of mepacrine for quinine both in suppression and in clinical cure abolished blackwater fever in West Africa among European military personnel (Findlay and Stevenson, 1945 ; Findlay, 1949a and b).

Mepacrine in its turn has the disadvantage that it is not without toxicity ; psychotic reactions, though rare, are alarming, and in addition it stains the skin and may in some instances be associated with severe skin reactions.

Accurate comparisons between proguanil and mepacrine have been made with only a small number of strains of *P. falciparum*. In tropical Africa, Arabia, and occasionally in India, however, there is general agreement that proguanil in doses of 300 mgm. daily is slightly slower in overcoming the fever and parasitæmia than mepacrine (Blackie, 1947 ; Abbott, 1949 ; Kay, 1949 ; Davey and Smith, 1949 ; Covell *et al.*, 1949b). In European non-immunes in East Africa, Handfield-Jones (1949) found no statistical difference between proguanil and mepacrine. In South-east Asia and New Guinea proguanil seems as rapid as mepacrine, but with some Arabian strains 900 mgm. daily fails to control fever and relapses occur within five days of a course of 3 gm. Proguanil also causes what has been termed " after fever," where the temperature again rises forty-eight hours after the last rigor. Earle *et al.* (1948) compared the total dosage and the plasma levels of mepacrine, proguanil, and chloroquine necessary to reduce fever and to keep the blood free from parasites for fourteen days (Class III effect). With the Costa strain of *P. falciparum* the doses were as follows :—

	Mepacrine.	Proguanil.	Chloroquine.
Total dose in mgm. .	>1,100	>750	650
Plasma level, μgm./l	65*	>100*	30*

* Six day mean plasma drug level.

In North Africa, Schneider and Méchali (1948) compared the effects of proguanil, chloroquine, sontoquine, and metachloridine in controlling acute attacks of *P. falciparum* infection. The results show that there is nothing to choose between proguanil, sontoquine, and chloroquine ; metachloridine, however, was slightly slower.

THE EFFECT OF DRUGS ON *P. falciparum* (NORTH AFRICAN STRAINS) (Schneider and Méchali, 1948)

Drug.	Dosage.	Number of cases.	Average duration of fever.	Average duration of parasitæmia.
Proguanil .	300 mgm. a day for 5 days	28	1·77	2·4
Sontoquine .	600 mgm. on the 1st day 500 mgm. ,, ,, 2nd day 300 mgm. ,, ,, 3rd, 4th and 5th days.	22	1·57	2·5
Chloroquine .	600 mgm. on the 1st day 500 mgm. ,, ,, 2nd day 300 mgm. ,, ,, 3rd, 4th and 5th days.	19	1·7	2·7
Metachloridine	2 or 6 gm. a day for 5 days	16	2·8	3·6

In Tunis, with partial immunes, a single dose of 0·6 gm. chloroquine caused disappearance of fever in 1·4 days and disappearance of parasitæmia in 1·6 days (Durand *et al.*, 1949).

In Indo-China, Canet (1948a, b) found proguanil slower in reducing fever and removing parasitæmia than chloroquine. The latter drug rendered 93·3 per cent. of 120 cases afebrile in forty-eight hours, the former only 66·6 per cent. : similarly 75·8 per cent. of cases treated with chloroquine had no parasitæmia in four days whereas only 60 per cent. of cases treated with proguanil were free from parasites. In East Africa, with European non-immunes, chloroquine is more rapid than proguanil (Handfield-Jones, 1949).

Thus in the acute stage of falciparum infections quinine, though rapid in its action, is ruled out because of the danger of inducing blackwater fever. The choice then lies between chloroquine, proguanil, mepacrine, and possibly sontoquine or camoquin; further information is required for these last two compounds. Mepacrine is probably the most toxic of these five drugs and also it stains the skin yellow. However, it does not predispose to blackwater fever. Proguanil is undoubtedly too slow with many African and some Indian strains of *P. falciparum* in non-immunes and requires reinforcement by mepacrine, as suggested by Covell *et al.* (1949b) : 300 mgm. proguanil should be given twice daily for ten days with 900 mgm. mepacrine on the first day. Chloroquine may be used in place of mepacrine. In partially immune subjects 300 mgm. proguanil is usually sufficient to produce clinical cure. Whether or not the administration of proguanil, chloroquine, camoquin or nivaquine is likely to precipitate blackwater fever is at present unknown, but it seems unlikely. Further investigations in regions where blackwater fever is common are required, but one case has already been described in which proguanil failed to prevent the onset of blackwater fever (Best, 1949).

The indiscriminate use of quinine in areas where *P. falciparum* is the prevailing parasite and all degrees of immunity are to be found in the population is to be condemned, more especially where, as in certain British Colonies in Africa, quinine has been obtainable at post offices, thus being available without medical supervision in uncontrolled doses to those who may be immune, non-immune or only partially immune to malaria.

Cerebral Malaria

In cerebral malaria due to *P. falciparum* intravenous quinine was formerly the only effective drug. If the systolic blood pressure is below 100 mm. Hg. intravenous saline or plasma should be given (Ransome, 1948). Machella *et al.* (1947b) have shown that, if given in very dilute solution, amounts up to 1 gm. of mepacrine hydrochloride can safely be given intravenously. The results of intravenous mepacrine as compared with quinine bisulphate and sontoquine are shown in the table on p. 460. The intravenous injection of mepacrine does not interfere with liver function, as shown by the bromsulphalein test (Machella *et al.*, 1947a), and it has already cured at least eight cases of cerebral malaria caused by *P. falciparum*. No patients treated with intravenous mepacrine died, but two developed temporary psychoses. Nevertheless the majority of workers prefer to give mepacrine intramuscularly in preference to the intravenous route in malarial emergencies if quinine is not available, or where for any reason the patient is unable to take the drug by mouth. The effects of proguanil, sontoquine, chloroquine, and camoquin in cerebral malaria require further study, but sufficient evidence is already available to show that proguanil is not a satisfactory drug for the treatment of cerebral malaria. As Black (1949) has pointed out, proguanil exerts its action on trophozoites only in the earliest stages of chromatin division. In cerebral malaria the parasites anchored within the cerebral capillaries are in the later stages of development, and much time will therefore be wasted in the treatment of a heavy falciparum infection if proguanil is the only drug to be used. Quinine and mepacrine both arrest parasites in the schizogonous stage, but proguanil does not prevent the parasites from developing to this stage when they may lodge in the brain capillaries. One instance is already known where a patient with a heavy falciparum infection

INTRAVENOUS MEPACRINE COMPARED WITH QUININE AND NIVAQUINE IN TREATMENT OF *P. falciparum* INFECTIONS
(Machella *et al.*, 1947b)

Drug dose route.	Number of cases.	Duration of fever in hours.		Day on which parasitæmia disappeared.		Number of failures.	Toxic reaction.
		Mean.	Range.	Mean.	Range.		
Quinine bisulphate, 1·2 gm., i.v.	10	45·6	8–88	3·2	2–4	5	0
Mepacrine, 400 mgm., i.v. .	10	21·8	8–44	2·3	1–3	1	0
600 mgm., i.v. .	20	29·1	8–64	2·3	2–3	0	0
800 mgm., i.v. .	20	24·2	8–48	2·0	1–3	0	0
1·0 gm., i.v. .	25	31·6	8–96	2·2	1–3	0	2
Mepacrine, 2·8 gm. in 4 days, per os	20	45·6	12–76	3·0	1–5	0	0
Sontoquine, 600 mgm. (base), i.v.	20	41·0	12–80	2·5	1–4	0	0

went into coma some time after the administration of proguanil, 400 mgm. over a period of two days. Deaths have also occurred in some heavy falciparum infections despite the intravenous injection of proguanil. Nicotin is said to be of value as a vasodilator.

Little information is available as to the effect of various drugs on the relapse rate of *P. falciparum* infections. Ferro-Luzzi (1948) found that of 112 cases from Eritrea treated with 300 mgm. proguanil daily for ten days no less than 43 per cent. had relapsed within thirty days. Bettini (1948) treated ninety-four cases in Sardinia with 100 mgm. three times daily for ten days followed by 100 mgm. weekly for twelve weeks : seventeen patients relapsed in this period. Covell *et al.* (1949b) noted relapses within three weeks of treatment in nine of ten neurosyphilitics infected with a Nigerian strain. Maegraith and Andrews (1949) reported that of thirty cases from various areas in West Africa treated with proguanil in England none had relapsed after an observation period of six months to four years. With quinine, short-term relapses occur, but after adequate and continued suppressive administration of mepacrine, chloroquine or sulphapyrazine the infection is totally eradicated.

Suppression and Causal Prophylaxis. Quinine, when taken regularly in doses of 5 or 10 gr. daily, will suppress falciparum malaria in a certain percentage of persons, but field experiments with large non-immune populations (Findlay and Stevenson, 1945 ; Bang *et al.*, 1946b ; Wynne-Griffith, 1947) showed that mepacrine taken daily is superior to quinine. Apart from its inefficiency and its relationship to blackwater fever quinine does not eradicate the infection rapidly or as certainly as does mepacrine. Mepacrine, though effective, is toxic, it stains the skin and it must be taken daily. It is possibly less effective in West Africa than in the Far East. Chloroquine has the advantage, in that it need be taken only once a week instead of every day, though experience with a large number of strains of *P. falciparum* is lacking. Packer (1947), using the Costa strain, found that 0·25 gm. weekly was insufficient unless a priming dose equal to twice the weekly dose were given. The toxicity of chloroquine is lower than that of mepacrine and though like mepacrine it is not a true causal prophylactic, it nevertheless eradicates the infection if continued for some weeks.

High hopes were at first aroused that in proguanil the ideal causal prophylactic had been found. It now seems probable that proguanil is a true causal prophylactic for many strains of *P. falciparum*, including those of African origin. With some strains it appears to eradicate infection and thus cause radical cure if continued over a considerable period, but information is lacking as to whether this is true for all African as opposed to New Guinea strains. On the other hand, at least 100 mgm. must be taken daily for suppression with tropical African strains. A number of cases have now been seen where clinical symptoms have occurred despite this daily dose (Davey and Smith, 1949 ; Jellife, 1949). The latter recommends at least 200 mgm. daily during and in convalescence from intercurrent infections. In some areas in Malaya the development of proguanil-resistant strains is interfering with widespread proguanil suppression (Field and Edeson, 1949). Haphazard proguanil suppression is a potential menace both with falciparum and vivax infections, and even under military discipline with intelligent troops it is not easy to ensure that a suppressive is regularly taken by all. With illiterate indigenous populations regular administration to all is practically impossible. It is doubtful therefore whether proguanil is suitable for civilian suppression. Edeson and Field (1950) suggest alternating proguanil with mepacrine or chloroquine : apart from administrative difficulties there is no guarantee that resistant strains would not thus be formed. For children the following doses have been advised : from birth to five years, 25 mgm. daily ; from six to twelve years, 50 mgm. daily (Col. Med. Res. Com., 1949). In Africa, although some groups of Europeans after two or more years of experience of proguanil as a suppressive have abandoned its use, comparative tests suggest that it is of considerable value.

The use of sulphapyrazine as a suppressive requires further study.

Whatever drug is used for suppression it is essential that a sufficient concentration to control infection should be present in the blood stream at the time the individual enters the malarial zone. In the case of mepacrine, where 0·1 gm. is taken daily, this will necessitate fourteen days' suppressive treatment before exposure to infection. However, as Parrot and Catanei (1949) point out, the supply of suppressive drugs to breast-fed children, and among indigenous peoples breast-feeding continues for two years or more, is a problem which has not yet been solved.

Gametocyticidal Action. None of the drugs commonly employed in the treatment or suppression of falciparum infections has any direct action on gametocytes. By their interference with the development of schizonts and by their eventual eradication of blood forms they have, however, an indirect action on gametocytes which do not appear in the peripheral blood stream. Although proguanil does not appear to have any direct action on gametocytes and fails to prevent fertilisation of the female gametes, it nevertheless inhibits the normal development of the oöcyst, so that the mosquito is unable to transmit infection by bite. This is a most important finding since it opens up a possibility of freeing considerable areas from falciparum infection by mass treatment over a short period, provided that strains do not become drug-resistant.

In view of this indirect gametocyticidal action on the part of drugs commonly used in dealing with *P. falciparum* and of the direct action of proguanil, it is doubtful whether the use of 8-aminoquinolines such as pamaquin or pentaquine is necessary.

INFECTIONS DUE TO *P. VIVAX*

It had been shown before the second World War that at any rate in Malaya mepacrine was more effective than quinine in controlling acute attacks due to *P. vivax* (Field, 1938). The community with which Field was dealing was, however, partially immune; nevertheless similar results have been obtained with non-immune troops treated by quinine and mepacrine (Hayman *et al.*, 1946b ; Gordon *et al.*, 1946, 1947 ; Bang *et al.*, 1947) and with non-immune volunteers experimentally infected with particular strains of vivax plasmodia (Pullman *et al.*, 1948b). Bang *et al.* (1946a) showed that the difference in the rate of disappearance of parasites from the blood in patients treated with mepacrine or quinine was statistically significant when mepacrine was given in a dose of 1·2 gm. on the first day, 0·8 gm. on the second day, and 0·4 gm. for the next four days, a total of 3·6 gm. in six days, and quinine was given as the dihydrochloride in solution in doses of 3 gm. per day for the first three days and 2 gm. per day for the next three. Whereas primary attacks, whether treated with quinine or mepacrine, tend to have a slower parasite clearance rate than secondary or later attacks, due to the development of immunity, primary attacks treated with quinine had a slower rate of parasite clearance than primary attacks treated with mepacrine.

In comparing the effects of mepacrine and quinine on the Chesson strain of vivax malaria, Pullman *et al.* (1948b) found that a total of 3·4 gm. of mepacrine hydrochloride in seven days abolished parasitæmia more quickly than 11 to 12 gm. of quinine (base) in seven days or 21 to 23 gm. of quinine base in fourteen days. The results were as follows :—

Drug.	Number of cases.	Number of days to end of parasitæmia.
Mepacrine . . .	9	2·77
Quinine (seven days) .	7	4·85
,, (fourteen days) .	15	3·46

Hayman *et al.* (1946b) obtained the following comparative figures for the disappearance of parasites from the peripheral blood stream following either mepacrine 2·8 gm. in seven days or quinine 20 gm. in fourteen days :—

Drug.	Number of cases.	Percentage of cases parasite-free in		
		24 hours.	48 hours.	72 hours.
Mepacrine .	391	26	77	96
Quinine . .	184	9	45	77

Figures obtained for the duration of fever in recurrent attacks showed little difference, for only 8 per cent. of those given mepacrine and 8·7 per cent. of those given quinine had fever for more than twenty-four hours.

Gordon *et al.* (1946, 1947) compared the action of quinine

sulphate and mepacrine in abolishing parasitæmia in vivax infections contracted in the Pacific and Mediterranean. Quinine sulphate was inferior not only to mepacrine but to chloroquine, sontoquine, and SN 8,137.

PERCENTAGE OF PATIENTS WITH BLOOD FILMS NEGATIVE FOR
P. vivax AFTER TREATMENT (Gordon *et al.*, 1947)

Drug.	Hours after treatment.			
	24	48	72	120
Quinine sulphate	9	59	80	100
Mepacrine .	53	95	99	100
Chloroquine .	66	98	99	100
Nivaquine. .	37	92	96	100
SN 8,137 . .	48	95	100	—

Mepacrine, however, was of equal value with the three other drugs.

Comparisons of chloroquine with mepacrine tend to show that the former is slightly the more active in reducing parasitæmia (Loeb *et al.*, 1946a). Hayman *et al.* (1946a) found that there was little difference in the therapeutic response when chloroquine was given in a dose of 1 gm. in one day, 1·5 gm. in four days or 2·0 gm. in seven days, but taking all their results together, 38 per cent. of their 244 patients were free from parasites after twenty-four hours, 86 per cent. after forty-eight hours and ninety-six after seventy-two hours. Of the same group of patients only five, or 2·1 per cent., had fever for more than twenty-four hours. Pullman *et al.* (1948b), whose general results on chloroquine agree with those of Most *et al.* (1946b), found little difference in the rate of parasite clearance with chloroquine and mepacrine ; among eight patients given chloroquine the average interval till the disappearance of parasites was 2·25 days and among nine patients given mepacrine 2·77 days. Earle *et al.* (1948) found that with the McCoy strain of vivax malaria a Class III effect could be produced with a total dose of 300 mgm. chloroquine and a plasma level of 10 *μ*gm. per litre, whereas the corresponding figures for mepacrine were 700 mgm. and 25 μgm. per litre. In Malaya, Wallace (1949, 1950) finds chloroquine or proguanil more effective than mepacrine in mass prophylaxis.

Comparison of the clinical effects of chloroquine with those produced by proguanil, sontoquine, and metachloridine have been made in North Africa by Schneider and Méchali (1948). The results are shown in the table :—

THE EFFECT OF DRUGS ON *Plasmodium vivax* (NORTH AFRICAN STRAINS) (Schneider and Méchali, 1948)

Drug.	Dosage.	Number of cases.	Duration of fever.	Duration of parasitæmia.
Chloroquine .	600 mgm. on the 1st day 500 mgm. ,, ,, 2nd day 300 mgm. ,, ,, 3rd, 4th and 5th days.	9	1·62	2·20
Proguanil .	300 mgm. for 5 days.	20	2·77	3·88
Sontoquine .	600 mgm. on the 1st day 500 mgm. ,, ,, 2nd day 300 mgm. ,, ,, 3rd, 4th and 5th days.	11	1·70	2·90
Metachloridine	2 or 6 gm. for 5 days.	10	3·4	4·4

Chloroquine was thus found to be the most rapid of the four drugs tested. Similar results were obtained by Durand *et al.* (1949). A single dose of 0·6 gm. of chloroquine caused among partial immunes a disappearance of fever and parasitæmia in an average of 1·5 days. In addition its toxicity is low.

A number of comparisons have been made of proguanil and other antimalarial drugs in the control of acute vivax attacks. Adams *et al.* (1945) found little significant difference between proguanil and mepacrine. Andrews *et al.* (1947) found that proguanil in doses of either 1·0 gm. or 500 mgm. a day for fourteen days was slightly slower when compared with mepacrine 600 mgm. for two days followed by 300 mgm. for ten days. The duration of parasitæmia was 3·2 days for proguanil (sixty-six cases) and 2·0 days for mepacrine (twenty-seven cases).

In India, Afridi (1947) has compared the effects of proguanil and mepacrine ; although he does not separate the various forms

of malaria a majority were apparently due to *P. vivax*. The results
on parasitæmia and temperature were as follows :—

THE EFFECT OF PROGUANIL AND MEPACRINE ON INDIAN STRAINS
OF MALARIA (Afridi, 1947)

Drug.	Number of cases.	Temperature.		Parasitæmia.	
		Number normal in three days.	Percentage normal in three days.	Number normal in three days.	Percentage normal in three days.
Proguanil, 100 mgm. . .	67	53	79	47	70
,, 400 mgm. daily up to 4 days .	66	57	86	53	80
Mepacrine, 300 mgm. daily up to 3 days.	34	25	74	26	76
,, 400 mgm. daily up to 4 days .	50	45	90	—	—

Among the foothills of the Himalayas, Srivastava (1947)
obtained the following comparative results on the fall of
temperature :—

Drug.	Number of cases.	Number of days for temperature to return to normal.				
		1	2	3	4	5
Proguanil, 300 mgm. . .	59	24	13	16	5	1
Mepacrine, 300 mgm. for 3 days	47	5	20	20	1	1

Among Europeans suffering from vivax infections contracted
in India, Burma, and the Far East, Johnstone (1946) found that
pamaquin 0·03 gm. and quinine 2 gm. given concurrently for ten
days reduced the temperature in an average of 0·98 days ; proguanil in a dose of either 500 or 50 mgm. daily brought the temperature down to normal in an average of 1·47 and 1·49 days
respectively. Woodruff (1947) similarly found that a single dose
of 100 mgm. proguanil was considerably slower in its action on
the temperature than quinine 30 gr. for three days followed by
mepacrine. The results in fifteen cases treated with both regimes
were :—

	Proguanil, 100 mgm.	Quinine and mepacrine.
Temperature normal in 12 hours	7	12
,, ,, ,, 24 ,,	3	1
,, ,, ,, 36 ,,	1	1
,, ,, ,, 48 ,,	1	1
,, ,, ,, 48 + ,,	3	0

The advantages of proguanil in treating a partially immune population such as is met with in India are that treatment of the acute attack can be confined to a single day, the toxicity of proguanil is less and the skin is not stained. On the other hand, after a single course the relapse rate is higher for proguanil than for mepacrine and it is in the relapse rate that the crux of the problem of the control of vivax infections is to be found.

Monk (1948a, c) has compared the duration of pyrexia in cases treated with proguanil with that following other courses, the patients being infected by *P. vivax* from India, Malaya, and the Far East.   The results are shown in the table :—

DURATION OF PYREXIA FOLLOWING VARIOUS TREATMENTS OF *P. vivax* INFECTIONS (Monk, 1948a, c)

	Course.		
	Pentaquine, 20 mgm., eight-hourly for ten days.	Pentaquine, 20 mgm., and quinine eight-hourly for ten days.	Quinine, 10 gr., pamaquin, 10 mgm., eight-hourly for ten days.
Number of cases . . .	25	26	168
Average duration of fever in days	1·2	0·73	1·44

	Course.		
	Proguanil, 250 mgm., pamaquin, 10 mgm., eight-hourly for ten days.	Pamaquin, 10 mgm., eight-hourly for ten days.	Proguanil, 250 mgm., twelve-hourly for ten days.
Number of cases . . .	179	22	24
Average duration of fever in days	2·1	2·8	2·1

Manfredi (1948), in Elba, found little difference in the activity of proguanil and mepacrine ; both compounds were given in doses of 300 mgm. daily for only four days.

Canet (1948a, b), in Indo-China, compared the effects of proguanil, 300 mgm. daily for ten days, with chloroquine in the same dosage : with chloroquine the disappearance of fever was rather more rapid than with proguanil for by the third day 95 per cent. of patients treated with chloroquine were afebrile whereas only 70 per cent. of those given proguanil were afebrile. The rate of disappearance of parasites showed no significant difference.

Relapses due to *P. vivax*

Infections due to *P. falciparum* can be eliminated either by prolonged chemotherapy or by removal from an endemic area for from eighteen months to two years. *P. vivax*, on the other hand, is a more difficult parasite to eradicate from the tissues owing to the persistence of its exo-erythrocytic forms. Cases are on record where it has remained latent in those who have gained some degree of immunity for periods of from fourteen to forty years. Mosquito-induced vivax malaria due to the Chesson strain tends, however, to burn itself out in eighteen months or less. Other South-West Pacific strains may continue to relapse for two or more years (Noe *et al.*, 1946) ; relapses after five years are rare.

After the cessation of mepacrine suppression, London *et al.* (1946) find that a primary attack usually occurs in a matter of a few weeks or months, but with some strains it may be delayed for a year or more. The Chesson strain, which comes from the South-West Pacific, tends to produce rapid and frequent relapses in a high percentage of cases in an average of thirty-two days ; other strains relapse after a longer interval (Young *et al.*, 1949). Mediterranean strains in patients treated with quinine and mepacrine tend to show a 30 per cent. relapse rate in 120 days. James *et al.* (1932) found 80·6 per cent. of relapses with their strains, Boyd (1941) only 8·3 per cent. Thus in assessing the value of drug-treatment in vivax infections it is essential to take into account a number of factors, some of which have been postulated by Sapero (1947) :—

(1) The strain of *P. vivax*.

(2) The frequency of reinfection.

(3) Density of the exo-erythrocytic infection.

(4) The immune response existing before drug therapy.

(5) The modification of the immune response produced by drug therapy.

(6) The toxicity of the drug.

It is also obviously of considerable importance to have the patient under observation for a period of at least one year, and preferably longer, after drug therapy has been completed.

While the symptoms and the parasitæmia consequent upon an acute attack can be rapidly controlled by a number of different drugs there is as yet no single drug which can be relied on to eradicate all vivax parasites from the tissues although greater efficiency is slowly being attained by combinations of drugs.

A considerable number of drugs and combinations of drugs have been investigated for their capacity to control the number of relapses due to *P. vivax*.

In determining the effects of drugs on relapses it is important to realise that strains of *P. vivax* fall into two groups. One group is characterised by an easily suppressed primary attack, followed by long latency and a series of late attacks after a period of six to eleven months from the date of exposure. These late attacks are not so easily controlled by drugs as the primary attack. The second group, on the other hand, tends to relapses in a few weeks. The St. Elizabeth strain is typical of Group I, the Chesson strain of Group II.

Relapse Rates

Quinine. The relapse rate with quinine alone in an adequate regime is well over 50 per cent. This figure was often exceeded during the 1914–18 war, despite the fact that fantastically large doses of quinine were given. In Macedonia and East Africa doses of 6 to 8 gm. (100 to 120 gr.) daily were not uncommonly prescribed. It is strange that quinine amblyopia was rare (Phear, 1920). A drug regime to be adequate should consist of not more nor less than 1·8 gm. (30 gr.) daily for not less than ten days. In a series treated by Most *et al.* (1946a) the relapse rate after a fourteen-day course was nearly 90 per cent. This is probably high, but when courses of quinine are self-administered, as so often happens, the relapse rate is almost certainly above 90 per cent. Quinine alone fails to produce a radical cure, and its use alone for the treatment of vivax malaria should be abandoned. On the other hand, there is no definite evidence that quinine precipitates blackwater fever in persons suffering from vivax infections.

THE RELATIVE EFFECT OF THE CINCHONA ALKALOIDS IN PREVENTING RELAPSE IN CHRONIC BENIGN TERTIAN MALARIA
(Sinton and Bird, 1929)

Alkaloid.	Number of patients.	Number lost sight of.	Number not re-lapsing.	Number relapsed.	Percentages of relapses.				
					Ob-served.	Possible maxi-mum.	Observed mini-mum.	Aver-age.	Devia-tion from average.
Quinine	667	66	184	417	69·4	72·4	62·6	68·0	− 3·2
Quinidine	208	14	30	164	84·5	85·6	78·8	83·0	+ 11·8
Cinchonine	72	3	22	47	68·1	69·4	65·3	67·6	− 3·6
Cinchonidine	107	24	23	60	72·3	78·5	56·0	68·7	− 2·5
Totaquina	110	25	19	66	77·6	82·7	60·0	73·1	+ 1·9
Totals	1,164	132	278	754	73·0	76·1	64·7	71·2	

The comparative effects of the cinchona alkaloids in preventing relapses due to vivax malaria were investigated by Sinton and Bird (1929). From the table it will be seen that the most active alkaloid in preventing relapse is cinchonine, the least powerful quinidine. These results were the opposite of those obtained by Acton *et al.* (1920), who found that cinchonine gave a relapse rate of 57 per cent. and quinidine a relapse rate of 37 per cent. Kligler *et al.* (1924) obtained a relapse rate of 26·6 per cent. with quinidine as compared with 28·5 per cent. with quinine.

Mepacrine. The relapse rate following mepacrine alone is rarely lower than 25 per cent. Most *et al.* (1946a) found it as high as 84 per cent., but this is probably exceptional. On the average two of every five cases treated relapse at some subsequent date. The actual amount of drug administered is relatively unimportant and not infrequently a higher total dosage of mepacrine is followed by a higher relapse rate than a smaller total dosage. An increase in the total duration of treatment also has little or no significant effect in improving the success rate. From the military point of view the value of mepacrine lies in the fact that the acute attack

Time Relationship of Relapses of *P. vivax* Malaria from the South-West Pacific Area following Treatment by Mepacrine or Chloroquine (Hill and Amatuzio, 1949)

Period of observation (days).	Mepacrine. 2·8 gm.			Chloroquine, 4·4 gm.		
	Number of cases treated: 169.	Number relapsed : 110.	Percentage relapses : 65.	Number of cases treated : 62.	Number relapsed : 35.	Percentage relapsed : 56.
	Occurrence of relapses.		Cumulative per cent.	Occurrence of relapses.		Cumulative per cent.
	Number of relapses.	Per cent.		Number of relapses.	Per cent.	
0–89	64	30	30	40	67	67
90–179	75	36	66	15	27	94
189–269	45	21	87	2	3	97
270–359	18	8	95	2	3	100
360–449	5	2	97	—	—	—
450–539	4	2	99	—	—	—
549–629	2	1	100	—	—	—
Total	213	100	100	59	100	100

can be completely controlled by a course of seven days' duration and that mepacrine suppression is not interrupted : also, owing to its slow excretion, relapses rarely occur within two to three months of treatment. With other forms of therapy, such as quinine and pamaquin, given concurrently, although the cure rate is higher, those patients who do relapse are apt to return in two to three weeks instead of two to three months. With South-West Pacific strains Hill and Amatuzio (1949) had a 60 per cent. relapse rate with mepacrine as compared with a 56 per cent. relapse rate for chloroquine, a difference which is not statistically significant. With mepacrine the average duration of fever was 22·4 hours as compared with 16·9 hours for chloroquine. Comparative results are shown in the table.

Proguanil. The relapse rate following treatment with proguanil alone is rarely less than 35 per cent. Andrews *et al.* (1947) showed that with 500 mgm. twice daily given to thirty-five patients ten had proved parasitological relapses and three had clinical relapses.

In a small series of patients from India and the Far East (Monk *et al.*, 1946) the relapse rate was 66·6 per cent. and relapses tended to occur after five to six weeks or longer. Johnstone (1946) had a relapse rate of 43·9 per cent. Ferro-Luzzi (1948), in Eritrea, gave 300 mgm. of proguanil for ten days to thirteen patients : three relapsed within thirty days. Thus the therapeutic value of proguanil alone is probably about the same as that of mepacrine.

Proguanil is remarkable for the fact that in a total amount as small as 50 mgm. it is capable of producing clinical cure of an overt attack of vivax malaria due to some strains, especially from the South Pacific. Maegraith *et al.* (1947) found that one patient continued to show parasites in the blood stream while taking 100 mgm. a week. It is therefore possible, but not yet proved, that this dose given once weekly for a period of six months or more may eradicate the infection due to certain strains.

A suppressive dose of 100 mgm. once or twice weekly was at first thought to be sufficient to suppress all manifestations of malaria (Fairley, 1946). In Dutch New Guinea, de Rook (1949) gave 100 mgm. twice weekly to 100 prisoners while the same number were kept as controls. Among the treated prisoners there were seven with relapsing vivax infection, among the controls fifteen. In Indo-China, Blanc (1949) found that 100 mgm. twice weekly controlled malaria in a mixed force of Europeans and indigenous inhabitants. It is now recognised that at least 300 mgm. a week, and with some strains possibly more, is required. It does not prevent the establishment of vivax infection although it inhibits to some extent the exo-erythrocytic forms (Fairley, 1946) which develop between the disappearance of sporozoites from the blood and the appearance of schizonts eight to ten days later. Smith *et al.* (1948), working in the Philippines, gave 200 mgm. once weekly to 104 persons, thirty had signs or symptoms of malaria within 280 days : of 106 controls given sodium bicarbonate fifty-four had malaria in the same time. If an attempt be made to eradicate vivax infection with proguanil alone the following course has been suggested : 100 mgm. three times a day for ten days followed by a single dose of 300 mgm. once weekly for a year. The value of such a course has yet to be proved.

Chloroquine. Although rapid clinical cure occurs with only small doses exhibited over short periods, relapses of vivax infection are common : they occur some weeks after discontinuing treatment since, like mepacrine, chloroquine is only slowly excreted. The interval till a relapse after treatment of a clinical attack is longer with chloroquine than with mepacrine or quinine (Pullman *et al.*, 1948b).

Given in doses of 300 mgm. once or twice weekly, it suppresses all forms of malaria, more especially among partially immune populations (Wallace, 1949). It does not, however, prevent the establishment of a vivax infection, having no action on the exo-erythrocytic forms, so that on discontinuing suppressive treatment an overt attack of vivax malaria will develop several weeks later. Smith *et al.* (1948) gave 0·5 gm. chloroquine diphosphate to 125 Philippinos : fifteen (12 per cent.) had signs and symptoms of malaria in the next thirty-nine to forty weeks, whereas 50 per cent. of controls had attacks in the same period. The comparative effects of chloroquine and mepacrine on strains of *P. vivax* from the Pacific area are shown in the table.

RELAPSE RATES IN *P. vivax* INFECTIONS FROM THE PACIFIC AREA AND PHILIPPINES AFTER TREATMENT WITH MEPACRINE OR CHLOROQUINE

Mepacrine.		Chloroquine.		Period of observation in months.	Author.
Number of attacks before treatment.	Relapse percentage.	Number of attacks before treatment.	Relapse percentage.		
—	74	—	—	7	Gordon *et al.* (1946)
—	82	—	75	3	Most *et al.* (1946a)
4·8	84	—	—	3	Most *et al.* (1946b)
—	67	—	75	3	Gordon *et al.* (1947)
—	84	—	84	1–12	Warthin *et al.* (1948)
2·8	65	4·4	56	24	Hill and Amatuzio (1949)
4·2	60	—	—	24	Hill and Amatuzio (1949)
—	—	—	12	10	Smith *et al.* (1948)

The relative effectiveness of chloroquine and proguanil in Indo-China with different dosages is shown in the table on p. 479. Chloroquine appears the more rapid on parasitæmia and fever.

In the Philippines, Smith *et al.* (1948) found 500 mgm. of chloroquine once a week superior to 200 mgm. of proguanil once a week. In 125 persons given chloroquine two had malarial attacks and thirteen had parasitæmia : among 104 given proguanil seventeen had malaria attacks and thirteen had parasitæmia. Among 106 given a placebo fifty-four had overt attacks.

Sontoquine, (SN 6,911), 3-methyl-4-[4'-diethylamino-1'-methyl-butylamino]-7-chloroquinoline, was used by Gordon *et al.* (1947). In vivax infections it is quicker than quinine in removing parasites from the blood stream but no more rapid in curing fever. The percentage of relapses is high, as it is also with SN 8,137. In Egypt, Halawani *et al.* (1947) claim to have treated ninety-three patients and only nine relapsed over an observation period of two to five months. In Indo China, Canet (1949a) obtained better results with prophylaxis by 500 mgm. of sontoquine weekly than with 100 or 200 mgm. of proguanil weekly. In Holland, Hulshoff (1949) treated thirty-two patients with 300 mgm. daily for five or seven days : seventeen relapsed.

Camoquin. Of thirty patients in the Philippines given only 10 mgm per kgm. one alone relapsed (Ejercito and Duque, 1948).

Pamaquin. Although pamaquin alone has the reputation of being of little value as a schizonticide it is, nevertheless, capable of producing a radical cure in an easily tolerated dosage. Thus Monk *et al.* (1946) found that 10 mgm. t.d.s. for ten days was followed by a relapse rate of only 27·6 per cent., a result comparing favourably with that of proguanil alone. Against artificially induced infection with the Chesson strain pamaquin proved ineffective in preventing relapses in all the five cases treated (Alving and Coggeshall, 1947).

Although there is only a small margin between the therapeutically effective dose and the toxic dose, an 8-aminoquinoline is likely to continue to be used in the treatment of vivax malaria, since in combination with other drugs it undoubtedly lowers the relapse rate.

Pentaquine. The relapse rate with pentaquine alone is not yet fully established. In a small series (Monk, 1948b) the relapse rate was only 12 per cent., but with the artificially induced Chesson strain three of five patients relapsed (Alving and Coggeshall, 1947).

Pentaquine is a very active schizonticide which produces rapid clinical cure. The recommended dose should not exceed 60 mgm. daily for ten to fourteen days.

Monk (1948b) records that in a series of twenty-five cases given 60 mgm. daily more than half had toxic symptoms. At the therapeutic dose rate the toxicity of pentaquine is qualitatively the same and quantitatively approximately one-half to three-fourths that of pamaquin in adult persons (Loeb *et al.*, 1946b). *iso*Pentaquine is less toxic than pentaquine and may therefore be the most satisfactory 8-aminoquinoline.

Quinine and Pamaquin. The specific action of pamaquin and quinine therapy in reducing the relapse rate was originally discovered by Sinton and Bird (1928), working on European soldiers infected in India. Pamaquin, 100 mgm. daily, was given concurrently with quinine for twenty-eight days and of twenty subjects eighteen showed no relapses, two being lost sight of. Control cases treated with quinine only suffered a relapse rate of 77 per cent. The actual salt of pamaquin employed was not stated. Later, Sinton, Smith, and Pottinger (1930) found that periods of treatment shorter than twenty-eight days and doses as small as 40 mgm. of the salt per day were satisfactory. Piebenga (1932) treated vivax malaria acquired naturally in the Netherlands with a fourteen-day course of quinine and pamaquin. Of sixty-seven patients treated only one relapsed, but controls given quinine only had a relapse rate of 60 to 70 per cent. Further confirmation of these results was obtained in India (Manifold, 1931 ; Kligler and Mer, 1931 ; Jarvis, 1932a, b ; Dixon, 1933 ; Drenowsky, 1943). The Malaria Commission of the League of Nations (1937) reported that a combination of quinine and pamaquin was most effective in reducing the number of relapses in benign tertian malaria, but owing to the supposed toxicity of pamaquin its use in the armed services of the United States was discontinued (Surgeon-General, U.S.A., 1943). Later Feldman *et al.* (1947) and Berliner *et al.* (1946) reinvestigated the whole question. With the Chesson strain pamaquin in the maximum tolerated dose, 90 mgm. of base a day for two weeks together with quinine, cured nine out of nine volunteers with sporozoite-induced infections. A dose of 30 mgm. a day with quinine, or 90 mgm. a day without quinine, failed to cure some of the patients.

Craige *et al.* (1947) used a variety of combinations of quinine and pamaquin against mosquito-induced malaria due to the Chesson strain. The daily administration of 63 mgm. of the base or 140 mgm. of the naphthoate concurrently with quinine for fourteen days failed to protect all but a few patients against relapse. No protection was afforded when the drugs were given serially. Similar results with the Chesson strain were reported by Alving and Coggeshall (1947). On the other hand, with natural infections acquired in the field much better results have been obtained. Hayman *et al.* (1946 b) found that 27 mgm. of pamaquin base with quinine for fourteen days caused a precipitous drop in the relapse rate. Spicknall and Terry (1948) observed no relapses over a period of eighteen months among twenty patients from the Pacific and South America. Similar good results have been reported by the Malaria Sub-Committee of the Medical Research Council (1945), where among 584 cases the relapse rate in six months was 10·3 per cent., by Innes and Fenton (1945), Johnstone (1946), Monk *et al.* (1946), Most *et al.* (1946a) and Fairley *et al.* (1946). These results are set out in the table (pp. 490–5). Strain differences may, however, be of importance. In Holland, Swellengrebel and De Buck (1932) showed that in one district only a single relapse occurred among sixty-six patients with vivax malaria given 0·03 gm. of pamaquin and 1·0 gm. daily of quinine, yet in another district the same treatment resulted in 50 per cent. of relapses (Malaria Commission of Holland, 1932). Similarly Bylmer (1947) found that of ninety-nine patients with vivax infections treated in Holland forty-seven relapsed, but of 123 given quinine and pamaquin only sixteen relapsed. The Malaria Commission of the Netherlands Health Council (1938, 1940) reported that in the town of Wormerveer, in Northern Holland, in 1936, a course of mepacrine was given to eighty-five patients for seven days ; thirty relapsed within the year. In the village of Vitgeest 452 patients were given hydroquinine for eight days ; 167 relapsed within the year. In Wormerveer 382 patients were given quinine and pamaquin for fourteen days ; fifty relapsed within the year. In the following year 500 relapsing patients were given the same course of quinine and pamaquin ; fifty-five only relapsed. Thus in the majority of naturally acquired vivax infections the combination of quinine and pamaquin has a rapid clinical action ; it rarely produces symptoms of toxicity ; it may be given to ambulant patients on light work, and as a rule it produces a radical cure in eight of ten patients. In fact so constant is this result that quinine 0·6 gm. given concurrently with pamaquin 10 mgm. three times a day for ten to fourteen days is now frequently used as a standard course by which other forms of treatment can be evaluated. Ruhe *et al.* (1949), working with the St. Elizabeth strain, have emphasised the importance of giving the pamaquin and quinine concurrently. No relapse occurred in twenty-three patients given either 0·65, 0·06 or 0·09 gm. of the base daily for twelve days concurrently with 2·0 gm. of quinine sulphate, but one in four relapsed if pamaquin followed the quinine.

Provided that the daily dose of pamaquin does not exceed 10 mgm. there is very little need to fear toxicity, but medical supervision and hospitalisation are still essential. Monk *et al.* (1946) found that of 168 patients given quinine and pamaquin combined, eighteen showed toxic signs and symptoms but of these seventeen were able to complete the course. Cyanosis and gastric distress do not *per se* necessitate termination of treatment and general malaise and anorexia require to be pronounced before desisting from treatment. Intravascular hæmolysis is of course a contra-indication ; it seems to be more common in dark-skinned races than in those of European or American origin. Methæm-albuminæmia is common but it does not produce cyanosis unless it exceeds 6 or 7 per cent. of the total hæmoglobin. Craige *et al.* (1947) used the average per cent. of total hæmoglobin converted to methæmalbumin for a group of patients as an objective numerical index for the toxicity of various pamaquin regimes. Granulocytopenia, not usually severe, may also occur, but the toxicity of the mixture is in general so low that it can be readily given even to elderly patients with brown atrophy of the heart.

It is by no means easy to determine why field strains of vivax malaria should be eradicated by a combination of quinine and pamaquin whereas the Chesson strain transmitted by the bites of infected mosquitoes is hardly affected. In field studies, however, many patients have been treated during late relapses when acquired immunity is already high. This immunity would necessarily aid the therapeutic effect. The intensity of the infection under field conditions is much more variable than in mosquito-induced therapeutic infections. Prolonged mepacrine suppression

TREATMENT OF VIVAX MALARIA, 1929–1948
(Cseh Firtos, 1949)

Treatment.	Total number of patients.	Number of patients with one or more relapses.	Percentage of patients relapsing.
Quinine sulphate 1 gm. daily for 7 or 14 days . .	264	130	49·2
Quinine sulphate 0·9 gm. and 30 mgm. pamaquin hydrochloride daily for 14 days	413	40	9·7
Quinine sulphate 0·9 gm. and 30 mgm. pamaquin hydrochloride daily for 21 days	115	2	1·7
Quinine sulphate 0·9 gm. and 30 mgm. pamaquin hydrochloride daily for 8 days	25	13	52
Quinine sulphate 0·9 gm. and 60 mgm. pamaquin naphthoate daily for 14 days	51	0	0
Mepacrine 0·3 gm. daily for 7 days. . . .	28	11	39·3
Various treatments	430	138	32·1

THE RATE OF DISAPPEARANCE OF FEVER AND PARASITÆMIA IN TONKINESE PEASANTS TREATED WITH CHLOROQUINE OR PROGUANIL (100 PATIENTS IN EACH GROUP) (Canet, 1949b)

Days.	Number of Cases without Fever.				Number of Cases without Parasitæmia.			
	Daily Dose Schedule.				Daily Dose Schedule.			
	0·1 gm. (1st day).	0·2 gm. (1st day).	0·3 gm. (1st day).	0·6 gm. (1st day).	0·1 gm. (1st day).	0·2 gm. (1st day).	0·3 gm. (1st day).	0·6 gm. (1st day).
	C. P.	C. P.	C. P.	C. P.	C. P.	C. P.	C. P.	C. P.
1	— —	— —	— —	— —	— —	— —	— —	— —
2	28 11	36 26	64 36	72 36	— —	— —	— —	2 —
3	37 37	32 28	30 31	24 40	6 —	21 11	23 20	46 24
4	26 31	25 28	3 19	4 16	11 9	27 26	51 38	42 44
5	6 9	5 11	2 11	— 8	29 16	30 34	22 27	6 24
6	3 9	2 4	1 3	— —	28 15	19 20	3 13	4 80
7	— 3	— 3	— —	— —	17 26	2 6	1 2	— —
8	— —	— —	— —	— —	6 23	1 3	— —	— —
9	— —	— —	— —	— —	3 11	— —	— —	— —

C = Chloroquine.   P = Proguanil.

may have altered the clinical course of the disease and may have assisted the therapeutic action, and finally the strains of infecting parasite are by no means uniform.   In Holland, Winckel (1949) believes that 30 mgm. of pamaquin daily combined with 0·9 gm. of quinine gives quite as good results as pamaquin and 2 gm. of quinine daily.   The results obtained by Cseh Firtos (1949) over a period of twenty years in Holland are of particular interest since the patients with whom he dealt, 1,326 in number, were all drawn from the same area and were thus presumably infected with similar strains of *P. vivax*.   The greater efficacy of pamaquin and quinine sulphate over quinine alone or mepacrine alone is well brought out by the table on p. 479, as is the greater effectiveness of 60 mgm. pamaquin naphthoate or 30 mgm. pamaquin hydrochloride for at least fourteen days.   Combinations of pamaquin and quinine are more effective than pamaquin and other cinchona alkaloids (Alving, 1948).

Proguanil and Pamaquin.   While treatment with proguanil alone gives a relapse rate of 35 to 40 per cent., the combination of proguanil and pamaquin has given results more closely resembling those obtained with quinine and pamaquin.

Monk (1948c) pointed out that success is just as great when quinine is combined with pamaquin in a small dose as when the dose is two and a half times as great and approaches the toxic level. When pamaquin is combined with a high dose of proguanil, however, approximately 40 per cent. of cases show cyanosis or gastric symptoms and, in addition, the majority of patients develop anorexia and general malaise.   This may be due to the fact that proguanil displaces pamaquin from the tissues and the toxic reactions are thus associated with a higher pamaquin level in the plasma.

The optimum eight-hourly dose of proguanil, when given concurrently with 10 mgm. of pamaquin, is probably not more than 100 mgm.   Further observation is required to determine whether such a course of treatment is as successful as quinine-pamaquin therapy.   The combination of proguanil and pentaquine or *iso*pentaquine requires extended study.

Pamaquin, Mepacrine, and other 8-aminoquinoline Derivatives with Pamaquin-like Action.   The combination of pamaquin or pentaquine and mepacrine is usually regarded as being too toxic for

VIVAX INFECTIONS

general use if the two drugs are given concurrently. Craige *et al.* (1947) found that with a daily dose of 0·3 gm. mepacrine and 31 mgm. of pamaquin for fourteen days there was considerable toxicity and 12·1 per cent. of the total hæmoglobin was converted into methæmoglobin : in addition, only one of five patients failed to relapse when infected with the Chesson strain. Combinations of pamaquin with chloroquine, metachloridine, SN 5,241 and SN 8,617 were also unsuccessful when patients were infected with the Chesson strain although the toxicity was not as high as with mepacrine and pamaquin. Wallace (1949, 1950), however, claims good results with tablets of neopremaline given to a relatively immune Indian population. Neopremaline tablets are said to contain 0·15 gm. of chloroquine base, 0·0075 gm. of pamaquin base, and 0·0075 gm. of rhodoquine base.

Pamaquin and Sontoquine. This combination was used in Holland by Hulshoff (1949) ; 138 patients were given 100 mgm. of sontoquine three times a day for five or seven days ; as the fever subsided 30 mgm. of pamaquin was begun and given daily for five or six days. The fever disappeared in an average of 1·8 days and the parasitæmia in 2·9 days. No toxic effects were noted. Relapses occurred after thirty to 268 days, on an average in eighty days, in 30 per cent. of cases.

THERAPEUTIC AND TOXIC EFFECTS OF ANTIMALARIAL DRUGS GIVEN WITH PAMAQUIN (31 MGM. PER DAY) FOR FOURTEEN DAYS (Craige *et al.*, 1947)

Drug.	Daily dose in gm.	Ratio of individuals relapsing to individuals treated.	Toxicity. Methæmoglobinæmia (per cent. of total hæmoglobin).
Mepacrine .	0·3	4/5	12·1
Chloroquine .	0·3	4/5	4·3
Metachloridine (SN 11,437).	1·0–1·7	5/5	4·9
SN 8,617 .	0·38	5/5	6·3
SN 5,241 .	2·0	3/3	8·8

Other 8-Aminoquinolines and Quinine. In association with quinine certain 8-aminoquinolines were tested by Alving *et al.*

(1948b) against the Chesson strain of vivax malaria. Acute attacks were terminated more rapidly than by quinine itself.

The following compounds were ineffective in doses which approached the maximum tolerated: SN 191; SN 11,191; SN 13,619; SN 13,697 and SN 14,011.

The quinine equivalents and the toxicity of those compounds which were effective are shown in the table in relation to their activity in preventing relapses of vivax malaria.

THE VALUE OF PAMAQUIN IN THE THERAPY OF *PLASMODIUM VIVAX*—ITALIAN STRAINS (Monk *et al.*, 1946)

Course.	Dosage.	Number of cases treated.	Number of relapses.	Relapse rate: percentage of all cases treated.	Relapse rate: percentage of cases followed up for six months.
Quinine, mepacrine, pamaquin.	Quinine, 90 gr. in 3 days; mepacrine 1·5 gm. in 3 days; pamaquin 90 mgm. in 3 days.	29	5	17·2	19·2
Mepacrine, pamaquin	Mepacrine 2·4 gm. in 7 days; pamaquin 90 mgm. in 3 days.	29	3	10·3	12·5
Quinine, pamaquin	Quinine 100 gr. in 10 days; pamaquin 100 mgm. in 10 days.	94	11	11·7	14·3
Mepacrine	Mepacrine 4·6 gm. in 12 days.	86	23	26·7	35·0
Mepacrine	Mepacrine 3·1 gm. in 7 days.	31	11	35·5	44·0
Mepacrine	Mepacrine 2·4 gm. n 7 days.	29	8	27·6	28·6
Quinine, mepacrine	Quinine 90 gr. in 3 days; mepacrine 2·5 gm. in 5 days.	21	5	23·8	26·3

Quinine and Pentaquine. The results so far obtained suggest that pentaquine, or more probably *iso*pentaquine, combined with quinine, forms the most satisfactory regime for the treatment of relapsing vivax malaria. With the Chesson strain the expected relapse rate is far lower than with any other mode of treatment yet tested (Alving and Coggeshall, 1947). Loeb *et al.*(1946b) also reported that quinine and pentaquine reduced the relapse rate of Pacific strains: Spicknall and Terry (1948) obtained similar results with Pacific and Indian strains.

In a series of twenty-six cases of naturally occurring vivax infections treated by Monk (1948b) three may have relapsed but in none were the symptoms definitely proved to be malarial in origin. Straus and Gennis (1948) treated forty-nine patients from the South Pacific area with pentaquine as the monophosphate (10 mgm. every eight hours) and 600 mgm. of quinine daily for fourteen days. None relapsed in an observation period of four to fourteen months. Coggeshall and Rice (1949) and Coggeshall (1949) found that of 185 patients given pentaquine and 1 or 2 gm. of quinine daily ten subsequently had parasitæmia and twelve fever but no parasitæmia. White *et al.* (1948) believed that in patients infected with the St. Elizabeth strain quinine and pentaquine brought about total eradication of parasites. In America, with the recommended dosage of 60 mgm. daily slight cyanosis and mild abdominal discomfort have been reported. Nausea, anorexia, and rarely drug fever from the seventh to eleventh days of treatment have been seen. Deafness has been noted with 2 gm. of quinine and two negroes are known to have had hæmolytic crises after pentaquine. In England these symptoms were noted in more than half those treated : one patient had such pyrexia and hepatic discomfort that treatment had to be abandoned, but on the whole the mixture of pentaquine or *iso*pentaquine and quinine is only half as toxic as that of pamaquin and quinine.

Quinine and *iso*Pentaquine have been shown by Alving (1948) to act synergistically in the same way as quinine and pamaquin and to be less toxic than the mixture of pamaquin and quinine. When 2 gm. of quinine sulphate was given daily for fourteen days the results depended on the dose of *iso*pentaquine base administered. The following results were obtained with the Chesson strain of vivax malaria ; the observation period was more than five months.

Daily dose of *iso*Pentaquine base.	Number of relapses.	
	Severe infections.	Moderate infections.
30	10 of 15 (67%)	—
45	7 of 15 (47%)	—
60	4 of 20 (20%)	0 of 5

Pentaquine and Chloroquine together have been employed by Wallace (1949) in the suppression of malaria among relative y immune Indians. Tablets contained 0·15 gm. of each base and two tablets a day were given to children. No evidence is provided to show whether plasmodia were actually eradicated by this treatment, but no undue toxicity was noted.

Quinine or Mepacrine and Sulphadiazine. The acute attacks were controlled with either quinine or mepacrine in thirty-three vivax patients from the S.W. Pacific area : sulphadiazine was then given for fourteen days to give blood levels of 4·7 to 10·7 mgm. per 100 ml. Within three months sixteen patients had relapsed (Coggeshall *et al.*, 1945).

Combinations of Quinine, Mepacrine, and Pamaquin. Quinine, mepacrine, and pamaquin have been given in various combinations. A commonly used combination during the war years was quinine, 10 gr. t.d.s. for three days, followed by 1·5 gm. of mepacrine for five days, followed by 10 mgm. of pamaquin eight-hourly for three days. Good results with moderately low relapse rates were obtained, but generally speaking it is less successful than combined quinine-pamaquin therapy. The possible toxic effects of combining mepacrine and pamaquin must also be considered.

Innes and Fenton (1945) treated several small series of cases at Rome with different combinations of quinine, mepacrine, and pamaquin ; they were followed up for six months or more by Monk *et al.* (1946) with the results shown in the table on p. 482.

It will be seen that the three courses containing pamaquin were more successful than the others, the relapse rate of all regimes containing pamaquin being 12·5 per cent. as against 28·2 per cent. when pamaquin was excluded.

It would seem preferable to administer pamaquin concurrently either with quinine or proguanil, for if mepacrine and pamaquin are given concurrently the plasma pamaquin level rises considerably and toxic reactions due to pamaquin are liable to occur.

Intermittent Therapy. Innes and Fenton (1945) treated a series of cases at Rome with intermittent regimes of either quinine and pamaquin or mepacrine alone. The cases were followed up for six months or more (Monk *et al.*, 1946).

The courses were as follows :—

(*a*) *Mepacrine.* An initial course of 2·5 mg in five days was followed by two courses of 3 gm. given over a period of six days with periods of " rest " of seven days between all courses.

(*b*) *Quinine and Pamaquin.* An initial course of quinine 10 gr. and pamaquin 10 mgm. is given eight-hourly for seven days followed by two similar courses of five days with " rest " periods of seven days between the courses. The results are seen in the table (pp. 492–3).

These results are remarkable and obviously further investigations are required.

The theory on which such treatment is based was put forward by Innes and Fenton (1945) and Monk *et al.* (1946). During treatment with quinine or mepacrine a drug-inhibited stage of development is believed to occur corresponding to the pre-schizont forms : if they persist in the host until the plasma level has fallen sufficiently low their development could be resumed during the periods of rest allowed for by intermittent therapy. Mepacrine is slowly excreted so that the " rest " periods are thought to be too short to allow the development of the drug-inhibited forms. This theory requires further investigation, but its practical application in eradicating vivax infection in forty-five cases is of considerable importance.

Thus the evidence suggests that in quinine combined with an 8-aminoquinoline a combination is available which can eradicate the majority of vivax infections. Of the 8-aminoquinolines available pentaquine and *iso*pentaquine are as effective as pamaquin and less toxic.

Suppression. It is obvious from what has been said that with vivax infections no drug can be guaranteed to ensure suppression unless it is taken regularly ; nor is there any instance of suppressive cure such as occurs with falciparum infections. Of the drugs available for suppression quinine is the least effective owing to the rapidity with which it disappears from the blood stream with vivax infections ; however, there is not the same risk of precipitating blackwater fever. Of the others, mepacrine has the same disadvantages as in falciparum suppression. Chloroquine is less toxic than mepacrine and has the advantage that it need be taken only once a week (Wallace, 1949, 1950). Proguanil also has low toxicity, but it must be taken at least three times weekly in a dose of 100 mgm., and even when this dosage is taken daily a certain number of failures have been reported. Whereas quinine and mepacrine have been taken for years by certain persons without toxic effects, sufficient time has not yet elapsed to show that chloroquine and proguanil can be similarly taken with the same impunity.

Gametocyticidal Action. While pamaquin and 8-aminoquinolines have a direct gametocyticidal action in vivax infections, this action is much less marked than in falciparum infections. The only drug treatment which can be reasonably guaranteed to destroy gametocytes is one which eradicates infection entirely, such as quinine and pamaquin or quinine and pentaquine.

INFECTIONS DUE TO *P. MALARIÆ*

Little work has been done to compare the action of antimalarial drugs on *P. malariæ*. Young and Eyles (1948), however, carried out comparative tests on patients infected therapeutically with two strains of *P. malariæ*, the U.S. Public Health Service and Trinidad strains. The drugs used were chloroquine, mepacrine hydrochloride, quinine sulphate, and totaquina. The dose schedules employed were as follows :—

Chloroquine   .   1·5 gm. total (eighteen patients) : first day 0·6 gm. followed in six to eight hours by 0·3 gm. ; second and third days 0·3 gm. daily.

2·4 gm. total (six patients) : as above with the single daily doses extended through the sixth day.

Mepacrine   .   1·5 gm. total (thirteen patients) : 0·1 gm. thrice daily for five days.

2·8 gm. total (six patients) : first day, 0·4, 0·3 and 0·3 gm. ; thereafter 0·3 gm. daily for six days.

Quinine sulphate   (seven patients) 0·67 gm. thrice daily for four
days, then 0·67 gm. daily for several weeks.

Totaquina   .   28 gm. total (four patients).
0·67 gm. thrice daily for fourteen days.

Chloroquine was the most effective in reducing the parasitæmia :
80 per cent. of chloroquine-treated patients (2·4 gm. course) were
free from parasites by the sixth day, whereas the same percentage
of patients treated by mepacrine (2·8 gm. course), quinine, and
totaquina was not reached till the seventh, ninth and tenth days
respectively. All patients treated with chloroquine were parasite-
free after nine days (2·4 gm. course) and eleven days (1·5 gm.
course) ; with mepacrine after eight days (2·8 gm. course) and
thirteen days (1·5 gm. course) and with quinine and totaquina
after ten days. Fever was controlled by chloroquine at least as
well as by the other drugs. In Tunis Durand *et al.* (1949) found
that in partial immunes a single dose of 0·6 gm. controlled
parasitæmia in three days, a dose of 1·2 gm. in twelve hours.

There is little to choose between these four drugs so far as
parasitæmia is concerned, though quinine and totaquina were
slightly slower.

Little or no evidence is available on the comparative effect of
other drugs, though there is a suggestion that proguanil acts
rather slowly on some strains of *P. malariæ*.

The effect of various drugs on the quartan relapse rate has been
insufficiently studied. Winckel (1949), however, finds that to
prevent relapses 1 gm. daily of quinine combined with 30 mgm. of
pamaquin daily for fourteen days is required. A daily dose of
2 gm. quinine is unnecessarily large.

MALARIA IN PREGNANCY

Untreated malaria is well known to be a frequent cause of
premature labour and threatened or incomplete abortion. *P. vivax*
and *P. falciparum* are equally responsible. If there is any clinical
suspicion that malaria exists, important signs being a leucopenia
and a relative mononucleosis, antimalarial treatment should be
given without delay. In the past there has been some fear that
quinine salts may assist in producing a miscarriage and for this

reason treatment has been withheld. It is very doubtful whether this fear of quinine was justified except when quinine was given in relatively enormous doses. Mepacrine is as a rule well tolerated by pregnant women and is undoubtedly more effective than quinine. Kulcsar (1947), for instance, found that mepacrine controlled the fever after one febrile attack in 50 per cent. of cases, quinine in only 22 per cent.

European babies born to mothers living in endemic areas occasionally show congenital infection with *P. falciparum*. Cord blood should be examined routinely and if parasites are present 0·03 gm. of mepacrine daily should be given at once. Intramuscular mepacrine causes convulsive seizures.

Ascoli's Treatment

In 1937 Ascoli claimed that doses of adrenaline given intravenously had a remarkably beneficial effect on chronic malaria associated with splenomegaly, anæmia and cachexia. The infection lingering in the spleen is said to be eliminated and relapses thus become impossible. The commencing dose is 0·01 mgm. and the daily dose is increased by this amount till 0·1 mgm. is being given daily. The total course is usually for twenty days. It has been claimed for this method, especially by Italian workers, that " resistance " to quinine often disappears, so that smaller doses of the drug can be given. The spleen is said to decrease in size and the general health to improve. In his original communication Ascoli claimed that of fifteen patients who had been treated for two years, and twenty who had been treated for one year none had shown a return of splenic enlargement and none had relapsed.

The adrenaline must be pure, the solution freshly prepared, and the injections given slowly. In very small children the injections may be given intramuscularly instead of intravenously (Marcialis and Cannas, 1937).

During the war attempts were made in infections due both to *P. vivax* and *P. falciparum* to substantiate these claims, mepacrine being given as the antimalarial drug. In certain hospitals control cases were given intravenous injections of sterile physiological saline. No difference in the course of an acute attack could be found in patients suffering from vivax infections and such patients treated with mepacrine and adrenaline are known to have relapsed at the same rate as those given mepacrine and saline. In patients with enlarged spleens due either to vivax or falciparum infections a decrease in the size of the spleen usually occurred during the course of the injections, but as a rule the spleen again enlarged a few weeks after the cessation of treatment. The symptoms of adrenalism are often unpleasant, the method is time-consuming and the results do not appear to warrant the procedure. In falciparum infections adrenaline does not influence in any way the formation or duration of existence of crescents (Nucciotti, 1938). Hasegawa (1949) claims that an injection of 0·1 to 0·4 mgm. of the alkaloid cepharanthin is more effective than adrenaline.

THE CONTROL OF MALARIA IN INDIGENOUS POPULATIONS

During the war of 1939–45 it was shown that even in hyper-endemic continental areas it was possible by a combination of anti-mosquito measures and chemotherapeutic suppression to reduce the malaria rate among non-immune European troops to a very low figure. Such a reduction in the malaria rate was attained only by extensive drainage and other engineering works, the use of Paris green, of insecticides such as D.D.T. and gammexane, and above all by the continuous taking of suppressive drugs. The time, money, and above all the discipline necessary to ensure the carrying out of these measures cannot be applied to an indigenous population even if they remain in completely urbanised areas. The vast majority of the inhabitants of the tropics lives in rural surroundings.

The results on the infection rate of an indigenous population of malaria control by drainage are sometimes disappointing. In Freetown, Sierra Leone, after four years of intensive malarial control by drainage, Walton (1948) has shown that half the child population still becomes infected every year. The parasite rate in school children in the area cannot be reduced below 10 per cent. and this parasite-rate implies that the number of infected mosquitoes biting each child per year is 0·4. Although the breeding of mosquitoes in a limited area can be abolished completely the seepage of mosquitoes into the periphery of this area cannot be

Relapse Rates in *P. vivax* Malaria Following Different Drug Treatments

Strain.	Drug.	Dosage.	Number of days' treatment.	Number of days' follow up.	Number of cases treated.	Number of cases relapsing.	Percentage of relapses.	Reference.
S.W. Pacific New Guinea	Quinine.	2·0 gm. daily for 3 days. 3·0 gm. daily for 2 days.	14	120	75	67	89·4	Most et al. (1946a). Trager et al. (1947).
	”	2·0 gm. daily for 2 days. 0·6 gm. daily for 21 days.	26	42	67	55	82·0	
S.W. Pacific: Chesson	”	2·0 gm. daily.	16	463	5	4	80·0	Berliner et al. (1948).
” ” ”	”	2·0 gm. daily.	14	365	13	12	92·3	Alving et al. (1948a).
” ” ”	”	11–12 gm. in 7 days.	7	} 221	7	7	100·0	Pullman et al. (1948b).
” ” ”	”	21–23 gm. in 14 days.	14		15	13	86·6	Pullman et al. (1948b).
St. Elizabeth	”	2·0 gm. daily.	14	547	5	5	100·0	White et al. (1948).
Totals					187	163	87·1	
S.W. Pacific: Chesson	Mepacrine hydrochloride	1·0 gm. for 1 day 0·4 gm. for 6 days.	7	334	9	9	100·0	Pullman et al. (1948b).
” ”	”	1·0 gm. for 1 day. 0·4 gm. for 6 days.	7	334	9	9	100·0	Jones et al. (1948).
Not stated	”	0·8 gm. daily for 2 days. 0·3 gm. for 10 days.	12	120	650	221	34·0	Army Med. Dept. (1945).
Mediterranean	”	0·8 gm. daily for 2 days. 0·3 gm. daily for 10 days.	12	180	86	23	26·7	Innes and Fenton (1945).
”	”	0·8 gm. daily for 2 days. 0·3 gm. daily for 5 days.	7	180	31	11	35·5	Monk et al. (1946).
S.W. Pacific	”	2·8 gm. in 7 days.	7	120	69	57	84·0	Most et al. (1946a). Innes and Fenton (1945).
Mediterranean.	”	2·4 gm. in 7 days.	7	180	29	8	27·6	Monk et al. (1946).
Far Eastern	”	0·6 gm. for 2 days. 0·3 gm. in 7 days.	12	180	27	8	29·6	Andrews et al. (1947).
Pacific	”	3·2 gm. in 7 days or 2·6 gm. in 6 days.	6 or 7	86 to 189 (mean 86)	22*	17	77	Gordon et al. (1947).
Pacific and Mediterranean	”	3·2 gm. in 7 days or 2·6 gm. in 6 days.	6 or 7	78 to 129 (mean 100)	39†	26	67	Gordon et al. (1947).

Area	Drug	Dose	No. of men	Days of observation	No. of attacks	No. of relapses	Per cent. relapse	Authority
Mediterranean	,,	3·2 gm. in 7 days or 2·6 gm. in 6 days.	6 or 7	96 to 141 (mean 128)	26†	15	58·0	Gordon et al. (1947).
New Guinea	,,	3·2 gm. in 6 days and 0·6 gm. weekly.	27–62	70	139	105	76·0	Trager et al. (1947).
Totals					1,136	509	44·8	
India-Burma	Proguanil	500 mgm. daily.	10	180	107	47	43·9	Johnstone (1946).
,,	,,	500 mgm. daily.	10	180	24	16	66·6	Monk et al. (1946).
,,	,,	50 mgm. daily.	10	180	108	46	42·6	Johnstone (1946).
Far Eastern	,,	1·0 gm. daily.	14	180	35	13	37·1	Andrews et al. (1947).
,,	,,	100 mgm. daily.	14	180	31	9	29·03	Andrews et al. (1947).
S.W. Pacific: Chesson	,,	97 mgm. daily.	14	335	10	7	70·0	Jones et al. (1948).
Totals					315	138	43·8	
S.W. Pacific: Chesson	Pamaquin	30 mgm. daily.	14	54	7	7	100·0	Pullman et al. (1948b).
S.W. Pacific: Chesson	Pentaquine (base)	30 mgm. daily.	14	40	5	5	100·0	Alving et al., (1948a).
,,	,,	60 mgm. daily.	14	274	5	2	40·0	Alving et al. (1948a).
,,	,,	60 mgm. daily.	14	423	5	3	60·0	Alving and Coggeshall (1947).
India-Burma	,,	60 mgm. daily.	10	180	25	3	12·0	Monk (1948b).
Totals					40	13	32·5	
S.W. Pacific: St. Elizabeth	Chloroquine diphosphate	0·9 gm. on 1st day, 0·3 gm. on 2nd and 3rd days.	3	120–425	46	14	30·4	Straus and Gennis (1948).
S.W. Pacific: Chesson	,,	3·2 gm. in 7 days.	7	241	8	8	100·0	Pullman et al. (1948b).
,,	,,	2·0 gm. in 14 days.	14	15–89	21	14	66·6	Alving and Coggeshall (1947).
Mediterranean	,,	5·0 gm. in 16 days.	16	66–166	40†	17	42·5	Gordon et al. (1947).
S.W. Pacific	,,	5·0 gm. in 16 days.	16	75–122	57*	42	73·7	Gordon et al. (1947).
Totals					172	95	55·2	

* Primary attacks.   † Secondary attacks.

RELAPSE RATES IN *P. vivax* MALARIA FOLLOWING DIFFERENT DRUG TREATMENTS (*Continued*)

Strain.	Drug.	Dosage.	Number of days' treatment.	Number of days' follow up.	Number of cases treated.	Number of cases relapsing.	Percentage of relapses.	Reference.
S.W. Pacific	Sontoquine	3·2 gm. in 7 days.	7	112	13*	12	92·3	Gordon et al. (1947).
Mediterranean	"	3·2 gm. in 7 days.	7	62–147	62†	37	50·6	Gordon et al. (1947).
"	"	3·2 gm. in 7 days.	7	183	15†	14	93·3	Gordon et al. (1947).
Netherlands	"	1·8 gm. in 5 days.	5	60–152	93	9	9·6	Halawani et al. (1947).
	"	300 mgm. daily.	5 or 7	30–268	32	17	53·0	Hulshoff (1949).
Totals					183	72	39·3	
India	Camoquin	200 mgm. daily or 500 mgm. on 1 day.	3} 1}	30–240	23	8	34·7	Chaudhuri (1948).
India-Burma	Quinine and pamaquin	Quinine sulphate 2·0 gm. daily. Pamaquin 30 mgm. daily.	10	180	168	35	20·8	Monk et al. (1946).
"	"	Quinine sulphate 2·0 gm. daily. Pamaquin 30 mgm. daily.	10	180	108	17	15·6	Johnstone (1946).
Not stated	"	Quinine sulphate 2·0 gm. daily. Pamaquin 30 mgm. daily.	10	150	584	60	10·3	Army Med. Dept. (1945).
Mediterranean	"	Quinine sulphate 2·0 gm. daily. Pamaquin 30 mgm. daily.	10	180	94	11	11·7	Innes and Fenton (1945).
S. Pacific	"	Quinine sulphate 2·0 gm. daily. Pamaquin 30 mgm. daily.	14	120	72	8	11·1	Monk et al. (1946).
"	"	Quinine sulphate 2·0 gm. daily. Pamaquin 30 mgm. daily.	10	30–180	223	31	13·5	Fairley et al. (1946).
"	"	Quinine sulphate 2·0 gm. daily. Pamaquin 40–60 mgm. daily.	10–12	60–547	10	5	50	Alving and Coggeshall (1947).
S.W. Pacific: Chesson	"	Quinine sulphate 2·0 gm. daily. Pamaquin 30 mgm. daily.	16} 12}	463	20	0	0	Spicknall and Terry (1948).
"	"	Quinine base 2·0 gm. daily. Pamaquin 30 mgm. daily.	14	54–355	18	2	11·1	Berliner et al., (1948).
"	"	Quinine base 2·0 gm. daily. Pamaquin 45 mgm. daily.	14	more than 152	21	14	66·6	Alving (1948).

Region	Drug	Treatment						Reference
„ „	„ „	Quinine base 2·0 gm. daily. Pamaquin 60 mgm. daily.	16 14	201–276	4	2	50	Berliner *et al.* (1948).
„ „	„ „	Quinine base 2·0 gm. daily.	16 14	508–555	10	5	50	Alving and Coggeshall (1947).
„ „	„ „	Quinine 90 mgm. daily. Pamaquin 90 mgm. daily followed by	16 14	459	9	0	0	Berliner *et al.* (1948).
„ „	„ „	Quinine base 2·0 gm. daily. Pamaquin 30 mg. daily.	10 17	120	5 17	2 1	40 5·8	Berliner *et al.* (1948). Bianco *et al.* (1947).
St. Elizabeth	„ „	Quinine sulphate 2·0 gm. daily. Pamaquin (base) 60 mgm. daily.	6	72–224	4	1	25	Ruhe *et al.* (1949).
„	„ „	Quinine sulphate 2·0 gm. daily. Pamaquin (base) 30, 60 or 90 mgm. daily.	12	174–250	19	0	0	Ruhe *et al.* (1949).
Totals .					1,486	194	13·1	
India and Burma	Quinine and pentaquine (base)	Quinine 2 gm. daily. Pentaquine 60 mgm. daily.	10	180	26	3	11·5	Monk (1948b).
Pacific .	„	Quinine 2 gm. daily. Pentaquine 60 mgm. daily.	14	365	22	0	0	Spicknall and Terry (1948).
S.W. Pacific: Chesson	„	Quinine 2 gm. daily. Pentaquine 60 mgm. daily.	14	523	76	6	7·9	Alving and Coggeshall (1947).
„ „	„	Quinine 2 gm. daily.	14	—	5	5	100	Alving *et al.* (1948a).
„ „	„	Pentaquine 15 mgm. daily.	14	187–192	14	13	93	Alving *et al.* (1948a) ; Alving (1948).
„ „	„	Quinine 2 gm. daily. Pentaquine 30 mgm. daily.	14	181–208	20	14	70	Alving *et al.* (1948a).
„ „	„	Quinine 2 gm. daily. Pentaquine 45 mgm. daily.	14	61–380	79	11	13·9	Alving *et al.* (1948a) ; Alving (1948).
S.W. Pacific (natural infections)	„	Quinine 2 gm. daily. Pentaquine 60 mgm. daily.	14	122	49	0	0	Straus and Gennis (1948).
S.W. Pacific: St. Elizabeth	„	Quinine 2 gm. daily. Pentaquine 30 mgm. daily.	14	547	10	0	0	White *et al.* (1948).
S.W. Pacific, Far East, Mediterranean and West Indies (natural infections).	„	Quinine 2 gm. daily. (67 patients had 1 gm. daily). Pentaquine 30 mgm. daily.	14	120 — 185 +	185	18	9·7	Coggeshall and Rice (1949).
Totals .					486	70	14·4	

* Primary attacks.   † Secondary attacks.

RELAPSE RATES IN *P. vivax* MALARIA FOLLOWING DIFFERENT DRUG TREATMENTS (*Continued*)

Strain.	Drug.	Dosage.	Number of days' treatment.	Number of days' follow up.	Number of cases treated.	Number of cases relapsing.	Percentage of relapses.	Reference.
S.W. Pacific: Chesson	Quinine and *iso*Pentaquine (base).	Quinine 2 gm. daily. *iso*Pentaquine 30 mgm. daily.	14	152 +	15	10	66·6	Alving (1948).
,, ,,	,, ,,	Quinine 2 gm. daily. *iso*Pentaquine 45 mgm. daily.	14	152 +	15	7	46·6	Alving (1948).
,, ,,	,, ,,	Quinine 2 gm. daily. *iso*Pentaquine 60 mgm. daily.	14	152 +	25	4	16·0	Alving (1948).
Totals .					55	21	38·1	
S. Pacific .	Proguanil and Pamaquin.	Proguanil 300 mgm. daily. Pamaquin 30 mgm. daily.	10	30–180	232	31	13·4	Fairley (1946).
India-Burma .	,, ,,	Proguanil 300 mgm. daily. Pamaquin 30 mgm. daily.	10	180	179	37	20·6	Monk (1948a).
Totals .					411	68	16·5	
S.W. Pacific: Chesson	Proguanil and pentaquine.	Proguanil 97 mgm. a day. Pentaquine 60 mgm. a day.	14	182	5	4	80	Alving *et al.* (1948a).
,, ,,	Proguanil and quinine.	Proguanil 97 mgm. a day. Quinine 1·3 gm.	14	182	10	9	90	Alving *et al.* (1948a).
Mediterranean .	Quinine, pamaquin, and mepacrine.	Quinine 2 gm. a day for 3 days. Mepacrine 0·3 gm. a day for 5 days. Pamaquin 30 mgm. a day for 3 days.	11	180	29	5	17·2	Innes and Fenton (1945). Monk *et al.* (1946).
New Guinea .	Pamaquin and mepacrine.	Mepacrine 3·2 gm. in 6 days. Pamaquin 0·1 to 0·15 gm. in 5 days. Mepacrine 0·6 gm. weekly for 21 to 56 days.	32–67	70	98	59	61	Trager *et al.* (1947).

Netherlands	Pamaquin and sontoquine.	Sontoquine 100 mgm. for 5 or 7 days. Pamaquin 30 mgm. daily for 5 or 6 days.	10–13	30–268	138	42	30	Hulshoff (1949).
New Guinea	Mepacrine and sulpha-merazine.	Mepacrine 3·2 gm. in 6 days. Sulphamerazine 15 to 20 gm. in 5 days. Mepacrine 0·6 gm. weekly for 3 to 8 weeks.	32–67	70	112	77	69	Trager et al. (1947).
Mediterranean	Intermittent quinine and pamaquin.	Quinine 2 gm. daily. Pamaquin 30 mgm. daily in 3 courses of 7, 5 and 5 days in 31 days.	31	130	45	0	0	Innes and Fenton (1945). Monk et al. (1946).
"	Intermittent mepacrine.	Mepacrine in 3 courses of 2·5 gm., 3·0 gm. and 3·0 gm. in 5, 6 and 6 days respectively during 31 days.	31	130	42	12	28·6	Innes and Fenton (1945). Monk et al. (1946).
S.W. Pacific: Chesson	Metachloridine.	44 to 82 gm. in 14 days.	14	31	5	4	80	Pullman et al. (1948a).
" "	Metachloridine and quinine.	Metachloridine 44 to 82 gm. in 14 days. Quinine sulphate 2 gm. daily.	14	31	5	4	80	Pullman et al. (1948a).
" "	Metachloridine and chloroquine.	Metachloridine 44 to 82 gm. in 14 days. Chloroquine 0·3 gm. (base) daily.	14	74	5	4	80	Pullman et al. (1948a).
" "	Metachloridine and pamaquin.	Metachloridine 44 to 82 gm. in 14 days. Pamaquin 0·031 gm.	14	113	5	5	100	Pullman et al. (1948a).

entirely prevented nor can the movement of people in and out of the control area be stopped. It is obvious that mosquito control measures throughout the tropical zone are at present difficult, and within uncontrolled zones the average African or Asiatic undoubtedly receives not less than five and probably many more than fifty infective mosquito bites each year. Even with anti-mosquito control, and certainly in its absence, the chief hope of reducing the ravages of malaria lies in suppression and in prompt control of acute attacks by chemotherapeutic means. The ideal chemotherapeutic drug for these purposes must be cheap, entirely non-toxic, and effective when taken in the absence of medical supervision. It is obvious that this ideal drug has not yet been found, but with chloroquine, proguanil or mepacrine, possibly camoquin, it is possible to reduce the frequency and virulence of acute attacks without interfering with the development of specific immunity or premunition. The periods for which suppressive treatment must be given to indigenous populations must depend on a number of factors such as the species of parasite and the seasonal incidence of the disease.

It must be fully recognised that there are certain sociological implications of extensive malarial suppression which must engage the attention of those engaged in antimalarial work.

Many African peoples are actively opposed to any extension of malarial control. They regard malaria as their main defence against the further intrusion of the European, and if malaria were abolished they consider that there would be nothing to prevent the European from settling in their lands and imposing segregation on the inhabitants who would thus find themselves compelled to live in reservations.

Intensive antimalarial control by suppression or rapid control of acute attacks removes an important cause of mortality in infancy and childhood and thus leads to an increase in the population. In many areas in the tropics the population is already pressing on the means of subsistence and the diet is deficient quantitatively and qualitatively. It would be ludicrous, if it were not tragic, that increased efficiency in the chemotherapeutic control of malaria should save children from dying of malaria in order to permit them to die later from malnutrition.

8-Aminoquinolines Capable of Preventing Relapses in Vivax Malaria when Given for Fourteen Days in Association with Quinine (Alving *et al.*, 1948b)

Survey No.	General formula of 8-(ω-aminoalkyl-amino) quinolines			Quinine equivalents.		Acute toxicity (pamaquin equivalent).	
	R'/R''>N	—(CH₂)ₙ—	Nuclear substituents.	P. gallinaceum in chicks.	P. lophuræ in ducks.	Rat.	Monkey.
SN 9,972	isopropylamino	1-methylbutyl	5, 6-dimethoxy	80	80	—	1
SN 12,325	methyl iso-propylamino	n-hexyl	6-methoxy	8–60	60	—	0·5
SN 12,352	amino	n-hexyl	6-methoxy	20	6	0·5	0·25+
SN 12,354	amino	n-hexyl	5, 6-dimethoxy	15–60	20	0·6	<0·25
SN 12,451	ethylamino	n-hexyl	6-methoxy	30	00	0 4	0 25
SN 13,232	isopropylamino	n-hexyl	6-methoxy	40	80	—	0·5
SN 13,233	n-propylamino	n-hexyl	6-methoxy	30	100	0·4	0·5
SN 13,274	isopropylamino	1-methylbutyl	5, 6-dimethoxy	20	40	—	0·5
SN 13,380	n-butylamino	n-hexyl	6-methoxy	20	40	0 2	0 5
SN 13,429	n-propylamino	1-methylbutyl	6-methoxy	80	80	0·3	0·5
SN 13,694	diethylamino	n-hexyl	5-chloro : 6-methoxy	3	10	—	0·5
DR 15,302	isopropylamino	n-amyl	4-methyl : 6-methoxy	—	256	—	—

	Daily dose (base), mgm.	Number of subjects.	Duration of follow-up in days.	Number of relapses.	Percentage of relapses.
SN 9,972	7·5	5	137	3	60
	15·0	12	81–214	2	16·6
SN 12,325	30	5	296–304	2	40
	60	5	216	3	60
SN 12,352	30	5	268	4	80
	60	5	227	3	60
SN 12,354	30	2	—	2	100
	60	5	262–328	3	60
SN 12,451	30	5	281	2	40
	60	5	245	3	60
SN 13,232	30	5	302–352	3	60
	60	5	236	4	80
SN 13,233	60	5	266	3	60
SN 13,274	30	5	222	3	60
	60	10	80–167	1	10
SN 13,380	60	5	282	4	80
SN 13,429	30	5	276	4	80
	60	5	120	2	40
SN 13,694	30	5	—	5	100
	60	5	126	4	80
DR 15,302	30	5	84–96	2	40
	60	5	91–93	2	40

References

ABBOTT, P. H., 1949, Proguanil in the Sudan. *Brit. med. J.*, i, 413.

ACTON, H. W., CURJEL, D. F., and DEWEY, J. O., 1920, The diagnosis and treatment of benign tertian and malignant tertian fevers. Section VII. The curative value of the total alkaloids (cinchona febrifuge) of cinchona bark on benign tertian infections. *Indian J. med. Res.*, 8, 861.

ADAMS, A. R. D., MAEGRAITH, B. G., KING, J. D., TOWNSHEND, R. H., DAVEY, T. H., and HAVARD, R. E., 1945, Studies on synthetic antimalarial drugs. XIII. Results of a preliminary investigation on the chemotherapeutic action of 4888 (paludrine) on acute attacks of benign tertian malaria. *Ann. trop. Med. Parasit.*, 39, 225.

AFRIDI, M. K., 1947, A critical review of therapeutic trials on paludrine carried out in India during 1946. *Indian J. Malariol.*, 1, 347.

ALVING, A. S., 1948, Pentaquine (SN 13,276) and *iso*pentaquine (SN 13,274), therapeutic agents effective in reducing relapse rate in vivax malaria. *Proc. 4th Int. Congr. trop. Med. Mal., Wash.*, p. 734.

ALVING, A. S., and COGGESHALL, L. T., 1947, Clinical testing of antimalarial drugs at Stateville Penitentiary. Malaria Rept. No. 30. National Institute of Health.

ALVING, A. S., CRAIGE, B., Jr., JONES, R., Jr., WHORTON, M., PULLMAN, T. N., and EICHELBERGER, L., 1948a, Pentaquine (SN 13,276), a therapeutic agent effective in reducing the relapse rate in vivax malaria. *J. clin. Invest.*, 27, Suppl. p. 25.

ALVING, A. S., PULLMAN, T. N., CRAIGE, B., Jr., JONES, R., Jr., WHORTON, C. M., and EICHELBERGER, L., 1948b, The clinical trial of eighteen analogues of pamaquin (plasmochin) in vivax malaria (Chesson strain). *J. clin. Invest.*, 27, Suppl. p. 34.

ANDREWS, W. H. H., GALL, D., and MAEGRAITH, B. G., 1947, Studies on synthetic antimalarial drugs. XIV. The effect of therapeutic courses of paludrine on the relapse-rate of vivax malaria. *Ann. trop. Med. Parasit.*, 41, 375.

ARMY MEDICAL DEPARTMENT, 1945, Drugs for relapsing vivax malaria. Bulletin No. 48, p. 6.

ASCOLI, M., 1937, Aspects théoriques et pratiques du traitement humoral de l'infection paludéenne. *Pr. méd.*, 45, 1827.

BANG, F. B., HAIRSTON, N. G., MAIER, J., and TRAGER, W., 1946a, Studies on atabrine (quinacrine) suppression of malaria. I. A consideration of the individual failures of suppression. *Amer. J. trop. Med.*, 26, 649.

BANG, F. B., HAIRSTON, N. G., MAIER, J., and TRAGER, W., 1946b, Studies on atabrine suppression of malaria. II. An evaluation of atabrine suppression in the field. *Amer. J. trop. Med.*, 26, 753.

BANG, F. B., HAIRSTON, N. G., TRAGER, W., and MAIER, J., 1947, Treatment of acute attacks of vivax and falciparum malaria. A comparison of atabrine and quinine. *Bull. U.S. Army med. Dept.*, 7, 75.

BERLINER, R. W., EARLE, D. P., Jr., TAGGART, J. V., WELCH, W. J., ZUBROD, C. G., KNOWLTON, P., ATCHLEY, J. A., and SHANNON, J. A., 1948, Studies on the chemotherapy of the human malarias. VII. The antimalarial activity of pamaquine. *J. clin. Invest.*, 27, Suppl. p. 108.

BERLINER, R. W., TAGGART, J. V., ZUBROD, J. V., WELCH, W. J., EARLE, D. P., Jr., and SHANNON, J. A., 1946, Pamaquin. I. Curative antimalarial activity in vivax malaria. *Fed. Proc.*, 5, 165.

BEST, A. M., 1949, Proguanil and blackwater fever. *Brit. med. J.*, i, 324.

BETTINI, S., 1948, Su alcuni casi di malaria trattati con il paludrine. *Riv. Parassit.*, 9, 107.

BIANCO, A. A., SAUNDERS, G. M., LEVINE, A. S., and COHN, R., 1947, Long-term observation of *Plasmodium vivax* malaria in returned service men. *Nav. med Bull. Wash.*, 47, 550.

BLACK, R. H., 1949, Observations on the treatment of falciparum malaria. *Trans. R. Soc. trop. Med. Hyg.*, **42**, 565.
BLACKIE, W. K., 1947, " Malaria with special reference to the African forms." Capetown. Postgraduate Press.
BLANC, F., 1949, Essais de traitement et de prophylaxie du paludisme par la paludrine en Indochine (Juillet-Novembre, 1947). *Med. trop.*, **9**, 143.
BOYD, M. F., 1941, The infection in the intermediate host : symptomatology, general considerations : in F. R. Moulton (editor), "A Symposium on Human Malaria," p. 163. Amer. Ass. Advance Sci., Pub. No. 15. Washington.
BOYD, M. F., and KITCHEN, S. F., 1948, On the homogeneity or heterogeneity of *Plasmodium vivax* infections acquired in highly endemic regions. *Amer. J. trop. Med.*, **28**, 29.
BRYANT, J., 1942, Heavy atebrin dosage in treatment of malaria. *E. Afr. med. J.*, **18**, 295.
BYLMER, H. J. T., 1949, Clinical and parasitic relapses of vivax malaria in the Netherlands : influence of various modes of treatment. *Doc. nederland. indon. Morb. trop.*, **1**, 97.
CANET, J., 1948a, Essais de traitement curatif du paludisme aigu dans la paludrine en Indochine. *Bull. Soc. Path. exot.*, **41**, 690.
CANET, J., 1948b, Efficacité comparée de la nivaquine dans le traitement curatif de l'accès palustre aigu en Indochine. *Bull. Soc. Path. exot.*, **41**, 661.
CANET, J., 1949a, Premiers essais de prophylaxie collective du paludisme en Indochine méridionale par la nivaquine B (résoquine) et la paludrine. *Bull. Soc. Path. exot.*, **42**, 165.
CANET, J., 1949b, Nivaquine et paludrine : posologie curative optima. *Bull. Soc. Path. exot.*, **42**, 278.
CHAUDHURI, R. N., 1948, Treatment of malaria. *Indian Med. Gaz.*, **83**, 225.
COGGESHALL, L. T., 1949, Cure of chronic vivax malaria with pentaquine and status of immunity thereafter. *Proc. Instit. Med. Chicago*, **17**, 357.
COGGESHALL, L. T., MARTIN, W. B., and BATES, R. D., Jr., 1945, Sulfadiazine in the treatment of relapsing malarial infections due to *Plasmodium vivax*. *J. Amer. med. Ass.*, **128**, 7.
COGGESHALL, L. T., and RICE, F. A., 1949, Cure by pentaquine of chronic vivax malaria. *J. Amer. med. Ass.*, **139**, 437.
COLONIAL MEDICAL RESEARCH COMMITTEE, 1949, Proguanil in prophylaxis and treatment. *Brit. med. J.*, **i**, 585.
COVELL, G., NICOL, W. D., SHUTE, P. G., and MARYON, M., 1949a, Paludrine (proguanil) in prophylaxis and treatment of malaria. *Brit. med. J.*, **i**, 88.
COVELL, G., NICOL, W. D., SHUTE, P. G., and MARYON, M., 1949b, Studies on a West African strain of *Plasmodium falciparum ;* the efficacy of paludrine as a therapeutic agent. *Trans. R. Soc. trop. Med. Hyg.*, **42**, 465.
CRAIGE, B., Jr., JONES, R., Jr., WHORTON, C. M., PULLMAN, T. N., ALVING, A. S., and EICHELBERGER, L., 1947, Clinical standardisation of pamaquin (plasmochin) in mosquito-induced vivax malaria, Chesson strain. *Amer. J. trop. Med.*, **27**, 309.
CSEH FIRTOS, S., 1949, Vivax malaria in the mental hospital, Franeker. *Doc. neerland. indon. Morb. trop.*, **1**, 258.
DAVEY, F., and SMITH, M., 1949, Malaria prophylaxis with proguanil. *Brit. med. J.*, **i**, 956.
DIXON, H. B. F., 1933, A report on 600 cases of malaria treated with plasmoquine and quinine. *J. R. Army med. Cps.*, **60**, 431.
DRENOWSKY, A. K., 1943, Einige Worte ueber die Chinoplasmin behandlung ambulanter Malariakranker. *Dtsch. tropenmed. Z.*, **47**, 51.
DURAND, P., SCHNEIDER, J., and DUPOUX, R., 1949, Traitément en un jour de l'accès de paludisme per la nivaquine. *Bull. Soc. Path. exot.*, **42**, 549.

EARLE, D. P., Jr., BERLINER, R. W., TAGGART, J. V., ZUBROD, C. G., WELCH, W. J., BIGELOW, F. S., KENNEDY, T. J., Jr., and SHANNON, J. A., 1948, Studies on the chemotherapy of the human malarias. X. The suppressive antimalarial effect of paludrine. *J. clin. Invest.*, 27, Suppl. p. 130.

EDESON, J. F. B., and FIELD, J. W., 1950, Proguanil-resistant falciparum malaria in Malaya. *Brit. med. J.*, i, 147.

EJERCITO, A., and DUQUE, M., 1948, Preliminary report on Cam-Aqi dihydro-chloride (miaquin, camoquin) in the treatment of human malaria. *J. Philipp. med. Ass.*, 24, 33.

FAIRLEY, N. H., 1945, Medicine in jungle warfare. *Proc. R. Soc. Med.*, 38, 195.

FAIRLEY, N. H., et. al., 1946, Researches on paludrine (M. 4888) in malaria. H. Appendix. Interim report on therapeutic trials in relapsing vivax malaria. Paludrine treatment followed by a maintenance dose (100 mgm.) twice weekly for six months. *Trans. R. Soc. trop. Med. Hyg.*, 40, 152.

FAIRLEY, N. H., BLACKBURN, C. R. B., BLACK, R. H., GREGORY, T. S., TONGE, J. I., POPE, K. S., DUNN, S. R., SWAN, M. S. A., AKHURST, T. A. F., MACKERRAS, M. J., LEMERLE, T. H., and ERCOLE, Q. N., 1946, Research on " paludrine " (M. 4888) in Australia. *Med. J. Aust.*, 1, 234.

FELDMAN, H. A., PACKER, H., MURPHY, F. D., and WATSON, R. B., 1947, Pamaquine naphthoate as prophylactic for malaria infections. *J. clin. Invest.*, 26, 77.

FERRO-LUZZI, G., 1948, La " paludrine " nella terapia della malaria in Eritrea. *Boll. Soc. ital. Med. Ig. trop.*, 8, 19.

FIELD, J. W., 1938, Notes on the chemotherapy of malaria. *Bull. inst. Med. Res.*, F.M.S. No. 2.

FIELD, J. W., and EDESON, J. F. B., 1949, Paludrine-resistant falciparum malaria. *Trans. R. Soc. trop. Med. Hyg.*, 43, 233.

FINDLAY, G. M., 1949a, Blackwater fever in West Africa, 1941–45. Part I. European troops. *Ann. trop. Med. Parasit.*, 43, 140.

FINDLAY, G. M., 1949b, Blackwater fever in West Africa, 1941–45. Part II. African troops. *Ann. trop. Med. Parasit.*, 43, 213.

FINDLAY, G. M., MARKSON, J. L., and HOLDEN, J. R., 1944a, Investigations in the chemotherapy of malaria in West Africa. I. Treatment with quinine and mepacrine. *Ann. trop. Med. Parasit.*, 38, 139.

FINDLAY, G. M., MARKSON, J. L., and HOLDEN, J. R., 1944b, Investigations in the chemotherapy of malaria in West Africa. II. Further investigations on treatment with quinine and mepacrine. *Ann. trop. Med. Parasit.*, 38, 201.

FINDLAY, G. M., and STEVENSON, A. C., 1945, Investigations in the chemotherapy of malaria in West Africa. Malaria suppression—quinine and mepacrine. *Ann. trop. Med. Parasit.*, 38, 168.

GORDON, H. H., CHRISTIANSON, H. B., and LIPPINCOTT, S. W., 1946, A comparison of quinine and quinacrine in the treatment of the clinical attacks of vivax malaria. *Sth. med. J.*, 39, 631.

GORDON, H. H., DIEUAIDE, F. R., MARBLE, A., CHRISTIANSON, H. B., and DAHL, L. K., 1947, Treatment of *Plasmodium vivax* malaria of foreign origin : a comparison of various drugs. *Arch. intern. Med.*, 79, 365.

HALAWANI, A., BAZI, I., and MORKOS, F., 1947, On the antimalarial activity of nivaquine C. *J. R. Egypt. med. Ass.*, 30, 665.

HANDFIELD-JONES, R. P. C., 1949, Chloroquine, proguanil, mepacrine and quinine in the treatment of malaria caused by *Plasmodium falciparum*. *Ann. trop. Med. Parasit.*, 43, 345.

HASEGAWA, S., 1949, Studies on the chemotherapy of tuberculosis. *Jap. J. exp. Med.*, 20, 69.

HAYMAN, J. M., Jr., MOST, H., LONDON, I. M., KANE, C. A., LAVIETES, P. H., and SCHROEDER, E. F., 1946a, Chloroquine (SN 7,618), a new highly effective antimalarial drug for routine use in the treatment of acute attacks of vivax malaria. *Trans. Ass. Amer. Phys.*, 59, 82.

HAYMAN, J. M., Jr., MOST, H., LONDON, I. M., KANE, C., LAVIETES, P. H., and SCHROEDER, E. F., 1946b, Combined quinine-plasmochine treatment of vivax malaria ; effect on relapse rate. Communication to the Assoc. Amer. Phys. 59th Ann. Meeting, Atlantic City, May 28th, quoted by Craige *et al.* (1947). *Amer. J. trop. Med.*, 27, 309.

HILL, E., and AMATUZIO, D. S., 1949, Southwest Pacific vivax malaria : clinical features and observations concerning duration of clinical activity. *Amer. J. trop. Med.*, 29, 203.

HULSHOFF, A. A., 1949, Nivaquine-plasmochinebehandeling bij M. tertiana. Een bijzonder geval van M. tertiana. *Ned. Tijdschr. Geneesk.*, 93i., 610.

INNES, J., and FENTON, J. C. B., 1945, A report on the work of No. 2 Malaria Research Team R.A.M.C., C.M.F., July. 1944–May, 1945. M.L.A. 87. (War Office D.M. (s) R.)

JAMES, S. P., NICOL, W. D., and SHUTE, P. G., 1932, A study of induced malignant tertian malaria. *Proc. R. Soc. Med.*, 25, 1153.

JARVIS, O. D., 1932a, Results of treatment of malaria by (a) plasmoquine and quinine and (b) atebrin, together with some observations on malaria convalescents. *J.R. Army med. Cps.*, 59, 190, 252.

JARVIS, O. D., 1932b, Further researches into the treatment of chronic benign tertian malaria with plasmoquine and quinine. *Indian J. med. Res.*, 20, 627.

JELLIFE, D. B., 1949, Proguanil prophylaxis and intercurrent infection. *Lancet, i*, 1052.

JOHNSTONE, R. D. C., 1946, Relapsing benign tertian malaria treated with paludrine. *Lancet, ii*, 825.

JONES, R., Jr., PULLMAN, T. N., WHORTON, C. M., CRAIGE, B., Jr., ALVING, A. S., and EICHELBERGER, L., 1948, The therapeutic effectiveness of large doses of paludrine in acute attacks of sporozoite-induced vivax malaria (Chesson strain). *J. clin. Invest.*, 27, Suppl. p. 51.

KAY, H. E. M., 1949, Resistance to proguanil. *Lancet, i*, 712.

KITCHEN, S. F., and PUTMAN, P., 1942, Observations on mechanisms in falciparum malaria. *Amer. J. trop. Med.*, 22, 361.

KLIGLER, I. J., and MER, G., 1931, Studies on malaria : relapse rate after quinine-plasmoquine treatment. *Trans. R. Soc. trop. Med. Hyg.*, 25, 121.

KLIGLER, I. J., SHAPIRO, J. M., and WEITZMAN, I., 1924, Malaria in rural settlements in Palestine. *J. Hyg., Camb.*, 23, 280.

KULCSAR, D. D., 1947, Effect of malaria on pregnancy. *Canad. med. Ass. J.*, 57, 32.

LEAGUE OF NATIONS MALARIA COMMISSION, FOURTH GENERAL REPORT, 1937, The treatment of malaria. Study of synthetic drugs, as compared with quinine, in the therapeutics and prophylaxis of malaria. *Bull. Health organ. L.o.N.*, 6, 895.

LOEB, R. F., CLARK, W. M., COATNEY, G. R., COGGESHALL, L. T., DIEUAIDE, F. R., DOCHEZ, A. R., HAKANSSON, E. G., MARSHALL, E. K., Jr., MARVEL, C. S., McCOY, O. R., SAPERO, J. J., SEBRELL, W. H., SHANNON, J. A., and CARDEN, G. A., Jr., 1946a, Activity of a new antimalarial agent, chloroquine (SN 7,618). *J. Amer. med. Ass.*, 130, 1069.

LOEB, R. F., CLARK, W. M., COATNEY, G. R., COGGESHALL, L. T., DIEUAIDE, F. R., DOCHEZ, A. R., HAKANSSON, E. G., MARSHALL, E. K., Jr., MARVEL, C. S., McCOY, O. R., SAPERO, J. J., SEBRELL, W. H., SHANNON, J. A., and CARDEN, G. A., Jr., 1946b, Activity of a new antimalarial agent, pentaquine (SN 13,276). Statement approved by the Board for Coordination of Malarial Studies. *J. Amer. med. Ass.*, 132, 321.

LONDON, I. M., KANE, C. A., SCHROEDER, E. F., and MOST, H., 1946, The delayed primary attack of vivax malaria. *New Engl. J. Med.*, 235, 406.

MACHELLA, T. E., FINE, R., and BURGOON, D. F., 1947a, The relationship of bromsulphalein retention to the fever of natural *P. falciparum* malaria. *Amer. J. med. Sci.*, 213, 81.

MACHELLA, T. E., KIMMELMAN, L. J., and LEWIS, R. A., 1947b, The intravenous administration of atabrine in falciparum malaria. *Bull. U.S. Army med. Dept.*, 7, 1000.

MAEGRAITH, B., ADAMS, A. R. D., ANDREWS, W. H. H., and TOTTEY, M., 1947, Relapse of benign tertian malaria during a course of 100 mgm. paludrine weekly. *Trans. R. Soc. trop. Med. Hyg.*, 40, 366.

MAEGRAITH, B., and ANDREWS, W. H. H., 1949, Proguanil and falciparum malaria. *Brit. med. J.*, i, 545.

MAIER, J., BANG, F. B., and HAIRSTON, N. G., 1948, A comparison of the effectiveness of quinacrine and quinine against falciparum malaria. *Amer. J. trop. Med.*, 28, 401.

MANFREDI, M., 1948, Prove di trattamento con paludrina (Farma 0105) nella malaria da vivax. *Acta med. ital.*, 3, 205.

MANIFOLD, J. A., 1931, Report on a trial of plasmoquine and quinine in the treatment of benign tertian malaria. *J. R. Army med. Cps.*, 56, 321, 410.

MARCIALIS, I., and CANNAS, E., 1937, Il metodo di Maurizio Ascoli nella cura della splenomegalia malarica nell' infanzia. *Pediatria.*, 45, 697.

MEDICAL RESEARCH COUNCIL, Malaria Sub-Committee, 1945, Report on relapsing vivax malaria. M.L.E., 30.

MONK, J. F., 1948a, Results of an investigation of the therapeutic action of paludrine and pamaquin on acute attacks of benign tertian malaria. *Trans. R. Soc. trop. Med. Hyg.*, 41, 657.

MONK, J. F., 1948b, Results of an investigation of the therapeutic action of pentaquin on acute attacks of benign tertian malaria. *Trans. R. Soc. trop. Med. Hyg.*, 41, 663.

MONK, J. F., 1948c, Modern therapy of benign tertian malaria. *Brit. med. J.*, i, 1221.

MONK, J. F., et al., 1946, A report on the work of No. 2 Malaria Research Team, R.A.M.C., at the Royal Herbert Hospital, Woolwich, October, 1945 —August, 1946. Unpublished Rept. War Office.

MOST, H., KANE, C. A., LAVIETES, P. K., LONDON, I. M., SCHROEDER, E. F., and HAYMAN, J. M., 1946a, Combined quinine-plasmochin treatment of vivax malaria effect of relapse rate. *Amer. J. med. Sci.*, 212, 550.

MOST, H., LONDON, I. M., KANE, C. A., LAVIETES, P. H., SCHROEDER, E. F., and HAYMAN, J. M., 1946b, Chloroquine for treatment of vivax malaria. *J. Amer. med. Ass.*, 131, 963.

NETHERLANDS HEALTH COUNCIL, 1932, REPORT OF MALARIA COMMISSION FOR 1930–31. *Versl. Med. Volksgezondh.*, p. 663.

NETHERLANDS HEALTH COUNCIL, 1938, REPORT OF MALARIA COMMISSION FOR 1936–7. *Versl. Med. Volksgezondh*, p. 435.

NETHERLANDS HEALTH COUNCIL, 1940, REPORT OF MALARIA COMMISSION FOR 1938–9. *Versl. Med. Volksgezondh*, p. 406.

NOE, W. L., GREENE, C. C., Jr., and CHENEY, G., 1946, The natural course of chronic southwest Pacific malaria. *Amer. J. med. Sci.*, 211, 215.

NUCCIOTTI, L., 1938, Ricerche sulla terapia adrenalinica nella malaria estivo-autunnale primitiva. *Riv. Malariol.*, 17, 131.

PACKER, H., 1947, Experimental field-type suppression with SN 7,618 (chloroquine), SN 8,137 and SN 12,837 (paludrine). *J. nat. mal. Soc.*, 6, 147.

PARROT, L., and CATANEI, A., 1949, La contamination palustre du nourrisson en milieu hyperendémique algérien. *Arch. Instit. Pasteur Algér.*, 27, 251.

PHEAR, A. G., 1920, The treatment of malaria in Macedonia. *Lancet*, i, 195.

PIEBENGA, P. J., 1932, De Malaria-Epidemieën in het Geneeskundig Gesticht te Franeker en de Gunstige invloed der Chinoplasminebehandeling. *Nedl. tjdschr. Geneesk.*, 76, 1564.

MALARIAL TREATMENT 503

PULLMAN, T. N., ALVING, A. S., JONES, R., Jr., WHORTON, C. M., CRAIGE,
B., Jr., and EICHELBERGER, L., 1948a, A study of the prophylactic, curative
and suppressive activity of SN 11,437 (metachloridine) in standardised
infections of vivax malaria. *Amer. J. trop. Med.*, **28**, 413.
PULLMAN, T. N., CRAIGE, B., Jr., ALVING, A. S., WHORTON, C. M., JONES,
R., Jr., and EICHELBERGER, L., 1948b, Comparison of chloroquine, quin-
acrine (atabrine), and quinine in the treatment of acute attacks of
sporozoite-induced vivax malaria (Chesson strain). *J. clin. Invest.*, **27**,
Suppl. p. 46.
RANSOME, G. A., 1948, Notes on the management of cases of cerebral malaria.
Proc. Alumni Ass. King Edward VII Coll. Med. Singapore, **1**, 23.
ROOK, H., DE., 1949, Prevention of malaria with proguanil in New Guinea.
Doc. nederdland. indon. Morb. trop., **1**, 160.
RUHE, D. S., COOPER, W. C., COATNEY, G. R., and JOSEPHSON, E. S., 1949,
Studies in human malaria. XV. The therapeutic action of pamaquine
(plasmochin) against St. Elizabeth strain vivax malaria. *Amer. J. Hyg.*,
49, 367.
SAPERO, J. J., 1947, New concepts in the treatment of relapsing malaria.
Amer. J. trop. Med., **27**, 272.
SCHNEIDER, J., and MÉCHALI, D., 1948, Traitement curatif du paludisme.
Etude de l'activité comparée de quatre nouveaux dérivés synthetiques.
Bull. Soc. Path. exot., **41**, 274.
SHANNON, J. A., 1945-46, The study of antimalarials and antimalarial activity
in the human malarias. *Harvey Lect.*, **41**, 43.
SINTON, J. A., 1939, Studies in immunity in malaria. Part VI. The effect of
drugs on the development of immunity and its relationship to the principles
of treatment. *J. Mal. Inst. India*, **2**, 191.
SINTON, J. A., and BIRD, W., 1928, Studies in malaria with special reference
to treatment. IX. Plasmoquine in the treatment of malaria. *Indian
J. med. Res.*, **16**, 159.
SINTON, J. A., and BIRD, W., 1929, Studies in malaria with special reference to
treatment. Part XI. The cinchona alkaloids in the treatment of benign
tertian malaria. *Indian J. med. Res.*, **16**, 725.
SINTON, J. A., SMITH, S., and POTTINGER, D., 1930, Studies in malaria with
special reference to treatment. Part XII. Further researches into the
treatment of chronic benign tertian malaria with plasmoquine and
quinine. *Indian J. Med. Res.*, **17**, 793.
SMITH, H. F., DY, F. J., and CABRERA, D. J., 1948, Studies on the efficiency
of chloroquine and chlorguanide as antimalarials. I. As suppressants.
Acta med. Philipp., **5**, No. 2, 1.
SPICKNALL, C. G., and TERRY, L. L., 1948, Combined quinine-plasmochin and
quinine-pentaquine treatment of relapsing vivax malaria. *Sth. med. J.*,
41, 338.
SRIVASTAVA, R. S., 1947, Final report on the field trials of " paludrine " in
selected hyperendemic malarious areas of Naini Tal Tarai in the United
Provinces (September 11th to December 31st, 1946). *Indian J. Malariol.*,
1, 361.
STRAUS, B., and GENNIS, J., 1948, Evaluation of pentaquine as a cure of
relapsing vivax malaria ; a controlled study of ninety-five cases. *Bull.
New York Acad. Med.*, **24**, 395.
SURGEON-GENERAL, UNITED STATES ARMY, 1943, The drug treatment of
malaria, suppressive and clinical. *J. Amer. med. Ass.*, **123**, 205.
SWELLENGREBEL, N. H., and BUCK, A. DE, 1932, Plasmoquine prophylaxis in
benign tertian malaria. *Proc. R. Acad. Sci. Amsterdam*, **35**, 911.
TRAGER, W., BANG, F. B., and HAIRSTON, N. G., 1947, The effect of four
different therapies on the relapse rate of vivax malaria. *Amer. J. Hyg.*,
45, 43.
WALLACE, R. B., 1949, Mass suppression with chloroquine : chloroquine and
pentaquine and neo-premaline. *J. trop. Med. Hyg.*, **52**, 93.

WALLACE, R. B., 1950, Mass suppression with chloroquine ; chloroquine and pentaquine and neo-premaline. *Med. J. Malaya*, 4, 190.
WALTON, G. A., 1948, Incidence of malaria in tropical Africa. *Nature, Lond.*, 162, 114.
WARTHIN, T. A., LEVINE, S. A., and EVANS, R. R., 1948, Observations on treatment with chloroquine (SN 7,618) and combined quinine and plasmochin. *New Engl. J. Med.*, 238, 467.
WHITE, W. C., COOPER, W. C., COATNEY, G. R., CULWELL, W. B., LINTS, H. A., and YOUNG, M. D., 1948, Studies on malaria in man. XXI. The cure of vivax malaria, St. Elizabeth strain, by the association of penta-quine-quinine administered during acute attacks or latent periods. *J. Nat. Mal. Soc.*, 7, 316.
WINCKEL, C. W. F., 1949, The efficacy of quinacrine and quinine in the treatment of *Plasmodium malariæ* infections. *Doc. nederdland. indon. Morb. trop.*, 1, 93.
WOODRUFF, A. W., 1947, The suppressive and schizonticidal value of palu-drine (100 mgm.) in vivax malaria. *Trans. R. Soc. trop. Med. Hyg.*, 41, 263.
WYNNE-GRIFFITH, G., 1947, Suppression of malaria by mepacrine. *J. R. Army med. Cps.*, 89, 112.
YOUNG, M. D., and EYLES, D. E., 1948, The efficacy of chloroquine, quinacrine, quinine and totaquine in the treatment of *Plasmodium malariæ* infections (quartan malariæ). *Amer. J. trop. Med.*, 28, 23.
YOUNG, M. D., EYLES, D. E., and BURGESS, R. W., 1949, Studies on imported malaria. 10. An evaluation of the foreign malarias introduced into the United States by returning troops. *J. nat. Mal. Soc.*, 7, 171.

CHAPTER XI
THE MODE OF ACTION OF ANTIMALARIAL DRUGS

As in the case of other chemotherapeutic drugs, the action of any antimalarial compound depends on the interaction of the parasite, the host, and the drug.

The Parasite. Attention has already been drawn to the differences in reaction to the same drug of different species of plasmodia, of different strains of the same species of plasmodia, and of the different stages of the same malarial parasite. The infecting dose of the parasite may also determine the therapeutic response ; in chickens aged three weeks, for instance, the maximal infecting dose of *P. gallinaceum* which can be controlled by intramuscular injections of 2-hydroxy-3-β-decalyl-propyl-1, 4-naphthoquinone, begun before the injection of the parasite, is twenty million parasitised red cells (Clarke and Theiler, 1948). The effect of pamaquin in the chick varies with the infecting dose of sporozoites (Greenberg *et al.*, 1950).

The Host may possess natural or acquired resistance or specific immunity which either inhibits the parasite from developing or prevents the appearance of clinical symptoms. The natural resistance of the negro to *P. vivax* infections is now well recognised. In addition there are well-marked differences in the response to treatment of primary and subsequent attacks of vivax malaria, whether the infection is therapeutically or naturally induced (Bang *et al.*, 1947). Some degree of immunity tends to occur whenever malarial parasites are introduced into the body unless the sporozoites are directly destroyed before any of the host's cells are infected. A drug which possibly has such an action on sporozoites is 2-hydroxy-3-β-decalyl-propyl-1, 4-naphthoquinone if it is present in the blood before the introduction of the sporozoites of *P. gallinaceum*.

The condition of the host's reticulo-endothelial system is probably of considerable importance. Kritschewski and Demidowa (1934), for instance, believe that the activity of malarial drugs is greatly reduced by blocking the reticulo-endothelial system with trypan blue. Such non-specific factors, of which little is yet known, may explain the widely differing reactions to malaria shown by persons infected with the same strain of plasmodium.

The Drug. The therapeutic potentialities of a drug are greatly influenced by such factors as its route of introduction. Intramuscular injection of hydroxynaphthoquinones leads to higher and longer-sustained plasma levels than oral administration and hence to greater efficiency. Quinine is three or four times as effective in one daily dose as when given continuously in lophuræ infection in ducks but not in cynomolgi malaria in monkeys (Marshall, 1949). Each individual tends to have a particular therapeutic pattern so that a similar blood concentration curve is repeated whenever the drug is administered. Dietary deficiencies may play some *rôle* in influencing the blood concentration curves of drugs and in affecting the development of the parasite. McKee and Geiman (1948) show that starving monkeys inhibit the growth of *P. knowlesi ;* the effects of fasting are counteracted by DL methionine but not by sucrose or sucrose and ascorbic acid. *In vitro* the growth of *P. knowlesi* is inhibited by methionine analogues such as methoxinine or ethionine. It should be noted that in man, unlike experimental animals, multiple food deficiencies are almost always present. Finally, the phenomenon of biological interference, well recognised in connection with viruses, may also play some part in influencing infection and therapeutic response. When *P. vivax* and *P. falciparum* are inoculated at the same time the vivax infection is suppressed and it is the falciparum infection which develops.

In an attempt to understand the way in which antimalarial drugs act on the parasite three techniques have been adopted :—

(1) The morphological changes induced in malarial parasites by drugs have been studied *in vivo* and *in vitro* : these changes can be correlated with the subsequent powers of development of the plasmodia.

(2) The chemical constitution of antimalarial drugs has been examined and the effect of changes in the molecular constitution of such drugs has been correlated with antimalarial action.

(3) The biochemical lesion has been sought by studying what links in the metabolic chain of malarial parasites are inhibited or depressed by antimalarial drugs. This involves a knowledge of the metabolic processes characteristic of all stages of malarial plasmodia.

Morphological Changes in Malarial Parasites

There is considerable evidence to show that antimalarial drugs have a direct action on the asexual erythrocytic stages of malarial parasites.

Mühlens and Kirschbaum (1924) found that blood containing *P. vivax* and quinine at a concentration of 1 in 5,000 was still infective for man after it had been incubated for five hours. Lourie (1934) similarly added quinine in the same concentration to canary blood containing *P. cathemerium* and incubated the mixture for one hour ; there was some delay in the development of infection when the blood was injected into canaries. Peter (1932) was probably the first to examine the effects of mepacrine on *P. vivax*. He believed that at first it destroyed rings, then schizonts, and finally gametocytes. Chopra *et al.* (1936) incubated monkey blood containing *P. knowlesi* trophozoites with mepacrine for twenty-four hours. When the incubated blood was injected into monkeys only one of three developed malaria. As, however, the concentration of mepacrine in the incubated blood was 20,000 μgm. per litre it was considerably in excess of any concentration which would normally be met with in the blood as a result of therapeutic dosage. The observations of Fischl and Singer (1934), and Bock and Oesterlin (1939) showed that the plasmodia of avian and simian malaria fix a number of fluorescent dyes, including mepacrine. Oesterlin (1936) thought that a strong basic group was essential for fixation of a dye, the subsequent lethal action being associated with the properties causing fluorescence.

Asexual Parasites. Morphological changes have been reported in the blood of patients or experimental animals given therapeutic doses of antimalarial drugs. Wenyon (1926), after quinine, noted decrease in size in the schizonts of *P. vivax* and a reduction in the number of merozoites produced. In canaries infected with *P.*

cathemerium quinine appears to cause a retardation in the growth rate of the parasites as well as the formation of a smaller number of merozoites. James (1934) showed that a single dose of 0·6 gm. mepacrine caused morphological changes in the erythrocytic forms of vivax and quartan malaria. The pigment becomes aggregated into clumps and rapidly disappears while the cytoplasm becomes ragged and also eventually disappears. The nuclear vacuole is distended, the chromatin opens up and becomes diffused till only a few stained dots remain. Bock (1939), Hühne (1942), and others confirmed these findings with mepacrine in human malaria, while Mosna (1936) and Chopra *et al.* (1936) observed similar morphological changes in *P. knowlesi*. Mosna showed that quinine had a very similar action to that of mepacrine on the blood forms of *P. knowlesi*, thus confirming the earlier work of Thomson and McLellan (1912) and Dudgeon and Clarke (1917) who, in discussing their cultivation of malaria parasites, believed that quinine in the patients' sera had adversely influenced the development of the parasites. Bass (1922) reported that by adding quinine in a dilution of 1 in 2,700 to a culture of *P. falciparum* he had prevented the growth of the parasites and caused their death. Hewitt and Richardson (1943) added drugs both in powder form and in solution to blood infected with *P. lophuræ* and incubated at 6° C. Degenerative changes were not seen when quinine or mepacrine were the drugs used, but were present when pamaquin was added. The degenerative changes were similar to those observed when infected ducks were treated with pamaquin.

The inhibitory action of quinine *in vivo* on the rate of reproduction of the asexual blood forms was studied also in *P. cathemerium* infections by Boyd and Dunn (1939) ; the inhibitory action of pamaquin was investigated by these observers and that of mepacrine by Boyd and Dunn (1941). With all these drugs there occurs a retardation in the rate of asexual reproduction and a reduction in the number of merozoites. No evidence of an increased rate of destruction by phagocytes was noted ; in fa ct treated birds exhibit a decreased rate of parasite destruction as compared with controls. Trager *et al.* (1945) showed that *P. vivax* lost its amœboid activity in an hour after an intramuscular injection of mepacrine into a patient. Some parasites regained their motility when the concentration of mepacrine in the plasma had fallen.

The most extensive studies on *P. vivax* have been made by Mackerras and Ercole (1949a) with quinine, mepacrine, and pamaquin, the drugs being given to volunteers infected with a New Guinea strain of *P. vivax*.

Quinine was given in doses of 2 gm. daily for three days. Young rings were reduced in numbers and their growth was retarded. Bizarre forms appeared and small degenerating parasites were closely applied to the edge of the red cell. After forty-four hours, when growth should have been complete, there remained half-grown amœboid forms, many without pigment. By seventy-six hours all asexual forms had disappeared. Larger trophozoites showed arrest of development and degenerative nuclear changes. No true schizonts were seen after the first dose of quinine and all large asexual forms had disappeared in sixteen hours. Normal and abnormal gametocytes were noted, but mosquitoes could be infected on each of the three days on which quinine was given, although the growth of young gametocytes was retarded. Daily doses of 0·66 gm. quinine merely diminished the rate of multiplication of the parasites.

Mepacrine. A dose of 1·0 gm. on the first day was followed by 0·4 gm. daily for six days. Two hours after the first dose of 0·5 gm. amœboid forms were still active but showed abnormal clumping of the pigment and occasional fragmentation of the cytoplasm. In a few young rings the cytoplasm was pale and indistinct. After four hours no amœboid movement was seen and at six hours all rings were abnormal. At eight hours some half-grown amœboids had extruded pigment from their cytoplasm or even from the red cell. At sixteen hours young rings were represented by marginal forms or pale wisps of cytoplasm detached from nuclei. Many parasites were extruded from red cells. Gametocytes at first increased in numbers and were infective for four days. The percentage of male gametocytes fell and by the fifth day none could be recognised.

Pamaquin was given in doses of 30 mgm. daily for five days. Schizogony occurred daily for four days and ceased on the fifth day in one patient but in another no schizogony was observed during treatment. Some rings contracted into small solid lumps, but more usually the vacuole increased in size until the parasite was only a thin ring of cytoplasm. In many amœboid forms the chromatin fragments had disappeared and the cytoplasm appeared pale and ragged. Similar changes were noted in the larger parasites, the nuclei, broken into ill-defined masses, merging with the cytoplasm. Some parasites which were not killed tended to round up and divide before reaching full size so that many very small schizonts were formed. A single dose of 10 mgm. of pamaquin appeared to cause gametocytes to lose their infectivity in forty-two hours ; before that, the percentage of cysts dying and becoming chitinised increased from batch to batch, but sufficient normal gametocytes remained to induce infection in mosquitoes. It would thus seem that quinine and mepacrine act similarly only on stages which are still metabolising hæmoglobin. It is uncertain what happens to schizonts under the influence of the drug between cessation of growth and sporulation ; some apparently may complete schizogony. Pamaquin, on the other hand, affects all stages, irrespective of whether they are metabolising hæmoglobin or not, and irrespective of growth. Gametocytes and pre-erythrocytic stages are also attacked. Pamaquin thus seems to act as a general protoplasmic poison.

Camoquin was shown by Thompson (1948) to produce morphological changes in the asexual stages of *P. lophuræ* when added to the diet in concentrations of 0·001 to 0·0013 per cent. Intracellular pigment became clumped to form a homogeneous greenish yellow mass. Chloroquine had a similar effect.

Hydroxynaphthoquinones, according to Clarke and Theiler (1948), appear to act in the same way as mepacrine on the asexual blood forms of *P. gallinaceum,* for they cause a pronounced retardation in the rate of transition from one form to another and a tendency towards the accumulation of a disproportionately large proportion of parasites of small and intermediate size. Very similar results were observed *in vivo* by Mackerras and Ercole (1947) from the action of proguanil on the trophozoites of *P. vivax.* The trophozoites may grow to full size and the lethal action is exerted only on the dividing nucleus in which the chromatin breaks up into irregular diffuse masses. With the trophozoites of *P.*

malariæ schizogony may occur up to the twentieth hour after beginning therapy, and on low doses of the drug the resulting merozoites may grow to full size before being destroyed. Young *et al.* (1943) found that thiobismol inhibited the further development of half-grown trophozoites of *P. vivax.*

These observations may be compared with those made by Black (1946a and b) in tissue cultures on the schizonts of *P. falciparum* with quinine, mepacrine, pamaquin, sontoquine (SN 6,911), chloroquine, proguanil, 4430, sulphadiazine, and sulphamerazine.

The results may be summarised as follows :—

Quinine. When the parasites were grown in serum containing between 6·0 and 8·8 mgm. of quinine base per litre the development of three strains of the parasite did not progress beyond the pre-schizont stage and the forms then present, ring, amœboid, and a few pre-schizonts, degenerated and fragmented with the formation of ghost cells from the containing red cells. Parasites of the fourth strain did undergo schizogony with re-entry of red cells by merozoites, but the cycle was retarded and the number of schizonts formed was less than in control cultures.

Mepacrine. When parasites were grown in serum mepacrine levels up to 120 μgm. per litre there was no effect on the development of parasites, but with higher concentrations up to 190 μgm. and 300 μgm. per litre there was no development beyond the amœboid stage. The amœboid forms degenerated with loss of definition in the staining of the cytoplasm and eventually underwent disintegration. Many ring forms degenerated without undergoing any development. The red cells containing these parasite fragments ruptured and became ghost cells.

Pamaquin. A donor was given 0·02 gm. of pamaquin, expressed as base, two-hourly for four doses. He was then bled three hours after the last dose. Two cultures with different strains of *P. falciparum* grown in this serum exhibited somewhat different results. One strain showed no development beyond a few amœboid forms, the other completed the cycle after considerable delay in the early stages.

Sontoquine, as the bisulphate, was given to a donor so that the concentration in the plasma was of the order of 300 μgm. per litre. The changes were similar to those seen with higher concentrations of mepacrine. A few amœboid forms appeared and then these and the ring forms degenerated leaving chromatin in the red cells.

Chloroquine as the diphosphate was given to donors to secure a calculated plasma concentration of 200 to 300 μgm. per litre. Very few amœboid forms developed ; these and the ring forms showed disintegration of the cytoplasm, leaving only chromatin material in the containing red cells.

Proguanil. With proguanil in the plasma the developmental cycle proceeded as in control cultures till the early stages of schizogony were reached ; then cultures containing proguanil ceased to develop. The scattered chromatin became rather granular instead of dividing into definite segments. The parasite and its containing red cell became swollen and vacuoles appeared in the cytoplasm.

Similar changes produced by proguanil have been noted in vivax parasites in the blood of patients given a therapeutic course of the drug.

Degenerate early schizonts may be seen in the red cells of the marrow when sternal puncture is performed on patients with falciparum malaria fifty-two hours after the commencement of proguanil therapy and occasionally in the circulation.

Trophozoites (ring forms) of *P. falciparum*, after exposure for about three hours to proguanil in a treated patient, develop normally when cultivated in normal serum but are arrested at the early schizont stage if grown in the serum of a patient who has received 100 mgm. of proguanil four hours before the cultures were set up.

Similar results with proguanil activated by the serum of fowl or monkeys were reported by Hawking and Perry (1948) on *P. cynomolgi*. In addition to their failure to develop into mature schizonts the parasites suffered a series of degenerative changes. A few of the parasites were small, with one piece of very darkly staining chromatin and having a minimum of cytoplasm, also darkly stained, closely packed round the chromatin. Other parasites had the same small mass of dense chromatin but poorly stained pinkish cytoplasm, thinned out and almost translucent ; many other parasites exhibited a different appearance. The cytoplasm was disrupted and often arranged in narrow dark-staining threads, the chromatin being represented by one or more dark-staining lumps. The cytoplasmic threads were scattered throughout the corpuscles and sometimes woven into fantastic patterns or completely separated from the chromatin mass, which was thus denuded of cytoplasm.

This series of changes was more common in samples withdrawn from culture tubes after incubation for forty-two hours than in samples withdrawn after only twenty hours.

The clinical importance of the fact that proguanil exerts its action on trophozoites only at the earliest stage of chromatin division of *P. falciparum* is emphasised by Black (1949). The trophozoites anchored within the cerebral capillaries and causing cerebral symptoms are in the later stages when they are not susceptible to proguanil.

M 4430. Similar results to those with proguanil were seen in tissue culture when serum was used from a patient given 400 mgm. of this drug per day.

Sulphonamides. With serum containing 13·7 mgm. of sulpha-diazine per 100 ml. parasites grew normally up to the stage of division of the chromatin into definite segments. Then the majority of the schizonts degenerated while the cytoplasm developed vacuoles and lost its blue colour with Leishman's stain. The chromatin segments became irregular and eventually ghosts of red cells were seen containing parasites only. A few rings of the second generation appeared showing that all schizonts had not disappeared. With sulphamerazine in the serum in a concentration of 16·9 mgm. per ml. parasites were slow in developing ; most schizonts degenerated and only a few rings of the second generation appeared.

It is therefore obvious that with a number of antimalarial drugs direct action on the parasites can be demonstrated ; in this action neither leucocytes, reticulo-endothelial cells nor immune bodies necessarily play any active part as shown in tissue culture, though they undoubtedly do so *in vivo*.

Thus quinine, mepacrine, chloroquine, and sontoquine exert an action on the early stages of the schizogonous cycle of *P. falciparum*, whereas proguanil and M 4430 act on a later stage when the chromatin of the schizont is dividing and the sulphonamides act on the divided schizont. If schizogony can occur in tissue culture, merozoites will invade fresh red cells and rings of the second generation will be seen.

Exo-erythrocytic Forms. The effect of drugs on the morphology of the exo-erythrocytic forms of human malarial parasites has not yet been reported, but the action of a number of drugs on the exo-erythrocytic forms of *P. gallinaceum* in chicken spleen cultures has been investigated by Tonkin (1946). The limitation to this method is that certain compounds such as mepacrine, stilbamidine, M 4430, chloroquine, pamaquin, and proguanil are very toxic to the cells and are inactive in the highest concentrations tolerated by the macrophages. Quinine had a slight action on the development of the exo-erythrocytic forms but was toxic to macrophages.

The drugs which inhibit the growth of the parasites and the minimum concentration inhibiting growth are shown in the table.

INHIBITION OF GROWTH OF EXO-ERYTHROCYTIC FORMS OF *Plasmodium gallinaceum* IN TISSUE CULTURE (Tonkin, 1946)

Drug	Minimum inhibitory concentration in mgm. per 100 ml.
Sulphathiazole	0·05
Sulphadiazine	0·1
m-Aminobenzenesulphonamidopyrimidine	0·1
Streptothricin	2·5 (10 units per ml.)
Streptomycin	250 (500 units per ml.)
p-Anisylguanidine nitrate . . .	0·5

p-Anisylguanidine nitrate is the most active of the series of guanidines and biguanidines made for testing on malarial infections (King and Tonkin, 1946). In addition to its inhibition of further growth in tissue culture the effect of sulphathiazole on parasites already grown in tissue culture was studied. Sulphathiazole has a gradual effect on the parasites, reducing their powers of division. The larger schizonts still remaining after three days' exposure show pathological changes for the chromatin coalesces into lumps, the parasite envelope becomes indistinct, and the cytoplasm develops vacuoles and loses its power to stain. In later stages the chromatin appears as indistinct collections of small granules.

With length of exposure from one to five days, the number of schizonts with eight nuclei gradually increases.

These changes are associated with loss of ability on the part of the parasites to infect chicks.

Coulston and Huff (1948) studied the effects of various drugs on the exo-erythrocytic forms of *P. gallinaceum*, distinguishing between cryptozoites and metacryptozoites. When sulphadiazine, sulphamerazine, sulphapyrazine, metanilamide and a naphthoquinone, 2-[3'-(decahydro-2 1-naphthyl)propyl]-3 hydroxy-1, 4-naphthoquinone, were fed to chickens in concentrations of from 0·05 to 4·0 per cent. the blood concentrations were many times that required to prevent the development of a blood infection. Despite this high concentration of drug, cryptozoite development occurred in the skin and spleen. Morphologically the cryptozoites appeared normal and only occasionally were abnormal forms seen ; these abnormal forms were vacuolar and irregular in size. Badly damaged cryptozoites were most common in animals treated with sulphadiazine and the naphthoquinone ; there was, however, no reduction in the number of cryptozoites. The effect of the drugs on the metacryptozoites was more apparent and it appeared as if the drugs acted on the cryptozoic merozoites just as they were released into the tissue spaces so that they died as they were being phagocytosed. The parasites appear vacuolated, are smaller in size than normal, and their numbers are greatly reduced.

Drugs which are merely suppressive only on *P. gallinaceum*, such as quinine, mepacrine, chloroquine, pamaquin, and pentaquine, also produce changes in the cryptozoites and metacryptozoites, but these are much less than those produced by drugs with a prophylactic action. Except for frequent abnormal schizonts they appeared similar to the exo-erythrocytic stages seen in control birds untreated by drugs.

Gametocytes. The effect of small doses of pamaquin on the gametocytes of *P. falciparum* and *P. cathemerium* was first described by Barber *et al.* (1929), Wampler (1930), and Jerace and Giovannola (1933). Mackerras and Ercole (1949b) found that after a single dose of 10 mgm. mosquitoes became infected three but not fifteen hours after administration. During the first six hours numerous oöcysts were formed but the sporozoite rate decreased ; at nine hours the number of oöcysts in the gut decreased and many of these failed to develop ; after fifteen hours very few oöcysts developed and no gland infections were detected. Missiroli and Mosna (1938) observed a similar action on the gametocytes of *P. falciparum* with certuna (cilional). When small doses are used exflagellation is prevented, and when very minute doses are used, though fertilisation of the gametes in the mosquito occurs, yet the formation of oöcysts is inhibited. The effect is similar to that observed with proguanil.

Mepacrine is known to have some slight action on the sexual forms of *P. vivax* and *P. malariæ*, but in the case of *P. falciparum* a number of observers have denied that mepacrine has any action on the gametocytes. This appears to be correct when the drug is given to a patient showing mature crescents in the peripheral blood stream, for no morphological changes are seen in the gametocytes and they are still capable of causing transmissible infection in mosquitoes. Sinton (1938), however, brought forward evidence to show that mepacrine has some action on gametocytes if it is present in the peripheral blood stream before the crescents appear. Morphological changes then appear in the immature stages of the sexual forms. The majority of the gametocytes as first seen show pigment aggregated into a single solid mass. Many crescents are immature, a few are normal, but others show signs of clumping of the pigment. After a day or two the forms with large pigment blocks become relatively scanty, their place being taken by crescents showing either very little pigment grouped as a few jet-black blocks or granules or a complete absence of pigment. Thereafter the number of pigmentless crescents tends to diminish, those with scanty pigment increase in relative frequency. Some pigment-free forms have a large block of extra-cellular pigment attached to one pole suggesting that it must have been extruded from the crescent. Mepacrine apparently causes clumping of the pigment in immature gametocytes and pigment-less forms ; these pigmentless forms are, however, quite capable of carrying on the sexual cycle in the mosquito and forming oöcysts.

Mackerras and Ercole (1949b) also studied the effects of quinine, mepacrine, and pamaquin on the gametocytes of *P. falciparum*.

The number of gametocytes produced when quinine is used for partial or full therapy is very much lower than when mepacrine is given. Similar results were obtained by Sinton (1938). With mepacrine a high proportion of the gametocytes are partially or wholly unpigmented but are otherwise normal and capable of infecting mosquitoes. The relatively mepacrine-resistant strain of *P. falciparum* from the Wewak area of New Guinea rarely produces more than 50 per cent. of unpigmented or lightly pigmented gametocytes. Sinton (1938) believed that the pigment was formed but was extruded under the influence of mepacrine, but Mackerras and Ercole (1949b) failed to find any actual extrusion of pigment. The unpigmented gametocytes behaved quite normally ; unpigmented zygotes developed at a normal rate, forming unpigmented vermicules which in turn produced unpigmented cysts.

The failure of proguanil to produce morphological changes in the gametocytes of human malarial parasites has already been mentioned (Mackerras and Ercole, 1947 ; Shute and Maryon, 1948), although oöcyst formation in the mosquito is inhibited to a very large extent, if not always completely. Terzian and Weathersby (1949) also observed inhibition of oöcyst formation by proguanil.

The Sexual Cycle in the Mosquito. Until recently there was little to show whether the developmental cycle of the malaria parasite in the mosquito could be influenced by drugs taken up by the insects themselves. Now, two techniques have been developed ; in the first chemotherapeutic drugs are given to the vertebrate host so that when the mosquito takes a blood meal it imbibes a concentration of the drug. By subsequent dissection of the mosquito it is possible to examine the developmental stages of the parasites in the insect's stomach wall and salivary glands. The second technique consists in adding the drug to the food of the insect subsequent to the infecting blood meal and dissecting insects at intervals (Johnson and Akins, 1948). By the former technique it has been possible to show that proguanil inhibits the development of the oöcyst but, as Johnson and Akins (1948) have proved, if proguanil is withheld till sporozoites have appeared in the salivary glands then its administration for five days produces no effect on the sporozoites. Geigy and Rahm

518 MODE OF ACTION OF ANTIMALARIAL DRUGS

(1949), however, claim that proguanil destroys sporozoites in fully-formed oöcysts. Mepacrine in a concentration of 0·09 per cent. in honey water fed to females is also said to inhibit oöcyst formation. One factor which has not been fully considered is the adequacy of the diet given to the mosquitoes after their infective blood meal. If the food consists only of carbohydrate there may be a reduction in the number of sporozoites produced (Mackerras and Ercole, 1948).

By incorporating drugs in the food for fourteen to twenty days after an infective blood meal, Johnson and Akins (1948) found that mepacrine dihydrochloride in concentrations of 0·15 to 1·3 gm. per litre, pamaquin naphthoate 11·2 to 67 mgm. per litre, and chloroquine base 0·25 to 2 gm. per litre had no effect on the development of sporozoites of *P. gallinaceum* in *Aëdes ægypti*: on the other hand, quinine sulphate in a concentration of 0·67 to 1·33 gm. per litre and proguanil hydrochloride, 0·218 to 0·435 gm. per litre, provided it was given immediately after the infecting blood feed, had a considerable inhibitory action. Chloroquine base was found to be very toxic for mosquitoes, but despite its toxicity it did not inhibit the development of sporozoites. These results, shown in the table opposite, are at variance with some of those obtained by Terzian *et al.* (1949), using both *P. gallinaceum* in *A. ægypti* and *P. falciparum* in *Anopheles quadrimaculatus*. Sulphadiazine, metachloridine, and proguanil, which have a true causal prophylactic action on *P. gallinaceum* in the vertebrate host, have a similar action in the insect host, since they permanently arrest the development of oöcysts and inhibit the formation of sporozoites. Quinine, mepacrine, and pamaquin, which are not true causal prophylactics in man, except in the case of pamaquin in toxic doses, do not act on the oöcyst, but pamaquin is effective only against sporozoites free from the oöcyst. *p*-Aminobenzoic acid given in sufficient concentration together with prophylactic concentrations of sulphadiazine and metachloridine antagonises their inhibitory action just as it does in the vertebrate host. As would be expected, the action of proguanil is not affected by the coincident administration of *p*-aminobenzoic acid. Quinine, mepacrine, sontoquine, and sulphadiazine have no effect on oöcyst development or sporozoite formation in *Anopheles quadrimaculatus* (Terzian and Weathersby, 1949).

The time of administration of the drugs in relation to the infective blood meal, the length of the period of administration, and the concentration are all factors influencing drug effectiveness.

THE EFFECT OF VARIOUS DRUGS ON THE SPOROGONOUS CYCLE OF *P. gallinaceum* IN *Aëdes ægypti* AS DETERMINED BY DISSECTION AND SUBSEQUENT INOCULATION INTO CHICKS (Terzian *et al.*, 1949)

Drug.	Sporozoite density in mosquitoes.	Drug concentration, gm. per 100 ml.	Average percentage of chick red cells parasitised (days after inoculation).					Number of survivors.
			8	10	12	14	16	
Quinine	4 +	0·05	+	20·2	28·0	2·0	—	1/6
Mepacrine	1 +	0·02	+	36·5	46·1	—	—	0/6
Sontoquine (SN 6,911) .	4 +	0·05	1·6	33·4	28·0	—	—	1/5
Chloroquine (SN 7,618) . .	4 +	0·03	3·2	11·8	23·0	—	—	0/6
1 - (7 - Chloro - 4' - quinolyl - amino) - 3 diethylamino - 2 - propanol (SN 8,137) . .	4 +	0·1	2·7	26·8	32·0	12·0	—	1/6
7 - Chloro - 4 - (3 - diethyl - aminopropylamino) quinoline (SN 9,584) . . .	4 +	0·05	+	15·9	26·2	—	—	0/6
4 - (7 - Chloro - 4 - quinolyl - amino) - α - diethylamino-*o*-cresol (SN 10,751) .	4 +	0·05	3·0	22·1	48·0	—	—	0/6
Pamaquin . . .	2 +	0·03	0	+	9·3	18·6	13·1	2/6
Metachloridine . .	0	0·01	0	0	0	0	0	6/6
Proguanil . . .	0	0·01	0	0	0	0	0	6/6
Sulphadiazine . . .	0	0·01	0	0	0	0	0	6/6
Controls	4 +	0·1	+	35·8	24·0	—	—	2/6

Chemical Constitution and Antimalarial Action

From what has been said it is obvious that the erythrocytic stages of malarial parasites can be influenced by a considerable number of drugs of widely differing chemical constitution. The exo-erythrocytic forms of certain malarial parasites can be destroyed by a smaller number of drugs, 8-aminoquinolines, sulphonamides, biguanides, and hydroxynaphthoquinones. The gametocytes are directly attacked only by 8-aminoquinolines and the sporozoites especially by 2-hydroxy-3-β-decalyl-propyl-1, 4-naphthoquinone and 8-aminoquinolines such as pamaquin : metachloridine, proguanil, and sulphadiazine affect particular stages of the oöcyst.

To attempt to correlate chemical constitution and antimalarial action has so far proved an impossible task. Many theories have been proposed which at first seemed to provide clues that might lead to an all-embracing explanation. Further studies and the discovery of ever-new antimalarial drugs have shown that these theories hold good, if at all, only in very limited fields.

At first attention was perforce focussed on the cinchona alkaloids. No obvious relationship between optical activity and antimalarial action could be deduced. It was soon realised, however, that small structural changes in the basic constitution of the cinchona alkaloids could cause inactivity, especially changes in the —CHOH— group, which links up the two parts of the cinchona alkaloids and involves changes in spatial distribution. These findings and the alteration in activity shown by successive members of homologous series merely led to the conclusion that there must obviously be a close " fit " between the drug and the enzyme groups in the malarial parasites.

The discovery of pamaquin, which is an 8-aminoquinoline, at first emphasised the importance of the quinoline nucleus for antimalarial action. At least five of the most effective antimalarials are quinolines : pamaquin, pentaquine, rhodoquine, chloroquine, and sontoquine. Among these five compounds three types of side-chain occur : δ-diethyl-amino-α-methyl-butylamino- for pamaquin, chloroquine and sontoquine, γ-diethylaminopropyl-amino- for rhodoquine and ω-*iso*propylamino- for pentaquine. Pamaquin, rhodoquine, and pentaquine are alike also in having the side-chain attached to position 8 of the nucleus and in possessing a methoxy group in position 6, an arrangement modified in chloroquine and sontoquine where the side-chain is in position 4 and no methoxy group is present. Thus, as Gray and Hill (1949) have emphasised, the range of structure among the quinoline antimalarials is undoubtedly limited.

The discovery of mepacrine, however, in which the dialkyl-aminoalkylamino side-chain is retained but the acridine is substituted for the quinoline nucleus prompted the views of Magidson *et al.* (1934) and Magidson and Grigorowsky (1936), who suggested that different parts of the molecule have different functions. The basic side-chain is primarily of pharmacological importance, controlling absorption and distribution of the drug in the host and aiding its penetration into the parasite and up to the particular point in the metabolic chain where toxic action is exerted : parasiticidal action is the function of the substituted acridine or quinoline nucleus.

The quinoline nucleus of pamaquin and the acridine nucleus of mepacrine are, however, heterocyclic systems which are foreign to the animal body. Curd and Rose (1946a) then considered that less toxic antimalarials might be prepared with a ring system of biological importance.

Pyrimidine derivatives were therefore selected on the ground that pyrimidines are important in building up nucleic acids, vitamins, and some coenzymes. Thus there might be some connection between pyrimidine derivatives and the synthesis of nucleoproteins by the malarial plasmodium. In addition, sulphonamides derived from 2-aminopyridine and 2-amino-4 : 6-dimethylpyrimidine attain very high blood levels. A study of the structural formulæ of certain of the pyrimidine compounds (III) prepared by Curd, Davey and Rose (1945b) showed that there is a formal similarity with mepacrine (I) and riboflavin (II).

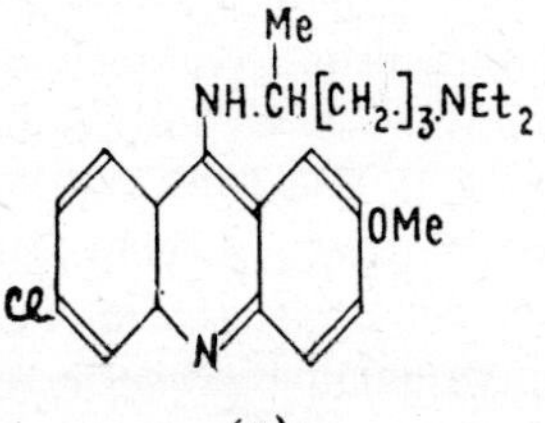

(I)

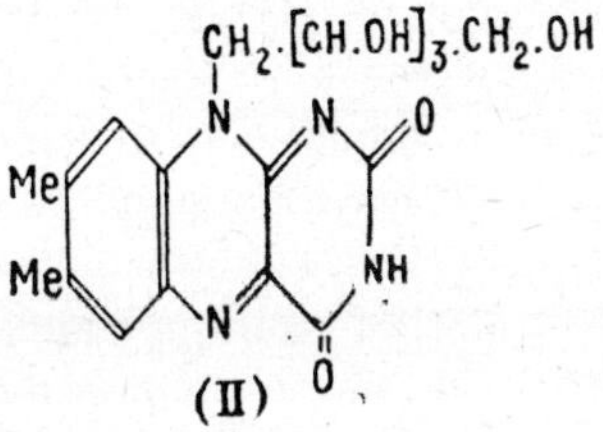

(II)

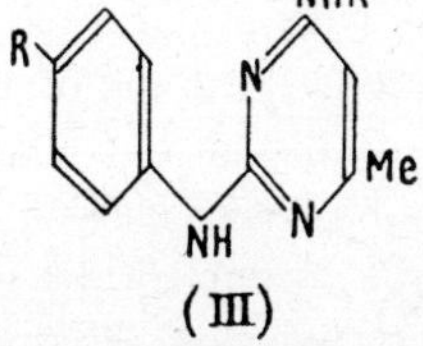

(III)

Oesterlin (1936) first suggested that mepacrine and pamaquin, by virtue of their ability to form hydro-derivatives, might act by interference with the functioning of a riboflavin nucleotide component of some enzyme essential to growth. Silverman and Evans (1944) showed that the bacteriostatic action of mepacrine on

Bacterium coli is reduced by riboflavin and this led to the suggestion that the activity of (I) is due to interference with one or more riboflavin enzyme systems in the malaria parasite. The hypothesis was further supported by the demonstration (Madinaveitia, 1946) that the growth-inhibitory action of mepacrine and 2-*p*-chloroanilino-4-β-diethylaminoethylamino-6-methylpyridine on *Lactobacillus casei* is antagonised by riboflavin.

The apparent necessity for substitution in the *para*-position of the anilino residue (Curd and Rose, 1946a) was, however, difficult to understand on the basis of such a riboflavin antagonism since substitution in the *meta*-position might be thought to lead to a similar result. In the case of mepacrine, the antagonism might be connected with the correspondence in position either of the chlorine with the 6-methyl group, or of the methoxyl group with 7-methyl group of riboflavin or partly with both, leading to a potentiation of the antagonistic effect. The observations of von Euler *et al.* (1935) that 6, 7-dimethyl-9-(D-1'-ribityl) *iso*alloxazine exhibited riboflavin activity indicated the importance of the 7-position and therefore probably of the *para*-position in the anilino group of (III) for riboflavin antagonism. The antimalarial activity of the 3 : 7-disubstituted acridines carrying an aminoalkylamino group in the 5-position (E.P. 411,132) and of the compounds corresponding to mepacrine but without the 8-substituent (E.P. 441,007) might be connected with this importance of the 7-methyl group in riboflavin. Although a *prima facie* case can be made out for supposing that mepacrine and quinine are riboflavin antagonists so far as bacterial growth is concerned, yet biochemical experiments with malaria parasites cannot be said to implicate the flavin enzyme systems of the plasmodia. Indeed, some of the enzymes inhibited by mepacrine and quinine in malaria parasites are not of this class. Evans (1946), however, noted that flavin adenine dinucleotides are actually present in red cells parasitised by *P. knowlesi*.

An added difficulty in determining the point of attack of antimalarial drugs is the inability to differentiate with certainty between primary and secondary inhibitory processes, concerned directly with the parasite or with the cells of the host. A further criticism of much theoretical speculation is that in many cases the drug concentrations required to produce inhibition of enzyme activity *in vitro* bear little or no relationship to those that must be found in the blood during the treatment of malaria. Ball (1946), however, claims that in the case of *P. knowlesi* the same concentrations of quinine and mepacrine are required to suppress growth *in vivo* and *in vitro*. At present therefore the biological evidence in favour of the view that mepacrine and other antimalarial drugs compete with riboflavin for certain enzyme systems cannot be said to be proved. Nevertheless, as Rose (1949) has pointed out, the demonstration *in vitro* of anti-bacterial activity of a type antagonised by riboflavin and also of antimalarial activity *in vivo*, with a sufficient number of compounds of distinct chemical types, each bearing some structural similarity to the vitamin, may well be accepted for the time at least as strong circumstantial evidence in favour of the hypothesis.

Curd *et al.* (1947) also compared the antimalarial activity of 2-*p*-toluidino-4-*β*-diethylaminoethylamino-6-methylpyrimidine and the corresponding *m*- and *o*-toluidino compounds, as derivatives showing a closer resemblance to riboflavin. Substitution in the *para*-position led to higher activity than *ortho*- or *meta*-substitution. The biochemical antagonism might be due to one or more of the major differences such as reducibility between the acridine and *iso*alloxazine ring systems or the substitution of chlorine for the two methyl groups.

In this connection the work of Kuhn, Weygand, and Möller (1943) on the anti-riboflavin activity of 6 : 7-dichloro-9-(D-1'-ribityl)*iso*-alloxazine and of Emerson and Tishler (1944) on the similar antagonistic effect of *iso*riboflavin (5 : 6-dimethyl-9-(D-1'-ribityl) *iso*alloxazine) is of interest. The opposite terminal ionic charge on the side-chain of the drug compared with that of the vitamin in its phosphorylated (mononucleotide) form may also be of significance.

Curd, Davis, and Rose (1946) also studied the effect of further variation in the side-chain (NHR') in (III ; R = Cl) since in other antimalarial types it has been shown that the permissible variation is fairly wide.

Madinaveitia (1946) found that using *Lactobacillus casei* as a test organism the growth inhibitory action of a number of antimalarials, mepacrine, quinine, and the 2-arylaminopyrimidine derivatives described by Curd and Rose (1946a), is antagonised by riboflavin : in addition such compounds are less anti-bacterial to strains of *Bact. coli* which have become adapted to mepacrine, thus suggesting a common point of attack on this organism.

However, an active antimalarial compound described by Hull *et al.* (1946) (IV ; R — CHMe . [CH$_2$]$_3$. NEt$_2$) is not inhibited by riboflavin as shown by the *L. casei* test.

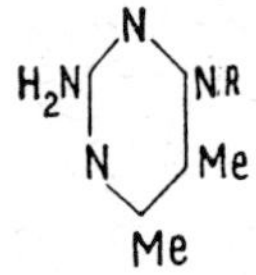

(IV)

The commonest known derivative of riboflavin exerting co-enzyme function is riboflavin-adenine-dinucleotide, believed to possess structure (V).

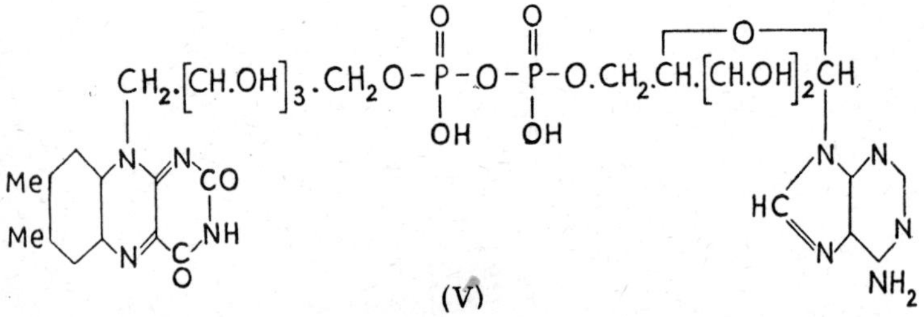

(V)

This compound is associated with specific proteins in a number of enzyme systems vital to cell metabolism, and interference with its synthesis or with its combination with the appropriate proteins in the parasites might well explain the action of an antimalarial drug. A riboflavin antagonist might interfere in one or both these ways. Interference might also be associated in the case of some agents with the adenosine rather than the riboflavin portion of the molecule.

Nucleoside synthesis is a general property of cells and interference with nucleoside synthesis is a possible mode of action of the simple pyrimidines shown to have antimalarial activity by Hull *et al.* (1946).

Hirst and Peat (1936) have pointed out that the structural

formulæ of riboflavin and the purine nucleosides show a striking similarity in the location of the carbohydrate residue relative to the pyrimidine nucleus. Baddiley, Lythgoe, and Todd (1944) believe that 5-amino-4-glycosidaminopyrimidines are intermediates in the biogenesis both of nucleosides and of riboflavin. It might therefore be expected that pyrimidine derivatives substituted in the 4 : 5-positions and in particular those bearing a side-chain of moderate size in position 4 would interfere with nucleoside and possibly riboflavin synthesis. Only compounds fulfilling these conditions were found by Hull *et al.* (1946) to exhibit antimalarial activity though in association with a rather high toxicity.

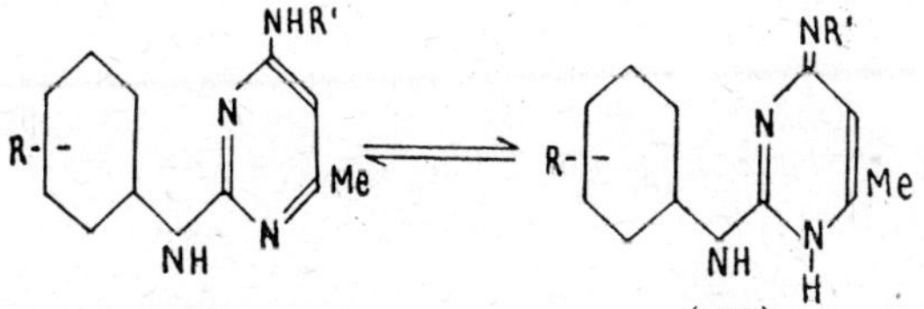

Schönhöfer (1942) thought the activity of mepacrine was associated with the possibility of tautomerism while Curd, Davey, and Rose (1945b) considered that the same might be true of drugs based on pyrimidine (VI) $\rightleftharpoons$ (VII) as well as their function as antagonists of riboflavin.

This tautomerism is largely independent of the nature of the amino substituent in the 2-position of the pyrimidine ring.

2-*p*- Chlorophenylguanidino - 4 - β - diethylaminoethylamino - 6 - methylpyrimidine (VI ; R = p — Cl, R' = CH_2 . CH_2 . NEt_2) (3349) has a high malarial activity against *P. gallinaceum* in chicken and is found to antagonise riboflavin as shown by the growth of *Lactobacillus casei*.

As shown by Magidson and Rubtsov (1937) and Schönhöfer

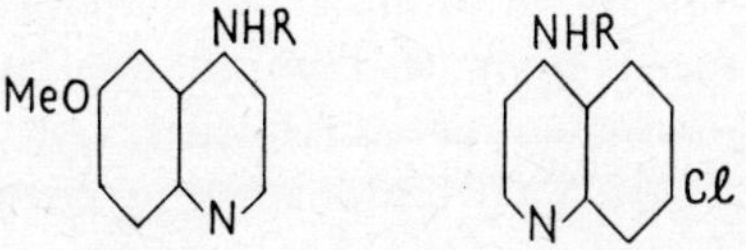

(1942), 4-dialkylaminoalkylamino derivatives of 6-methoxyquino-line (VIII) have antimalarial activity, as well as the 7-halogeno-substituted-4-dialkylaminoalkylaminoquinolines (IX) of D.R.P. 683,692. These compounds represent portions of the mepacrine molecule (I) and possibly owe their activity to this relation-ship, acting in a similar manner to mepacrine. Curd, Raison and Rose (1946) believe that the mode of action of the 2-β-naphthylamino compounds of type (X) also involves a riboflavin antagonism.

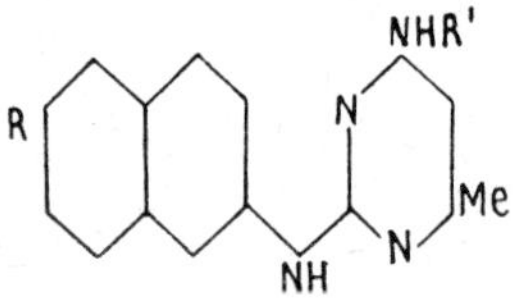

(X) 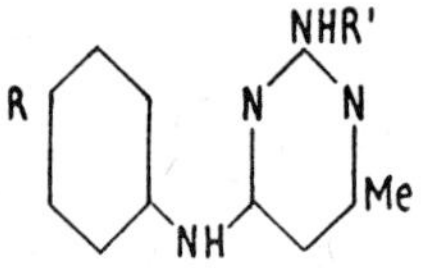   (XI)

The inactivity of 2-aminoalkylamino-6-methoxyquinolines (Schönhöfer, 1942 ; Magidson and Rubtsov, 1937) may be due to their inability to function as riboflavin antagonists rather than to the fact that tautomerism to give a p-quinonoid structure is not possible. Compounds of type (XI) are also incapable of exhibiting the p-quinonoid type of tautomerism.

Quite apart from the possibility that the antimalarial activity of compounds of type XII is associated with their capacity to function as riboflavin antagonists, Curd and Rose (1946a) had found that for antimalarial activity it was essential for the aryl and pyrimidine nuclei to be linked by groupings capable of prototropic change. Compounds of type XIII are similarly constituted, but while type XII conforms to the hypothesis of Schönhöfer (1942), whereby antimalarial activity is associated with an aminoalkylamino group in the γ-position relative to a heterocyclic nitrogen atom, thereby allowing tautomerism to a p-quinonoid structure, type XIII does not conform. With type XIII only o-quinonoid tautomerism is possible. Types XII and XIII do, however, possess a common tautomeric feature. The possibilities in type XII are as follows :—

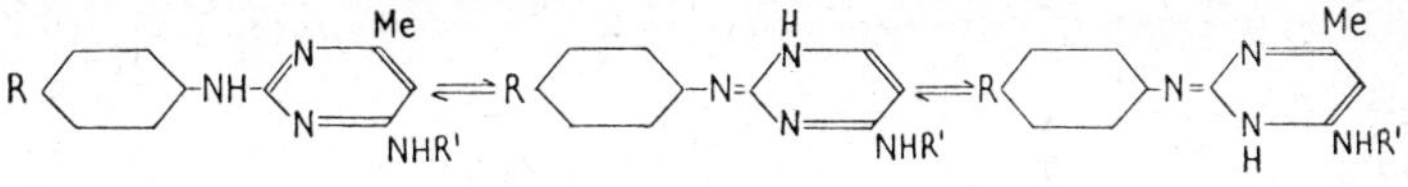

(XII)

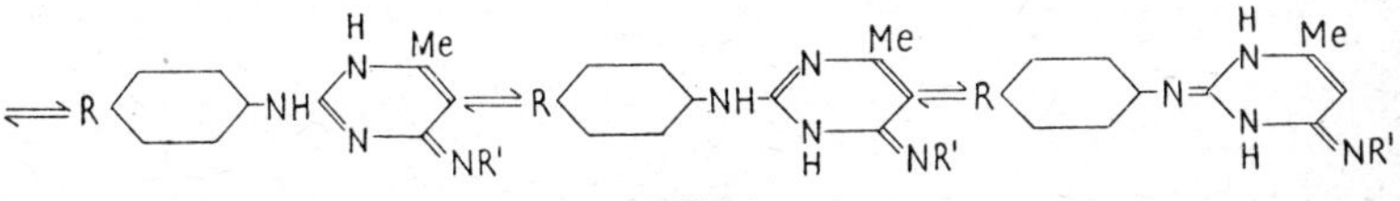

(XIIa)

Similar possibilities exist in type **XIII** so that in both types the **NH**-groups linking the phenyl and aminoalkyl residues to the pyrimidine nucleus are simultaneously capable of prototropy as in (**XIIa**) and (**XIIIa**). In contrast to this

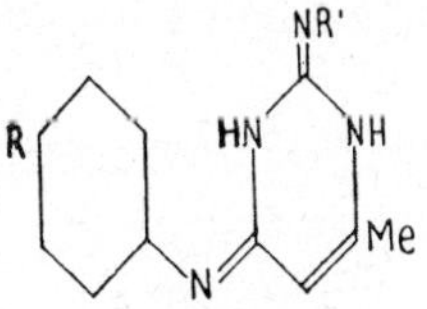

(XIIIa)

4-arylamino-6-aminoalkylamino-2-methyl-pyrimidines of type (**XIV**) which are inactive against *P. gallinaceum,* while capable of tautomerism to give the *p*-quinonoid structures (**XIVa**) and (**XIVb**), do not permit further prototropic change involving the second heterocyclic nitrogen atom analogous to (**XIIa**) and (**XIIIa**).

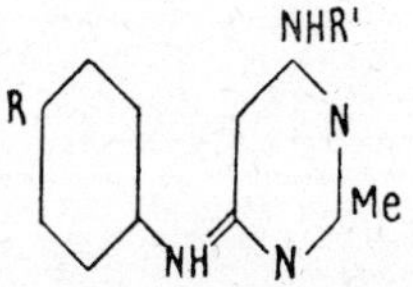

(XIV) 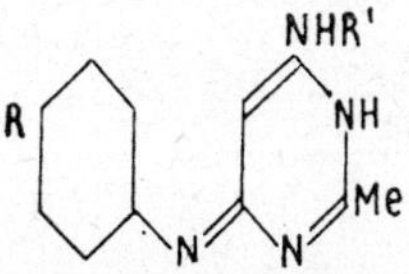   (XIVa) 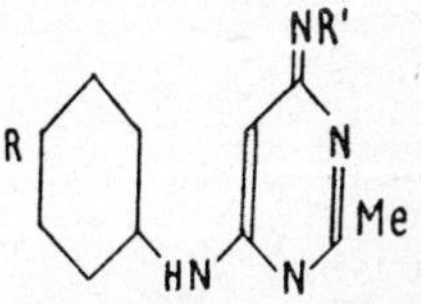   (XIVb)

Basford, Curd, and Rose (1946) therefore examined a number of compounds of type (**XIV**) to throw further light on the relationship between antimalarial activity and structure. Substances of type (**XIV**) and also of type (**XV**) showed no significant antimalarial action, in this respect differing entirely from compounds of types (XIIa) and (XIIIa).

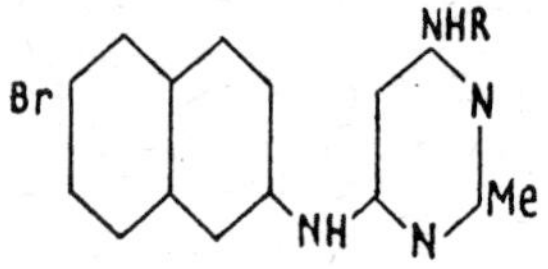

(XV)

The question of the inhibition of riboflavin by mepacrine and pyrimidine derivatives has also been studied by Madinaveitia (1946), employing *Bacterium coli* adapted to withstand higher concentrations of mepacrine than the normal strain. This mepacrine-resistant strain is also protected against 4-*p*-chloroanilino-2-*γ*-di-*n*-butylaminopropylamino-6-methylpyrimidine. This affords evidence that compounds of type (XIII) share with mepacrine a common point of attack on *Bact. coli* which may extend to other micro-organisms, including the parasites of malaria. This is perhaps a flavine enzyme, since mepacrine inhibits liver aldehyde oxidase (Madinaveitia, 1946) and *d*-amino-acid oxidase (Wright and Sabine, 1944).

Emerson and Tishler (1944) have shown the riboflavin antagonistic effect of 5 : 6-dimethyl-9-(D-1'-ribityl)*iso*alloxazine (*iso*riboflavin) and a comparison of the formula of this compound (XVI) with that of 4-arylamino-2-aminoalkylamino-6-methylpyrimidines carrying a 5-alkyl group (XVII ; R″ = alkyl) may explain their anti-malarial activity

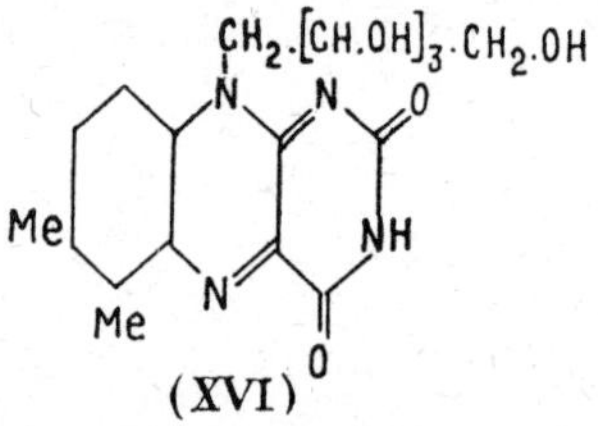

(XVI) 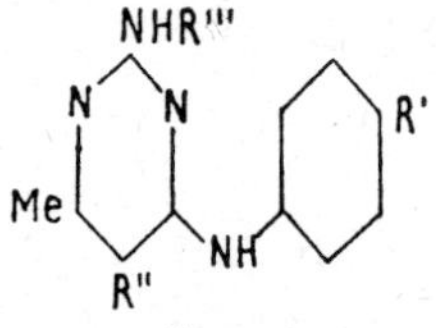   (XVII)

Too much emphasis must not, however, be placed on the inactivation of mepacrine action by riboflavin for it is now recognised that several substances can antagonise the inhibitory effects of mepacrine on the growth of *Bacterium coli*, in addition to the naturally occurring polyamines, such as spermine and spermidine (Silverman and Evans, 1943, 1944 ; Miller and Peters, 1945). Certain synthetic polyamines as well as pantothenic acid are active but monoamines and amino acids are inactive. Enzymatically digested lactalbumin, however, acts in the same way ; this is due to its content of calcium for both calcium and magnesium chloride will produce the same results. Calcium will also antagonise the growth inhibition of *Bact. coli* by the cyanine dye 1, 1′-dimethyl-2, 2′-cyanine chloride (Silverman, 1948a). Little is yet known of the *rôle*, if any, of spermine or spermidine in the metabolism of malarial plasmodia.

Finally, a chemical link in the hypothesis relating antimalarial structure to antagonism of some flavin system is provided by Ing (1949), who has synthesised compounds of type XVIII.

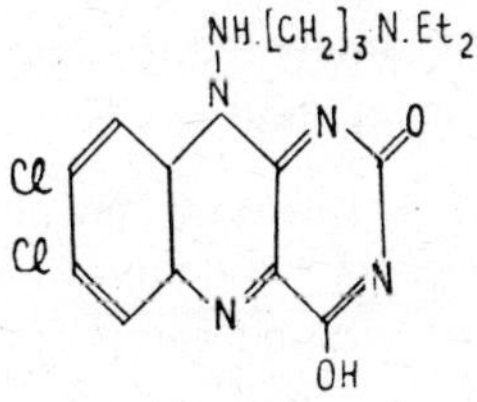

(XVIII)

In these the *iso*alloxazine system of the growth factor has been retained but the 6 : 7-methyl groups have been replaced by 6 : 7-dichloro substituents and the carbohydrate group by a basic side-chain. The resultant molecule is a riboflavin antagonist with respect to the growth of *Lactobacillus casei* and it also possesses slight therapeutic activity against *P. gallinaceum* in chicks.

On the other hand, a series of 6 : 7-dichloro-9-dialkylamino-alkyl*iso*alloxazines and some related compounds containing the same side chain as mepacrine are inactive as antimalarials though they possess trypanocidal activity (Barlow and Ing, 1950).

The possibility that antimalarial compounds might inhibit adenosine has been already mentioned.

This alternative hypothesis that an interference with an

adenosine-containing enzyme system may result in antimalarial activity has already led to the preparation of antimalarial compounds (Hull *et al.*, 1946, 1947). The effects of antimalarial compounds on adenosine activity have been studied by Madinaveitia and Raventós (1949), using the action of adenosine on the isolated hen's cæcum as one test and the lengthening of the auriculo-ventricular block produced by adenosine in the anæsthetised guinea-pig as the other.

With all groups of antimalarials, except one group of anilinopyrimidines (2666 type), there seems to be a close parallelism between antimalarial action and the power to antagonise adenosine, as expressed by the dose which halves the sensitivity of animals to this substance. The results are shown in the tables. Mepacrine, it will be seen, is one of the best antagonists of adenosine but is one of the weakest antimalarials in chicks.

In heart-lung preparations of the guinea-pig proguanil is not as effective in acute as in chronic experiments ; this is probably because proguanil in the body is rapidly metabolised into some as yet unknown active compound.

MINIMAL DOSES WHICH ANTAGONISE THE ACTION OF ADENOSINE
IN ACUTE EXPERIMENTS * ON THE GUINEA-PIG'S HEART
(Madinaveitia and Raventós, 1949)

Compound.	Minimum antagonistic dose. mgm./kgm./minute.	Dose which halves sensitivity to adenosine. mgm./kgm./minute.
Quinine hydrochloride	0·75	0·8
Mepacrine hydrochloride	0·25	0·35
Proguanil hydrochloride	too toxic at 0·25	
Chloroquine H_3PO_4	0·25	0·45
Proguanil lactate	1·25	1·25
3349	3·0 (?)	3·0 (?)
2666	0·6	0·9
Procaine	Inactive at 2·0	—
Suramin	,, ,, 5·0	—
Methylene blue	,, ,, 2·0	—
Trypan blue	,, ,, 2·0	—
Trypan red	,, ,, 2·0	—
Sulphadimethylpyrimidine	,, ,, 8·5	—

* Compounds introduced by slow intravenous injection.

RELATIVE ANTIMALARIAL ACTIVITY AGAINST *P. gallinaceum* IN
THE CHICK AND POWER TO ANTAGONISE ADENOSINE
(Madinaveitia and Raventós, 1949)

Antagonism, " Acute." *	Antagonism, " Chronic." †	Antimalarial activity.
Mepacrine.	Pamaquin.	Pamaquin.
Chloroquine.	Chloroquine.	Chloroquine.
Quinine.	Mepacrine.	Proguanil.
2666.	Proguanil.	3349.
Proguanil.	3349.	Mepacrine.
3349.	Quinine.	Quinine.
	2666.	2666.

* Compounds given intravenously.
† Compounds given in two doses daily for 3½ days.

A biochemical relationship between adenosine derivatives and
antimalarials may be found in the fact that adenylic acid and
adenosine triphosphate prevent the inhibition which mepacrine
causes in the recovery of oxygen uptake by washed *Plasmodium
lophuræ* in the presence of glucose (Hellerman, Bovarnick, and
Potter, 1946).   Since some enzymes contain both adenosine and
riboflavin these suggestions as to the mode of action of antimalarial substances are not incompatible.   As Madinaveitia and
Raventós (1949) point out, it is unlikely that *L. casei* uses riboflavin as such in its metabolic processes ; it is more probable
that the micro-organism builds up some coenzyme from the free
riboflavin present in the medium, possibly by combining it
through a polyphosphate group with adenosine.   It is conceivable
that the antagonistic effect of riboflavin in *L. casei* assays is not
due to the vitamin itself but to an adenosine-containing coenzyme
into which the free riboflavin is incorporated.   The prosthetic
group of D-amino-acid oxidase is such a flavin-adenine dinucleotide
(Corran, Green, and Straub, 1939) and is known to antagonise the
inhibitory action of mepacrine on the enzymatic deamination of
D-amino-acids (Wright and Sabine, 1944).   On the other hand,
Haas (1944) has shown that mepacrine also inhibits cytochrome
reductase by an irreversible reaction with the protein ; here the
drug competes with the prosthetic group of the enzyme since its

action is prevented by the addition of alloxazine mononucleotide. In this coenzyme riboflavin is not combined with adenosine.

Thus, according to Madinaveitia and Raventós (1949), antimalarial drugs have the property in common of antagonising adenosine and the intensity of this antagonism is proportional to their antimalarial action as measured in chicks harbouring the blood forms of *P. gallinaceum*.

Irvin *et al.* (1949) suggest that cationic acridines and quinolines interact with polyvalent nucleate anions. Such an interaction involves coulombic forces, hydrogen-bonding, and van der Waal's forces. The interaction of quinoline and acridine antimalarials appears to be dependent on the molecular size of the nucleic acids involved. Irvin and Irvin (1949) show that the proton-acceptor species of 2-methoxy-6-chloro-9-(1'-methyl-8'-diethylamino-octyl-amino)-acridine and of mepacrine combine reversibly with bovine plasma albumin and with the proteins of fraction III–1 of bovine plasma. It is possible that an interaction takes place between a cationic species of these acridines and sodium ribonucleate or desoxyribonucleate.

A possible relationship between antimalarial action and antagonism of purines and pteroylglutamic acid has been suggested by Falco *et al.* (1949). The growth of *Lactobacillus casei* with pteroylglutamic acid, in the absence of purine, is inhibited by nearly all 2 : 4-diaminopyrimidines (Lampen and Jones, 1947). Many of the inhibitions are reversible by (*a*) pteroylglutamic acid or (*b*) purines, or (*c*) both. Members of the 2 : 4-diamino-5-aryloxy-pyrimidines (I) are extremely strong inhibitors of pteroylglutamic acid. There is, however, a formal analogy between the 2 : 4-diamino-5-*p*-chlorophenoxypyrimidine (I, Ar $= - C_6H_4Cl(p)$) and proguanil and Falco *et al.* (1949) have shown that proguanil is an antagonist of pteroylglutamic acid whereas 2 : 4-diamino-5-*p*-chlorophenoxypyrimidine is active against *P. gallinaceum* infection in chicks. The inhibition of *L. casei* by proguanil is reversed by pteroylglutamic acid and purines such as hypoxanthine, xanthine, and adenine : purines similarly reverse the inhibition of *L. casei* growth by 2 : 4-diamino-5-*p*-chlorophenoxypyrimidine. The inhibition by quinine of the same system is readily reversed by adenine but only partially inhibited by pteroylglutamic acid.

The correlation between anti-pteroylglutamic acid activity and antimalarial activity is, however, somewhat obscure : 2 : 4-diamino-5-p-chlorophenoxypyrimidine is a much stronger pteroylglutamic acid antagonist than is proguanil but is less active against *P. gallinaceum* in chicks. In addition, several 2-amino-4-dialkylamino-alkyaminopyrimidines which are active antimalarially do not show any anti-pteroylglutamic acid activity in the *L. casei* system. Hull *et al.* (1946) suggested that the antimalarial activity of the pyrimidine derivatives might be due to interference with nucleoside synthesis, a view supported by the observations of Madinaveitia and Raventós (1949) and Hellerman *et al.* (1946). If the findings of Falco *et al.* (1949) are correct both purines and pteroylglutamic acid may be involved in the systems affected by antimalarial drugs : in neither case, however, is the antagonism definitely of a competitive nature.

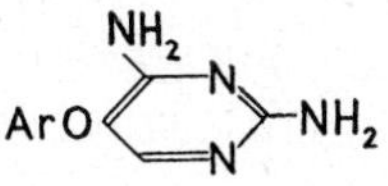

2 : 4-*Diamino*-5-p-*chloro-phenoxypyrimidine.*   *Proguanil.*

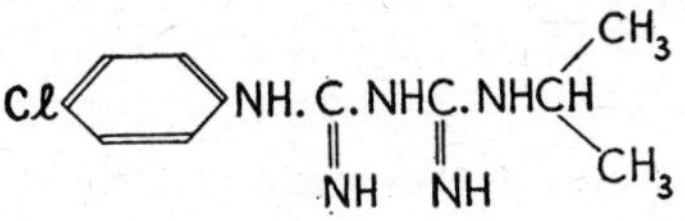

Calcium metabolism has also been considered in relation to the antimalarial action of mepacrine and other antimalarial compounds. Silverman (1948b) showed that in descending order of activity Ca^{++}, Mg^{++}, Mn^{++}, and Ba^{++} antagonise the bacteriostatic effects of mepacrine on the growth of *Bact. coli*. The inhibitory effect of mepacrine is intensified by sodium citrate and there is undoubtedly a stoichiometric relationship between mepacrine concentration and the concentration of Ca^{++} ions required to relieve the mepacrine inhibition on *Bact. coli*. The exact nature of the relationship between calcium and mepacrine in biological systems is not yet apparent ; however, the Ca^{++} : drug ratios for quinine, mepacrine, and proguanil on *Bact. coli* roughly parallel the relative activities of these compounds in suppressing blood-induced infections of *P. lophuræ* in the duck. Cations, it may be noted, compete with acridines for adsorption on cellular ribonucleoproteins (Massart *et al.*, 1947).

The possible mode of action of proguanil is discussed on pp. 546–548.

ANTIMALARIAL DRUGS AND THE METABOLISM OF PLASMODIA

Despite the fact that the specific action of quinine in malaria has been recognised for so long, it is curious that so little is known for certain of the precise action on malarial parasites, not only of quinine but of other more recent antimalarials such as mepacrine.

Quinine and Mepacrine. Before discussing the action of quinine and mepacrine on the metabolism of malarial parasites it is necessary to discuss very briefly the action of these two compounds on the enzymes of tissue cells.

Action on Tissue Enzymes

The effect of mepacrine on enzyme systems of the vertebrate host has received attention in view of the action of the drug in interfering with the respiration of malaria parasites.

Martin *et al.* (1939) believed that at a concentration of 3 mgm. per 100 mgm. of tissue, or approximately 2×10^{-3} M, mepacrine had no effect on the oxygen consumption of the tissues. Wright and Sabine (1944), in reinvestigating the question, found almost complete inhibition of brain respiration at a concentration of mepacrine less than 5×10^{-4} M. In investigating this inhibition they were able to show that tissues, after thorough treatment with mepacrine, are able to catalyse rapidly the oxidation of *p*-phenylene-diamine or succinate, thus proving that the inhibition of oxygen consumption is probably not due to interference with the cytochrome or the cytochrome oxidase of the respiratory mechanism. The oxidation of succinate also proves that succinic dehydrogenase is not blocked by the concentrations of mepacrine in therapeutic use. Evidence brought forward by Haas (1944) shows that triphosphopyridine nucleotide and cytochrome C are not inhibited, while cytochrome oxidase is only affected to a minor degree by mepacrine. The activity of cytochrome reductase and glucose-6-phosphate dehydrogenase is inhibited by low concentrations of mepacrine. The inhibition of cytochrome reductase is brought about by an irreversible reaction of mepacrine and the free protein, whereby the drug competes with the prosthetic group of the enzyme. Antagonism between the prosthetic group and mepacrine can be demonstrated by adding increasing amounts of the drug to a constant amount of alloxazine mononucleotide or inhibition can be prevented by supplying increasing amounts of prosthetic group at a constant drug concentration. The enzyme protein has a much greater affinity for the prosthetic group alloxazine mononucleotide than for mepacrine, since 1 μgm. of riboflavin phosphate will neutralise about 500 μgm. of mepacrine. In this connection it might be expected that if the respiratory mechanism of malaria parasites is similar to that of mammalian cells, some of the alloxazine derivatives would prove to be effective antimalarials by combining with specific enzyme proteins of malaria parasites. A riboflavin analogue might compete with riboflavin thus preventing respiration and growth of the parasites. However, Bovarnick *et al.* (1946b) believe that if indeed respiration of malaria parasites is actually mediated through a flavoprotein, the latter may be like the flavoprotein from heart muscle, not subject to dissociation by mepacrine (Straub, 1939). Since the *in vitro* action of mepacrine on respiratory enzymes can be counteracted by riboflavin phosphate the efficiency of the drug *in vivo* might conceivably be considerably enhanced by avoiding an excess of riboflavin in the diet during the treatment of an attack. As the diet of the African is normally deficient in riboflavin, the success of mepacrine in treating his attacks of malaria may thus in part be explained. However, one molecule of riboflavin phosphate neutralises approximately 500 molecules of mepacrine so that the latter is hardly " the ideal antagonist " of riboflavin.

Mepacrine also inhibits glucose-6-phosphate dehydrogenase by reacting with the protein moiety of this enzyme. Addition of glucose-6-phosphate partially prevents and even reverses the inhibition by mepacrine thus again indicating competition between a substrate and the drug.

Quinine is much less effective than mepacrine as an inhibitor of respiratory catalysts, as shown in the table, thus rendering it doubtful whether the antimalarial action of quinine is due to interference with the respiratory processes of the malaria parasite.

COMPARISON OF INHIBITION OF RESPIRATORY ENZYMES BY MEPACRINE AND QUININE : DRUG CONCENTRATION 5×10^{-4} M (Haas, 1944)

Enzyme.	Temperature, °C.	Inhibition by	
		Mepacrine, per cent.	Quinine, per cent.
Cytochrome oxidase . .	25	40	17
,, reductase . .	25	73	14
Zwischenferment (protein I)	25	78	0
Respiration of *Plasmodium knowlesi* . . .	38	80	26

Thus among the known components of the respiratory system only cytochrome reductase and Zwischenferment need to be considered as possible points of interference by mepacrine.

EFFECT OF MEPACRINE ON ISOLATED RESPIRATORY ENZYMES, ON TISSUE RESPIRATION, AND ON THE RESPIRATION OF *Plasmodium knowlesi* (Haas, 1944)

Enzymes.	Temperature, °C.	Mepacrine, concentration M.	Inhibition, per cent.
Cytochrome oxidase . .	25	10×10^{-4}	60
,, C . . .	25	10×10^{-4}	0
,, reductase . .	25	2×10^{-4}	49
,, ,, . .	*(38)	*$(0\cdot3) \times 10^{-4}$	*(50)
Triphosphopyridine nucleotide.	25	10×10^{-4}	0
Zwischenferment (protein I) .	25	5×10^{-4}	77
Respiration of mammalian tissue	38	1×10^{-4}	61
,, ,, malaria parasites	38	5×10^{-4}	61

* Figures obtained by extrapolation.

Wolf (1949) from experiments with mepacrine on *Pseudomonas fluorescens* believes that mepacrine inhibits the transport of hydrogen. This does not exclude the hypothesis of Haas (1944) that mepacrine acts by inhibiting the cytochrome-reductase system by competition with the prosthetic group of the enzyme. Moulder (1948a, b), in summarising the effects of quinine given intravenously to chickens infected with *P. gallinaceum* believes that (1) the rate of glucose utilisation is increased, (2) the rate of pyruvate utilisation is decreased ; (3) the oxygen : glucose ratio is lowered and (4) the increase in oxygen uptake on addition of glucose, lactate or pyruvate is decreased. Whereas anaerobic breakdown of glucose to pyruvate is unaffected by quinine, aerobic oxidation of pyruvate is inhibited : this effect is irreversible.

Antimalarial drugs inactivate cholinesterases (Ammon, 1935 ; Richter and Croft, 1942 ; Waelsch and Nachmansohn, 1943 ; Vincent and Beaujard, 1945 ; Blaschko *et al.*, 1947). This applies both to the cholinesterase of human plasma and of human red cells (Wright and Sabine, 1948). Chloroquine, mepacrine, pamaquin, and quinidine exhibit a typical competitive inhibition for human plasma cholinesterase, proguanil a combination of competitive and non-competitive action, whereas quinine fails to fit the theoretical curves. None of the drugs is destroyed during the reaction, and equilibrium between inhibitor and enzyme is reached very rapidly, certainly within five minutes in the case of mepacrine and quinidine. Proguanil, according to Blaschko *et al.* (1946), has little

INHIBITION OF CHOLINESTERASES BY PROGUANIL
(Blaschko *et al.* 1946)

Tissue.	Substrate and concentration.	Inhibition in per cent. by proguanil.	
		10^{-3}M.	10^{-4}M.
Dog's caudate nucleus . .	6×10^{-3} M—acetylcholine	22	0
Human red cells (hæmolysed) .	6×10^{-3} M—acetylcholine	49	0
Horse serum	6×10^{-3} M—benzoylcholine	67	35
Guinea-pig's liver . . .	6×10^{-3} M—benzoylcholine	94	79
Ox kidney	6×10^{-3} M—benzoylcholine	0	—
Rabbit serum . . .	1 per cent. atropine	48	—

affinity for the cholinesterase of the central nervous system and this is in accordance with its low toxicity. Some of the other cholinesterases are more strongly inhibited by proguanil. No clear-cut correlation appears to exist between the relative inhibiting action on cholinesterase and either the antimalarial activity or chemical constitution of the more commonly employed anti-malarials.

As morphine and physostigmine also inhibit the hydrolysis of acetyl choline by cholinesterase but are devoid of antimalarial action, it is difficult to correlate inhibition of cholinesterase with antimalarial activity.

Action on Malarial Parasites

In an attempt to determine how antimalarial drugs work numerous studies have been made on the metabolism of malarial parasites under normal conditions and in the presence of quinine and mepacrine. The normal metabolism of malarial parasites has been studied either in parasitised red blood cells or, following the lead of Christophers and Fulton (1939), after separation of the parasites from red cells by treatment with saponin. Before discussing the effect of quinine and mepacrine on the metabolism of malaria parasites it is necessary to describe briefly what is at present known of the metabolism of these parasites under normal conditions.

Christophers and Fulton (1938) first showed that the blood of monkeys parasitised by *Plasmodium knowlesi* exhibited a rapid oxygen consumption in the presence of glucose ; this was inhibited in the presence of cyanides. Even when separated from the red cells by saponin, utilisation of oxygen by the parasites still occurred in the presence of oxygen (Fulton and Christophers, 1938).

Fulton (1939) showed that both with parasitised red cells and saponised parasites of *P. knowlesi* an increased oxygen uptake was brought about not only by glucose but by lævulose, maltose, mannose and, above all, glycerol. Aldopentoses such as arabinose and xylose and various other sugars, alcohols, and glycosides failed to increase oxygen uptake which was thus affected only by sugars containing the group

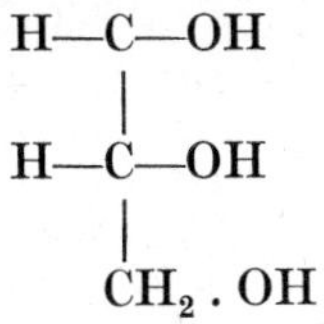

$$\begin{array}{c} \text{H—C—OH} \\ | \\ \text{H—C—OH} \\ | \\ \text{CH}_2 \text{ . OH} \end{array}$$

Estimation of the different phosphorus fractions during metabolism of glucose by *P. knowlesi* did not produce clear evidence of phosphorylation of this sugar by the parasites.

Maier and Coggeshall (1941) confirmed the fact that mannose and glycerol could be substituted for glucose ; they also obtained increased oxygen uptake when fructose and sodium D-lactate were used as a substrate though maltose and sodium α-β-glycerophosphate were far less active. Citrate, malate, fumarate, and succinate did not appear to be metabolised.

The red cells infected with malaria parasites are able also to metabolise lactate, pyruvate, and amino acids. Glutamic acid and tyrosine are not oxidised (Marshall, 1948). Glucose appears to be converted to lactic acid by phosphorylation, as in muscle (Evans *et al.*, 1945 ; Evans, 1946 ; Ball, 1946 ; Bovarnick *et al.*, 1946a and b ; McKee *et al.*, 1946).

Wendel (1943) also found that infected monkey blood destroyed glucose aerobically with far greater rapidity than did unparasitised red cells. About half the glucose destroyed appeared as lactic acid. Under anaerobic conditions the glycolysis of parasitised red cells was stimulated while normal monkeys' cells were unaffected. Under comparable conditions of *p*H, lactate, and glucose appear to be equally good substrates for the respiration of infected red cells. Later Speck and Evans (1945a) studied the individual enzymes of *P. gallinaceum*. It was concluded that cell-free extracts of malarial parasites formed lactic acid from glucose by a path similar to the phosphorylating glycolysis exhibited by bacteria, yeasts, and mammalian cells. *P. gallinaceum* was found to contain enzymes capable of catalysing the phosphorylation of glucose by adenosine triphosphate, the splitting of fructose-1, 6-diphosphate to form 3-phosphoglyceraldehyde, and the dismutation between 3-phosphoglyceraldehyde and pyruvic acid.

Further studies on washed parasites of *Plasmodium lophuræ*

separated from duck red cells by saponin were made by Bovarnick *et al.* (1946a). The parasites had an oxygen uptake which averaged 70 per cent. of that of the parasitised intact blood. When the parasites were washed free of glucose, lactate or pyruvate restored the oxygen uptake to the level attained with glucose as a substrate. With succinate or fumarate as a substrate the oxygen uptake was only a third that with glucose. The oxygen uptake was inhibited by cyanide but was partially restored by the addition of cresyl blue, although cresyl blue itself inhibited normal respiration to some extent.

Silverman *et al.* (1944), as a result of adding quinine *in vitro* to chicken red cells parasitised by *P. gallinaceum*, came to the conclusion that quinine affects the carbohydrate metabolism of *P. gallinaceum* by inhibiting the oxidation of pyruvate. Moulder (1948b), by intravenous administration of 20 mgm. quinine per kgm. body weight to chickens infected with *P. gallinaceum*, showed that there were marked changes in the metabolism of parasitised red cells of chickens twenty-four hours after quinine injection. The complete oxidation of glucose to carbon dioxide and water is inhibited by quinine, whereas the anaerobic breakdown of glucose to lactate and pyruvate is unaffected. Thus *in vivo* also it appears that quinine inhibits the oxidation of pyruvate by *P. gallinaceum*. The effect of quinine on the carbohydrate metabolism of erythrocyte-free parasites of *P. gallinaceum* has been studied by Moulder (1949). The known course of pyruvate oxidation in *P. gallinaceum* has been examined by Speck *et al.* (1946) and is shown in the following schema:—

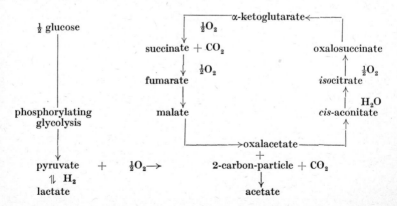

Pyruvate may be reduced to lactate, oxidised to carbon dioxide and water by way of the tricarboxylic acid cycle, or oxidised to acetate and carbon dioxide. With pyruvate as substrate, there is no significant lactate formation, aerobically or anaerobically. In parasitised red cells, acetate is not formed from pyruvate under normal conditions but it accumulates when the tricarboxylic acid cycle is blocked by addition of malonate which inhibits the succinic dehydrogenase. In free parasites about half of the utilised pyruvate is completely oxidised by way of the tricarboxylic acid cycle and about half is oxidised to acetate. When malonate is added to free parasites pyruvate is converted almost quantitatively into acetate. In the light of current concepts of pyruvate metabolism, as set out by Vennesland (1948), it seems probable that pyruvate is oxidised to carbon dioxide and a highly reactive two-carbon particle which is not acetate or any other compound yet tested. This two-carbon particle may condense with oxalacetate to enter the tricarboxylic acid cycle or may irreversibly decompose to acetate. When the first path is inhibited, as in the presence of malonate, more pyruvate is diverted into the second path and acetate formation is increased. Moulder (1949) finds that in free parasites from quinine-treated chicks pyruvate oxidation is marked by equal suppression of both pathways of metabolism, oxidation by way of the tricarboxylic acid cycle and oxidation to acetate. This suppression can be explained by assuming that quinine interferes with the only step common to both pathways, the formation of the two-carbon particle. Quinine, it is suggested, inhibits pyruvate oxidation in free parasites by irreversibly removing some unknown factor necessary for conversion of pyruvate into a reactive two-carbon particle. In *Bacterium coli*, it may be noted, streptomycin apparently interferes with the condensation of pyruvate and oxalacetate but does not inhibit the oxidation of pyruvate to acetate (Umbreit, 1949). Quinine does not interfere with the oxidation of any acid of the tricarboxylic acid cycle to nearly the same degree as it interferes with the oxidation of pyruvate.

The effects of antimalarial drugs on the respiration of *P. knowlesi* were first studied in a Warburg manometer by Fulton and Christophers (1938) and Fulton (1939), using intact parasitised red cells and parasites freed from extraneous matter by saponin. Inhibition of oxygen consumption by the parasites was brought about by quinine, mepacrine, and pamaquin ; mepacrine was considerably more active than quinine even though concentrations of the latter drugs were active in dilutions as low as 10^{-5} M. Methylene blue and acriflavine also inhibited oxygen uptake *in vitro*, their *in vitro* action on parasites thus corresponding to their *in vivo* activity. Inhibition of oxygen consumption led to an accumulation of lactic acid, though the rate of glucose utilisation was unaffected (Silverman *et al.*, 1944), thus suggesting that the action of these antimalarial drugs is to inhibit the oxidative removal of lactic acid rather than to prevent its formation by the process of glycolysis. Inhibition of the respiration of plasmodia by quinine or mepacrine is delayed until the third or fourth hour of incubation with the drug.

The action of mepacrine as an antimalarial was thought by Speck and Evans (1945b) to be due to its inhibitory action on the hexokinase activity and the enzymic lactic dehydrogenase of *P. gallinaceum* : quinine was much less active than mepacrine in inhibiting these enzymes. The enzyme 3-phosphoglyceraldehyde dehydrogenase was not affected by either drug. Lactic dehydrogenase from extracts of plasmodia and from ox heart is inhibited more by mepacrine than by quinine. Further studies on the action of antimalarial drugs were made with *P. lophuræ* by Bovarnick *et al.* (1946a and b). Both mepacrine and quinine were again found to inhibit the oxygen uptake of the parasites but only at a concentration of 0·001 M was inhibition approximately 50 per cent. No selective inhibition of oxidation occurred when lactate, pyruvate, succinate or fumarate were substituted for glucose as a substrate. In addition, the cyanide-cresyl blue respiration of the parasites was entirely unaffected by mepacrine or quinine. This means that if under these conditions respiration is mediated by a flavoprotein it must be one that is not dissociated by mepacrine. Further observations showed that if saponised parasites first had their substrate completely exhausted they oxidised glucose only after a considerable interval, oxygen uptake being resumed only slowly. If in these circumstances mepacrine is added the oxygen uptake is strongly inhibited at concentrations considerably lower than those effective in the case of cells not first deprived of glucose. A mepacrine concentration of 0·0001 M, for instance, will produce a 75 to 90 per cent. inhibition of oxygen uptake as contrasted with a 20 per cent. reduction in the rate of oxygen uptake by cells not first deprived of glucose. This very considerable inhibition is not observed when other substrates are substituted for glucose, but a similar increased inhibition is produced by quinine and pamaquin but not by sulphanilamide, sulphathiazole or 6-methoxyquinoline.

In plasmodia thoroughly exhausted of substrates by washing and preliminary incubation the sensitivity to antimalarial drugs is increased. Recovery of respiration after addition of glucose to exhausted parasites is strongly inhibited by mepacrine. Inhibition of glycolysis by mepacrine is antagonised by adenylic acid or adenosine triphosphate. It seems reasonable to attribute the induction period in the oxidation of glucose by substrate-depleted malarial parasites to the necessity for the phosphorylation of glucose before the substrate can be utilised. If this supposition be correct, then it would seem that mepacrine, and to a lesser extent quinine, interferes with some phosphorylation reactions necessary before glucose can be utilised, possibly by competing with adenylic acid, adenosine triphosphate, or both. Marshall (1948) demonstrated that while quinine inhibits glucose utilisation of *P. gallinaceum* to a greater degree than mepacrine, the latter gives a more pronounced inhibition of hexokinase in *P. gallinaceum*. In the presence of mepacrine the accumulation of glucose-1-phosphate was inhibited, presumably because the formation of glucose-6-phosphate was reduced. Both mepacrine and quinine show a slight iodoacetate-like inhibitory effect. Quinine caused lactate and pyruvate to accumulate and therefore inhibited lactate as well as pyruvate oxidation. All the evidence is thus in favour of the view that glucose metabolism in plasmodia proceeds by way of the Embden-Meyerhof-Parnas system characteristic of yeast and muscle metabolism. Following Marshall (1948), it is possible to draw up a scheme for the glucose metabolism of *P. gallinaceum* and to suggest that mepacrine and quinine exert an inhibitory action at several points in this scheme. Ball *et al.* (1948) find that the pattern of carbohydrate metabolism in *P. knowlesi* is essentially similar to that of *P. gallinaceum*. Each parasitised cell uses up from twenty-five to seventy-five times the oxygen and glucose required by the normal cell. Flavin-adenine-dinucleotide causes a six to fifteen-fold increase, and, without bringing forward any direct experimental evidence, Ball and his colleagues suggest that mepacrine may function by blocking the synthesis of flavin-adenine-dinucleotide rather than by competing with it for the enzyme molecule.

It is of course possible that not all or even the greater part of the inhibition is against carbohydrate metabolism. The similarity in structure of mepacrine and riboflavin has suggested that mepacrine may compete with flavin nucleotides for one or more essential enzyme proteins (Wright and Sabine, 1944 ; Haas, 1944). However, Hellerman *et al.* (1946), as the result of flavo-enzyme studies, do not find evidence of a specific antagonism between mepacrine and flavin-adenine-dinucleotide ; mepacrine, quinine, and the sulphonamides all belong to a class capable of combining reversibly or irreversibly with proteins. The combination might, with certain enzymes, result in competition for a prosthetic group. Such competition would not necessarily be related to a close structural similarity between inhibitor and prosthetic group. Hellerman *et al.* (1946) also find that, though sodium *p*-chloromercuribenzoate (0·0001 M) stops oxidation of glucose and of pyruvate in separated parasites, no reversal is realised with glutathione (0·001 M), though the latter reagent itself does not affect the rate.

It is doubtful whether the action of antimalarial drugs on lipase is of any significance. Fulton (1936), using tributyrin as substrate, found that cinchona alkaloids depressed the lipase activity of human and monkey sera. Hellerman *et al.* (1946) obtained similar results with tributyrin both with cinchona alkaloids and mepacrine. The presence of the quinoline or acridine nucleus seems to be essential for lipase inhibition, but methylene blue is also slightly depressant.

Further work is required to determine how far the same mechanisms hold good for malarial parasites within red cells in the body as for washed, saponised parasites *in vitro*, and whether the ratio of intracellular to extracellular drugs is such, in the absence of a special mechanism for concentrating drugs within the red cells, as to permit a sufficient concentration of drug to come in contact with the parasite. Speck *et al.* (1946), for instance, found that in the case of *P. gallinaceum* freed from chick red cells by hæmolytic serum the parasites require various co-factors for the oxidation of pyruvate whereas these substances were not needed when parasites were within intact red cells. Free parasites form appreciable acetate from pyruvate whereas in the intact cell pyruvate is oxidised by parasites almost entirely to CO_2 and water. The oxidation of pyruvate is probably catalysed by the dicarboxylic acids and involves the tricarboxylic acid cycle : glucose and lactate are oxidised in the same way as pyruvate.

SCHEME OF GLUCOSE METABOLISM OF *Plasmodium gallinaceum,* SHOWING POSSIBLE POINTS OF ACTION BY QUININE AND MEPACRINE (Marshall, 1948)

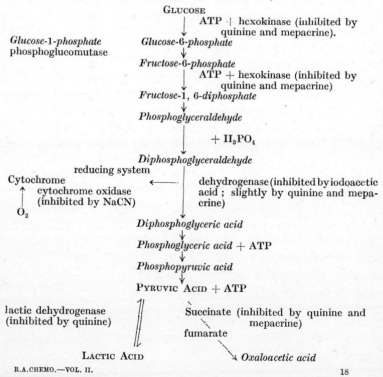

GLUCOSE
$\qquad$ ATP + hexokinase (inhibited by quinine and mepacrine).

Glucose-1-phosphate   *Glucose-6-phosphate*
phosphoglucomutase

Fructose-6-phosphate
$\qquad$ ATP + hexokinase (inhibited by quinine and mepacrine)
Fructose-1, 6-diphosphate

Phosphoglyceraldehyde

$\qquad$ + H_3PO_4

Diphosphoglyceraldehyde
              reducing system
Cytochrome $\qquad\longleftarrow$ dehydrogenase (inhibited by iodoacetic
$\uparrow$ cytochrome oxidase   acid ; slightly by quinine and mepa-
O_2 (inhibited by NaCN)   crine)

Diphosphoglyceric acid

Phosphoglyceric acid + ATP

Phosphopyruvic acid

PYRUVIC ACID + ATP

lactic dehydrogenase   Succinate (inhibited by quinine and
(inhibited by quinine)   mepacrine)
                    fumarate

LACTIC ACID   *Oxaloacetic acid*

In this connection it is of interest to note that Oldham *et al.* (1944) observed that in chickens infected with malaria the concentration of quinine was invariably higher than in normal birds in the plasma, red cells, spleen, bone marrow, and liver; higher values in infected birds were occasionally found in brain, lungs, and leg muscle, while no significant differences were found in the concentrations in pancreas, kidney, heart, and spinal cord. In addition, Wendel (1946) has found that the antimalarial action of hydroxynaphthoquinones on *P. lophuræ* in ducks parallels very closely their *in vitro* action in depressing the oxygen uptake and carbohydrate metabolism of the parasites.

Proguanil. Very little is yet known of the way in which proguanil acts on malaria. Tonkin (1946), in studying the effects on the exo-erythrocytic forms of *P. gallinaceum* grown in tissue culture, found that proguanil had no action on the parasites even in concentrations of 2 to 5 mgm. per litre, which were the highest concentrations tolerated by macrophages. Yet *in vivo* its concentration is only about 0·3 mgm. per litre. It was therefore concluded that in the body proguanil must be converted into some active compound (Geiman, 1948). Evidence that such a conversion occurred was brought forward by Black (1946b), who showed that the serum of a patient treated with proguanil arrested the development of the trophozoites of *P. falciparum* when cultured *in vitro*. Similar results were obtained by Hawking (1947), who treated cultures of the blood forms of *P. cynomolgi* and the exo-erythrocytic forms of *P. gallinaceum* with the sera of monkeys which had received 50 mgm. of proguanil acetate five and twenty-one hours before bleeding. The development of the parasites was inhibited and they underwent degenerative changes. Hawking and Perry (1948) found that the sera of fowls and minced liver also activated proguanil *in vitro*. The nature of this transformation is still unknown, but Acheson *et al.* (1947) have excluded one possibility. The biguanidine molecule was approached because of the possibilities of tautomerism shown by the guanidino group and the activities of compounds 2666 and 3349 against *P. gallinaceum* in the chick. The following skeletal configurations were thought necessary for activity,

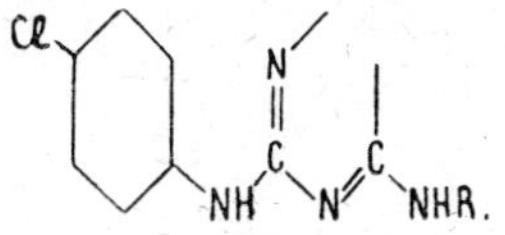

(I) 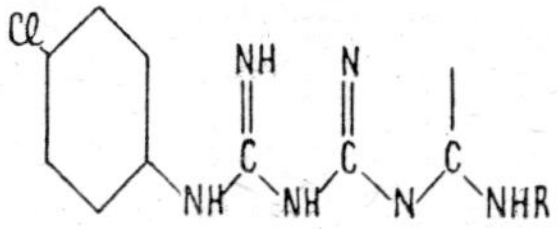   (II)

since X-ray crystallographic studies of proguanil hydrochloride show that it exists as a pseudo-triazole involving a hydrogen bond.

2666 (I) then appears as a derivative of biguanidine

$$\underset{NH_2-C-NH-C-NH_2,}{\overset{NH \qquad\quad NH}{\overset{\|\qquad\qquad\|}{}}}$$

and 3349 (II) as a derivative of an extended biguanidine, actually of the hypothetical triguanidine system. Consideration of the proguanil molecule (III) shows that without introducing any appreciable strain it is possible for N^2 to approach the benzene ring and by the loss of two hydrogen atoms to form a new bond. If this oxidation were a step in the metabolism of proguanil then the related guanidinobenziminazole (IV, $R = CHMe_2$) would be expected to show comparable biological activity. According to Woolley (1944), the growth of certain micro-organisms can be inhibited by benziminazole, which interferes with the utilisation of guanine and adenine. Proguanil might thus conceivably function as a competitor with some purine essential to the growth of the malaria parasite.

The benziminazole (IV, $R = CHMe_2$) has many of the properties of proguanil and can be readily converted into a chelate copper derivative, a reaction implying the formation of a dimolecular complex similar in outline to that of the porphyrin ring-system. Curd and Rose (1946b) suggested that proguanil may interfere with the porphyrin metabolism of the parasite, for proguanil forms a copper derivative in which two molecules of the drug combine with one atom of copper and the probable spatial formula of this copper complex bears a striking resemblance to the formula of the metal porphyrins. It is therefore remarkable that the

guanidinobenziminazole (IV, R = CHMe$_2$) and several analogous benziminazoles, none of which is more toxic than proguanil,
are at their maximum tolerated doses without action on infections
in chicks due to *P. gallinaceum.*

(III)   (IV)

Rose (1949), however, has pointed out that whatever chemical
variations are made either in the aromatic portion of the molecule,
or along the diguanide chain, optimum antimalarial activity,
where present, always requires a terminal *iso*propyl group. Proguanil shows very little interference with a root peroxidase
system, nor does it specifically inhibit the growth of *Hæmophilus
influenzæ*, an organism which requires a source of hæmatin. Some
inhibition occurs but this is due to the formation of a sparingly
soluble compound between proguanil and hæmatin. The pigment
of *P. knowlesi* and *P. gallinaceum* is, however, undoubtedly
hæmatin (Rimington, Fulton, and Sheinman, 1947).

Although further speculation is idle, Rose (1949) has suggested
that the flavin systems also bear some structural resemblance to
those of the porphyrin group. The close association of the two
types in enzymic dehydrogenases would thus be of significance.
One potential point of resemblance is that the riboflavin molecule
contains a system in the 4-hydroxy*iso*alloxazine residue potentially
able to chelate a metal atom.

Another possibility which also seems unlikely is indicated by
Marshall (1947), who has pointed out that *in vitro* proguanil
inhibits the oxidation of glucose, pyruvate, and lactate by washed
cells infected with *P. gallinaceum* more powerfully than does
quinine. The inhibition produced by proguanil is different from
that produced by iodoacetate. While the latter inhibits both
oxygen consumption and glycolysis and causes the accumulation
of hexose phosphates, proguanil, on the other hand, shows less
than 50 per cent. inhibition of glucose utilisation, although oxygen
consumption is inhibited to a greater extent. In comparative

experiments with quinine the greater inhibitory action of proguanil is much more striking at high than at low concentrations. Thus with the low concentrations necessary for activity *in vitro* it is rather doubtful whether inhibition of oxidative processes can be responsible for antimalarial action. Massart (1949) has pointed out that proguanil causes a progressive inhibition of the respiration of yeast cells. This inhibition is reversed by metallic cations such as magnesium.

It has been suggested by Laser (1946, 1948) that the development of the hæmolytic unsaturated monocarboxylic fatty acid normally present in human blood plasma and probably produced also by the development of malarial parasites is inhibited both *in vivo* and *in vitro* by antimalarial drugs. If this hæmolytic acid is a normal metabolic product of malarial parasites inhibition of its formation may destroy the parasites. Further investigations are required. It seems doubtful whether this lytic agent can be lysolecithin (Laser and Friedman, 1945), though lysolecithin can be extracted from human blood serum (de Vries, 1948).

Sulphonamides. The mode of action of sulphonamides on malarial parasites was first elicited by Marshall, Litchfield, and White (1942), who showed that *p*-aminobenzoic (PABA) acid inhibited the action of sulphanilamide against *P. lophuræ*. These results were confirmed by Maier and Riley (1942) in the case of sulphanilamide and *P. gallinaceum* in the chick, and by Seeler *et al.* (1943) in the case of sulphamethyldiazine and *P. lophuræ* in ducklings, *p*-aminobenzoic acid being given by mouth. PABA also inhibits the action of sulphonamides on *P. knowlesi* infections in rhesus monkeys (Richardson *et al.*, 1946). Considerable interest attaches to the fact that whereas sulphonamides are relatively ineffective against *P. relictum* and *P. cathemerium* in the canary yet N^1-$3'$: $5'$-dibromosulphanilamide and the dichloro- compound analogously named are active against *P. cathemerium* and probably against *P. relictum* (U.S. Patent 2,238,911, July 8th, 1941) and their action is not inhibited by *p*-aminobenzoic acid.

Tonkin (1946) has shown that PABA inhibited the action of sulphathiazole on the exo-erythrocytic forms of *P. gallinaceum* in tissue culture ; *ortho-* and *meta*-amino benzoic acids had no such action.

It is therefore probable that PABA is an essential metabolite for plasmodia just as it appears to be for certain bacteria and for viruses of the lymphogranuloma psittacosis group. The antimalarial action of sulphonamides is then due to competition of sulphonamides with this essential metabolite for certain enzymes in the parasites, possibly, as Henry (1944) suggests in the case of bacteria, respiratory enzymes. In view of the relationship of sulphonamides to reductone, shown by O'Meara *et al.* (1947), studies on reductone in malaria parasites are required. The action of sulphonamides and of proguanil on the malaria parasite has been linked up by the work of Bishop and McConnachie (1948) and Greenberg (1948, 1949a, b) and Greenberg *et al.* (1948). In the first place it was shown that a strain of *P. gallinaceum* made resistant to proguanil by passage in chicks was resistant to sulphonamides, and *vice versâ*. Greenberg (1948), however, showed that a proguanil strain had become hypersensitive to sulphadiazine and this hypersensitivity to sulphadiazine, an increased sensitivity of four to eight times, was still present after five passages in the absence of proguanil. The sensitivity to sulphadiazine was not associated with any increased sensitivity to pamaquin, quinine or chloroquine. Greenberg *et al.* (1948) found that proguanil and sulphadiazine act synergistically on *P. gallinaceum* in the chick. The same is true of sulphanilamide. The ability to potentiate proguanil is, however, independent of substituents on the aliphatic amino group of sulphonamides but is related to the capacity to be inhibited by PABA. Thus, according to Greenberg (1949b), all sulphonamides known to be inhibited by PABA are able to potentiate the antimalarial action of proguanil. Thus, in addition, phosphanilic acid, sulphanilic acid, *p,p'*-sulphonyldianiline and *p,p'*-sulphenyldianiline are inactivated by PABA and potientiate proguanil : on the other hand, dibromo- and dichloro-phenylsulphanilamide are not inactivated by PABA and do not potentiate proguanil. Proguanil is not inhibited by PABA but the presence of proguanil, mixed with sulphadiazine at a concentration well below that necessary by itself to achieve antimalarial action, increases by 150-fold the amount of PABA required to inhibit the sulphadiazine present. One of the products of PABA metabolism is pteroylglutamic acid

(Lampen and Jones, 1946) and Greenberg (1949a) has found that pteroylglutamic acid inhibits the antimalarial activity of both sulphadiazine and proguanil. However, while the antimalarial activity of sulphadiazine is completely inhibited by pteroylglutamic acid that of proguanil is only partially inhibited. Proguanil might therefore interfere either with the synthesis or utilisation of pteroylglutamic acid by some other means than competition with PABA. The first suggestion appears the more probable, thus proguanil would interfere with the utilisation by the malaria parasite either of pteroylglutamic acid or of some closely allied product of PABA metabolism. If this hypothesis is correct the synthetic antimalarial proguanil is far more effective than the natural metabolite pteroylglutamic acid in whatever linkages they undergo.

The only other known example of inhibition of an antimalarial drug is the finding by Seeler (1945) that an excess of pyridoxine inhibits the action of quinine and mepacrine on *P. lophuræ* and *P. cathemerium* in ducks. Further studies are required to determine at what point in the metabolic chain pyridoxine inhibits these drugs.

The *rôle* of pantothenic acid and its analogues is discussed on p. 407.

Nitrogen Metabolism and Antimalarial Compounds

From studies on the respiration and carbohydrate metabolism of malarial parasites it is possible to indicate certain points where this metabolism may be deranged by antimalarial drugs, although it must be emphasised that the discovery that certain enzymes are inhibited under *in vitro* conditions does not necessarily mean that it is this particular enzyme inhibition which is all important *in vivo*. There are still many lacunæ in our knowledge of the carbohydrate metabolism of particular stages of the malarial parasite. The question is very fully discussed by Moulder (1948a).

Similarly, it is possible, at least to indicate that certain vitamins if deficient or in excess may influence antimalarial action. Very little, however, is yet known of the nitrogen requirements or nitrogen metabolism of malarial parasites. The need of *P. knowlesi* for methionine is discussed on p. 432. Possibly other amino acids are required. In addition, Moulder and Evans (1946) found that hen red cells infected with *P. gallinaceum* produce considerable amounts of amino nitrogen if incubated aerobically in the presence of glucose. If glucose is absent much of the amino nitrogen appears as ammonia. Uninfected hen red cells produce only a small amount of amino nitrogen or ammonia. It thus seems probable that *P. gallinaceum* can deaminate amino acids. Anaerobiosis strongly inhibits the formation of amino nitrogen by infected red cells. Cell-free extracts of malaria parasites hydrolyse hæmoglobin at a very slow rate but denatured globin is split much more rapidly, and in addition the production of amino nitrogen from denatured globin in cell-free extracts is not inhibited by anaerobiosis. These observations suggest that while the malaria parasite relies on the red cell for its protein metabolism, protein hydrolysis is probably linked up with oxidative processes.

Further intensive studies are obviously necessary before the possible *rôle* of antimalarial drugs in protein metabolism can be explained on a satisfactory basis.

One other action of antimalarial drugs is not without interest. It has been known for some time (Pinelli, 1929 ; Velick and Scudder, 1940 ; Overman and Feldman, 1947) that in malaria the extracellular fluid volume increases, the cell permeability is altered, and the red cell content of potassium decreases while that of sodium increases. This change is reflected in an increased urinary output of K ions and a decreased output of sodium ions. Treatment of falciparum malaria by mepacrine or chloroquine has been shown by Overman *et al.* (1949) to reduce, though slowly, the sodium content of the red cells.

It must therefore be confessed that the mode of action of the majority of antimalarial drugs is still obscure. In the case of the sulphonamides the mode of action is possibly similar to that exercised by these drugs on bacteria, for in the case of plasmodia also the action of sulphonamides is inhibited by *p*-aminobenzoic acid (Marshall *et al.*, 1942 ; Maier and Riley, 1942). Phenyl-pantothenone as an analogue of pantothenic acid presumably interferes with the employment of this substance, for though pantothenic acid is known to exist in animals in the form of coenzyme A, a more complex molecule, micro-organisms, though carrying out a similar elimination of pantothenic acid, do not seem to be able to make use of animal coenzyme A to supply their own requirements.

Although theoretically quinine, mepacrine, and pamaquin might interfere with a number of reactions essential for the metabolism of malaria parasites there is still uncertainty as to how far any such inhibition is responsible for their antimalarial action. There is evidence both biological and chemical that they may act, as possibly do the anilinopyrimidines, as inhibitors of reactions involving the metabolism of riboflavin, at any rate in so far as bacteria are concerned. However, the fact that a substance chemically related to a growth factor can compete with that growth factor does not necessarily imply that an associated growth inhibition can be correlated with the metabolite analogue. Thus the final biological proof that these antimalarials are active solely because they may interfere with the action of flavin derivatives is not yet forthcoming and recent observations by King and Wright (1948) give no support to the view that the antimalarial action of quinine is due to riboflavin antagonism. Although proguanil was developed by logical chemical steps from mepacrine, yet in no system has it yet been shown to act as a riboflavin competitor. There is in fact as yet little clear evidence of the mode of action of proguanil. The view that it might act by chelating a metal has not commanded general assent nor has the view that by reason of the intrinsic size and shape of its cation (there is evidence that it exists as a pseudo-triazole involving a hydrogen bond) it may possess a structure similar enough to that of the porphyrins to interfere with their metabolism. The other suggestion is that proguanil interferes with the utilisation of pteroylglutamic acid or some closely related product of p-aminobenzoic acid metabolism.

References

ACHESON, R. M., KING, F. E., and SPENSLEY, P. C., 1947, Benziminazoles related to paludrine. *Nature, Lond.*, **160**, 53.

AMMON, R., 1935, Die Cholinesterase. *Ergebn. Enzymforsch.*, **4**, 102.

BADDILEY, J., LYTHGOE, B., and TODD, A. R., 1944, Experiments on the synthesis of purine nucleosides. Part VI. The synthesis of 9-D-xylosido-2-methyladenine and of 6-D-xylosidamino-2-methylpurine. *J. chem. Soc.*, 318.

BALL, E. G., 1946, Chemical and nutritional observations on malarial parasites grown *in vitro*. *Fed. Proc.*, **5**, 397.

BALL, E. G., MCKEE, R. W., ANFINSEN, C. B., CRUZ, W. D., and GEIMAN, Q. M., 1948, Studies on malarial parasites. IX. Chemical and metabolic changes during growth and multiplication *in vivo* and *in vitro*. *J. biol. Chem.*, **175**, 547.

BANG, F. B., HAIRSTON, N. G., TRAGER, W., and MAIER, J., 1947, Treatment of acute attacks of vivax and falciparum malaria. A comparison of atabrine and quinine. *Bull. U.S. Army med. Dept.*, **7**, 75.

BARBER, M. A., KOMP, W. H. W., and NEWMAN, B. M., 1929, Effect of small doses of plasmochin on viability of gametocytes of malaria as measured by mosquito infection experiments. *Publ. Hlth Rept., Wash.*, **44**, 1409.

BARLOW, R. B., and ING, H. R., 1950, A series of 9'-dialkylaminoalkyl*iso*-alloxazines. *J. chem. Soc.*, 713.

BASFORD, F. R., CURD, F. H. S., and ROSE, F. L., 1946, Synthetic anti-malarials. Part VIII. Some 4-arylamino-6-aminoalkylamino-2-methyl-pyrimidines. *J. chem. Soc.*, 713.

BASS, C. C., 1922, Some observations on the effect of quinine upon the growth of malaria plasmodia *in vitro*. *Amer. J. trop. Med.*, **2**, 289.

BISHOP, A., and MCCONNACHIE, E. W., 1948, Resistance to sulphadiazine and " paludrine " in the malaria parasite of the fowl (*P. gallinaceum*). *Nature, Lond.*, **162**, 541.

BLACK, R. H., 1946a, The effect of antimalarial drugs on *Plasmodium falciparum* (New Guinea strains) developing *in vitro*. *Trans. R. Soc. trop. Med. Hyg.*, **40**, 163.

BLACK, R. H., 1946b, The behaviour of New Guinea strains of *Plasmodium falciparum* and *Plasmodium vivax* when cultivated *in vitro*. *Med. J. Aust.*, **2**, 109.

BLACK, R. H., 1949, Observations on the treatment of falciparum malaria. *Trans. R. Soc. trop. Med. Hyg.*, **42**, 565.

BLASCHKO, H., CHOU, T. C., and WAJDA, I., 1946, The inhibition of esterases by paludrine. *Biochem J.*, **40**, Proc. LXVII.

BLASCHKO, H., CHOU, T. C., and WAJDA, I., 1947, The inhibition of esterases by paludrine. *Brit. J. Pharmacol.*, **2**, 116.

BOCK, E., 1939, Ueber morphologische Veränderungen menschlicher Malaria-parasiten durch Atebrineinwirkung. *Arch. Schiffs-u. Tropenhyg.*, **43**, 209.

BOCK, E., and OESTERLIN, M., 1939, Ueber einige fluoreszenmikroskopische Beobachtungen. *Zent. Bakt. (Abt. 1, Orig.)*, **143**, 306.

BOVARNICK, M. R., LINDSAY, A., and HELLERMAN, L., 1946a, Metabolism of the malarial parasite with reference particularly to the action of anti-malarial agents. I. Preparation and properties of *Plasmodium lophurœ* separated from the red cells of duck blood by means of saponin. *J. biol. Chem.*, **163**, 523.

BOVARNICK, M. R., LINDSAY, A., and HELLERMAN, L., 1946b, Metabolism of the malarial parasite with reference particularly to the action of anti-malarial agents. II. Atabrine (quinacrine) inhibition of glucose oxidation in parasites initially depleted by substrate : reversal by adenylic acid. *J. biol. Chem.*, **163**, 535.

BOYD, G. H., and DUNN, M., 1939, Effects of quinine and plasmochin upon parasite reproduction and destruction in avian malaria. *Amer. J. Hyg.*, **30C**, 1.

BOYD, G. H., and DUNN, M., 1941, The method of action of atabrine upon the avian malaria parasite, *Plasmodium cathemerium*. *Amer. J. Hyg.*, **34C**, 129.

CHOPRA, R. N., GANGULI, S. K., and ROY, A. C., 1936, Studies on the action of antimalarial remedies on monkey malaria. The relationship between the concentration of atebrin in the circulating blood and parasite count. *Indian med. Gaz.*, **71**, 443.

CHRISTOPHERS, S. R., and FULTON, J. D., 1938, Observations on the respiratory metabolism of malaria parasites and trypanozomes. *Ann. trop. Med. Parasit.*, 32, 43.

CHRISTOPHERS, S. R., and FULTON, J. D., 1939, Experiments with isolated malaria parasites (*Plasmodium knowlesi*) free from red cells. *Ann. trop. Med. Parasit.*, 33, 161.

CLARKE, D. H., and THEILER, M., 1948, Studies on parasite-host interplay between *Plasmodium gallinaceum* and the chicken as influenced by hydroxynaphthoquinones. *J. infect. Dis.*, 82, 138.

CORRAN, H. S., GREEN, D. E., and STRAUB, F. B., 1939, On the catalytic function of heart. *Biochem. J.*, 33, 793.

COULSTON, F., and HUFF, C. G., 1948, The chemotherapy and immunology of pre-erythrocytic stages in avian malaria. *J. Parasit.*, 34, 290.

CURD, F. H. S., DAVEY, D. G., and ROSE, F. L., 1945a, Studies on synthetic malarials. II. General chemical considerations. *Ann. trop. Med. Parasit.*, 39, 157.

CURD, F. H. S., DAVEY, D. G., ROSE, F. L., 1945b, Studies on synthetic malarials. X. Some biguanide derivatives as new types of antimalarial substances with both therapeutic and causal prophylactic activity. *Ann. trop. Med. Parasit.*, 39, 208.

CURD, F. H. S., DAVIS, M. I., HOGGARTH, E., and ROSE, F. L., 1947, Synthetic antimalarials. Part XV. Some aryloxy- and arylthio-dialkyamino-alkylamino-pyrimidines. *J. chem. Soc.*, 783.

CURD, F. H. S., DAVIS, M. I., and ROSE, F. L., 1946, Synthetic antimalarials. Part II. 2-Substituted-anilino-4-aminoalkylamino-6-methylpyrimidines. *J. chem. Soc.*, 351.

CURD, F. H. S., RAISON, C. G., and ROSE, F. L., 1946, Synthetic antimalarials. Part V. 2-Naphthylamino-4-aminoalklyamino-6-methylpyrimidines. *J. chem. Soc.*, 366.

CURD, F. H. S., and ROSE, F. L., 1946a, Synthetic antimalarials. Part I. Some derivatives of arylamino and aryl-substituted pyrimidines. *J. chem. Soc.*, 343.

CURD, F. H. S., and ROSE, F. L., 1946b, A possible mode of action of " paludrine." *Nature, Lond.*, 158, 707.

DUDGEON, L. S., and CLARKE, C., 1917, On the cultivation of the malarial parasite *in vitro*. *Lancet, i*, 530.

EMERSON, G. A., and TISHLER, M., 1944, The antiriboflavin effect of *iso*-riboflavin. *Proc. Soc. exp. Biol., N.Y.*, 55, 184.

EULER, H. VON, KARRER, P., MALMBERG, M., SCHÖPP, K., BENZ, F., BECKER, B., and FREI, P., 1935, Synthese des Lactoflavins (vitamin B_2) und anderer Flavine. *Helv. chim. Acta*, 18, 522.

EVANS, E. A., Jr., 1946, Enzyme systems operating within the malarial parasite. *Fed. Proc.*, 5, 390.

EVANS, E. A., Jr., CEITHAML, J., SPECK, J. F., and MOULDER, J. W., 1945, Biochemistry of the malarial parasite, *Plasmodium gallinaceum*. *Fed. Proc.*, 4, 89.

FALCO, E. A., HITCHINGS, G. H., RUSSELL, P. B., VAN DER WERFF, H., 1949, Antimalarials as antagonists of purine and pteroylglutamic acid. *Nature, Lond.*, 164, 107.

FISCHL, V., and SINGER, E., 1934, Die Wirkungsweise chemotherapeutisch verwendeter Farbstoffe. *Z. Hyg. InfektKr.*, 116, 348.

FULTON, J. D., 1936, Studies in the chemotherapy of malaria. The inhibitory action of antimalarial drugs on blood lipases. *Ann. trop. Med. Parasit.*, 30, 491.

FULTON, J. D., 1939, Experiments on the utilisation of sugars by malarial parasites (*Plasmodium knowlesi*). *Ann. trop. Med. Parasit.*, 33, 217.

556 MODE OF ACTION OF ANTIMALARIAL DRUGS

FULTON, J. D., and CHRISTOPHERS, S. R., 1938, The inhibitive effect of drugs upon oxygen uptake by trypanosomes (*Trypanosoma rhodesiense*) and malaria parasites (*Plasmodium knowlesi*). *Ann. trop. Med. Parasit.*, 32, 77.
GEIGY, R., and RAHM, U., 1949, Testen von Antimalaria-Mitteln an *Plasmodium-gallinaceum* im Darm von *Aëdes œgypti*. *Acta trop.*, 6, 153.
GEIMAN, Q. M., 1948, Cultivation and metabolism of malarial parasites. *Proc. 4th internat. Congr. trop. Med. Mal. Wash. D.C.*, 1, 618.
GRAY, A., and HILL, J., 1949, Antimalarial studies in the quinoline series. *Ann. trop. Med. Parasit.*, 43, 32.
GREENBERG, J., 1948, Hypersensitivity to sulfadiazine of a chlorguanide-resistant strain of *Plasmodium gallinaceum*. *J. nat. Mal. Soc.*, 8, 80.
GREENBERG, J., 1949a, Inhibition of the antimalarial activity of chlorguanide by pteroylglutamic acid. *Proc. Soc. exp. Biol., N.Y.*, 71, 306.
GREENBERG, J., 1949b, The potentiation of the antimalarial activity of chlorguanide by *p*-aminobenzoic acid competitors. *J. Pharmacol.*, 97, 238.
GREENBERG, J., BOYD, B. L., and JOSEPHSON, E. S., 1948, Synergistic effect of chlorguanide and sulfadiazine against *Plasmodium gallinaceum* in the chick. *J. Pharmacol.*, 94, 60.
GREENBERG, J., TREMBLEY, H. L., and COATNEY, G. R., 1950, Effects of drugs on *Plasmodium gallinaceum* infections produced by decreasing concentrations of a sporozoite inoculum. *Amer. J. Hyg.*, 51, 194.
HAAS, E., 1944, The effect of atabrine and quinine on isolated respiratory enzymes. *J. biol. Chem.*, 155, 321.
HAWKING, F., 1947, Activation of paludrine *in vitro*. *Nature, Lond.*, 159, 409.
HAWKING, F., and PERRY, W. L. M., 1948, Activation of paludrine. *Brit. J. Pharmacol.*, 3, 320.
HELLERMAN, L., BOVARNICK, M. R., and POTTER, C. C., 1946, Metabolism of the malarial parasite. Action of antimalarial agents upon separated *Plasmodium lophuræ* and upon certain isolated enzyme systems. *Fed. Proc.*, 5, 400.
HENRY, R. J., 1944, "The mode of action of the sulfonamides." New York. Josiah Macey Foundation.
HEWITT, R. I., and RICHARDSON, A. P., 1943, The direct plasmodicidal effect of quinine, atabrine and plasmochin on *Plasmodium lophuræ*. *J. infect. Dis.*, 73, 1.
HIRST, E. L., and PEAT, S., 1936, Carbohydrates—Monosaccharides, Disaccharides and Glycosides. *Rep. Progr. Chem.*, 33, 245.
HÜHNE, W., 1942, Ueber atebrineinwirkungen auf das morphologische Verhalten von *Plasmodium falciparum*. *Dtsch. tropenmed. Z.*, 46, 385.
HULL, R., LOVELL, B. J., OPENSHAW, H. T., PAYMAN, L. C., and TODD, A. R., 1946, Synthetic antimalarials. Part III. Some derivatives of mono- and di-alkylpyrimidines. *J. chem. Soc.*, 357.
HULL, R., LOVELL, B. J., OPENSHAW, H. T., PAYMAN, L. C., and TODD, A. R., 1947, Synthetic antimalarials. *J. chem. Soc.*, 41.
ING, H. R., 1949, quoted by F. L. ROSE. *Proc. roy. Soc. Lond. B.*, 136, 109.
IRVIN, J. L., and IRVIN, E. M., 1949, Interaction of 9-aminoacridines with proteins and nucleic acids. *Fed. Proc.*, 8, 209.
IRVIN, J. L., IRVIN, E. M., and PARKER, F. S., 1949, The interaction of antimalarials with nucleic acids. I. Acridines. II. Quinolines. *Science*, 110, 426.
JAMES, S. P., 1934, The direct effect of atebrine on the parasites of benign tertian and quartan malaria. *Trans. R. Soc. trop. Med. Hyg.*, 28, 3.
JERACE, F., and GIOVANNOLA, A., 1933, L'azione sterilizzante della plasmochina sui gameti dei parassiti malarigeni e sua importanza profilattica. *Riv. Malariol.*, 12, 457.

JOHNSON, H. A., and AKINS, H., 1948, The effect of one plant extract and of certain drugs on the development of *Plasmodium gallinaceum* in *Aëdes ægypti*. *J. nat. Mal. Soc.*, **7**, 144.

KING, H., and TONKIN, I. M., 1946, Antiplasmodial action and chemical constitution. Part VIII. Guanidines and diguanidines. *J. chem. Soc.*, 1063.

KING, H., and WRIGHT, J., 1948, Antiplasmodial action and chemical constitution. IX. Carbinolamines derived from 6 : 7-dimethylquinoline. *Proc. roy. Soc. B.*, **135**, 271.

KRITSCHEWSKI, I. L., and DEMIDOWA, L. W., 1934, Ueber eine noch unbekannte Funktion des reticuloendothelialen Systems. XXII. Ueber die Bedeutung des retikuloendothelialen Systems in der Therapie der Malaria. *Z. ImmunForsch.*, **84**, 14.

KUHN, R., WEYGAND, F., and MÖLLER, E. F., 1943, Über einen antagonisten des lactoflavins. *Ber. dtsch. chem. Ges.*, **76**, 1044.

LAMPEN, J. O., and JONES, M. J., 1946, The antagonism of sulfonamides by pteroylglutamic acid and related compounds. *J. biol. Chem.*, **164**, 485.

LAMPEN, J. O., and JONES, M. J., 1947, The growth-promoting and anti-sulfonamide activity of p-aminobenzoic acid, pteroylglutamic acid and related compounds for *Lactobacillus arabinosus* and *Streptobacterium plantarum*. *J. biol. chem.*, **170**, 133.

LASER, H., 1946, A method of testing the antimalarial properties of compounds *in vitro*. *Nature, Lond.*, **157**, 301.

LASER, H., 1948, Hæmolytic system in the blood of malaria-infected monkeys. *Nature, Lond.*, **161**, 560.

LASER, H., and FRIEDMANN, E., 1945, Crystalline hæmolytic substance from normal blood. *Nature, Lond.*, **156**, 507.

LOURIE, F. M., 1934, Studies on chemotherapy in bird malaria. II. Observations bearing on the mode of action of quinine. *Ann. trop. Med. Parasit.*, **28**, 255.

McKEE, R. W., and GEIMAN, Q. M., 1948, Methionine in the growth of the malarial parasite *Plasmodium knowlesi*. *Fed. Proc.*, **7**, 172.

McKEE, R. W., ORMSBEE, R. A., ANFINSEN, C. B., GEIMAN, Q. M., and BALL, E. G., 1946, Studies on malarial parasites. VI. The chemistry and metabolism of normal and parasitised (*P. knowlesi*) monkey blood. *J. exp. Med.*, **84**, 569.

MACKERRAS, M. J., and ERCOLE, Q. N., 1947, Observations on the action of paludrine on malarial parasites. *Trans. R. Soc. trop. Med. Hyg.*, **41**, 365.

MACKERRAS, M. J., and ERCOLE, Q. N., 1948, Observations on the development of human malarial parasites in the mosquito. *Aust. J. exp. Biol. med. Sci.*, **26**, 439.

MACKERRAS, M. J., and ERCOLE, Q. N., 1949a, Some observations on the action of quinine, atebrin and plasmoquine on *Plasmodium vivax*. *Trans. R. Soc. trop. Med. Hyg.*, **42**, 443.

MACKERRAS, M. J., and ERCOLE, Q. N., 1949b, Observations on the action of quinine, atebrin and plasmoquine on the gametocytes of *Plasmodium falciparum*. *Trans. R. Soc. trop. Med. Hyg.*, **42**, 465.

MADINAVEITIA, J., 1946, The antagonism of some antimalarial drugs by riboflavin. *Biochem. J.*, **40**, 373.

MADINAVEITIA, J., and RAVENTÓS, J., 1949, Antimalarial compounds as antagonists of adenosine. *Brit. J. Pharmacol.*, **4**, 81.

MAGIDSON, O. Y., DELEKTORSKAYA, N. M., and LIPOWITSCH, I. M., 1934, Die Derivate des 8-Aminochinolins als Antimalariapräparate. Mitt. III : Der Einfluss der Verzweigung der Kette in Stellung 8. *Arch. Pharm. Berl.*, **272**, 74.

MAGIDSON, O. Y., and GRIGOROWSKY, A. M., 1936, Acridin-Uerbin dungen und ihre Antimalaria-Wirkung. (I. Mitteil.) *Ber. dtsch. chem. Ges.*, **69**, 396.

MAGIDSON, O. Y., and RUBTSOV, M. V., 1937, [Quinoline compounds as sources of medicinal products. VI. Antimalarial compounds with the side chain in the four-position]. *J. gen. Chem. Russ.*, **7**, 1896.

MAIER, J., and COGGESHALL, L. T., 1941, Respiration of malaria plasmodia. *J. infect. Dis.*, **69**, 87.

MAIER, J., and RILEY, E., 1942, Inhibition of antimalarial action of sulfonamides by p-aminobenzoic acid. *Proc. Soc. exp. Biol.*, *N.Y.*, **50**, 152.

MARSHALL, E. K., Jr., 1949, The significance of drug concentration in the blood as applied to chemotherapy, in " Evaluation of chemotherapeutic agents," edited by C. M. Macleod, Symposia of the Section on Microbiology, No. 2, p. 3. New York. Columbia Univ. Press.

MARSHALL, E. K., Jr., LITCHFIELD, J. T., Jr., and WHITE, H. J., 1942, Sulfonamide therapy of malaria in ducks. *J. Pharmacol.*, **75**, 89.

MARSHALL, P. B., 1947, Mode of action of paludrine. *Nature, Lond.*, **160**, 463.

MARSHALL, P. B., 1948, The glucose metabolism of *Plasmodium gallinaceum*, and the action of antimalarial agents. *Brit. J. Pharmacol.*, **3**, 1.

MARTIN, S. J., COMINOLE, B., and CLARK, B. B., 1939, Chronic oral administration of atabrine. *J. Pharmacol.*, **65**, 156.

MASSART, L., 1949, Paludrine and cation exchange. *Arch. int. Pharmacodyn.*, **80**, 470.

MASSART, L., PETERS, G., VAN HOUKE, A., and LAGRAIN, A., 1947, The uptake of acridines by cell substances. *Arch. int. Pharmacodyn.*, **75**, 141.

MILLER, A. K., and PETERS, L., 1945, The antagonism by spermine and spermidine of the antibacterial action of quinacrine and other drugs. *Arch. Biochem.*, **6**, 281.

MISSIROLI, A., and MOSNA, E., 1938, La sterilizzazione dei gametociti dei plasmodi malarici. *Riv. Parassit.*, **2**, 55.

MOSNA, E., 1936, L'azione della chinina e dell'atebrin sul' *Plasmodium knowlesi*. *Riv. Malariol. Sez.* 1, **15**, 99.

MOULDER, J. H., 1948a, The metabolism of malarial parasites. *Ann. Rev. Microbiol.*, **2**, 101.

MOULDER, J. H., 1948b, Effect of quinine treatment of the host upon the carbohydrate metabolism of the malarial parasite *Plasmodium gallinaceum*. *J. infect. Dis.*, **83**, 262.

MOULDER, J. W., 1949, Inhibition of pyruvate oxidation in the malarial parasite *Plasmodium gallinaceum* by quinine treatment of the host. *J. infect. Dis.*, **85**, 195.

MOULDER, J. W., and EVANS, E. A., Jr., 1946, The biochemistry of the malaria parasite. VI. Studies on the nitrogen metabolism of the malaria parasite. *J. biol. Chem.*, **164**, 145.

MÜHLENS, P., and KIRSCHBAUM, W., 1924, Weitere parasitologische Beobachtungen bei Künstlichen Malariainfectionen von Paralytikern. *Arch. Schiffs-u. Tropenhyg.*, **28**, 131.

OESTERLIN, M., 1936, Chemotherapie, Fluorescenz und Krebs. *Klin. Wschr.*, **15ii**, 1719.

OLDHAM, F. K., KELSEY, F. E., CANTRELL, W., and GEILING, E. M. K., 1944, Studies on antimalarial drugs. The effect of malaria (*Plasmodium gallinaceum*) and of anæmia on the distribution of quinine in the tissues of the fowl. *J. Pharmacol.*, **82**, 349.

O'MEARA, R. A. Q., McNALLY, P. A., and NELSON, H. G., 1947, The intracellular mode of action of the sulphonamide derivatives. *Lancet, ii*, 747.

OVERMAN, R. R., and FELDMAN, H. A., 1947. The effect of fatal *P. knowlesi* malaria on simian circulatory and body fluid compartment physiology. *J. clin. Invest.*, **26**, 1049.

OVERMAN, R. R., HILL, T. S., and WONG, Y. T., 1949, Physiological studies in the human malaria host. I. Blood plasma, " extracellular " fluid volumes and ionic balance in therapeutic *P. vivax* and *P. falciparum* infections. *J. nat. Mal. Soc.*, **8**, 14.

PETER, F. M., 1932, Zur Weiterentwicklung synthetisch dargestellter Malaria-mittel : über die wirkung des Atebrin gegen natürliche malaria infektion. *Dtsch. med. Wschr.*, **58**, 533.

PINELLI, L., 1929, La potassiema nella malaria. *Riv. Malariol.*, **8**, 310.

RICHARDSON, A. P., HEWITT, R. I., SEAGER, L. D., BROOKE, M. M., MARTIN, F., and MADDUX, H., 1946, Chemotherapy of *Plasmodium knowlesi* infections in *Macaca mulatta* monkeys. *J. Pharmacol.*, **87**, 203.

RICHTER, D., and CROFT, P. G., 1942, Blood esterases. *Biochem. J.*, **36**, 746.

RIMINGTON, C., FULTON, J. D., and SHEINMAN, H., 1947, The pigment of the malarial parasites *Plasmodium knowlesi* and *Plasmodium gallinaceum*. *Biochem. J.*, **41**, 619.

ROSE, F. L., 1949, Some anti-malarial agents as possible growth factor antagonists : in a discussion on antibiotic activity of growth factor analogues. *Proc. roy. Soc. B.*, **136**, 109.

SCHÖNHÖFER, F., 1942, Ueber die Bedeutung der chinoiden Bindung in Chinolinverbindungen für die Malariawirkung. *Z. physiol. Chem.*, **274**, 1.

SEELER, A. O., 1945, The inhibiting effect of pyridoxine on the activity of quinine and atebrin against avian malaria. *J. nat. malar. Soc.*, **4**, 13.

SEELER, A. O., GRAESSLE, O., and DUSENBERRY, E. D., 1943, The effect of para-aminobenzoic acid on the chemotherapeutic activity of the sulfon-amides in lymphogranuloma venereum and in duck malaria. *J. Bact.*, **45**, 205.

SHUTE, P. G., and MARYON, M., 1948, The gametocytocidal action of paludrine upon infections with *Plasmodium falciparum*. *Parasitology*, **38**, 264.

SILVERMAN, M., 1948a, The antagonism of antibacterial action of atabrine. *J. biol. Chem.*, **172**, 849.

SILVERMAN, M., 1948b, Metal antagonism of the antibacterial action of atabrine and other drugs. *Arch. Biochem.*, **19**, 193.

SILVERMAN, M., CEITHAML, J., TALIAFERRO, L. G., and EVANS, E. A., Jr., 1944, The *in vitro* metabolism of *Plasmodium gallinaceum*. *J. infect. Dis.*, **75**, 212.

SILVERMAN, M., and EVANS, E. A., Jr., 1943, Effects of spermidine and other polyamines on growth inhibition of *Escherichia coli*. *J. biol. Chem.*, **150**, 265.

SILVERMAN, M., and EVANS, E. A., Jr., 1944, The effect of spermine, spermidine, and other polyamines on growth inhibition of *Escherichia coli* by atebrine. *J. biol. Chem.*, **154**, 521.

SINTON, J. A., 1938, Action of atebrin upon the gametocytes (crescents) of *Plasmodium falciparum*. *Trans. R. Soc. trop. Med. Hyg.*, **32**, 11.

SPECK, J. F., and EVANS, E. A., Jr., 1945a, The biochemistry of the malaria parasite. II. Glycolysis in cell-free preparations of the malaria parasite. *J. biol. Chem.*, **159**, 71.

SPECK, J. F., and EVANS, E. A., Jr., 1945b, The biochemistry of the malaria parasites. III. The effects of quinine and atabrine on glycolysis. *J. biol. Chem.*, **159**, 83.

SPECK, J. F., MOULDER, J. W., and EVANS, E. A., Jr., 1946, The biochemistry of the malaria parasite. V. Mechanism of pyruvate oxidation in the malaria parasite. *J. biol. Chem.*, **164**, 119.

STRAUB, F. B., 1939, Isolation and properties of flavoprotein from heart muscle tissue. *Biochem. J.*, **33**, 787.

TERZIAN, L. A., STAHLER, N., and WEATHERSBY, A. B., 1949, The action of anti-malarial drugs in mosquitoes infected with *Plasmodium gallinaceum*. *J. infect. Dis.*, **84**, 47.

TERZIAN, L. A., and WEATHERSBY, A. B., 1949, The action of anti-malarial drugs in mosquitoes infected with *Plasmodium falciparum*. *Amer. J. trop. Med.*, **29**, 19.

THOMPSON, P. E., 1948, On the ability of *Plasmodium lophuræ* to acquire resistance to chlorguanide, " Camoquin " and chloroquine. *J. infect. Dis.*, 83, 250.

THOMSON, J. G., and MCLELLAN, S. W., 1912, The cultivation of one generation of malarial parasites (*Plasmodium falciparum*) *in vitro* by Bass's method. *Ann. trop. Med. Parasit.*, 6, 449.

TONKIN, I. M., 1946, The testing of drugs against exoerythrocytic forms of *P. gallinaceum* in tissue culture. *Brit. J. Pharmacol.*, 1, 163.

TRAGER, W., BANG, F. B., and HAIRSTON, N. G., 1945, Relation of plasma level of atabrine to morphology and motility of *Plasmodium vivax*. *Proc. Soc. exp. Biol.*, N.Y., 60, 257.

UMBREIT, W. W., 1949, A site of action of streptomycin. *J. biol. Chem.*, 177, 703.

VELICK, S. F., and SCUDDER, J., 1940, Plasma potassium level in avian malaria. *Amer. J. Hyg.*, 31, 92.

VENNESLAND, B., 1948, Carbohydrate metabolism. *Ann. Rev. Biochem.*, 17, 227.

VINCENT, D., and BEAUJARD, P., 1945, La détection des alcaloïdes inhibiteurs de la cholinesterase. (Esérine en particulier.) Applications toxicologiques *Ann. pharm. franç.*, 3, 22.

VRIES, S. I. DE, 1948, Experimentele hæmolytische anæmie. *Ned. Tijdschr. Geneesk.*, 92iii, 2013.

WAELSCH, H., and NACHMANSOHN, D., 1943, On the toxicity of atabrine. *Proc. Soc. exp. Biol.*, N.Y., 54, 336.

WAMPLER, F. J., 1930, A preliminary report on the early effects of plasmochin on *P. cathemerium*. *Arch. Protistenk.*, 69, 1.

WENDEL, W. B., 1943, Respiratory and carbohydrate metabolism of malaria parasites (*Plasmodium knowlesi*). *J. biol. Chem.*, 148, 21.

WENDEL, W. B., 1946, The influence of naphthoquinones upon the respiration and carbohydrate metabolism of malarial parasites. *Fed. Proc.*, 5, 406.

WENYON, C. M., 1926, " Protozoology. A manual for medical men, veterinarians and zoologists." London. Baillière, Tindall & Cox.

WOLF, P., 1949, Action anti-anaerobique de la quinacrine sur des cultures de *Pseudomonas fluorescens*. *Schweiz. Z. Path. Bakt.*, 12, 608.

WOOLLEY, D. W., 1944, Some biological effects produced by benzimidazole and their reversal by purines. *J. biol. Chem.*, 152, 225.

WRIGHT, C. I., and SABINE, J. C., 1944, The effect of atabrine on the oxygen consumption of tissues. *J. biol. Chem.*, 155, 315.

WRIGHT, C. I., and SABINE, J. C., 1948, Cholinesterases of human erythrocytes and plasma and their inhibition by antimalarial drugs. *J. Pharmacol.*, 93, 230.

YOUNG, M. D., MCKENDON, S. B., and SMARR, R. G., 1943, The selective action of thiobismol on induced malaria. *J. Amer. med. Ass.*, 122, 492.

AUTHOR INDEX

Lidz, T., 214, 218, 220, 263, 266
Liebig, H., 214, 269
Lillie, R. D., 198, 269
Lind, J., 271, 283, 361, 418, 419
Lindsay, A., 554
Lindsay, D. K., 280, 361
Lind van Wijngaarden, C. de, 152, 183, 236, 263
Linnell, W. H., 109, 120
Lints, H. A., 354, 504
Lipkin, I. J., 184
Lipowitsch, I. M., 120, 183, 557
Lippard, V. W., 200, 264
Lippincott, S. W., 124, 136, 183, 356, 500
Lips, M., 17, 32
Litchfield, J. T., Jr., 120, 402, 549, 557
Liu, Shao-Kwang, 416
Livados, G., 382, 402
Livingood, C. S., 201, 222, 264
Lobato Paraense, W., 272, 361
Loeb, R. F., 245, 246, 264, 292, 339, 361, 465, 476, 482, 501
Löken, A. C., 240, 243, 264
Loewenstein, A., 189, 264
Loewenthal, L. J. A., 199, 201, 202, 264
Lomax, P. H., 325, 361
London, I. M., 186, 262, 265, 268, 344, 358, 361, 363, 366, 469, 500–502
Lorant, S., 422
Lorenz, F. W., 435
Losee, K., 118, 399
Lott, W. A., 118, 399
Lourdenadin, S., 217, 264
Lourie, E. M., 179, 371, 375, 411, 413, 438–42, 444, 445, 450, 453, 507, 557
Love, W. R., 370, 374
Lovell, B. J., 115, 120, 556
Lowe, J., 355, 372, 375
Lu, G., 418
Lucherini, T., 226, 264
Lucena, D. T., 295, 361
Ludovici, H. L., 262
Lum, L. C., 208, 264
Lutterloh, C. H., 200, 264
Lutz, R. E., 38, 76
Lynch, P. P., 188, 264
Lyons, C., 405, 407
Lythgoe, B., 525, 553

MacBRIDE, D., 278, 361, 437
McCain, B. E., 412, 413
MacCallum, F. O., 363
McCarrison, R., 195, 264, 280, 361
McConnachie, E. W., 442, 444, 550, 554
McCoy, O. R., 264, 361, 501
McCreight, W. G., 297, 360
McDaniel, G. E., 367
MacDonald, D. R., 217, 264
MacDonald, I. C., 357
MacDuffie, K., 181
McEwen, M. M., 76, 183

Macey, P. E., 117, 119
McFadzean, A. J. S., 223, 264
Macfie, J. W. S., 12, 32, 43, 75, 272, 368, 376, 446, 450, 451, 453
McGhee, R. B., 17, 30, 435–37, 446, 453
McGibben, J. M., 269
MacGilchrist, A. C., 282, 361
McGinn, S., 349, 361
McGinty, D. A., 376
McGregor, I. S., 189, 264
Machella, T. E., 349, 361, 459, 460, 501
McIlwain, H., 408, 411
MacIntosh, F. C., 163, 183
McKee, R. W., 28, 432, 434, 506, 539, 554, 557
McKendon, S. B., 560
MacKerras, I. M., 349, 361
MacKerras, M. J., 26, 30, 325, 330, 356, 357, 361, 401, 500, 509, 510, 515–18, 557
McKibbin, J. M., 262
McLay, K., 128, 183
M'Lean, Hector, 369, 375
McLean, I. W., Jr., 405, 407
McLean, N., 3, 5
McLellan, G. W., 508, 559
McLendon, S. B., 377, 383, 400
McMartin, R. B., 238, 259
McNally, P. A., 558
McWilliam, J. O., 284, 361
Madajewa, O. S., 77
Maddux, H., 364, 403, 558
Madinaveitia, J., 39, 77, 87, 91, 120, 176, 177, 183, 433, 434, 522, 523, 528, 530–33, 557
Maegraith, B. G., 29, 156–58, 166, 177, 183, 185, 186, 257, 311, 312, 315, 316, 326, 327, 350, 351, 361, 362, 378, 401, 461, 473, 498, 502
Magidson, O. Y., 38, 45, 54, 57, 58, 68, 76, 77, 80, 83, 88, 89, 94, 120, 130, 173, 183, 520, 525, 526, 557
Magnusson, A. B., 72
Maier, J., 132, 133, 183, 214, 215, 232, 258, 262, 264, 342, 351, 354, 378, 383–87, 398, 400, 402, 452, 457, 498, 502, 539, 549, 552, 554, 557
Malamos, B., 10, 32, 342, 362
Malanga, C., 407, 419
Malmberg, M., 555
Mamou, H., 194, 264
Manfredi, M., 325, 362, 469, 502
Manifold, J. A., 476, 502
Manifold, M. C., 220, 264
Mann, F. G., 70, 73, 114, 120
Mann, I., 223, 264
Mann, W. N., 238, 264
Mannhardt, J., 405, 407
Manoliu, E., 354
Manwell, R. D., 17, 26, 27, 30, 31, 272, 335, 342, 362, 375, 387, 402

Maranon, J., 288, 362
Marchoux, E., 373, 375
Marcialis, I., 488, 502
Marble, A., 183, 262, 356, 358, 500
Mariani, F., 128, 183
Marini, C., 355
Marino, P., 237, 265
Marino-Assereto, P., 240, 266
Maritschek, M., 194, 264
Markowicz, H., 194, 264
Markson, J. L., 29, 193, 197, 220, 261, 264, 357, 378, 401, 500
Marousek, A. A., 498
Marshall, E. K., Jr., 12, 13, 20–21, 27–29, 31, 38, 77, 80, 120, 264, 281, 335, 342, 343, 355, 361, 369, 387, 388, 401, 402, 501, 506, 549, 552, 557
Marshall, L. E., 202, 259
Marshall, P. B., 21, 31, 122, 125, 126, 130, 183, 184, 276, 277, 281, 362, 388, 402, 539, 543, 545, 558
Marson, H. W., 401
Martin, F., 364, 403, 558
Martin, S. J., 534, 558
Martin, T. A., 76
Martin, W. B., 383, 400, 499
Marvel, C. S., 264, 361, 501
Maryon, M., 317, 354, 365, 499, 517, 559
Masen, J. M., 143, 184
Mason, S. F., 60, 75, 140, 181
Massart, L., 163, 184, 534, 549, 558
Massias, C., 50, 77
Más y Guindal, J., 437
Mathieson, D. W., 43, 77
Matson, E. J., 70, 76, 431
Matthews, J., 284, 362
Matzner, M. J., 143, 144, 183
Mauss, H., 54, 77, 184
May, E. L., 42, 77, 420, 422
Mayer, M., 240, 266
Maynard, J. T., 74
Mazza, S., 335, 362
Mead, J., 95, 120, 124, 184
Mead, J. F., 78, 125, 184, 418, 419
Méchali, D., 295, 300, 312, 313, 324, 329, 365, 397, 398, 403, 458, 466, 503
Medical Consultants' Division, 205, 265
Medical Research Council, 282, 362, 477, 502
Mehta, J. M., 305, 363
Mein, R. M., 297, 305, 325, 362
Melamed, S., 74
Melnotte, P., 351
Melville, K. I., 138, 184
Menk, W., 377, 382, 402
Mer, G., 476, 501
Mergener, J. C., 217, 265
Messerlin, A., 346, 365
Meyer, P. F., 280, 355
Meythaler, F., 137, 184
Mietzsch, F., 54, 77, 131, 184
Mighton, H. R., 73, 74, 180, 186
Miller, A. K., 529, 558

SUBJECT INDEX

The names of proprietary compounds are placed in inverted commas.

Abortion and quinine, 192
4-Acetamido-α-diethylamino-*o*-cresol, 303
Acetarsol, 373, 374
5-Acetylamino-2-hydroxyphenylarsinic acid, quinine salt of, 373
Acetylcholine, 161
Acetyldihydroquinine, activity, 36
Acetyl-β-methyl-choline, 161
Acridanes, and mepacrine, 140
Acridine dyes, action on brain tissue, 220
Acridone derivatives, 61–64
Acriflavine, and *P. knowlesi*, 542
Acriquine, formula, 54
Adenine, mode of action, 532
Adenosine derivatives, mode of action, 530, 531
Adenosine triphosphate, mode of action, 531
Adenylic acid, mode of action, 531
Adrenaline, 161, 488, 489
and quinine administration, 279, 280
toxicity, 127
Aëdes ægypti and M2279, 428
and *P. gallinaceum*, 25, 390, 438, 439, 440, 442, 518
Agranulocytosis, and quinine, 188
and mepacrine, 222, 223
Alkalis, and mepacrine excretion, 140
8-(5'-Alkylamino-1'-methylpentylamino)-derivatives of quinoline, 52
Alkylquitenines, antimalarial activities, 43
and *Padda oryzivora*, 45
Allium sativum, 418
*iso*Alloxazines, 39, 40
3-Allyl-4-hydroxy-2-methylquinoline,63
Alstonia scholaris F. Br., activity, 416
Aluminium *para*-aminobenzene sulphonate, 392
Amaryllidaceæ activity, 418
Amblyopia, and quinine, 188
2-Amino-6-acetylamidopyridine, activity, 109
2-Aminoalkylamino-6-methoxyquinolines, antimalarial activity, 94
mode of action, 526
p-Aminobenzenesulphonamide, activity, 393

m-Aminobenzenesulphonamidopyrimidine, mode of action, 514
2-(*m*-Aminobenzenesulphonamido)-pyrimidine, 25
p-Aminobenzoic acid, activity, 437
and malaria in monkeys, 386
mode of action, 518, 549–51
N¹-(4-Amino-5-bromo-2-pyrimidyl) sulphanilamide, activity, 394
5-Amino-N-(5-bromo-2-pyrimidyl)-*o*-toluene-sulphonamide, activity, 394
9-Amino-6-chloro-2-hydroxy-acridine, 140
α-Aminocresols, 66–67
2-Amino-4-dialkylaminoalkylamino-5 : 6-dialkyl-pyrimidines, antimalarial activity, 107
2-Amino-4-β-diethylaminoethyl-amino-5-methylpyrimidine, 107
2-Amino-4-(δ-diethylamino-α-methyl-butylamino)-5 : 6-dimethylpyrimidine, 83
4-Amino-6-γ-diethylamino-propyl-amino-2 : 5-dimethylpyrimidine, activity, 108
2-Amino-4-γ-diethylamino-propylamino-5 : 6-dimethyl-pyrimidine, 83, 107
5-Amino-4-glycosidaminopyrimidines, mode of action, 525
2-Amino-5-iodopyridine, and *P. lophuræ*, 109
4'-Aminomethyl-8-benzylamino-6-methoxyquinoline (2409F), chemotherapeutic index, 61
8-(4'-Amino-1'-methylbutylamino)-6-methoxyquinoline, 53
8-γ-Aminopropylamino-6-*n*-butoxyquinoline, 49
8-γ-Aminopropylamino-6-ethoxyquinoline, chemotherapeutic index, 48
8-γ-Aminopropylamino-6-methoxyquinoline, 48
8-γ-Aminopropylamino-6-methoxyquinoline hydrochloride, 52, 53, 137
8-γ-Aminopropylamino-6-methoxyquinoline dihydrochloride, 27, 52

7-Chloro-2-phenyl-α-2-piperidyl-4-
quinolyl-2'-piperidyl methanol
dihydrochloride, and avian malaria,
27
7-Chloro-2-phenyl-4-quinolyl-
dihexylamino-methyl carbinol, and
P. vivax, 38
N₁-*p*-Chlorophenyl-N₅-
*iso*propylbiguanide. *See* Proguanil.
4-*p*-Chlorophenylguanidino-2-γ-di-*n*-
butylaminopropylamino-6-
methylpyrimidine, activity, 113
2-*p*-Chlorophenyl-guanidine-4-β-
diethylaminoethylamino-6-
methylpyrimidine, antimalarial
activity, 87
4-*p*-Chlorophenylguanidino-2-β-
diethylaminoethylamino-6-
methylpyrimidine, activity, 113
2-*p*-Chlorophenylguanidino-4-γ-
diethylaminopropylamino-5 : 6-
dimethylpyrimidine, activity, 112
2-*p*-Chlorophenylguanidino-4-β-
diethylaminoethyl-amino-6-
methylpyrimidine, 167, 307
pharmacology, 168–70
and *P. gallinaceum,* 442
2-*p*-Chlorophenylguanidine-4-β-
diethylaminoethylamino-6-
methylpyrimidine, and *P. gallinaceum,*
525
4-*p*-Chlorophenylguanidino-6-γ-
diethylaminopropyl-amino-2-
methylpyrimidine, activity, 113
2-*p*-Chlorophenylguanidino-4 : 6-
dimethylpyrimidine, activity. 112
2-*p*-Chlorophenylguanidino-4-β-
piperidino-α-methyl-ethyl-amino-6-
methyl-pyrimidine, activity, 112
N¹-(5-Chloro-2-pyrazinyl)metanilamide,
activity, 394
N¹-(5-Chloro-2-
pyrazinyl)sulphanilamide, activity,
393
N¹-(6-Chloro-2-
pyrazinyl)sulphanilamide, activity,
393
N¹-(5-Chloro-2-pyrimidyl)metanilamide,
activity, 22, 27, 394, 399
pharmacological tests, 20
quinine equivalent, 21
N¹-(5-Chloro-2-pyrimidyl)-*m*-
nitrobenzene-sulphonamide, activity,
394
m-(5-Chloro-2-
pyrimidylsulphamyl)acetanilide,
activity, 394

3'-(5-Chloro-2-
pyrimidylsulphamyl)benzanilide,
activity, 394
m-[(5-Chloro-2-
pyrimidyl)sulphamyl]phenylurea,
activity, 394
N¹-(5-Chloro-2-
pyrimidyl)sulphanilamide, activity,
394
Chlorguanide. *See* Proguanil.
Chloroquine, 58, 230, 291–98
and cerebral malaria, 460, 461
chemical constitution and
antimalarial action, 520
and dermatitis, 233
dosage, 293, 294
mode of action, 510, 512, 515, 518,
530, 531, 550
and pentaquine in relapsing *P. vivax,*
484
pharmacology, 140, 144, 145, 147,
537
and *P. berghei,* 291
and *P. cathemerium,* 291
and *P. cynomolgi,* 291
and *P. falciparum,* 14 ,279, 292, 295–
97, 316, 456–59, 552
and *P. gallinaceum,* 13, 26, 59, 302,
519
and *P. lophuræ,* 291, 442
and *P. malariæ,* 231, 295, 486, 487
and *P. vivax,* 14, 231, 292, 293, 295–
97, 465, 466, 469, 479
and pregnancy, 296, 488
relapses with *P. vivax,* 472–75
resistance, 438
suppression and causal prophylaxis,
296, 461, 462
toxicity, 227, 236, 292, 293
Chloroquine diphosphate, and avian
malarias, 27
4-(7'-Chloro-4'-quinolyl-amino)-
diethyl-amino-*o*-cresol, and *P.
gallinaceum,* 26, 519
toxicity, 229, 230
1-(7'-Chloro-4'-quinolyl)-3-
diethylamino-2-propanol and *P.
gallinaceum,* 26
1-(7-Chloro-4-quinolylamino)-3-
diethylamino-2-propanol, and *P.
gallinaceum,* 519
toxicity, 230, 234
1-(7'-Chloro-4'-quinolylamino)-3-
diethylamino-2-propanol
diphosphate, and avian malarias, 27
N¹-(5-Chloro-2-pyrimidyl)
metanilamide, and avian malaria, 27

19*

PRINTED IN GREAT BRITAIN BY THE WHITEFRIARS PRESS LTD
LONDON AND TONBRIDGE